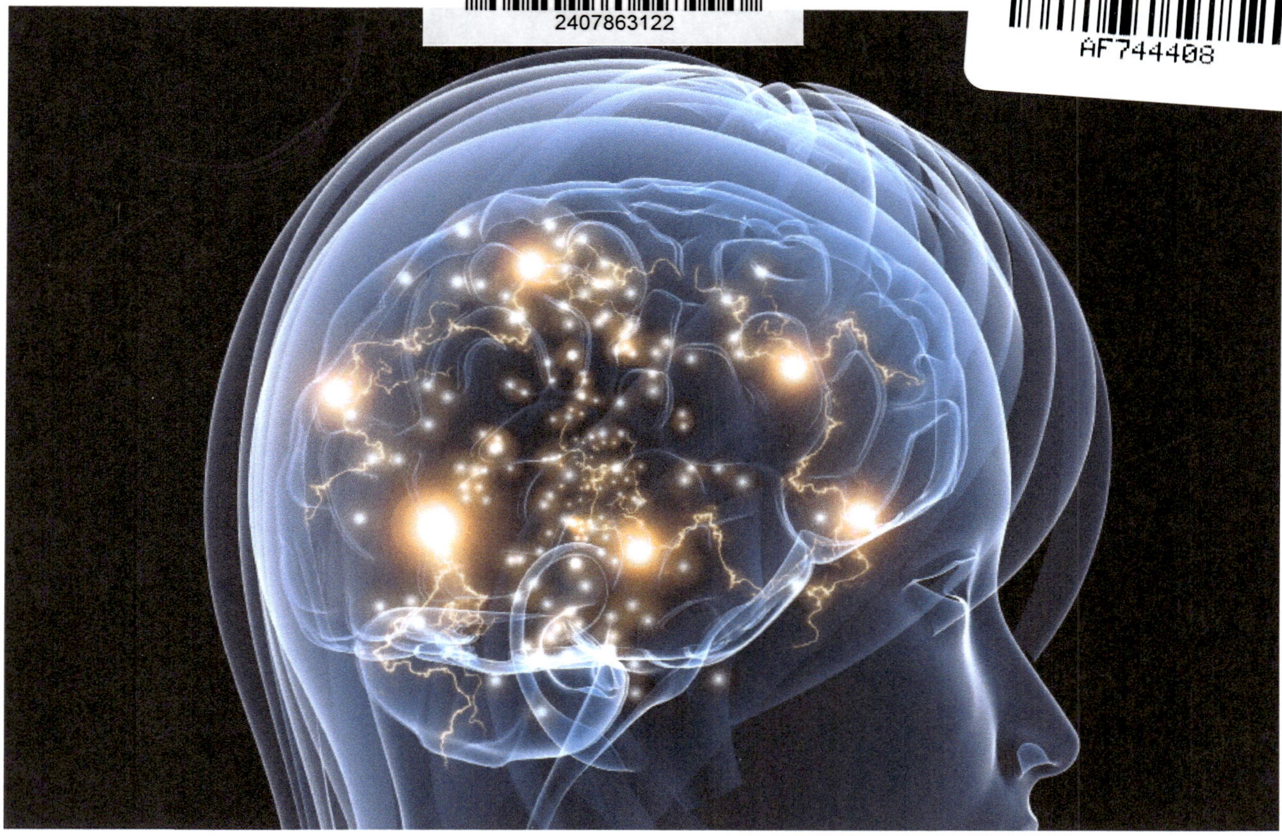

BMJ Clinical Review:

Neurology and Pain

by
Babita Jyoti and Michail A. Karvelis

BPP
UNIVERSITY
SCHOOL OF HEALTH

First edition May 2016

ISBN 9781 4727 4728 0
eISBN 9781 4727 4331 2
eISBN 9781 4727 4327 5

British Library Cataloguing-in-Publication Data
A catalogue record for this book is available from the British Library

Published by
BPP Learning Media Ltd
BPP House, Aldine Place
London W12 8AA

www.bpp.com/health

Printed in the United Kingdom by
Ashford Colour Press Ltd.

Unit 600, Fareham Reach,
Fareham Road,
Gosport, Hampshire,
PO13 0FW

Your learning materials, published by BPP Learning Media Ltd, are printed on paper sourced from sustainable, managed forests.

About the publisher

BPP Learning Media is dedicated to supporting aspiring professionals with top quality learning material. BPP Learning Media's commitment to success is shown by our record of quality, innovation and market leadership in paper-based and e-learning materials. BPP Learning Media's study materials are written by professionally-qualified specialists who know from personal experience the importance of top quality materials for success.

About The BMJ

The BMJ (formerly the British Medical Journal) in print has a long history and has been published without interruption since 1840. The BMJ's vision is to be the world's most influential and widely read medical journal. Our mission is to lead the debate on health and to engage, inform, and stimulate doctors, researchers, and other health professionals in ways that will improve outcomes for patients. We aim to help doctors to make better decisions. BMJ, the company, advances healthcare worldwide by sharing knowledge and expertise to improve experiences, outcomes and value.

BPP UNIVERSITY SCHOOL OF HEALTH BMJ

Contents

About the editors

Dr Babita Jyoti is a Radiation Oncologist with a special interest in Paediatric Proton Therapy. She graduated in Medicine in India followed by training in UK and obtained MRCP (UK) & FRCR (UK). She trained as a Clinical Oncologist at Clatterbridge Cancer Centre. She is currently working at the University of Florida Health Proton Therapy Institute in Paediatric Proton Therapy. She has been a PBL tutor and an OSCE examiner at Manchester Medical School.

Dr Michail A. Karvelis is a Locum Consultant in Anaesthesia and Pain Medicine at the Royal Liverpool and Broadgreen University Hospitals. He qualified from the Medical School of the Aristotle University of Thessaloniki, Greece in 2003. He trained as an anaesthetist both in Greece and the UK and he obtained his CCT in 2011. He was awarded a Masters degree in Pain management from Leicester University in 2011. He has worked as a Consultant Anaesthetist in the Naval Hospital of Athens and since 2014 he has been developing his special interest in regional anaesthesia and pain medicine in the NHS.

Introduction to Neurology and Pain

There are many examples in everyday clinical practice where the Science of Neurology overlaps with that of Pain Medicine. Neurologists commonly manage patients with chronic headaches but some of them can be treated as well in general pain clinics. Some cases of neuropathic pain are tackled by neurosurgeons or spine surgeons, whereas others can be managed conservatively by pain physicians and neurologists. Chronic pain affects approximately 20% of the European population occurring either as a pain syndrome or secondary to other conditions such as cerebrovascular accidents or cancer. The prevalence of diabetic neuropathy and fibromyalgia is constantly rising and the use of previously accepted treatments such as opioids is becoming nowadays more infrequent due to the now acknowledged long-term side effects.

Diagnosis and management of epilepsy as well first seizure prevention in adult patients is increasingly becoming a difficult task not only for the uninitiated but also the expert. All these reasons pose an arduous challenge to the physician who is keen to stay abreast of the latest developments in research. New pharmaceutical products are being trialed and relevant guidelines as well as diagnostic criteria are constantly under review. In this book, we have made every effort to contribute to the advancement of knowledge by carefully selecting clinical reviews on neurology and chronic pain from the past 6 years, as those were published in The BMJ.

Clinical reviews from The BMJ provide a clear, up to date account of the topic from highly esteemed colleagues. This book is a collaborative venture including general physicians and general practitioners, anaesthetists, neurologists and neurosurgeons, rheumatologists as well as psychologists.

Each review includes a broad update of recent developments and their likely clinical applications in primary and secondary care. Its aim is to stimulate professionals as well as patients to elaborate further on the subject and therefore each article additionally indicates other sources of information. Articles are written in a question-answer format using simple language in order to make it easy for then non-expert to apprehend.

We have attempted to select and include the clinical reviews that provide a thorough, useful, ready-to-use knowledge on common neurological and chronic conditions. Our intention was to try and cover some of the major topics in the field and to provide answers to everyday raised clinical questions. However, there is no book that can compete with the pace of literature. New data is being published everyday and knowledge becomes obsolete unimaginably fast. The reader should use this book as a stimulus to look further into the published literature, rather than an answer to every clinical question. In addition, The BMJ reviews tend to be treated as the "common knowledge" in the field, as it is something that most of your peers as well as patients will be reading. From that perspective, healthcare professionals should use this book as their starting point of their challenging journey into the world of evidence based medicine. We do hope that you will find this book useful.

Diagnosis and management of transient ischaemic attack and ischaemic stroke in the acute phase

K S McArthur, clinical research fellow, T J Quinn, lecturer in geriatric medicine, J Dawson, lecturer in clinical pharmacology and stroke, M R Walters, professor of clinical pharmacology and stroke

Institute of Cardiovascular and Medical Sciences, University of Glasgow, Western Infirmary, Glasgow G116NT, UK

Correspondence to: K S McArthur kate.mcarthur@glasgow.ac.uk

Cite this as: *BMJ* 2011;342:d1938

DOI: 10.1136/bmj.d1938

http://www.bmj.com/content/342/bmj.d1938

The care of people with acute ischaemic stroke has improved dramatically in recent years. Both stroke and transient ischaemic attack (TIA) are now recognised as medical emergencies that must be treated with the same urgency as myocardial infarction. Treatments such as thrombolysis are now widely adopted and underpinned by a robust evidence base. Rapid and accurate recognition of cerebral ischaemia, prompt treatment, and referral to specialist services can reduce the risk of further events.

Although cautious optimism has replaced therapeutic nihilism, stroke remains an important cause of death and disability and improvements in stroke services are still sorely needed. There are an estimated 900 000 stroke survivors in England, half of whom are dependent on others for care at an estimated cost of £8bn per year (about €9bn or $13bn).[1] This burden will increase as population demographics change. We review the diagnosis and acute management of cerebral ischaemia drawing on evidence from original research (particularly multicentre randomised clinical trials), registry data, and systematic review and meta-analysis, and with particular attention to national and international clinical guidelines. Further discussion of the epidemiology and economical aspects of contemporary stroke care are available elsewhere[1 2w1]; the management of intracerebral haemorrhage was reviewed in a previous *BMJ* article (2009;339:b2586) and is not discussed here. We will review care in hospital, rehabilitation, and secondary prevention of stroke in a second paper.

What is an acute cerebrovascular event?

The World Health Organization defines stroke as the sudden onset of focal neurological signs, of presumed vascular origin, lasting longer than 24 hours or causing death. It can be further classified as ischaemic, due to interruption of blood supply, or haemorrhagic, due to rupture of a cerebral artery. The term cerebrovascular accident is now discouraged, because there is nothing "accidental" about cerebrovascular disease. In recognition of stroke as a medical emergency the term "brain attack" has been used and seems appropriate. Symptoms of a TIA are similar to those of stroke but last less than 24 hours. Indeed, a truly "transient" ischaemic event, with no cerebral infarction, will usually manifest as a symptom complex lasting only minutes. Longer events are typically associated with infarction and should be considered "stroke"; definitions are likely to change to reflect this.[3]

Various clinical, radiological, and pathological classification systems have been proposed to further classify stroke. The Oxford clinical classification is often used because it is simple to apply and is of prognostic use.[4] It describes four subtypes of stroke; total anterior circulation stroke (TACS), partial anterior circulation stroke (PACS), lacunar stroke (LACS), and posterior circulation stroke (POCS) (box 1).

Once an ischaemic cause is confirmed, the nomenclature can be altered to convey greater specificityfor example, a partial anterior circulation infarct (PACI). The underlying cause in most cerebral ischaemic events is cardioembolic or atherosclerotic arterial disease, which can cause either in situ thrombosis or distal embolism. Other causes are much rarer. Common sources of cardiac emboli are atrial fibrillation, mural thrombus, and valvular heart disease and these typically involve the territory of the large intracerebral arteries, particularly the middle cerebral artery. Atherosclerotic disease typically affects the extracranial

SUMMARY POINTS

- Education of patients and their relatives to recognise signs of stroke and transient ischaemic attack (TIA) is crucial to promote early presentation to medical services
- TIA and stroke are medical emergencies; refer for urgent specialist opinion
- The risk of further cerebrovascular event following TIA is substantial, immediate, quantifiable, and preventable; do not be reassured by resolution of symptoms
- Effective treatments for selected stroke patients include: aspirin within first 48 hours; intravenous thrombolysis; surgical decompression of cerebral oedema
- Admission to a dedicated stroke unit offers mortality and functional benefits to all patients with stroke
- Deranged physiology is common in acute stroke and associated with poor prognosis

BOX 1 OXFORD SYSTEM OF STROKE CLASSIFICATION[4]

Total anterior circulation stroke (TACS)
All three of:
- Contralateral motor or sensory deficit
- Homonymous hemianopia
- Higher cortical dysfunction*

Partial anterior circulation stroke (PACS)
Two of:
- Contralateral motor or sensory deficit
- Homonymous hemianopia
- Higher cortical dysfunction

Posterior circulation stroke (POCS)
Any one of:
- Isolated homonymous hemianopia
- Brain stem signs
- Cerebellar ataxia

Lacunar stroke (LACS)
Any one of:
- Pure motor deficit
- Pure sensory deficit
- Sensorimotor deficit

**Higher cortical dysfunction includes dysphasia/visiospatial disturbance.*

internal carotid artery but also the vertebral and basilar arteries. Lacunar infarction results from occlusion of deep perforating arteries, which arise from both the anterior and posterior circulation, and supply the white matter of the cerebral hemispheres and brainstem.

Is it an acute cerebrovascular event?

Clinical diagnosis

It is important to rapidly distinguish stroke from one of the numerous conditions that resemble it ("stroke mimics", box 2). In a UK observational study of 350 consecutive suspected stroke presentations to a teaching hospital at least 30% of referrals resulted in a non-stroke diagnosis.[5] This distinction is important to allow evidence based treatment to be started early and to refer alternative conditions to the appropriate team. It may be useful to consider the definition of stroke "sudden onset, focal neurology, of presumed vascular cause". Thus, for patients with gradual onset of symptoms, who have no focal symptoms (such as those who have lost consciousness), or who give a history that suggests a non-vascular basis for the episode (seizure, migraine), stroke can probably be excluded, albeit with a few exceptions.

Formal assessment tools are available to facilitate diagnosis and are based on these simple principles. Box 3 outlines two tools commonly used in routine practice. The Face Arm Speech Test (FAST) is suitable for use by the general public and has a positive predictive value of 78% (95% confidence interval 72 to 84) for stroke[6] while the ROSIER scale, designed for emergency department use, functions similarly well and includes a screen for common stroke mimics (but can still be administered in less than five minutes[7]). Similar tools are available for the diagnosis of TIA but have yet to be widely adopted.[8]

BOX 2 FREQUENCY OF COMMON CONDITIONS THAT MIMIC STROKE[5]

- Seizure 21%
- Sepsis 13%
- Toxic/metabolic 11%
- Space occupying lesion 9%
- Syncope 9%
- Delirium 7%
- Vestibular 7%
- Mononeuropathy 6%
- Functional 6%
- Dementia 4%
- Migraine 3%
- Spinal cord lesion 3%
- Other 3%

BOX 3 CLINOMETRIC PROPERTIES OF TOOLS TO AID RECOGNITION AND DIAGNOSIS OF A CEREBROVASCULAR EVENT[34]

Recognition of Stroke in Emergency Room (ROSIER) scale

- Loss of consciousness or syncope? Yes: −1 point
- Seizure activity? Yes: −1 point
- New acute onset:
- Asymmetric facial weakness? Yes: +1 point
- Asymmetric arm weakness? Yes: +1 point
- Asymmetric leg weakness? Yes: +1 point
- Speech disturbance? Yes: +1 point
- Visual field defect? Yes: +1 point
- Total −2 to +5
- Stroke likely if score >0 in the absence of hypoglycaemia
- Sensitivity for stroke diagnosis 82%
- Specificity for stroke diagnosis 42%

The Fast Arm Speech Test (FAST) scale

- Facial asymmetry? Yes: +1 point
- Arm (or leg) weakness? Yes: +1 point
- Speech disturbance? Yes: +1 point
- Total 0 to 3
- Suspect stroke if score >0
- Sensitivity for stroke diagnosis 82%
- Specificity for stroke diagnosis 37%

For comparison, diagnosis of stroke by clinical staff's first impression had sensitivity 77% and specificity 58%.

Imaging

Brain imaging is indicated to help confirm the diagnosis, identify the causes, and help initiation of evidence based treatment. The usual imaging modality is non-contrast computed tomography (CT) and this remains useful particularly in excluding intracerebral haemorrhage and important mimics such as brain metastasis. However, sensitivity for detection of ischaemia is low in the very early stages of stroke and differentiating ischaemic from haemorrhagic strokes can be difficult on CT after a period of several days. More advanced CT imaging techniques such as CT perfusion and angiography are available and are likely to be used in the future to help better select patients for some of the acute treatments discussed below. At present, however, magnetic resonance imaging (MRI) is the modality of choice. In a study of 217 sequential acute stroke patients who underwent imaging using both non-contrast CT and MRI, CT demonstrated sensitivity of 26% (95% CI 20% to 32%) compared with 83% (78% to 88%) for MRI in the detection of early ischaemia. Further, concerns that MRI may not detect intracerebral haemorrhage or proves impractical for "emergency" imaging were not supported.[w2]

Imaging of the extracranial carotid arteries is required for patients with anterior circulation stroke. Carotid endarterectomy is of proved benefit for those with at least moderate carotid stenosis ipsilateral to an ischaemic stroke in the carotid artery (?).[9 10] This procedure should be performed early; further details on patient selection will be discussed in a future review. Carotid duplex ultrasonography is well tolerated and non-invasive but substantial interobserver variability limits its accuracy.[w3] Most surgical teams will require corroborative imaging, often with CT or MR angiography, before surgical intervention and many specialist centres use these as modalities of choice.

Other investigations

Electrocardiogram abnormalities may suggest a cardiac origin for thrombus. Where brain imaging and clinical presentation fit with embolic stroke, or where clinical findings suggest cardiac disease, cardiac imaging and more detailed telemetry are indicated. Routine screening for vasculitides or thrombophilia is not justified.

How should I approach suspected TIA?

Remember that all patients who have ongoing symptoms, however mild, are considered to have had stroke and urgent transfer to hospital should be arranged. Where symptoms have resolved before presentation urgent hospital transfer may not be required but rapid assessment and treatment if TIA has occurred is mandatory.

A substantial risk of stroke exists in the early period after TIA. The magnitude of risk is greater and the time to event shorter than previously recognised. A recent systematic review reported an overall 7 day stroke risk of 5.2% after TIA.[11]

Simple stratification scores can be used to better estimate a patient's individual risk. The most commonly used (and best validated) tool is the $ABCD^2$ score[12] (table 1). $ABCD^2$ estimates risk of recurrence at two days from 1% for patients with "low risk" to 8.1% for those patients with "high risk". $ABCD^2$ scoring is recommended in UK national guidelines and many centres offer same day assessment of patients at highest risk of stroke. $ABCD^2$ may also be useful in diagnosis. Single centre registry data (3646 patients) showed that few referrals with an $ABCD^2$ score of 0 were subsequently found to have a cerebrovascular diagnosis.[13]

The fact that the increased risk occurs so soon after TIA tells us that same day assessment should be the aim for patients with TIA, although the practicalities of referral and investigation of stroke will vary according to the local facilities available. UK guidelines (National Institute for Health and Clinical Excellence and Scottish Intercollegiate Guidelines Network)[14 15] suggest starting all patients on antiplatelet treatment (aspirin 300 mg) and referring them for urgent specialist assessment. NICE recommends that patients with $ABCD^2$ scores greater than 4 be assessed within 24 hours. Delivery of these targets on a nationwide and fully inclusive basis will require substantial investment in services.

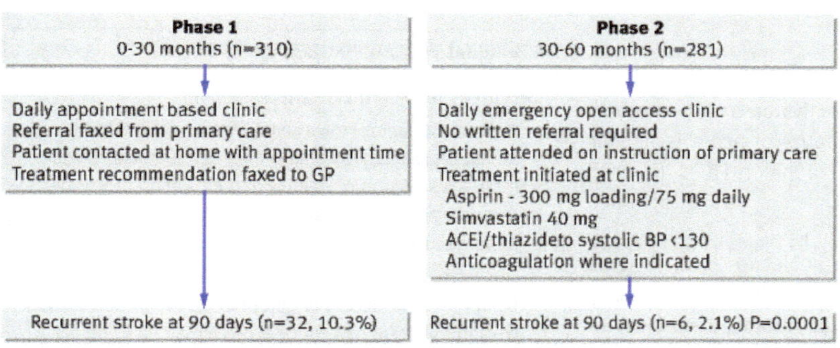

Fig 1 EXPRESS study protocol[16]

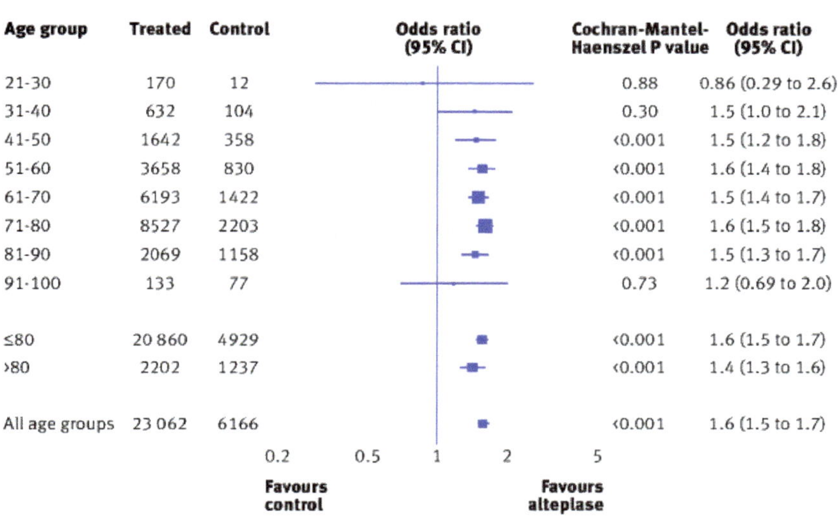

Fig 2 Shift towards better outcomes on modified Rankin scale at three months adjusted for age and baseline severity (defined by National Institutes of Stroke scale)[23]

The landmark EXPRESS study compared stroke events in Oxford, UK, before and after a move from their standard to an immediate access, comprehensive, TIA assessment service.[16] An 80% reduction in recurrent stroke at 90 days was demonstrated with no increase in adverse events (fig 1). Although we extrapolate these results from a single centre with caution, it is worth noting that if outcomes were replicated across all UK stroke centres 10 000 stroke events could be prevented annually.

How will specialist services manage the patient with suspected stroke or TIA?

The aim of specialist stroke assessment is confirmation of stroke diagnosis, identification of the causes, and timely initiation of evidence based treatment.

Brain imaging should be performed with minimal delay to distinguish ischaemic from haemorrhagic stroke. Even when the patient is not eligible for thrombolysis, imaging within 24 hours (although ideally as soon as possible) is the most cost effective strategy. The need for imaging in transient ischaemic attack is more contentious. In our unit we routinely scan anyone with symptoms lasting more than one hour before starting secondary prevention.

Patients with TIA

Treatments are aimed at preventing a further event, similar to the secondary treatments given to patients following acute stroke. In those with confirmed atrial fibrillation or mural thrombus anticoagulants are warranted. Antiplatelet or anticoagulant drugs may be considered in all patients, as may lipid lowering therapy, antihypertensive therapy, carotid surgery, treatment of diabetes, and advice about diet, lifestyle, and smoking cessation. A recent focus

Table 1 $ABCD^2$ score and risk of stroke[12]

	$ABCD^2$ score	Risk of stroke	
		2 days	7 days
Characteristic			
Age ≥60 years	1 point	-	-
Blood pressure ≥140/90 mm Hg	1 point	-	-
Clinical features			
Focal weakness	2 points	-	-
Speech disturbance without weakness	1 point	-	-
Duration			
≥60 minutes	2 points	-	-
1-59 minutes	1 point	-	-
Diabetes	1 point	-	-
Total $ABCD^2$ score			
Low risk	<4 points	1%	1.2%
Moderate risk	4-5 points	4.1%	5.9%
High risk	>5 points	8.1%	11.7%

SOURCES AND SELECTION CRITERIA

The review is based on the authors' clinical and research experience and informed by a search of published literature. Electronic databases (Medline and Embase) were searched from inception to December 2010 inclusive, using truncated keywords: "transient ischaemic attack"; "thrombolytic"; "stroke or cerebrovascular". In addition, key reference works; national and international guidelines; and key journals were searched for relevant papers. Particular attention was given to large randomised controlled trials, systematic reviews, and meta-analyses. The intention was not to offer a comprehensive systematic review, rather to give a narrative overview and critique of published literature.

of research has been the potential benefits of early antiplatelets, statins, and antihypertensives. The marked reduction in stroke rate seen in EXPRESS may have been caused by immediate delivery of these therapies (patients were given medication at clinic review). We await results of ongoing trials, although emergent stroke data suggest that "acute" prescription of antihypertensives may have no clinical benefit.[17]

Patients with acute ischaemic stroke

Within the first hours to days, proved treatments for acute ischaemic stroke include admission to a dedicated stroke unit; administration of intravenous tissue plasminogen activator (rt-PA); antiplatelet agents; and surgical decompression of massive cerebral oedema (table 2).

Aspirin

A systematic review of antiplatelets after ischaemic stroke (n=43 041) demonstrated that for every 1000 patients treated acutely with aspirin (160-300 mg) 13 fewer deaths occurred by the end of follow-up, which is a modest but important effect at a population level.[18] UK guidelines recommend that patients with acute ischaemic stroke are prescribed aspirin 300 mg daily for two weeks, followed by a long term secondary preventative antiplatelet strategy.[14 15] Aspirin should be withheld for 24 hours after thrombolysis. Where a patient's swallowing is impaired to a degree that precludes oral administration, rectal preparations may be used. In patients unable to take aspirin, alternatives such as clopidogrel may be used. There is no evidence to support the use of early anticoagulation as a treatment for acute ischaemic stroke.[19]

Thrombolysis

Intravenous tissue plasminogen activator (rt-PA) alteplase is beneficial if given within 4.5 hours of acute ischaemic stroke in selected patients. In Europe, rt-PA is licensed for the treatment of acute ischaemic stroke provided it is administered within three hours of symptom onset, but many centres will administer it up to 4.5 hours based on evidence.[20] The benefits of rt-PA are in reducing longer term disability and not in improved survival or in immediate improvement in neurological impairment (although anecdotally this has been observed). Two recent pooled meta-analyses of the major thrombolysis trials (n=2775[21] and n=3670[22]) have demonstrated clear benefit of thrombolysis with significantly better outcomes seen with early treatment (table 3) In the larger analysis the odds ratios of a favourable outcome with rt-PA were 2.55 (95% CI 1.44 to 4.52) for 0-90 minutes, 1.64 (1.12 to 2.4) for 91-180 minutes, 1.34 (1.06 to 1.68) for 181-270 minutes, and 1.22 (0.92 to 1.61) for 271-360 minutes in favour of the rt-PA group.[22] Trials have reported that mortality rates at three months are equivalent to placebo.

The limited time window for delivery of thrombolytic therapy is a major barrier to its delivery. The risk:benefit ratio beyond 4.5 hours has not been fully established and ongoing clinical trials aim to provide further evidence. Patients older than 80 years were excluded from most of the clinical trials. Non-randomised observational data suggest that their risk:benefit ratio is similar to that of other patients[23] (fig 2) and many centres will give thrombolysis to selected older patients. However, data from randomised studies are lacking and we await results of the third international stroke trial.[w4].

Many clinicians fear the potential for iatrogenic intracerebral haemorrhage after thrombolysis and patient selection guidance is designed to minimise this risk. A list of contraindications to thrombolysis is shown in table 4. For many of these, as we have gained more experience with thrombolysis, conditions that were previously "absolute" contraindications to rt-PA are now deemed "relative" contraindications. Because this is an evolving landscape, we advise referral of all hyperacute suspected strokes to a specialist team unless there is substantial premorbid disability. As the benefits of rt-PA are in reducing disability, this approach is not routinely used in patients who are already functionally impaired.

The Safe Implementation of Thrombolysis in Stroke-Monitoring Study (SITS-MOST) registry of clinical practice was conducted in accordance with the terms of the

Table 2 Effective treatments for stroke

	Aspirin	Stroke unit	rt-PA	Surgery
Number needed to treat	100	20	10	2
Proportion eligible	70-80%	100%	10%*	5%†

Based on UK data; some European centres have achieved far higher rates of thrombolysis within licence.
†Based on European data; values vary depending on demographics (particularly age) of population served.

Table 3 Benefit of rt-PA treatment at 90 days[22]

Time between event and treatment	Odds ratio in favour of favourable outcome (95% CI)	Estimated number needed to treat for favourable outcome
0-90 minutes	2.55 (1.44 to 4.52)	4.5
91-180 minutes	1.64 (1.12 to 2.40)	9.0
181-270 minutes	1.34 (1.06 to 1.68)	14.1
271-360 minutes	1.22 (0.92 to 1.61)	21.4

Favourable outcome defined as modified Rankin score of 0-1 at 90 days.

ADDITIONAL EDUCATIONAL RESOURCES

Resources for healthcare professionals

- Stroke Association Professional Training (www.stroke.org.uk/professionals/training_and_development/index.html)– A selection of training and education programmes offered by the stroke association, suitable for all healthcare professionals
- European Stroke Organisation (www.eso-stroke.org)–Comprehensive access to European stroke guidelines and educational resources for health professionals and lay people
- UK Stroke Research Network (www.uksrn.ac.uk)–Provides an infrastructure to facilitate stroke research and improve communication between academics, stroke clinicians, stroke service users, and research funders
- Stroke Training and Awareness Resources (STARS) project (www.stroketraining.org)–Commissioned by the Scottish Government to provide an e-learning resource for all healthcare professionals and social care staff working with patients affected by stroke

Resources for patients

- The Stroke Association (www.stroke.org.uk)–Produces a number of publications to help educate and inform and increase awareness of stroke, including patient leaflets, and *Stroke News* (a quarterly magazine)
- Act FAST campaign (www.nhs.uk/actfast/Pages/stroke.aspx)–Public awareness campaign to improve community recognition of stroke symptoms and encourage those affected to seek urgent medical help
- Connect (www.ukconnect.org/index.aspx)–communication disability charity for patients and carers affected by aphasia
- Carers UK (www.carersuk.org)–charity providing support for home carers

restricted European licence for alteplase use and has helped to assuage some concerns about the potential for iatrogenic intracerebral haemorrhage.[24] Across 285 European centres (and 6483 patients), rates of "good" outcome (independence) were comparable or improved compared to those seen in clinical trials and likewise for rates of haemorrhagic transformation. Importantly, outcomes were similar regardless of levels of experience of the centre.

Provision of a comprehensive thrombolysis service demands substantial economic investment and infrastructural change. Despite endorsement by guideline and national targets, geographical disparity in availability and use of rt-PA are apparent within the UK and internationally. In an era of increasing financial scrutiny it is reassuring that the (limited) economic data on use of rt-PA suggest overall cost benefit, driven by prevention of longer term disability.[25]

Surgical intervention

"Malignant" swelling of an infarcted cerebral hemisphere can arise in the days following occlusion of the carotid or middle cerebral artery, and although uncommon it is associated with a very high mortality.[26] However, surgical intervention saves lives and reduces disability in selected patients younger than 60. In this group, meta-analysis of three randomised controlled trials showed superiority of surgical craniotomy compared to standard medical care with a number needed to treat of two to reduce disability.[26] Reducing mortality at the expense of substantial disability remains a possibility and improved data on selecting patients for surgery are urgently needed.

Physiological monitoring and other treatments

Failure of homoeostasic mechanisms during the acute phase of stroke is common and supportive care delivered through a specialist stroke unit is crucial. However, evidence to support taking measures to "correct" deranged physiology is lacking; even simple interventions such as supplementary hydration and oxygen therapy are of unproved benefit and are currently being investigated. Regular observation of level of consciousness is useful as change in Glasgow coma scale can herald potentially treatable complications such as development of cerebral oedema or haemorrhage.

The role of blood pressure control in the immediate phase after stroke is unclear. Arterial hypertension is found in 80% of patients following acute stroke and is associated with a poor outcome.[27] The ACCESS study suggested that early use of angiotensin receptor blockade was safe in acute ischaemic stroke;[28] however, recent publication of a larger phase III efficacy trial (SCAST) has demonstrated no benefit and a suggestion of increased harm.[29] Routine lowering of blood pressure is not recommended in UK or international guidelines. Treatment may be appropriate in specific circumstances such as hypertensive encephalopathy or aortic dissection; however, guidance on agent to use and target blood pressure varies across guidelines.

A meta-analysis of observational studies showed that the acute phase of stroke carries a high risk of infection and pyrexia is associated with a poor outcome, possibly because of adverse effects on free radical production or intracerebral metabolism.[30] Limited data support the use of anti-pyretic medication and cooling[31] but no adequately powered randomised trial has investigated their benefits. Standard treatment of pyrexia is recommended and should prompt an assessment for a possible underlying source of sepsis.

Raised blood glucose is also common in the acute phase after ischaemic stroke, often in the absence of pre-existing diabetes, which may represent a stress response. Despite its association with increased mortality and poor functional outcome,[32] the largest randomised controlled trial of blood glucose reduction in stroke reported no benefit of insulin infusion compared with placebo;[33] although some have argued that the study was underpowered to detect a true effect. Lowering of abnormally high blood

TIPS FOR NON-SPECIALISTS

- Sudden onset focal neurological symptoms represent a medical emergency and should be treated as such
- Eligibility for acute treatments is constantly evolving, discuss any patient with possible acute stroke with the local stroke team
- A sudden change in consciousness of an acute stroke patient may indicate a treatable complication and warrants urgent investigation.

QUESTIONS FOR FUTURE RESEARCH

- What factors influence a patient's decision to seek medical help following stroke or TIA, and how can we use this to improve rates of early presentation?
- Should secondary prevention be initiated by the referring clinician before assessment in TIA clinic?
- Is routine screening for cardioembolic disease cost effective?
- How can we improve access to thrombolysis in remote or rural areas?
- How safe and effective is thrombolysis in elderly patients or those with a previous stroke?
- Is intervention to correct deranged physiology of clinical benefit in acute stroke patients?

Table 4 Contraindications to use of rt-PA in acute ischaemic stroke

General contraindications to any use of rt-PA	Specific contraindications to use in ischaemic stroke
Severe bleeding within past six months	Evidence of intracranial haemorrhage
Known bleeding diathesis	Onset of symptoms >4.5 hours
Oral anticoagulant use (INR >1.4)	Unclear time of onset
History of intracranial haemorrhage	Age <18 or >80 years
Recent (<10 days) cardiopulmonary resuscitation	Mild stroke (NIHSS <5) or rapid improvement
Bacterial endocarditis or pericarditis	Severe stroke (NIHSS >25 or imaging)
Acute pancreatitis	Seizure at onset of stroke
Recent (<3 months) peptic ulcer disease	Symptoms indicating subarachnoid haemorrhage
Neoplasm with bleeding risk	Platelet count < 100 $\times 10^6$/L
Recent puncture of non-compressible vessel	Heparin within last 48 hours with raised PTT
Major surgery or trauma (<3 months)	Previous stroke within past three months
Severe liver disease	Previous stroke and concomitant diabetes
Recent obstetric delivery	Systolic BP >185 mm Hg or diastolic BP >110 mm Hg

INR=international normalised ratio, NIHSS=National Institute of Health Stroke Scale, PTT: prothrombin time, BP=blood pressure.

glucose (>11 mmol/L) with titrated insulin remains common practice to maintain normoglycaemia. Aggressive treatment of hyperglycaemia in critically ill patients was found to increase mortality in the NICE SUGAR study.[w5] Although this study was not specific to stroke patients, we must be cautious in the use of intravenous insulin in any severely unwell group of patients.

Contributors: KSMcA, TJQ, JD, and MRW all contributed to conception, design, literature searching, interpretation of data, drafting the article or revising it critically for important intellectual content, and final approval of the version to be published. KSMcA is guarantor.

Competing interests: All authors have completed the Unified Competing Interest form at www.icmje.org/coi_disclosure.pdf (available on request from the corresponding author) and declare: KSMcA, TJQ, JD, MRW have no external support for the submitted work; KSMcA and MRW have no relationships with companies that might have an interest in the submitted work in the previous three years, JD and TQ have received speaker fees for educational meetings sponsored by Bristol Myers Squibb and Pfizer; KSMcA, TJQ, JD, MRW have no non-financial interests that may be relevant to the submitted work.

Provenance and peer review: Commissioned, externally peer reviewed.

1 National Audit Office. Department of Health: progress in improving stroke care. National Audit Office, 2010.
2 The Intercollegiate Stroke Working Party. National sentinel stroke audit organisational audit 2009; report for England, Wales and Northern Ireland. 2010.
3 Albers GW, Caplan LR, Easton JD, Fayad PB, Mohr JP, Saver JL, et al. Transient ischemic attack—proposal for a new definition. *N Engl J Med* 2002;347:1713-6.
4 Bamford J, Sandercock P, Dennis M, Warlow C, Burn J. Classification and natural history of clinically identifiable subtypes of cerebral infarction. *Lancet* 1991;337:1521-6.
5 Hand PJ, Kwan J, Lindley RI, Dennis MS, Wardlaw JM. Distinguishing between stroke and mimic at the bedside: the Brain Attack Study. *Stroke* 2006;37:769-75.
6 Stroke Association. Suspect a stroke? Act FAST. Stroke Association, 2010.
7 Nor AM, Davis J, Sen B, Shipsey D, Louw SJ, Dyker AG, et al. The Recognition of Stroke in the Emergency Room (ROSIER) scale: development and validation of a stroke recognition instrument. *Lancet Neurol* 2005;4:727-34.
8 Dawson J, Lamb KE, Quinn TJ, Lees KR, Horvers M, Verrijth MJ, et al. A recognition tool for transient ischaemic attack. *QJM* 2009;102:43-9.
9 Rothwell PM, Eliasziw M, Gutnikov SA, Warlow CP, Barnett HJM. Sex difference in the effect of time from symptoms to surgery on benefit from carotid endarterectomy for transient ischemic attack and nondisabling stroke. *Stroke* 2004;35:2855-61.
10 Barnett HJ, Taylor DW, Eliasziw M, Fox AJ, Ferguson GG, Haynes RB, et al. Benefit of carotid endarterectomy in patients with symptomatic moderate or severe stenosis. *N Engl J Med* 1998;339:1415-25.
11 Giles MF, Rothwell PM. Risk of stroke early after transient ischaemic attack: a systematic review and meta-analysis. *Lancet Neurol* 2007;6:1063-72.
12 Johnston SC, Rothwell PM, Nguyen-Huynh MN, Giles MF, Elkins JS, Bernstein AL, et al. Validation and refinement of scores to predict very early stroke risk after transient ischaemic attack. *Lancet* 2007;369:283-92.
13 Quinn TJ, Cameron AC, Dawson J, Lees KR, Walters MR. ABCD[2] scores and prediction of noncerebrovascular diagnoses in an outpatient population: a case-control study. *Stroke* 2009;40:749-53.
14 National Collaborating Centre for Chronic Conditions, National Institute of Health and Clinical Excellence. Stroke: National clinical guideline for diagnosis and initial management of acute stroke and transient ischaemic attack (TIA). Royal College of Physicians, 2008.
15 Management of patients with stroke or TIA: assessment, investigation, immediate management and secondary prevention. A national clinical guideline. Edinburgh: Scottish Intercollegiate Guidelines Network, 2008.
16 Rothwell PM, Giles MF, Chandratheva A, Marquardt L, Geraghty O, Redgrave JN, et al. Effect of urgent treatment of transient ischaemic attack and minor stroke on early recurrent stroke (EXPRESS study): a prospective population-based sequential comparison. *Lancet* 2007;370:1432-42.
17 Robinson TG, Potter JF, Ford GA, Bulpitt CJ, Chernova J, Jagger C, et al. Effects of antihypertensive treatment after acute stroke in the Continue or Stop Post-Stroke Antihypertensives Collaborative Study (COSSACS): a prospective, randomised, open, blinded-endpoint trial. *Lancet Neurol* 2010;9:767-75.
18 Sandercock P, Gubitz G, Foley P, Counsell C. Antiplatelet therapy for acute ischaemic stroke. *Cochrane Database Syst Rev* 2008;3:CD000029.
19 Hart RG, Palacio S, Pearce LA. Atrial fibrillation, stroke, and acute antithrombotic therapy: analysis of randomized clinical trials. *Stroke* 2002;33:2722-7.
20 Hacke W, Kaste M, Bluhmki E, Brozman M, Davalos A, Guidetti D, et al. Thrombolysis with alteplase 3 to 4.5 hours after acute ischemic stroke. *N Engl J Med* 2008;359:1317-29.
21 Hacke W, Donnan G, Fieschi C, Kaste M, von KR, Broderick JP, et al. Association of outcome with early stroke treatment: pooled analysis of ATLANTIS, ECASS, and NINDS rt-PA stroke trials. *Lancet* 2004;363:768-74.
22 Lees KR, Bluhmki E, von Kummer R, Brott TG, Toni D, Grotta JC, et al. Time to treatment with intravenous alteplase and outcome in stroke: an updated pooled analysis of ECASS, ATLANTIS, NINDS, and EPITHET trials. *Lancet* 2010;375:1695-703.
23 Mishra NK, Ahmed N, Andersen G, Egido JA, Lindsberg PJ, Ringleb PA, et al. Thrombolysis in very elderly people: controlled comparison of SITS International Stroke Thrombolysis Registry and Virtual International Stroke Trials Archive. *BMJ* 2010;341:c6046.
24 Wahlgren N, Ahmed N, Davalos A, Ford GA, Grond M, Hacke W, et al. Thrombolysis with alteplase for acute ischaemic stroke in the Safe Implementation of Thrombolysis in Stroke-Monitoring Study (SITS-MOST): an observational study. *Lancet* 2007;369:275-82.
25 Sandercock P, Berge E, Dennis M, Forbes J, Hand P, Kwan J, et al. Cost-effectiveness of thrombolysis with recombinant tissue plasminogen activator for acute ischemic stroke assessed by a model based on UK NHS Costs. *Stroke* 2004;35:1490-7.
26 Vahedi K, Hofmeijer J, Juettler E, Vicaut E, George B, Algra A, et al. Early decompressive surgery in malignant infarction of the middle cerebral artery: a pooled analysis of three randomised controlled trials. *Lancet Neurol* 2007;6:215-22.
27 Leonardi-Bee J, Bath PMW, Phillips SJ, Sandercock PAG. Blood pressure and clinical outcomes in the International Stroke Trial. *Stroke* 2002;33:1315-20.
28 Schrader J, Luders S, Kulschewski A, Berger J, Zidek W, Treib J, et al. The ACCESS study: Evaluation of acute candesartan cilexetil therapy in stroke survivors. *Stroke* 2003;34:1699-703.
29 Sandset EC, Bath PM, Boysen G, Jatuzis D, Kõrv J, Lüders S, et al. The angiotensin-receptor blocker candesartan for treatment of acute stroke (SCAST): a randomised, placebo-controlled, double-blind trial. *Lancet* 2011;337:741-50.
30 Hajat C, Hajat S, Sharma P. Effects of poststroke pyrexia on stroke outcome : a meta-analysis of studies in patients. *Stroke* 2000;31:410-4.
31 Correia M, Silva M, Veloso M. Cooling therapy for acute stroke. *Cochrane Database Syst Rev* 2009;1:CD001247.
32 Capes SE, Hunt D, Malmberg K, Pathak P, Gerstein HC. Stress hyperglycemia and prognosis of stroke in nondiabetic and diabetic patients: a systematic overview. *Stroke* 2001;32:2426-32.
33 Gray CS, Hildreth AJ, Sandercock PA, O'Connell JE, Johnston DE, Cartlidge NE, et al. Glucose-potassium-insulin infusions in the management of post-stroke hyperglycaemia: the UK Glucose Insulin in Stroke Trial (GIST-UK). *Lancet Neurol* 2007;6:397-406.
34 Whiteley W, Wardlaw J, Thomas R, Dennis M, Sandercock P. Oral presentations of 5th UK Stroke Forum. A comparison of stroke screening tools with the clinical diagnosis of emergency room staff: a prospective cohort study. *Int J Stroke* 2010;5:3-13.

Post-acute care and secondary prevention after ischaemic stroke

K S McArthur, clinical research fellow, T J Quinn, lecturer in geriatric medicine, P Higgins, clinical research fellow, P Langhorne, professor of stroke care

Institute of Cardiovascular and Medical Sciences, University of Glasgow, Western Infirmary, Glasgow G11 6NT, UK

Correspondence to: K S McArthur kate.mcarthur@glasgow.ac.uk

Cite this as: *BMJ* 2011;342:d2083

DOI: 10.1136/bmj.d2083

http://www.bmj.com/content/342/bmj.d2083

In the first part of this two part review (*BMJ* 2011;342:d1938) we discussed acute diagnosis and management of cerebrovascular events. Much of the focus of recent research, public health initiatives, and health policy has been around acute and hyperacute management of stroke. However, important goals of stroke care are to maximise functional recovery and prevent recurrent events. Here we draw on evidence from randomised trials and meta-analyses to discuss models of care, rehabilitation, and secondary prevention in stroke.

An important aspect of post-acute stroke care is rehabilitation. Rehabilitation research remains a "young" science, although an evidence base is emerging. As we make progress in this field, we need a common language to describe this important intervention. In the box we offer our own definition of stroke rehabilitation, although others may offer differing suggestions. Many questions remain unanswered regarding timing, optimal components, and frequency and intensity of rehabilitation. Further discussion of rehabilitation as a concept or rehabilitation theory specific to stroke is beyond the scope of this article, but recent high quality publications on the subject are available.[w1 w2]

This review will focus on the early period after stroke. Effective early intervention may affect longer term outcomes,[w3] with combined analysis of three UK stroke cohorts (n=7710 patients) showing that long term survival is predicted by functional outcome at six months.[w4] Most interventional research in stroke has focused on these first days to months after a stroke event, whereas health needs and management of stroke survivors outside of this period has received little attention. This is unfortunate in a cohort with high incidence of residual disability and often complex comorbidity, and more work is needed to inform practice and policy.

SOURCES AND SELECTION CRITERIA

This review is based on the authors' clinical and research experience and informed by a search of published literature. Electronic databases (Medline and Embase) were searched from inception to December 2010 inclusive, using truncated keywords: "stroke or cerebrovascular"; "rehabilitation"; "prevention". In addition key reference works, national and international guidelines, and journals were searched for relevant papers. Particular attention was given to large randomised controlled trials, systematic reviews, and meta-analyses. The intention was not to offer comprehensive systematic review but to give a narrative overview and critique of published work.

SUMMARY POINTS

- The management of stroke patients within dedicated stroke units prevents disability and saves lives for patients of all ages, with all types and severities of stroke
- Venous thromboembolism prophylaxis with compression stockings is not routinely recommended and may cause harm.
- Early mobilisation and physiotherapy are recommended by guidelines and appear to be safe, although definitive data on efficacy are awaited
- Medical complications after stroke are common and affect functional outcomes as well as mortality; infection, delirium, and dysphagia are potentially treatable
- Early artificial feeding with percutaneous gastrostomy tube has not shown longer term benefit for stroke survivors with impaired swallow and nasogastric feeding is recommended for initial management
- Secondary prevention with anti-hypertensive, anti-thrombotic, and lipid lowering drugs reduces likelihood of recurrent stroke

How should I assess a patient who has survived a stroke?

Assessment in the first days after stroke will guide subsequent management. The aims are to ascertain the pathology and mechanism of the stroke, identify post-stroke complications, and describe initial impairments.

"Acute" brain imaging was discussed in the first part of this review and will not be covered here. Further investigation to identify a possible origin and guide treatment may include assessment of extracranial carotid arteries, heart structure, or arrhythmia. The potential deleterious effects of deranged "physiology" (temperature, blood pressure, glycaemic control) were also discussed in the previous review. Evidence for intervention remains inconclusive, although routine frequent monitoring of these parameters in the first 72 hours remains usual practice.

Regular (at least daily) assessments of neurological function are important in planning effective ongoing medical care and early rehabilitation. Longitudinal cohort studies suggest that early measures of disability predict longer term outcomes.[w5] In the first days after stroke, neurological findings are dynamic. The National Institutes of Health Stroke Scale[w6] and Glasgow Coma Scale[w7] are often used initially as global measures. Deterioration suggests that further investigation is needed to exclude hemispheric oedema or haemorrhage. Therapists will plan intervention on the basis of early functional assessments of visuospatial awareness, sitting balance, and mobility. Later the focus of assessment will move to activity measures, using validated tools such as the Barthel index[w8] or modified Rankin scale.[w9]

Post-stroke dysphagia is common—occurring in up to half of patients—and is associated with an increased risk of aspiration pneumonia and poor outcomes related to disability, increased length of stay, and death.[w10] Meanwhile, withholding oral intake presents a risk of dehydration and malnutrition. Routine early assessment of swallow is recommended by national guidelines.[1 2] Assessment should be frequent; most patients with early dysphagia will regain swallow by the second week.[w11] A bedside water swallow test (where a patient is asked to swallow a small volume of water) is a reasonable screening test[w12] and will determine the need for formal assessment of swallowing. Such assessment is performed by speech and language therapists and is often complemented by functional imaging, such as video fluoroscopy.

What kind of care should be delivered in hospital?

Evidence of benefit of stroke units

In the past two decades many single centre trials highlighted poor outcomes associated with generic care compared with care undertaken in dedicated stroke units. A Cochrane review from 2007 of 31 trials (n=6936 participants) confirmed the benefits of organised specialist care for patients with stroke.[3] Compared with general wards, the number needed to treat in a specialist unit was 22 to prevent one death and 16 to prevent one patient losing their independence, which compares favourably with other interventions for stroke (tables 1 and 2). The benefits of being cared for in a stroke unit extend to all ages, subtypes, and severities of stroke, and studies with longer follow-up suggest that benefits endure.[w3, w13] An economic analysis alongside a randomised trial found that care in a dedicated stroke unit was cost effective.[w14] The evidence clearly suggests that such a service should be available for all patients who experience a stroke.

What makes a stroke unit?

To tease out the components of an effective complex intervention can be a challenge.[4] Although a systematic review has highlighted the importance of monitoring and treating complications,[5] traditional medical input is unlikely to be the sole factor contributing to the success of a stroke unit. A survey of recent trials suggests that an essential component is the multidisciplinary team with a specialist interest in stroke, who provide an organised package of care coordinated through regular team meetings. The setting and achievement of goals requires collaboration of medical, nursing, and therapy staff in hospital and in the community and should be guided by the patient and carers.

Within this generic description, care in the stroke unit varies, and the definition of the "ideal" stroke unit is flexible. Many countries are pushing towards direct admission to stroke units, although other models of care were included in the Cochrane review[3] Although the benefits of immediate admission to stroke care seem intuitive (early specialist input, prompt intervention), robust supporting evidence is not available.

Opening the 'black box' of stroke unit care

Important components of stroke unit care

Staff with specialist interest	Early discharge planning
Early mobilisation	Multidisciplinary team
Prompt investigation	Goal setting approach
Prompt pharmacotherapy	Positioning and handling
Physiological monitoring	

Potentially important components

Management of:	Oral care
Pyrexia	Assessment of dysphagia
Hyperglycaemia	Bladder and bowel care
Hypoxia	Information provision
Hypertension	Involvement of carers
Hydration/nutrition	

Components with no evidence of efficacy

Routine use of compression stockings
Early percutaneous gastronomy feeding
Routine use of nutritional supplements

Components of effective stroke unit care subject to randomised trials (based on Langhorne et al[5])

Recent research has focused on opening the "black box" of stroke unit care. The individual components that have been investigated and shown to be beneficial, potentially beneficial, or of uncertain benefit are summarised in the figure. Robust evidence is emerging for specific areas of stroke care and those with recent data have been selected for further discussion here.

Prevention of venous thrombosis

Stroke survivors are at substantially increased risk of developing deep vein thrombosis because they are immobile and often dehydrated.[w15 w16] An open label randomised trial compared prophylactic low molecular weight heparin and unfractionated heparin for the prevention of venous thromboembolism after acute ischaemic stroke, and showed that enoxaparin was effective and relatively safe in reducing ultrasound detected deep vein thrombosis, although whether a clinical benefit exists is uncertain.[6] The trial did not compare heparin with placebo. The available data do not allow definitive advice on use of heparin, and further research about targeting this treatment to those at greatest risk is needed.[w17]

The recently published Clots in Legs Or sTockings after Stroke (CLOTS) trials provided pragmatic data about use of thromboembolic prevention stockings. Compared with no stockings, thigh or knee length stockings did not significantly reduce the risk of deep vein thrombosis.[7] There was a trend towards increased deep vein thrombosis in the group that used knee length stockings, and substantial rates of skin complications were reported with both types of stocking.[8] Although the clinical implications of the CLOTS trials continue to be debated, routine use of stockings cannot be recommended on the basis of current evidence.

Feeding patients

The Feed Or Ordinary Diet (FOOD) family of large randomised trials assessed different aspects of nutrition after stroke. The first assessed routine oral supplementation in stroke survivors with intact swallow (n=4023)[9] compared with normal diet, and found that routine supplementation

STROKE REHABILITATION—A WORKING DEFINITION

Stroke rehabilitation is not (usually) a single intervention; rather, it is an active process with a holistic, individualised focus. It usually involves teams made up of various professionals, the patient, and other relevant parties (such as carers), all with a final common goal of enhancing functioning to enable patients and carers to live their lives to the fullest potential.

Based on Quinn and Langhorne, Oxford Desk Reference Geriatric Medicine, 2011.

TIPS FOR NON SPECIALISTS

- Refer all patients with suspected stroke to the local dedicated stroke unit
- Stroke survivors with ipsilateral carotid disease may benefit from revascularisation. Outcomes are best when intervention is performed early; liaise with a vascular multidisciplinary team
- Look out for common post-stroke complications such as infection, delirium, depression, pain, incontinence, and falls
- Treat hypertension aggressively and ensure that patients receive long term thromboprophylaxis
- Consider anticoagulation for all stroke survivors with atrial fibrillation, remembering that age alone is not a contraindication to anticoagulation

did not improve outcomes or reduce complications (absolute risk reduction in mortality 0.7%, 95% confidence interval -1.4 to 2.7; overall mortality rates were 12% in groups receiving supplements and 13% in those with no supplements). However, these findings do not preclude the targeted use of supplements where there is evidence or risk of malnutrition. The second and third studies examined the relative merits of early feeding by nasogastric tube (n=859) or percutaneous gastrostomy tube (n=321) after stroke.[10] Early tube feeding was associated with a trend towards reduction in risk of death (absolute risk reduction 5.8%, 95% confidence interval -0.8 to 12.5). By contrast, early feeding by percutaneous gastrostomy tube was associated with a trend towards increased risk of death or poor outcome (7.8%, 0 to 15.5). This finding is partly explained by the severity of stroke that requires artificial feeding; however, use of percutaneous gastrostomy tube is not a benign intervention and has associated short and longer term morbidity.[w18 w19] Patients' preferences and quality of life after percutaneous gastrostomy tube feeding are poorly researched, but available data suggest no improvement in quality of life.[w20] Based on these findings, early placement of percutaneous gastrostomy tubes is not advisable. Options for long term feeding are limited and percutaneous gastrostomy tube feeding may have a role in selected individuals, after discussion with the patient, relatives, and multidisciplinary team.

Mobilisation: how soon?

UK guidelines recommend by consensus that patients should sit out of their bed and become mobile as soon as their clinical condition permits. It seems intuitive that early mobilisation should reduce the sedentary complications of stroke (muscle wasting, thrombosis, pressure sores, hypostatic pneumonia) but there is limited evidence to support the practice. A Very Early Rehabilitation Trial (AVERT) is currently assessing the value of early mobilisation in a multicentre randomised controlled trial. Fears that early mobilisation may be harmful seem to be unfounded; initial results suggest that mobilisation within the first day is well tolerated and may prevent complications.[w21]

Facilitating discharge

Patients and their carers have reported feeling afraid and unsupported at the time of discharge, and an interview questionnaire study has shown that inadequate provision of information is associated with poor satisfaction for stroke survivors and carers.[w22] However, a recent systematic review and meta-analysis of randomised controlled trials that evaluated dedicated stroke liaison services found no evidence of efficacy compared with standard care in improving measures of extended activities of daily living and patient/carer subjective health status.[11]

A prolonged inpatient stay is costly, and services are increasingly encouraged to facilitate an early return to the community. A 2005 meta-analysis of data from studies of early supported discharge concluded that a multidisciplinary, appropriately trained early supported discharge service can significantly reduce days in bed for stroke survivors with mild to moderate impairments, with no corresponding increase in readmission or morbidity[12] and with overall cost benefit.[w23]

In view of the sound evidence base for stroke unit admission and early supported discharge for selected patients, it is unfortunate that recent UK audit data suggest continuing inequity of access to these services. It seems reasonable to speculate that universal delivery of evidence based post-acute stroke care would, through its impact on disability, result in lower incidence of stroke survivors needing institutional or additional domiciliary care, and ultimately would offer cost savings.

Antithrombotic following ischaemic stroke

The preventive efficacy of aspirin, clopidogrel, dipyridamole, and the coumarin anticoagulant warfarin have been evaluated, as monotherapy and (because of their differing mechanisms of action) in combination. (table 3)

For monotherapy, a large meta-analysis showed a 15% reduction in risk of vascular events with aspirin compared with placebo over two years.[w41] A randomised trial showed a modest benefit of clopidogrel over aspirin in reducing vascular events, in a population that included patients with stroke related disease.[w42] Dipyridamole has similar efficacy to aspirin but is associated with frequent adverse effects, mainly headache and gastrointestinal disturbance.[w43]

A meta-analysis of trials showed that the combination of aspirin and modified release dipyridamole is better than aspirin monotherapy[15] and equivalent to clopidogrel monotherapy for stroke prevention.[16] Dipyridamole has little effect on non-stroke vascular events, suggesting that it has specific cerebrovascular efficacy. Combinations of aspirin and clopidogrel have been studied in two large trials, both of which found that any reduction in vascular events was outweighed by increased haemorrhagic adverse events.[17 18] Bleeding rates with aspirin and clopidogrel in combination are similar to those with warfarin and the risks should not be underestimated.[w44] Some patients at high risk may benefit from short term combination antiplatelet therapy; in a trial of 107 patients with carotid stenosis and active embolisation, dual antiplatelet therapy was associated with reduced embolic burden and a trend towards reduced events.[19]

Interpretation of antiplatelet trial data to guide clinical practice is complex. While current Scottish guidance suggests aspirin and modified release dipyridamole as routine therapy, the most recent National Institute for

Table 1 Potential population impact of acute stroke interventions for a hypothetical population of one million with 2500 strokes per year[34]

Treatment	Efficacy (extra independent survivors (n))*	Eligibility (proportion stroke population)	Effectiveness (number of extra independent survivors†)
Aspirin in acute ischaemic stroke	25	80%	20
Thrombolysis in ischaemic stroke			
rt-PA within 3 hours	280	10%	28
rt-PA within 3-4.5 hours	125	10%	12
Basic stroke unit care	125	80%	100
Early supported discharge teams and home rehabilitation	120	35%	42

*rt-PA=tissue plasminogen activator. Calculations indicate number of extra independent survivors (modified Rankin score 0-2) resulting from an intervention during a one year period. *Assuming all stroke patients are eligible for treatment. †Taking into account population eligible for treatment.*

Health and Clinical Excellence assessment recommends clopidogrel because of its better tolerability. For example, in one large study, premature discontinuation of aspirin plus extended release dipyridamole was substantially higher than with clopidogrel (1650 patients [16.4%] versus 1069 [10.6%], P<0.001).[w45]

Warfarin has been studied in patients with sinus rhythm and with atrial fibrillation. For those with sinus rhythm a series of trials has shown that any benefit of anticoagulation is outweighed by an increased risk of bleeding for all levels of stroke risk.[20] Patients with cardioembolic stroke face a particularly high risk of recurrence. Stroke risk in patients with atrial fibrillation can be stratified and scoring systems have been developed (webfigure) to guide choice of therapy. Regardless of the scoring system used, where a patient has sustained a cerebrovascular event, the risk of subsequent stroke is sufficiently high to warrant the use of warfarin where possible. In patients with atrial fibrillation treated with aspirin, the risk of first stroke is 2.7% per annum and risk of recurrent stroke 10%. Treatment with warfarin has been shown to reduce these risks to 1.5% and 4% respectively in a meta-analysis.[21] A Cochrane review confirmed the benefit of warfarin compared with aspirin (odds ratio 0.49, 95% confidence interval 0.33 to 0.72), calculating 60 fewer annual recurrent strokes per 1000 patients treated with warfarin.[22]

The timing of anticoagulant initiation after stroke is unclear. Large infarcts or major clinical deficits raise concerns about haemorrhage and decisions should be based on individual patients' characteristics. Some guidelines suggest starting therapy within 14 days. Although this is a reasonable general approach, patients must be considered individually—these data are from a single study (n=225) where less than half of the participants started warfarin within the first two weeks.[w46]

Despite its clear efficacy, clinicians may avoid warfarin, perhaps fearing risk of haemorrhage and problems with monitoring and adherence. Risk of warfarin related bleeding complications can also be stratified (webfigure). Oral anticoagulation shows the classic "inverse care law", with those at greatest risk of stroke least likely to receive therapy. For example, older cohorts have a raised prevalence of atrial fibrillation and greater risk of stroke, yet underuse of anticoagulation remains prevalent,[w47] despite compelling evidence from a UK general practice based study that showed the efficacy and relative safety of warfarin in selected older patients.[23] A new generation of oral anticoagulants are showing promise in clinical trials and may widen delivery of anticoagulation.[24]

Table 2 Summary of patient outcomes in the stroke unit trials[3]

Outcome	Stroke unit	Conventional care	Extra events per 100 patients (95% CI)
Home (independent)	44%	38%	5 (1 to 8)*
Home (dependent)	16%	16%	0 (−2 to 3)
Institutional care	18%	20%	−2 (−5 to 0)*
Dead	22%	26%	−3 (−6 to −1)*

Proportion (%) of patients with various outcomes at the end of scheduled follow-up (median one year), based on data from Stroke Unit Review (n=6900).
** P<0.05 for difference between groups.*

How are common complications treated after stroke?

Common complications in the longer term after stroke include delirium, infection, depression, post-stroke pain, falls, and incontinence. All these complications may be underdiagnosed and have little evidence available to guide treatment, although they affect rehabilitation negatively and are strong predictors of poor functional outcome and mortality.[13 w24]

Delirium is a common complication after stroke; observational studies suggest an incidence of around 13-48% of patients[w25] but assessment is complicated by the prevalence of concomitant communication deficits and dementia. The stroke insult itself may cause delirium, but infection is often a precipitant. The rate of nosocomial infection after stroke can be as high as 30%.[w26] Pneumonia and urinary tract infections remain the most common infections, although they may be prevented by regular assessment of swallow and avoidance of urinary catheters.[w27]

Post-stroke depression has been reported in a third of patients[w28] but the validity of estimates is questionable because the best method for screening or diagnosis is uncertain. A systematic review found that drug treatment can improve mood and reduce excessive emotions but had frequent side effects, and there was no robust evidence of benefit for non-drug treatments.[w29]

Post-stroke pain is multifactorial in origin, with important components including neuropathic pain and spasticity. Treatments that have been assessed for specific causes of pain include tricyclics, anticonvulsants, and botulinum toxin; evidence of their benefit is emerging but high costs and side effects may limit their widespread use. Shoulder pain in a paretic limb is increasingly recognised.[w30] Robust evidence to guide management of such pain is lacking,[w31] although suggestions are available for best practice in assessment and intervention.[w32]

Falls are common both in the acute setting and in the longer term after stroke.[w33] Putative risk factors include dementia, depression, polypharmacy, and sensory

Table 3 Evidence for antiplatelets in stroke prevention[w57-w59]

Antiplatelet and comparison		Comparator	Result for stroke	Comments
Aspirin	>	Placebo	RR 0.78 95% CI 0.61 to 0.99	AT secondary prevention analysis
Dipyridamole	>	Placebo	RR 0.88(95% CI 0.81 to 0.95)	SR (n=23.19 with ischaemic stroke)
Aspirin + dipyridamole MR	>	Thienopyridines (clopidogrel)	RR 0.76 95% CI 0.65 to 0.89	SR 4 RCT (n=1611)
Aspirin	<	Clopidogrel	OR 0.91, 95% CI 0.84 to 0.98	SR 4 RCT (n=86 865)
Aspirin + dipyridamole MR	≈	Aspirin	HR 1.01 (95% CI 0.92 to 1.11)	RCT (n=20 332)
Aspirin + clopidogrel	≈		RR 0.93 (95%CI 0.83 to 1.05)	SR (n=15 603 with risk factors)
Aspirin + clopidogrel	≈ *	Clopidogrel	RRR 6.4% 95% CI −4.6 to 16.3)	RCT (n=7599 with risk factors)
(Aspirin +) dipyridamole + clopidogrel		–	–	On-going multicentre trials

Data are for ischaemic stroke secondary prevention unless otherwise stated; references for individual trials and analysis within main body of text.
> indicates greater efficacy than; < indicates lesser efficacy than; ≈ indicates equivalent efficacy; RR=relative risk; OR=odds ratio; HR=hazard ratio; RRR=relative risk reduction; AT=antiplatelet trialists; SR=systematic review; RCT=randomised controlled trial.
**Increased risk of life threatening or major bleeding seen with addition of aspirin.*

impairment.[w34] The incidence of fracture is substantial (twofold increase in risk of hip/femur fracture[w35]) in the post-stroke population.[w36] Interventions to reduce risk of fracture are extrapolated from studies in older people that were not limited to those who had had a stroke; no stroke specific data are available. Preventive treatments may include bisphosphonates and preparations of calcium vitamin D, and multidisciplinary prevention packages that focus on personal and environmental factors. A recent systematic review and meta-analysis has highlighted the need for future randomised controlled trials in this area; it found evidence only to support vitamin D supplementation in a female population in hospital.[w37]

Prevalence of urinary incontinence is estimated at 40-60% in an acute stroke population, with 15% remaining incontinent at one year.[w38] Causes may include abnormalities of normal central control of voiding, lower urinary tract infection, and functional incontinence. A Cochrane review evaluated the limited evidence on physical interventions such as bladder retraining and pelvic floor exercises, and drug treatment, which may have a role in selected patients.[w39]

What measures help to prevent another stroke?

The risk of recurrent vascular events after a stroke or TIA is substantial. Recurrent stroke has been reported in 17.3% of patients after TIA and 18.5% after minor stroke at three months.[w40] National guidelines suggest that secondary preventive strategies be commenced early and continue indefinitely.[1 14]

Management of carotid disease

International guidelines recommend that survivors of stroke are investigated for large artery atherosclerosis, particularly ipsilateral extracranial carotid artery disease.[25] Where imaging confirms stenotic carotid disease, patients with non-disabling events may benefit from surgical carotid endarterectomy. As a general rule, all patients with greater than 50% symptomatic internal carotid stenosis should be considered for intervention in the setting of a neurovascular multidisciplinary team. The benefits of intervention vary with degree of stenosis and time since event. A pooled analysis of data from randomised controlled trials of endarterectomy for symptomatic carotid stenosis (6092 patients) showed that for severe symptomatic stenosis (>70%), surgery afforded a 15.6% absolute risk reduction in ipsilateral ischaemic stroke over five years versus medical treatment alone, with a smaller 4.5% absolute risk reduction for moderate (50-69%) stenosis.[26] Surgery carried no benefit in less severe disease or in cases of complete occlusion. Greater benefit is seen with early surgery. Treatment within two weeks of symptoms afforded an absolute risk reduction of 23%, by comparison with absolute risk reduction of 7.4% for those treated after 12 weeks. In order to prevent one ipsilateral stroke at five years, the number needed to treat is five within two weeks and 125 if surgery is delayed beyond 12 weeks.[27] The benefits of early treatment are particularly pronounced in women, where significant efficacy of revascularisation is seen only in the first two weeks.[w48]

Percutaneous stenting of carotid vessels has been proposed as a less invasive method of revascularisation, but studies have failed to show that stenting has the long term benefits of traditional endarterectomy. Risk and benefit may change as technical expertise develops but present guidelines do not recommend stenting outside clinical trials.[28]

How to manage hypertension

Management of hypertension in the acute phase was discussed in the first part of this review. Long term management of hypertension significantly reduces the risk of recurrent events. Meta-analysis of secondary prevention trials showed a 24% reduced odds of recurrent stroke with antihypertensive treatment (odds ratio 0.76, 95% confidence interval 0.63-0.92; absolute rate of recurrent stroke 10%).[w49] Risk reduction is related to change in blood pressure and substantial benefit is seen even with a modest change in pressure. An overview of published reviews including more than 188 000 participants, showed that for each 10 mm Hg reduction in systolic pressure, risk was reduced by one third. This finding was consistent across sex, region, and stroke subtypes.[29]

QUESTIONS FOR FUTURE RESEARCH

- What is the optimal model for deep vein thrombosis prophylaxis for patients with ischaemic stroke?
- What is the optimal timing and intensity of multidisciplinary intervention? Can this be targeted?
- Is there a role for screening stroke survivors for common complications; do we have adequate tools to inform a screening approach?
- Can we develop novel drugs to minimise recurrent disease and provide alternative strategies for intolerant patients; are novel anticoagulation treatments cost effective?
- What is the role of short duration, high potency antithrombotic therapy following ischaemic stroke?
- What happens to stroke survivors' functional status in the longer term (years) post-event; is there a role for ongoing or opportunistic intervention and rehabilitation?

ADDITIONAL EDUCATIONAL RESOURCES

Resources for healthcare professionals

- Stroke Association Professional Training (www.stroke.org.uk/professionals/training_and_development/index.html)– A selection of training and education programmes offered by the stroke association, suitable for all healthcare professionals
- European Stroke Organisation (www.eso-stroke.org)–Comprehensive access to European stroke guidelines and educational resources for health professionals and lay people
- UK Stroke Research Network (www.uksrn.ac.uk)–Provides an infrastructure to facilitate stroke research and improve communication between academics, stroke clinicians, stroke service users, and research funders
- Stroke Training and Awareness Resources (STARS) project (www.stroketraining.org)–Commissioned by the Scottish Government to provide an e-learning resource for all healthcare professionals and social care staff working with patients affected by stroke

Resources for patients

- The Stroke Association (www.stroke.org.uk)–Produces a number of publications to help educate and inform and increase awareness of stroke, including patient leaflets, and *Stroke News* (a quarterly magazine)
- Act FAST campaign (www.nhs.uk/actfast/Pages/stroke.aspx)–Public awareness campaign to improve community recognition of stroke symptoms and encourage those affected to seek urgent medical help
- Connect (www.ukconnect.org/index.aspx)–communication disability charity for patients and carers affected by aphasia
- Carers UK (www.carersuk.org)–charity providing support for home carers

Evidence clearly indicates that all patients should be considered for antihypertensive therapy to prevent recurrent stroke. UK guidelines suggest a target blood pressure of 130/80 mm Hg; for most patients this will require at least two agents, one of which should be a diuretic.[28]

The large PROGRESS trial has been pivotal in guiding post-stroke blood pressure management.[30] Treatment with the ACE inhibitor perindopril, in combination with the thiazide indapamide, showed a 26% reduced risk of stroke (95% confidence interval 16% to 34%) compared with placebo. Patients were considered for inclusion regardless of baseline blood pressure and benefits were seen even in those traditionally defined as normotensive.

Choice of antihypertensive agent may be important. In one pooled analysis the strongest evidence was for diuretic based therapy (odds ratio 0.63, 95% confidence interval 0.55 to 0.73).[w50] Theoretical benefits of angiotensin receptor antagonists in stroke prevention have not been supported by large scale trials.[w51 w52]

Treating high cholesterol, diabetes and lifestyle risks

The stroke related benefits of statin treatment were originally described through sub-analyses data relating to ischaemic heart disease. In a large pooled analysis of data from coronary disease trials, statin treatment significantly reduced the risk of incident stroke (odds ratio 0.79, 95% confidence interval 0.73 to 0.85).[31] The SPARCL trial (n=4731), a stroke specific placebo controlled study of statins (atorvastatin 80 mg), showed a reduction in incident ischaemic stroke (number needed to treat 45 over five years) and other vascular events, but a rise in incident haemorrhagic stroke (number needed to harm 107 over five years).[w53] UK guidelines recommend treating to a total cholesterol of less than 4.0 mmol/L and LDL less than 2.0 mmol/L.[28] Statins are not recommended after intracerebral haemorrhage unless indicated for other vascular disease.

Observational studies have suggested a high prevalence of occult diabetes in stroke cohorts, which suggests that screening for diabetes may be useful after stroke. Although diabetes is an important risk factor for vascular events, no specific guidelines are available for optimal therapy in patients with stroke. A subgroup analysis of the PROactive trial described a reduced incidence of stroke with pioglitazone in selected patients[32] but the findings must be interpreted in the light of other risks associated with thiazolidinediones. Several large randomised controlled trials have compared aggresive glycaemic control with standard therapy. Although these studies were not designed to measure stroke outcomes, they did not show reduced incidence of stroke with tight glycaemic control.[w54]

No data from randomised controlled trials are available to guide lifestyle modification in patients with stroke. Compelling observational data support cessation of smoking.[w55] The relation between alcohol and cerebrovascular risk is controversial. Meta-analysis of 84 observational studies described a "J-shaped curve" where lowest vascular risk was associated with modest intake, but specific stroke risk was increased at intakes of more than one unit daily.[w56] Controlled weight reduction in overweight patients and physical activity have been associated with improvements in blood pressure, cholesterol, and diabetes. There are no stroke specific data on dietary modification, although routine vitamin supplementation probably has no benefit.[33]

Contributors: All authors contributed to writing the manuscript and have approved the final version. KSMcA is guarantor.

Competing interests: All authors have completed the Unified Competing Interest form at www.icmje.org/coi_disclosure.pdf (available on request from the corresponding author) and declare: no external support for the submitted work; KSMcA, PH, PL have no relationships with companies that might have an interest in the submitted work in the previous three years. TJQ has received modest speakers' fees and travel assistance from Bristol Myers Squibb, Sanofi, and Pfizer; no non-financial interests that may be relevant to the submitted work.

Provenance and peer review: Commissioned, externally peer reviewed.

1 National Collaborating Centre for Chronic Conditions. Stroke: national clinical guideline for diagnosis and initial management of acute stroke and transient ischaemic attack (TIA). Royal College of Physicians, 2008.

2 Scottish Intercollegiate Guideline Network. Management of patients with stroke: identification and management of dysphagia. A national clinical guideline. 2010.

3 Stroke Unit Trialists' Collaboration. Organised inpatient (stroke unit) care for stroke. *Cochrane Database Syst Rev* 2007;4:CD000197.

4 Govan L, Langhorne P, Weir CJ, Stroke Unit Trialists' Collaboration. Does the prevention of complications explain the survival benefit of organized inpatient (stroke unit) care? Further analysis of a systematic review. *Stroke* 2007;38:2536-40.

5 Langhorne P, Pollock A, Stroke Unit Trialists' Collaboration. What are the components of effective stroke unit care? *Age Ageing* 2002;31:365-71.

6 Sherman DG, Albers GW, Bladin C, Fieschi C, Gabbai AA, Kase CS, et al. The efficacy and safety of enoxaparin versus unfractionated heparin for the prevention of venous thromboembolism after acute ischaemic stroke (PREVAIL Study): an open-label randomised comparison. *Lancet* 2007;369:1347-55.

7 CLOTS Trials Collaboration, Dennis M, Sandercock PA, Reid J, Graham C, Murray G, et al. Effectiveness of thigh-length graduated compression stockings to reduce the risk of deep vein thrombosis after stroke (CLOTS trial 1): a multicentre, randomised controlled trial. *Lancet* 2009;373:1958-65.

8 CLOTS Trial Collaboration. Thigh-length versus below-knee stockings for deep venous thrombosis prophylaxis after stroke. *Ann Intern Med* 2010;153:553-62.

9 Routine oral nutritional supplementation for stroke patients in hospital (FOOD): a multicentre randomised controlled trial. *Lancet* 2005;365:755-63.

10 Effect of timing and method of enteral tube feeding for dysphagic stroke patients (FOOD): a multicentre randomised controlled trial. *Lancet* 2005;365:764-72.

11 Ellis G, Mant J, Langhorne P, Dennis M, Winner S. Stroke liaison workers for stroke patients and carers: an individual patient data meta-analysis. *Cochrane Database Syst Rev* 2010;5:CD005066.

12 Langhorne P, Taylor G, Murray G, Dennis M, Anderson C, Bautz-Holter E, et al. Early supported discharge services for stroke patients: a meta-analysis of individual patients' data. *Lancet* 2005;365:501-6.

13 Quinn TJ, Paolucci S, Sunnerhagen KS, Sivenius J, Walker MF, Toni D, et al. Evidence-based stroke rehabilitation: an expanded guidance document from the European Stroke Organisation (ESO) guidelines for management of ischaemic stroke and transient ischaemic attack 2008. *J Rehab Med* 2009;41:99-111.

14 Scottish Intercollegiate Guidelines Network. Management of patients with stroke or TIA: assessment, investigation, immediate management and secondary prevention. A national clinical guideline. 2008.

15 Verro P, Gorelick PB, Nguyen D. Aspirin plus dipyridamole versus aspirin for prevention of vascular events after stroke or tia: a meta-analysis. *Stroke* 2008;39:1358-63.

16 Sacco RL, Diener HC, Yusuf S, Cotton D, Ounpuu S, Lawton WA, et al. Aspirin and extended-release dipyridamole versus clopidogrel for recurrent stroke. *N Engl J Med* 2008;359:1238-51.

17 Bhatt DL, Fox KA, Hacke W, Berger PB, Black HR, Boden WE, et al. Clopidogrel and aspirin versus aspirin alone for the prevention of atherothrombotic events. *N Engl J Med* 2006;354:1706-17.

18 Diener HC, Bogousslavsky J, Brass LM, Cimminiello C, Csiba L, Kaste M, et al. Aspirin and clopidogrel compared with clopidogrel alone after recent ischaemic stroke or transient ischaemic attack in high-risk patients (MATCH): randomised, double-blind, placebo-controlled trial. *Lancet* 2004;364:331-7.

19 Markus HS, Droste DW, Kaps M, Larrue V, Lees KR, Siebler M, et al. Dual antiplatelet therapy with clopidogrel and aspirin in symptomatic carotid stenosis evaluated using doppler embolic signal detection: the clopidogrel and aspirin for reduction of emboli in symptomatic carotid stenosis (CARESS) trial. *Circulation* 2005;111:2233-40.

20 Algra A, De Schryver EL, van GJ, Kappelle LJ, Koudstaal PJ. Oral anticoagulants versus antiplatelet therapy for preventing further vascular events after transient ischaemic attack or minor stroke of presumed arterial origin. *Cochrane Database Syst Rev* 2006;3:CD001342.

21 van WC, Hart RG, Singer DE, Laupacis A, Connolly S, Petersen P, et al. Oral anticoagulants vs aspirin in nonvalvular atrial fibrillation: an individual patient meta-analysis. *JAMA* 2002;288:2441-8.

22 Saxena R, Koudstaal P. Anticoagulants versus antiplatelet therapy for preventing stroke in patients with nonrheumatic atrial fibrillation and a history of stroke or transient ischemic attack. *Cochrane Database Syst Rev* 2004;4:CD000187.

23 Mant J, Hobbs FD, Fletcher K, Roalfe A, Fitzmaurice D, Lip GY, et al. Warfarin versus aspirin for stroke prevention in an elderly community population with atrial fibrillation (the Birmingham Atrial Fibrillation Treatment of the Aged Study, BAFTA): a randomised controlled trial. *Lancet* 2007;370:493-503.

24 Connolly SJ, Ezekowitz MD, Yusuf S, Eikelboom J, Oldgren J, Parekh A, et al. Dabigatran versus warfarin in patients with atrial fibrillation. *N Eng J Med* 2009;361:1139-51.

25 European Stroke Organisation (ESO) Executive Committee, ESO Writing Committee. Guidelines for management of ischaemic stroke and transient ischaemic attack 2008. *Cerebrovasc Dis* 2008;25:457-507.

26 Rothwell PM, Eliasziw M, Gutnikov SA, Fox AJ, Taylor DW, Mayberg MR, et al. Analysis of pooled data from the randomised controlled trials of endarterectomy for symptomatic carotid stenosis. *Lancet* 2003;361:107-16.

27 Rothwell PM, Gutnikov SA, Warlow CP. Reanalysis of the final results of the European Carotid Surgery Trial. *Stroke* 2003;34:514-23.

28 Intercollegiate Stroke Working Party. National clinical guideline for stroke. Third ed. Royal College of Physicians, 2008.

29 Lawes CM, Bennett DA, Feigin VL, Rodgers A. Blood pressure and stroke: an overview of published reviews. *Stroke* 2004;35:776-85.

30 PROGRESS Collaborative Group. Randomised trial of a perindopril-based blood-pressure-lowering regimen among 6105 individuals with previous stroke or transient ischaemic attack. *Lancet* 2001;358:1033-41.

31 Amarenco P, Labreuche J, Lavalle P, Touboul PJ. Statins in stroke prevention and carotid atherosclerosis: systematic review and up-to-date meta-analysis. *Stroke* 2004;35:2902-9.

32 Dormandy JA, Charbonnel B, Eckland DJ, Erdmann E, Massi-Benedetti M, Moules IK, et al. Secondary prevention of macrovascular events in patients with type 2 diabetes in the PROactive Study (PROspective pioglitAzone Clinical Trial In macroVascular Events): a randomised controlled trial. *Lancet* 2005;366:1279-89.

33 VITATOPS Trial Study Group. B vitamins in patients with recent transient ischaemic attack or stroke in the VITAmins TO Prevent Stroke (VITATOPS) trial: a randomised, double-blind, parallel, placebo-controlled trial. *Lancet Neurology* 2010;9:855-65.

34 Langhorne P, Sandercock P, Prasad K. Evidence-based practice for stroke. *Lancet Neurology* 2009;8:308-9.

Posterior circulation ischaemic stroke

Áine Merwick, stroke and metabolic medicine clinical fellow[1],
David Werring, reader in clinical neurology[2]

[1]National Hospital for Neurology and Neurosurgery, London, UK

[2]Stroke Research Group, UCL Institute of Neurology, National Hospital for Neurology and Neurosurgery, London WC1N 3BG, UK

Correspondence to: D Werring d.werring@ucl.ac.uk

Cite this as: *BMJ* 2014;348:g3175

DOI: 10.1136/bmj.g3175

http://www.bmj.com/content/348/bmj.g3175

About 20-25% (range 17-40%) of the 150 000 ischaemic strokes in the United Kingdom each year affect posterior circulation brain structures (including the brainstem, cerebellum, midbrain, thalamuses, and areas of temporal and occipital cortex), which are supplied by the vertebrobasilar arterial system.[1] Early recognition of posterior circulation stroke or transient ischaemic attack (TIA) may prevent disability and save lives, but it remains more difficult to recognise and treat effectively than other stroke types. Delayed or incorrect diagnosis may have devastating consequences, including potentially preventable death or severe disability, if acute treatment or secondary prevention is delayed.[2] The annual adjusted incidence of posterior circulation infarction was estimated at 18 per 100 000 person years (95% confidence interval 10/100 000 to 26/100 000) in an Australian study.[3] Preceding posterior circulation TIA or other transient brainstem symptoms, particularly if recurrent, signal a high risk of impending ischaemic stroke and should prompt specialist urgent referral for further management.[4] New acute treatment options and stroke prevention strategies specific to the posterior circulation are important areas of active research.

This review aims to demonstrate the importance and challenges of recognising and treating posterior circulation stroke, including the key differences between posterior and anterior circulation stroke.

What is posterior circulation ischaemic stroke?

Posterior circulation ischaemic stroke is a clinical syndrome associated with ischaemia related to stenosis, in situ thrombosis, or embolic occlusion of the posterior circulation arteries—the vertebral arteries in the neck, the intracranial vertebral, basilar, and posterior cerebral arteries, and their branches (fig 1). Common sites of occlusion cause characteristic clinical patterns and syndromes (figs 1 and 2).

There are important differences between posterior and anterior circulation stroke. The differences include the value of screening instruments, optimum diagnostic modalities, and clinical features (table).[5 6 7 8 9] The face arm speech test (FAST), a widely used prehospital stroke recognition screening instrument, is less sensitive for detecting posterior circulation stroke than for anterior circulation stroke (the carotid territory, including the anterior and middle cerebral arteries and their branches).[5] It can be difficult to determine the vascular territory of an acute ischaemic clinical syndrome on purely clinical grounds, but this knowledge may be needed to determine the most appropriate acute treatment and prevention strategy.[10] However, computed tomography (CT), the standard brain imaging modality in hyperacute stroke, has limited sensitivity in posterior circulation stroke. Although in the past posterior circulation ischaemia was considered to have a lower recurrence risk than anterior circulation ischaemia, current data suggest that the risk is at least as high, if not higher.[1]

What causes posterior circulation stroke?

The most common causes of posterior circulation stroke are occlusion or embolism from large artery vertebrobasilar atherosclerosis or dissection, and embolism from the heart.[11 12] In a large US hospital registry study of 407 patients with posterior circulation stroke, embolism was the most common mechanism (40% of patients); large artery occlusive lesions caused haemodynamic brain ischaemia in 32%; and the remainder of strokes were attributed to in situ small vessel occlusion, other identified mechanisms, or unknown causes.[12] Of the strokes attributed to embolism 24% had cardiac source, 14% were caused by to artery-to-artery embolism, and 2% had multiple sources of potential embolism.[12]

Recent population based and hospital observational studies have shown a threefold increased risk of stroke after posterior circulation TIA or minor stroke in patients

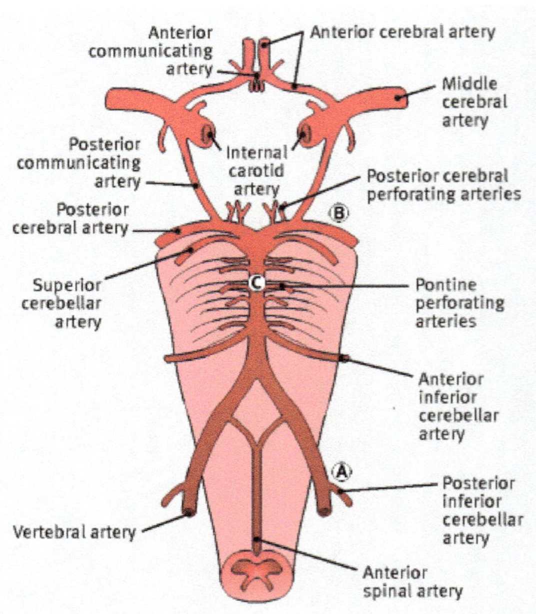

Fig 1 Anatomy of the vertebral and basilar arterial circulation and circle of Willis. (A) Site of posterior inferior cerebellar artery occlusion; (B) site of posterior cerebral artery occlusion; (C) site of pontine perforating artery occlusion

SUMMARY POINTS

- Posterior circulation stroke accounts for 20-25% (range 17-40%) of ischaemic strokes
- Posterior circulation transient ischaemic attacks may include brief or minor brainstem symptoms and are more difficult to diagnose than anterior circulation ischaemia
- Specialist assessment and administration of intravenous tissue plasminogen activator are delayed in posterior circulation stroke compared with anterior circulation stroke
- The risk of recurrent stroke after posterior circulation stroke is at least as high as for anterior circulation stroke, and vertebrobasilar stenosis increases the risk threefold
- Acute neurosurgical input may be needed in patients with hydrocephalus or raised intracranial pressure
- Basilar occlusion is associated with high mortality or severe disability, especially if blood flow is not restored in the vessel; if symptoms such as acute coma, dysarthria, dysphagia, quadriparesis, pupillary and oculomotor abnormalities are detected, urgently seek the input of a stroke specialist

with symptomatic vertebrobasilar stenosis than in those without stenosis.[6 13 14] Dissection of the extracranial vertebral artery is also an important cause of stroke, especially in young patients; it may be painless and usually occurs without a clear history of trauma. In a systematic review of vertebral artery dissection the most common symptoms were dizziness or vertigo (58%), headache (51%), and neck pain (46%). The annual incidence of spontaneous vertebral artery dissection is estimated at 1-1.5 per 100 000 per year.[15] Less common causes include vasculitis and dolichoectasia (elongation and tortuosity) of the vertebral and basilar arteries. In younger people, dolichoectasia may be a clue to Fabry's disease, a rare X linked inherited multisystem lysosomal storage disorder.[16]

Similar to other forms of cerebrovascular and cardiovascular disease, the risk factors for posterior circulation strokes include hypertension, smoking, hypercholesterolaemia, atrial fibrillation, and coronary artery disease.

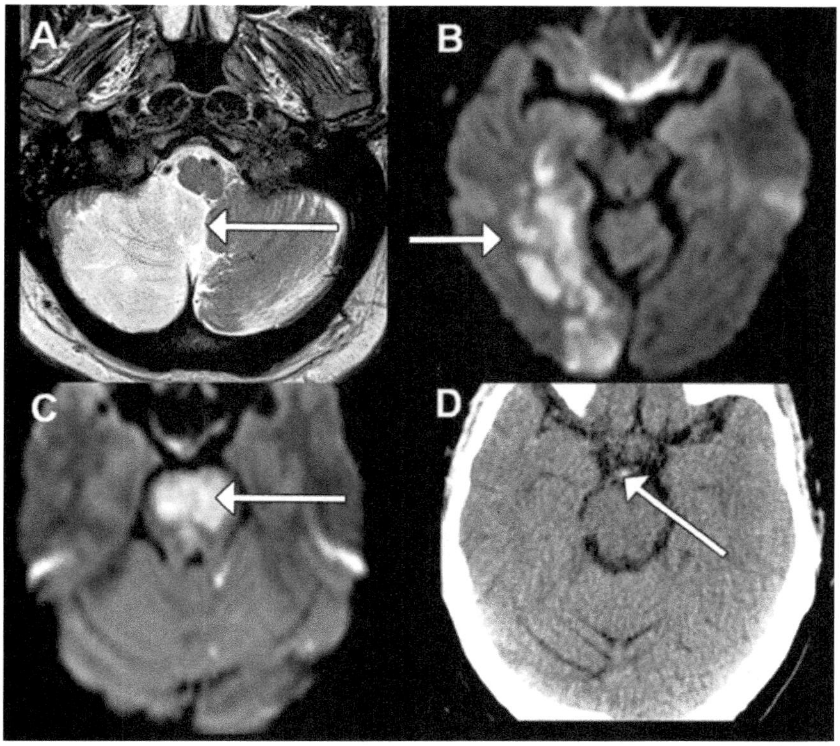

Fig 2 Imaging findings associated with the sites of occlusion shown in fig 1. (A) Full right posterior inferior cerebellar artery territory infarct (arrow) shown on T2 weighted magnetic resonance imaging (MRI); (B) acute right posterior cerebral artery territory infarct (arrow) shown on diffusion weighted MRI; (C) acute bilateral pontine infarction (arrow) as a result of acute basilar occlusion shown on diffusion weighted MRI; (D) axial computed tomography scan showing bright (hyperdense) region (arrow) consistent with an acute basilar thrombus

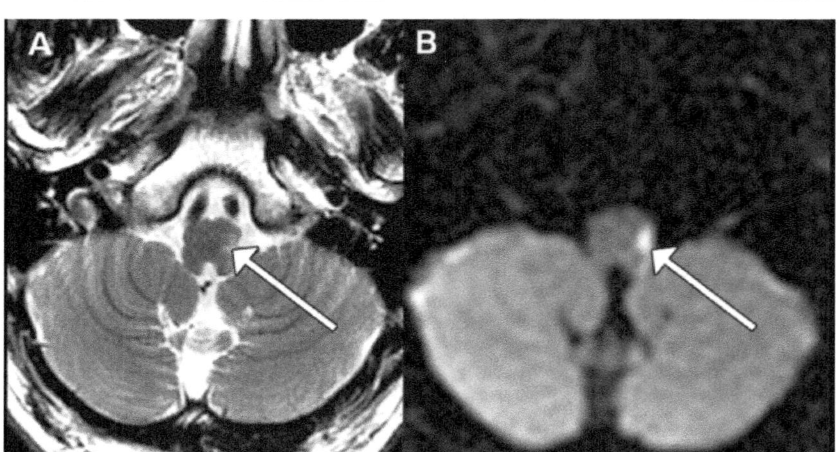

Fig 3 Left lateral medullary infarction (arrows) shown on (A) T2 weighted axial magnetic resonance imaging (MRI) scan; (B) MRI scan with diffusion weighted imaging. Note the infarct is more conspicuous with diffusion weighted imaging

What are the clinical symptoms and signs of posterior circulation ischaemia?

Posterior circulation ischaemia can be challenging to recognise, particularly in patients with a TIA, which may have resolved by the time of presentation. However, there are some characteristic clinical patterns (box 1).

Because the posterior circulation supplies the brainstem, cerebellum, and occipital cortex, symptoms often include dizziness, diplopia, dysarthria, dysphagia, disequilibrium, ataxia, and visual field deficits. Acute onset "crossed" deficits—cranial nerve territory symptoms on one side and sensory or motor deficits of the opposite arm and leg—are virtually diagnostic of posterior circulation ischaemia.[7] In a large single centre observational study of 407 patients, the most common posterior circulation symptoms were dizziness (47%), unilateral limb weakness (41%), dysarthria (31%), headache (28%), and nausea or vomiting (27%). The most common signs were unilateral limb weakness (38%), gait ataxia (31%), unilateral limb ataxia (30%), dysarthria (28%), and nystagmus (24%).[18]

In a large Chinese registry observational study of patients with posterior or anterior circulation stroke on confirmed magnetic resonance imaging, the signs with the highest predictive values favouring a diagnosis of posterior circulation stroke were crossed sensory deficits (3.0% *v* 0%; P<0.001; positive predictive value (PPV) 100%; odds ratio 3.98), crossed motor deficits (4.0% *v* 0.1%; P<0.001; PPV 92.3%; 36.04), oculomotor (third) nerve palsy (4.0% *v* 0%; P<0.001; PPV 100%; 4.00), and quadrantanopia (1.3% *v* 0%; P<0.001; PPV 100%; 3.93). However, all of these signs had a low sensitivity, ranging from 1.3% to 4.0%.[7]

In practice it can be difficult to distinguish between posterior and anterior circulation stroke because some common syndromes (such as hemiparesis) are not specific for one or the other (table).[7 10]

Vertigo (a feeling of true movement relative to the environment) and "dizziness" are common symptoms in general practice and the emergency room and present a particular challenge.[19] It is crucial to elicit exactly what a patient means by dizziness (true feeling of rotation, dissociation between the patient and the environment, or presyncopal symptoms). Urgently refer all patients with acute vertigo and any other focal neurological symptoms for specialist assessment. New neck pain or new headache with focal neurological symptoms should also prompt urgent referral.[15] TIAs, often with minor symptoms such as dysarthria or diplopia, may precede devastating basilar stroke syndromes, so they need to be promptly recognised and patients referred for specialist evaluation.[20 21] This can be a real challenge because some of these attacks are very brief, may seem minor, and do not fulfil traditional TIA criteria ("transient neurological attacks").[4 17] Transient brainstem symptoms that do not fully meet the traditional definition of TIA (such as isolated vertigo) have also recently been associated with the risk of subsequent stroke in the posterior circulation, although they may also be due to alternative non-ischaemic disease.[4]

Which other disorders can mimic posterior circulation ischaemic stroke?

Acute peripheral vestibular dysfunction can mimic stroke in general practice or the emergency department. It typically causes isolated vertigo with no other brainstem symptoms or signs and is more common than stroke. The head impulse or Dix-Hallpike tests may help in the diagnosis of peripheral vestibular disturbance.[19] Acute intracranial haemorrhage, subarachnoid haemorrhage, and tumour can mimic ischaemic stroke, further highlighting the importance of prompt imaging. Basilar migraine, which may have aura features including vertigo and diplopia, as well as severe occipital headache, can resemble acute stroke, and should always be excluded, especially if it is the patient's first presentation.[21]

Toxic or metabolic disturbances may initially present with features resembling cerebrovascular disease. These include drugs of misuse or prescribed drugs (such as anticonvulsants), hypoglycaemia, central pontine myelinolysis, and post-infectious disorders, such as antibody associated disorders (for example, Miller Fisher syndrome, which causes ophthalmoplegia, ataxia, and areflexia).[21]

Posterior reversible encephalopathy syndrome can cause posterior circulation ischaemia, which results in visual disturbance, seizures, and other focal symptoms. This syndrome has a predilection for the posterior circulation and is usually associated with hypertension.

Neuroinflammatory or chronic infectious disorders, such as sarcoidosis, Behçet's disease, and Whipple's disease, which may affect the brainstem and present acutely, often have preceding or systemic clinical features. Infection of the medulla, pons, and cerebellum (rhomboencephalitis) by viruses (for example, Epstein Barr virus or West Nile virus), bacteria (for example, *Listeria monocytogenes*), or fungi may mimic stroke by direct effects and by causing para-infectious vasculitis.[21]

Stroke chameleons

Stroke chameleons are disorders that look like other disorders but are actually stroke syndromes. Bilateral thalamic ischaemia is such a disorder and may cause reduced consciousness level or a global amnesic syndrome; bilateral occipital stroke may present as confusion or delirium; and infarcts limited to the medial vermis in medial posterior inferior cerebellar artery (PICA) territory usually cause a vertiginous syndrome that resembles peripheral vestibulopathy.[2 19] Rarely acute brainstem ischaemia can cause bilateral rhythmic leg movements that can resemble fasciculations or convulsive seizures.[22]

Which clinical syndromes are caused by posterior circulation stroke?

Although ischaemia can occur anywhere in the vertebrobasilar territory, a large registry study from the United States suggested that infarcts most often include

Comparison of anterior and posterior circulation ischaemic stroke[5-9]

Aspects	Anterior circulation (carotid territory)	Posterior circulation (vertebrobasilar territory)
Clinical recognition tools		
Prehospital triage tools and scores, such as FAST*	High sensitivity: >90%	Moderate sensitivity: ~60%
Imaging		
Computed tomography	Moderate sensitivity	Poor sensitivity
Magnetic resonance imaging	Very good to excellent sensitivity (>95%)	Very good sensitivity (>80%)
Clinical features†		
Isolated hemianopia	+	++
Quadrantanopia	+	++
Pupil abnormalities	+ (Horner's syndrome)	+++ (may be bilateral)
Diplopia	–	+++
Focal (unilateral) sensorimotor	+++	++
Bilateral sensorimotor	–	+++
Unsteadiness/ataxia	+	++
Vertigo	±	+++
Dysarthria	++	++
Dysphasia	+++	+ (thalamic infarcts)
Coma	+	+++
	Coma unusual, unless there is mass effect and raised intracranial pressure (for example, as a result of large middle cerebral artery stroke); rare as an initial hyperacute presenting symptom; somnolence may occur	Coma well recognised in thalamic and brainstem ischaemia and may be an acute presenting symptom
Acute management		
Intravenous tissue plasminogen activator time window (h)	4.5	4.5 (but used up to 24 in basilar occlusion)
Endovascular treatment	Benefit not proved	Benefit not proved but often considered for basilar occlusion, especially if it has not responded to intravenous treatment
Neurosurgical intervention	Hemicraniectomy indicated for malignant middle cerebral artery syndrome	External ventricular drainage or posterior decompression indicated for hydrocephalus in acute infarction with mass effect
Stroke risk in symptomatic large vessel disease by 90 days after transient ischaemic attack or stroke	18%	Almost 25%

**FAST=face arm speech test.*

†Scores represent the estimated relative likelihood of each symptom being present in anterior and posterior circulation ischaemic stroke.

the distal territory (rostral brainstem, superior cerebellum, occipital and temporal lobes).[12] Several posterior circulation clinical syndromes are highly localising and are important for all doctors who look after acute stroke patients to recognise (fig 2; box 2).

A large single centre series of 1000 patients in Switzerland reported that 48% of vertebrobasilar territory infarcts were in the brainstem (mainly the pons in 27%, mainly the medulla in 14%, mainly the midbrain in 7%), 7% in the cerebellum, 36% in the posterior inferior cerebellar artery territory, and 9% in multiple locations.[23]

Lateral medullary infarction (Wallenberg syndrome) (fig 3) is the most common syndrome related to intracranial vertebral artery occlusion, in which blood flow through perforating branches to the lateral medulla is impaired.[12,20] It is often missed or misdiagnosed. If this syndrome is suspected, diagnostic signs include reduced pin prick sensations and temperature in the face, contralateral limbs, and body; box 2 shows other clinical features.[17] PICA territory infarcts typically cause ataxia, and full PICA territory infarcts (fig 2A) cause occipital headache or neck pain on the same side owing to swelling and mass effect.[12,18] The combination of hemianopia and sensory loss on the same side without paralysis is virtually diagnostic of posterior cerebral artery territory infarction (fig 2B). Occlusion of the rostral (distal) portion of the basilar artery can cause ischaemia of the midbrain, thalamuses, and temporal and occipital lobe territories supplied by the posterior cerebral artery branches of the basilar artery.[18] The major abnormalities associated with rostral brainstem infarction affect alertness as well as behavioural, memory, oculomotor, and pupillary functions.[18] Complete pontine infarction (fig 2C and 2D) causes the "locked in syndrome" of quadriplegia and anarthria with preserved consciousness. Patients may be able to communicate using eye or facial movements.[18,22]

Numerous eponymous posterior circulation stroke syndromes exist, many of which present in an incomplete form.[20] Furthermore, variations are common in the well described clinical syndromes, particularly in the pattern of sensory changes (for instance in PICA syndromes, facial pain may be an initial feature and hypoalgesia can affect either side of the face).[18] Coma is a rare initial feature in posterior circulation stroke (2% in one registry study), but it is important to distinguish coma as a result of basilar thrombosis.[7,18] Useful methods of identifying basilar artery occlusion as a cause of coma include a history suggestive of preceding TIA episodes and sudden onset of coma. Clinical examination findings including eye movement abnormalities, focal lateralising signs, pupil abnormalities, a dense appearance of the basilar artery vessel on CT as well as basilar occlusion on CT angiography or magnetic resonance angiography.[18,21,22]

BOX 1 COMMON SYMPTOMS SEEN IN POSTERIOR CIRCULATION ISCHAEMIA

- Motor deficits (weakness, clumsiness, or paralysis of any combination of arms and legs, up to quadriplegia, sometimes changing from one side to another in different attacks)[17]
- "Crossed" syndromes, consisting of ipsilateral cranial nerve dysfunction and contralateral long motor or sensory tract dysfunction are highly characteristic of posterior circulation stroke[18]
- Sensory deficits (numbness, including loss of sensation or paraesthesia in any combination of extremities, sometimes including all four limbs or both sides of the face or mouth)
- Homonymous hemianopia—a visual field defect affecting either the two right or the two left halves of the visual fields of both eyes
- Ataxia, imbalance, unsteadiness, or disequilibrium
- Vertigo, with or without nausea and vomiting
- Diplopia as a result of ophthalmoplegia
- Dysphagia or dysarthria
- Isolated reduced level of consciousness is not a typical stroke symptom but can result from bilateral thalamic or brainstem ischaemia (especially from rostral basilar artery occlusion)

How is posterior circulation ischaemic stroke diagnosed?

The diagnosis of posterior circulation ischaemic stroke is based on rapidly developing clinical signs of focal (or occasionally global) disturbance of cerebral function, with no apparent cause other than that of vascular origin.[24]

An index of suspicion for posterior circulation stroke should be maintained in patients presenting with acute neurological symptoms. In the initial assessment phase it is important to establish the onset and tempo of symptoms and establish whether the patient has experienced typical or characteristic posterior circulation stroke symptoms such as acute diplopia, visual field disturbance, or swallowing difficulties.

BOX 2 KEY CLINICAL FEATURES OF POSTERIOR CIRCULATION INFARCTION ACCORDING TO ANATOMICAL LOCATION AND VASCULAR TERRITORY AFFECTED[12,17,18,22]

Lateral medulla (intracranial vertebral artery infarct, also known as Wallenberg syndrome)

- Nystagmus, vertigo, ipsilateral Horner's syndrome, ipsilateral facial sensory loss, dysarthria, hoarseness, and dysphagia
- Contralateral hemisensory loss in the trunk and limb—pain and temperature

Medial medulla

- Ipsilateral tongue weakness and later hemiatrophy of the tongue
- Contralateral hemiparesis of the arm and leg
- Hemisensory loss—touch and proprioception

Pons

- Hemiparesis or hemisensory loss, ataxic hemiparesis, dysarthria, horizontal gaze palsy
- Complete infarction causes "locked-in syndrome" with quadriparesis, loss of speech, but preserved awareness and cognition, and sometimes preserved eye movements

Top of the basilar (distal basilar occlusion)

- Somnolence, confusion (from thalamic infarction)
- Bilateral loss of vision, unawareness or denial of blindness (from bilateral occipital infarction)

Posterior inferior cerebellar artery

- Truncal ataxia, vertigo (limb ataxia may occur, especially if the inferior cerebellar peduncle is affected)

Posterior cerebral artery

- Contralateral homonymous hemianopia (from occipital infarction)
- Hemisensory loss—all modalities (from thalamic infarction)
- Hemi-body pain—pain (usually with a burning quality) down one side of the body (face, arm, and leg) as a result of thalamic infarction
- If bilateral, may have poor visual-motor coordination, inability to understand visual objects

Diagnostic tools such as the recognition of stroke in the emergency room (ROSIER) scale may help medical staff in the emergency department rapidly recognise acute stroke because this tool includes assessment of visual fields.[25]

Posterior circulation stroke is diagnosed on the basis of history and clinical examination, assisted by imaging. Assessment by a specialist stroke team with admission to a stroke unit is the optimum approach. Assessment in the emergency department for homonymous visual field deficits; eye movement abnormalities (including simple labyrinthine tests such as the head thrust/impulse test (http://content.lib.utah.edu/cdm/singleitem/collection/ehsl-dent/id/6)); and looking for Horner's syndrome (ptosis, small pupil (miosis), and anhydrosis on the same side), bilateral small or fixed pupils, and ataxia may aid early diagnosis.[18 19]

All cases of suspected stroke require urgent brain imaging with CT or magnetic resonance imaging (MRI) to exclude haemorrhage. If a patient is a candidate for thrombolysis therapy, brain and vessel imaging with a technique such as CT angiography is essential to identify basilar artery occlusion. It should be performed without delay, because minimising the time between stroke onset and the start of thrombolysis is associated with a good outcome.

Acute phase CT imaging may allow identification of large vessel occlusion or dissection. In many centres CT and CT angiography is more readily available in the acute phase than MRI, and is helpful if MRI is contraindicated or unavailable. On the basis of a patient series that compared each modality to digital subtraction angiography of all intracranial vessel territories, CT angiography and time-of-flight magnetic resonance angiography had high sensitivity for identifying vessel occlusion—100% and 87% sensitivity, respectively.[26]

MRI with diffusion weighted imaging is the brain imaging modality of choice for suspected posterior circulation stroke, although it is difficult to access at most UK hospitals and in many other countries, especially in the hyperacute phase.

MRI is far more sensitive than CT in the diagnosis of acute ischaemic stroke for all vascular territories, with study results indicating 80-95% sensitivity in the first 24 hours when diffusion weighted imaging is used, versus 16% sensitivity with CT.[27 28] Sensitivity may be lower in the posterior circulation and false negatives can occur with early MRI—a 19% false negative rate was reported in one single centre case series of 31 patients with vertebrobasilar stroke.[7 28] MRI or magnetic resonance angiography with dedicated fat saturated sequences may help identify vertebral dissection, but this is more challenging than in the carotid artery.

Current international guidelines recommend MRI for assessing TIA, including those in the posterior circulation. It can help diagnose disorders that mimic stroke and TIA, can help verify vascular territory, and diffusion weighted imaging abnormalities independently predict early stroke risk after TIA.[29 30] MRI provides the greatest diagnostic yield when performed as soon as possible (certainly within a few days) of symptom onset, especially in minor stroke or TIA.[31] To help differentiate stroke from rare mimic disorders, such as encephalitis, further investigation with lumbar puncture (if no clinical or radiological contraindications are present) may be necessary if fever or atypical imaging features are identified.

How is posterior circulation stroke managed?

Similar to other stroke and acute neurological emergencies, stabilisation and resuscitation of patients with acute phase posterior circulation stroke are crucial. Careful assessment of airway, breathing, and circulation is also crucial before transfer in patients who may be at risk of deterioration during inter-hospital transportation, with input from an anaesthetics team if indicated.

Thrombolysis

The large ECASS3 randomised controlled trial found that intravenous tissue-type plasminogen activator (tPA) may be used in patients with posterior circulation stroke who meet the eligibility criteria, within 4.5 hours of symptom onset.[32] Results from randomised controlled trials in ischaemic stroke showed that intravenous alteplase (recombinant tPA) improves functional outcome using the modified Rankin score (a functional outcome score) at three months. Unfortunately, specialist assessment and intravenous administration of tPA are slower in patients with posterior circulation stroke compared with those with anterior circulation stroke, probably because of delayed or missed diagnosis.[33 34] Case series have shown prolonged door to needle time in patients with posterior circulation stroke; one observational study of 237 patients showed a mean time of 156.2 min (standard deviation 23.2) in the posterior circulation group versus 141.1 min (30.7) in the anterior circulation group; P=0.01.[33] Another study showed a prolonged door to needle time, but no prolonged stroke specialist to needle time.[34]

As with anterior circulation events, the administration of tPA in the posterior circulation carries a risk of haemorrhage, anaphylaxis, or angio-oedema. On the basis of its licence for use, contraindications to tPA include any intracerebral haemorrhage, known or suspected central nervous system lesion with high likelihood of haemorrhage after tPA (such as brain tumour, abscess, vascular malformation, aneurysm, contusion, or endocarditis), and clinical presentation suggestive of subarachnoid haemorrhage even with normal CT results. Other contraindications are uncontrolled hypertension (systolic blood pressure >180 mm Hg or diastolic blood pressure >110 mm Hg at start of tPA treatment), history of intracranial haemorrhage, active internal bleeding, fracture, acute trauma, stroke, serious head trauma, intracranial or intraspinal surgery in past three months, or bleeding disorder.[32]

Acute endovascular therapy

Acute endovascular therapy (intra-arterial clot removal or lysis) has been used in acute basilar occlusion because of the high likelihood of death or severe disability in the absence of recanalisation.[35 36 37] Evidence from a systematic review of published case series reporting the outcome of basilar artery occlusion after intravenous or intra-arterial thrombolysis showed that only 2% of 420 patients had a good outcome in the absence of basilar artery recanalisation.[38] However, intra-arterial therapy has not been proved to be of benefit. In a large international registry study of 592 patients with basilar occlusion, no significant difference was detected in outcome, as defined by modified Rankin score at one month after intravenous versus intra-arterial therapy.[35] Data from the Basilar Artery International Cooperation Study BASIC registry found similar outcomes in 347 patients with a severe deficit (coma, locked-in syndrome, or tetraplegia) when treated with intra-arterial thrombolysis or intravenous thrombolysis (relative risk 1.06, 95% confidence interval 0.91 to 1.22).[35] An ongoing randomised controlled trial is investigating the value of early intra-arterial therapy in basilar occlusion (www.basicstrial.com).

The time window for treatment for basilar occlusion may be longer than for other stroke types, and although treatment within 4.5 hours is desirable, it may be reasonable to consider treatment (intravenous or endovascular) up to 24 hours from onset.[39] An observational series of 184 consecutive patients with angiography confirmed basilar artery occlusion treated with intravenous thrombolysis at a Finnish specialist centre found that onset to treatment time was not significantly associated with outcome measured on the modified Rankin score.[40] It has been hypothesised that salvageable tissue in the territory of the posterior circulation exists well beyond the time window for anterior circulation stroke thrombolysis. This might be because a high proportion of white matter in the brainstem makes it more resistant to ischaemia than other brain tissue, and better collaterals in the posterior than in the anterior circulation allow for slower progression of ischaemic tissue damage.[22 38] Thrombolysis may be most effective in patients who have had stuttering symptoms with preceding TIA(s) or do not show radiological evidence of extensive infarction.[40] The usefulness of emergency angioplasty or stenting of the extracranial vertebral arteries in unselected patients is not yet well established.[39]

Neurosurgery

Neurosurgical intervention (including external ventricular drainage or decompression) may be lifesaving in large volume cerebellar infarction with falling level of consciousness attributable to raised intracranial pressure or acute hydrocephalus.[41 42 43] A large infarction of the cerebellum is often followed by delayed swelling. Although the early symptoms may be limited to impaired function of the cerebellum, oedema can cause brain stem compression and can rapidly progress to loss of brain stem function. Emergency posterior fossa decompression with partial removal of the infarcted tissue may be lifesaving. However, data come from case series—evidence from randomised controlled trials is lacking. In a case series of 52 patients with space occupying cerebellar infarction defined by computed tomographic criteria, 39 patients developed signs of brain stem compression and 41 developed a disturbance of consciousness.[42] Twenty one of the patients with decompressive surgery who were in an advanced clinical state (stuporous or comatose with posturing and cardiovascular or respiratory instability) before surgery were reported to recover well, compared with none of the patients who did not have surgery.[42]

Which investigations are needed after treatment of posterior circulation stroke?

Identification of the underlying mechanism or risk factors is an important aspect of stroke prevention because it has implications for optimum preventive treatment—such as anticoagulation for atrial fibrillation. Therefore, general and cardiac investigations recommended by international stroke guidelines should be carried out to help identify modifiable risk factors and guide secondary prevention strategies. Tests include electrocardiography, renal and liver function tests, full blood count including platelets, and the measurement of glucose, lipids, serum electrolytes, prothrombin time, international normalised ratio, and activated partial thromboplastin time.[29 43 44]

Some stroke patterns, specifically isolated posterior cerebral artery infarction and top of the basilar syndrome, are often associated with cardioembolism—more than 40% of posterior cerebral artery infarcts were attributed to a cardioembolic mechanism in the New England registry. These clinical syndromes therefore merit detailed assessment for a cardioembolic source including atrial fibrillation through cardiac rhythm monitoring.[12] Prolonged monitoring (with a prolonged ambulatory tape or an implantable device) increases the rate of detecting atrial fibrillation in patients in whom no other stroke mechanism or risk factor is identified but a cardioembolic source is suspected.[45] Echocardiography is recommended in selected patients, such as those with evidence of cardiac disease or suspected cardiac, aortic, or paradoxical embolism.[29 44] Further specialist serum investigations for systemic disease that predisposes to arterial thrombosis may be needed in patients in whom no clear cause is identified.[43 44]

What treatment is recommended after posterior circulation stroke?

Current international guidelines recommend secondary prevention with lifestyle modification and drugs, including antiplatelet agents, lipid lowering drugs, and blood pressure control to a target of less than 140 mm Hg/80 mm Hg.[29 44 46] Antiplatelet agents should be started once haemorrhage has been excluded and 24 hours has elapsed in patients who have received thrombolysis. Clopidogrel alone (or aspirin and dipyridamole) is recommended for long term secondary prevention of thromboembolic events.[44] In patients with indications for anticoagulation (such as atrial fibrillation), treatment should be started when the potential benefit outweighs the risk of harm by haemorrhagic transformation of the infarct generally about two weeks after an acute ischaemic stroke.[44] In patients at high risk of ischaemic stroke, such as those with symptomatic vertebrobasilar stenosis, dual antiplatelet treatment should be considered. A recent randomised trial in 5170 Chinese patients found that short term use of clopidogrel and aspirin when given within 24 h of minor stroke in any territory or onset of high risk TIA reduced the risk of recurrent stroke.[47]

The SPARCL randomised controlled trial included all subtypes of ischaemic stroke and showed that atorvastatin 80 mg per day reduced non-fatal or fatal stroke after stroke and TIA; however, there is a paucity of randomised controlled trial data for the hyperacute phase in the hours and days after TIA or stroke.[9 48]

Antihypertensive treatment and targets should be in accordance with guidelines for comorbid diseases such as diabetes. Evidence to support the use of antihypertensives

SOURCES AND SELECTION CRITERIA

We searched PubMed up to November 2013 with the terms "posterior circulation," "stroke," "ischaemic," and "vertebrobasilar," targeting full text English language studies published since 1990. We also searched the reference lists of the identified articles and our own files. Only papers published in English, or with an English abstract, were reviewed. The final selection of references was based on our judgment of relevance to the topic of this review.

in patients with stroke comes from the PROGRESS study, a randomised controlled trial of a perindopril based regimen in 6105 patients (including those with and without hypertension) with previous stroke or TIA, which showed a 28% relative risk reduction for stroke.[46]

Which patients are at highest risk of deterioration or recurrence after posterior circulation minor stroke or TIA?

Patients with basilar occlusion may have a stuttering onset, with fluctuating or resolving symptoms that initially present as TIA but progress after vessel occlusion to devastating brainstem stroke.[21] Between 55% and 63% of patients with basilar artery occlusion have prodromal TIAs, minor strokes, or other symptoms, which are more common with atherosclerotic than embolic occlusions.[22] Patients with acute basilar artery occlusion have high mortality rates of 41-95% in natural history studies or studies of intravenous thrombolysis, with mortality rates being highest when there is no recanalisation.[22 32] In survivors with poor recanalisation, severe disability (for example, the locked-in syndrome) is common. In a single centre case series of 50 consecutive patients with angiographically confirmed basilar artery occlusion treated with intravenous thrombolysis, none of those with failed recanalisation who survived were living independently at three months.[49] For patients with symptomatic vertebrobasilar stenosis, the risk of recurrent stroke is almost 25% in the first 90 days.[6]

It is therefore crucial to be able to identify which patients are at highest risk of early recurrent stroke, both for triage purposes and for optimum management. If ongoing studies of vertebrobasilar stenosis demonstrate the efficacy of endovascular treatment, identification of high risk patients may be increasingly necessary.[50 51] Unfortunately, no specific dedicated prediction rule for identifying patients at highest risk of stroke after posterior circulation TIA or minor stroke currently exists. The ABCD2 clinical prediction score (Age, Blood pressure, Clinical symptoms (such as speech disturbance or weakness), Duration of symptoms and Diabetes) for use in TIA has not been specifically validated in vertebrobasilar territory TIA. However, one observational hospital based series showed that 30% of patients with recurrent posterior circulation events within the first 90 days after stroke or TIA were not identified as being high risk using the ABCD2 score.[5 52 53]

To improve risk prediction in posterior circulation TIA, further research may focus on external validation of the ABCD2 score in posterior circulation events or the post-investigation phase ABCD3-I score. The ABCD3-I score is an externally validated risk prediction tool, which incorporates abnormalities on diffusion weighted imaging MRI, multiple preceding TIAs, carotid stenosis, and the components of the ABCD2 score into a risk prediction score.[30] Substituting vertebrobasilar stenosis in posterior circulation cases for the 2 points scored for carotid stenosis in the ABCD3-I score, or incorporating the clinical features vertigo, visual

ADDITIONAL EDUCATIONAL RESOURCES

Resources for healthcare professionals

- European Stroke Organisation (www.eso-stroke.org)—Useful source of European stroke guidelines (free, registration not required)
- Virtual Stroke University (www.stroke-university.com)—Useful source of expert lectures on all aspects of stroke (free, registration not required)
- Internet Stroke Centre (www.strokecenter.org/professionals)—Independent source of educational and clinical trial information (free, registration not required)
- Royal College of Physicians (www.rcplondon.ac.uk/resources/stroke-guidelines)—UK national clinical guidelines for stroke (free, registration not needed)
- American Heart Association (http://stroke.ahajournals.org/content/44/3/870)—Guidelines for the early management of patients with acute ischemic stroke (free, registration not needed)

Resources for patients

- Stroke Association (www.stroke.org.uk)—Important source of information about stroke for patients and carers; provides an online patient forum
- National Institute for Health Research Stroke (www.crn.nihr.ac.uk/focus_on/stroke)—Research information
- UK Stroke Forum (www.ukstrokeforum.org)—A coalition of more than 30 organisations committed to improving stroke care in the UK
- Bauby J-D. The diving bell and the butterfly: a memoir of life in death. Random House, 1997. Autobiographical short book written by a journalist using his eye movements to communicate his account of life after he had a pontine stroke that caused quadriparesis, leaving him "locked in"
- ARNI Institute (www.arni.uk.com/)—Focuses on functional rehabilitation and exercise training after stroke
- Different Strokes (www.differentstrokes.co.uk)—A charity specifically for young patients with stroke

QUESTIONS FOR FUTURE RESEARCH

- What are the optimal secondary prevention strategies for posterior circulation stroke, including pharmacological treatments, or endovascular approaches for symptomatic vertebrobasilar stenosis?
- Does acute endovascular therapy have a role in basilar artery occlusion?
- Should a longer time window be used for thrombolysis in the posterior circulation?

TIPS FOR NON-SPECIALISTS

- Careful history taking is needed to identify patients with posterior circulation stroke, who may present with recurrent, stuttering, or progressive symptoms, which may include altered level of awareness (not a typical stroke symptom but seen in bilateral thalamic ischaemia)
- Clinical signs that may help identify a posterior circulation stroke include the presence of homonymous visual field deficits, eye movement abnormalities, Horner's syndrome, or gait ataxia
- Previously ambulant patients with acute focal neurological symptoms leading to acute loss of balance should never be discharged without ensuring they can walk if stroke is a possible explanation. Always consider a posterior circulation stroke if a patient is uncharacteristically disabled for the amount of alcohol reportedly consumed
- Investigate posterior circulation transient ischaemic attack symptoms urgently to avoid preventable disability or death. Use rapid access transient ischaemic attack services or stroke specialist assessment if available, and use magnetic resonance imaging in the acute phase, especially if the diagnosis is unclear, because this modality has high sensitivity for identifying ischaemic lesions
- Consider transferring patients at risk of deterioration in the acute phase of posterior circulation ischaemic stroke to a neuroscience centre because they may need urgent neurosurgery for mass effect or hydrocephalus

symptoms, or ataxia into a risk prediction score, may refine the prediction of stroke after posterior circulation TIA.[5 30]

Registry data from New England in the US have shown an overall 30 day mortality of 3.6% in posterior circulation stroke, with embolic mechanism, distal territory location, and basilar artery occlusive disease carrying the worst prognosis.[12]

What is on the horizon for posterior circulation stroke?
Outstanding research questions remain regarding acute phase management, secondary prevention, and risk prediction.

Treatment time windows in acute basilar occlusion and different treatment strategies should be tested against each other in randomised trials. The BASICS trial—a randomised controlled multicentre open label phase III intervention trial with blinded outcome assessment, investigating the efficacy and safety of additional intra-arterial treatment (within six hours of symptom onset) after intravenous thrombolysis in patients with basilar artery occlusion—is currently recruiting patients.

The management of posterior circulation large artery disease in patients with vertebrobasilar stenosis, especially among patients with TIA and minor stroke, is an area of active research and interest. Current studies include a multi-centre randomised controlled open prospective clinical trial of vertebral artery stenting versus best medical treatment.[50 51]

Thanks to Annemarie O'Flynn (general physician) for her comments on the review article.

Contributors: Both authors helped plan and write the article and in the literature search. DW is also responsible for the illustrations and is guarantor.

Competing interests: We have read and understood BMJ policy on declaration of interests and declare the following interests: ÁM reports salary funding from the Health Service Executive (HSE) Ireland/Dr Richard Steeven's scholarship, and has received unrestricted educational grants towards travel and accommodation costs for attendance at conferences from Boehringer Ingelheim, Pfizer Healthcare, Lundbeck, and Biogen Idec. DW reports educational grants from Allergan; he also receives research support from the Stroke Association and the British Heart Foundation. Part of this work was undertaken at UCLH/UCL which received a proportion of funding from the Department of Health's NIHR Biomedical Research Centres funding scheme.

Provenance and peer review: Commissioned; externally peer reviewed.

1 Flossmann E, Rothwell PM. Prognosis of vertebrobasilar transient ischaemic attack and minor stroke. *Brain* 2003;126:1940-54.
2 Kuruvilla A, Bhattacharya P, Rajamani K, Chaturvedi S. Factors associated with misdiagnosis of acute stroke in young adults. *J Stroke Cerebrovasc Dis* 2011;20:523-7.
3 Dewey HM, Sturm J, Donnan GA, Macdonell RA, McNeil JJ, Thrift AG; North East Melbourne Stroke Incidence Study. Incidence and Outcome of Subtypes of Ischaemic Stroke: Initial Results from the North East Melbourne Stroke Incidence Study (NEMESIS). *Cerebrovasc Dis* 2003;15:133-9.
4 Paul NL, Simoni M, Rothwell PM; Oxford Vascular Study. Transient isolated brainstem symptoms preceding posterior circulation stroke: a population-based study. *Lancet Neurol* 2013;12:65-71.
5 Gulli G, Markus HS. The use of FAST and ABCD2 scores in posterior circulation, compared with anterior circulation, stroke and transient ischemic attack. *J Neurol Neurosurg Psychiatry* 2012;83:228-9.
6 Gulli G, Marquardt L, Rothwell PM, Markus HS. Stroke risk after posterior circulation stroke/transient ischemic attack and its relationship to site of vertebrobasilar stenosis: Pooled data analysis from prospective studies. *Stroke* 2013;44:598-604.
7 Tao WD, Liu M, Fisher M, Wang DR, Li J, Furie KL, et al. Posterior versus anterior circulation infarction: how different are the neurological deficits? *Stroke* 2012;43:2060-5.
8 Oppenheim C, Stanescu R, Dormont D, Crozier S, Marro B, Samson Y, et al. False-negative diffusion-weighted MR findings in acute ischemic stroke. *AJNR Am J Neuroradiol* 2000;21:1434-40.
9 Merwick Á, Albers GW, Arsava EM, Ay H, Calvet D,Coutts SB, et al. Reduction in early stroke risk in carotid stenosis with transient ischemic attack associated with statin treatment. *Stroke* 2013;44:2814-20.
10 Flossmann E, Redgrave JN, Briley D, Rothwell PM. Reliability of clinical diagnosis of the symptomatic vascular territory in patients with recent transient ischemic attack or minor stroke. *Stroke* 2008;39:2457-60.
11 Savitz SI, Caplan LR. Vertebrobasilar disease. *N Engl J Med* 2005;352:2618.
12 Caplan LR, Wityk RJ, Glass TA, Tapia J, Pazdera L, Chang HM, et al. New England Medical Center posterior circulation registry. *Ann Neurol* 2004;56:389.
13 Gulli G, Khan S, Markus HS. Vertebrobasilar stenosis predicts high early recurrent stroke risk in posterior circulation stroke and TIA. *Stroke* 2009;40:2732-7.
14 Marquardt L, Kuker W, Chandratheva A, Geraghty O, Rothwell PM. Incidence and prognosis of ≥50% symptomatic vertebral or basilar artery stenosis: prospective population-based study. *Brain* 2009;132:982-8.
15 Schievink WI. Spontaneous dissection of the carotid and vertebral arteries. *N Engl J Med* 2001;344:898-906.
16 Lou M, Caplan LR. Vertebrobasilar dilatative arteriopathy (dolichoectasia). *Ann N Y Acad Sci* 2010;1184:121-33.
17 Ad Hoc Committee National Institute of Neurological and Communicative Disorders and Stroke. A classification and outline of cerebrovascular diseases. II. *Stroke* 1975;6:564-616.
18 Searls DE, Pazdera L, Korbel E, Vysata O, Caplan LR. Symptoms and signs of posterior circulation ischemia in the New England Medical Center posterior circulation registry. *Arch Neurol* 2012;69:346.
19 Kattah JC, Talkad AV, Wang DZ, Hsieh YH, Newman-Toker DE. HINTS to diagnose stroke in the acute vestibular syndrome: three-step bedside oculomotor examination more sensitive than early MRI diffusion-weighted imaging. *Stroke* 2009;40:3504-10.
20 Caplan L. Posterior circulation ischemia: then, now, and tomorrow. The Thomas Willis lecture-2000. *Stroke* 2000;31:2011-23.
21 Von Campe G, Regli F, Bogousslavsky J. Heralding manifestations of basilar artery occlusion with lethal or severe stroke *J Neurol Neurosurg Psychiatry* 2003;74:1621-6.
22 Mattle HP, Arnold M, Lindsberg PJ, Schonewille WJ, Schroth G. Basilar artery occlusion. *Lancet Neurol* 2011;10:1002-14.
23 Bogousslavsky J, Van Melle G, Regli F. The Lausanne stroke registry: analysis of 1000 consecutive patients with first stroke. *Stroke* 1988;19:1083-92.
24 Hatano S. Experience from a multicentre stroke register: a preliminary report. *Bull World Health Organ* 1976;54:541-53.
25 Nor AM, Davis J, Sen B, Shipsey D, Louw SJ, Dyker AG et al. The recognition of stroke in the emergency room (ROSIER) scale: Development and validation of a stroke recognition instrument. *Lancet Neurol* 2005;4:727-34.
26 Bash S, Villablanca JP, Jahan R, Duckwiler G, Tillis M, Kidwell C, et al. Intracranial vascular stenosis and occlusive disease: evaluation with CT angiography, MR angiography, and digital subtraction angiography. *AJNR Am J Neuroradiol* 2005;26:1012-21.
27 Chalela JA, Kidwell CS, Nentwich LM, Luby M, Butman JA, Demchuk AM, et al. Magnetic resonance imaging and computed tomography in emergency assessment of patients with suspected acute stroke: a prospective comparison. *Lancet* 2007;369:293-8.
28 Edlow JA, Newman-Toker DE, Savitz SI. Diagnosis and initial management of cerebellar infarction. *Lancet Neurol* 2008;7:951-64.
29 Easton JD, Saver JL, Albers GW, Alberts MJ, Chaturvedi S, Feldmann E, et al. Definition and evaluation of transient ischemic attack: a scientific statement for healthcare professionals from the American Heart Association/American Stroke Association Stroke Council; Council on Cardiovascular Surgery and Anesthesia; Council on Cardiovascular Radiology and Intervention; Council on Cardiovascular Nursing; and the Interdisciplinary Council on Peripheral Vascular Disease. *Stroke* 2009;40:2276-93.
30 Merwick A, Albers GW, Amarenco P, Arsava EM, Ay H, Calvet D, et al. Addition of brain and carotid imaging to the ABCD^2 score to improve identification of patients at high early stroke risk after transient ischaemic attack. *Lancet Neurol* 2010;9:1060-9.
31 Moreau F, Modi J, Almekhlafi M, Bal S, Goyal M, Hill MD, et al. Early magnetic resonance imaging in transient ischemic attack and minor stroke: do it or lose it. *Stroke* 2013;44:671-4.
32 Hacke W, Kaste M, Bluhmki E, Brozman M, Dávalos A, Guidetti D, et al. Thrombolysis with alteplase 3 to 4.5 hours after acute ischemic stroke. *N Engl J Med* 2008;359:1317-29.
33 Förster A, Gass A, Kern R, Griebe M, Hennerici MG, Szabo K. Thrombolysis in posterior circulation stroke: stroke subtypes and patterns, complications and outcome. *Cerebrovasc Dis* 2011;32:349-53.
34 Sarraj A, Medrek S, Albright K, Martin-Schild S, Bibars W, Vahidy F, et al. Posterior circulation stroke is associated with prolonged door-to-needle time. *Int J Stroke* 2013; published online 22 Mar.
35 Schonewille WJ, Wijman CA, Michel P, Rueckert CM, Weimar C, Mattle HP, et al. Treatment and outcomes of acute basilar artery occlusion in the Basilar Artery International Cooperation Study (BASICS): a prospective registry study. *Lancet Neurol* 2009;8:724-30.
36 Lutsep HL, Rymer MM, Nesbit GM. Vertebrobasilar revascularization rates and outcomes in the MERCI and multi-MERCI trials. *J Stroke Cerebrovasc Dis* 2008;17:55-7.
37 Hacke W, Zeumer H, Ferbert A, Bruckmann H, del Zoppo GJ. Intra-arterial thrombolytic therapy improves outcome in patients with acute vertebrobasilar occlusive disease. *Stroke* 1988;19:1216-22.

38 Lindsberg PJ, Mattle HP. Therapy of basilar artery occlusion: a systematic analysis comparing intra-arterial and intravenous thrombolysis. *Stroke* 2006;37:922-8.

39 Levy EI, Siddiqui AH, Crumlish A, Snyder KV, Hauck EF, Fiorella DJ, et al. First Food and Drug Administration-approved prospective trial of primary intracranial stenting for acute stroke: SARIS (stent-assisted recanalization in acute ischemic stroke). *Stroke* 2009;40:3552-6.

40 Strbian D, Sairanen T, Silvennoinen H, Salonen O, Kaste M, Lindsberg PJ. Thrombolysis of basilar artery occlusion: impact of baseline ischemia and time. *Ann Neurol* 2013;73:688-94.

41 Horwitz NH, Ludolph C. Acute obstructive hydrocephalus caused by cerebellar infarction: treatment alternatives. *Surg Neurol* 1983;20:13-9.

42 Hornig CR, Rust DS, Busse O, Jauss M, Laun A. Space-occupying cerebellar infarction: clinical course and prognosis. *Stroke* 1994;25:372-4.

43 Jauch EC, Saver JL, Adams HP Jr, Bruno A, Connors JJ, Demaerschalk BM, et al; American Heart Association Stroke Council; Council on Cardiovascular Nursing; Council on Peripheral Vascular Disease; Council on Clinical Cardiology. Guidelines for the early management of patients with acute ischemic stroke: a guideline for healthcare professionals from the American Heart Association/American Stroke Association. *Stroke* 2013;44:870-947.

44 Intercollegiate Stroke Working Party. National clinical guideline for stroke. 4th ed. Royal College of Physicians, 2012. www.rcplondon.ac.uk/sites/default/files/national-clinical-guidelines-for-stroke-fourth-edition.pdf.

45 Cotter PE, Martin PJ, Ring L, Warburton EA, Belham M, Pugh PJ. Incidence of atrial fibrillation detected by implantable loop recorders in unexplained stroke. *Neurology* 2013;80:1546-50.

46 PROGRESS Collaborative Group. Randomised trial of a perindopril-based blood-pressure lowering regimen among 6105 individuals with previous stroke or transient ischaemic attack. *Lancet* 2001;358:1033-41.

47 Wang Y, WangY, Zhao X, Liu L, Wang D, Wang C, et al. Clopidogrel with aspirin in acute minor stroke or transient ischemic attack. *N Engl J Med* 2013;369:11-9.

48 Amarenco P, Bogousslavsky J, Callahan A III, Goldstein LB, Hennerici M, Rudolph AE, et al; Stroke Prevention by Aggressive Reduction in Cholesterol Levels (SPARCL) Investigators. High-dose atorvastatin after stroke or transient ischemic attack. *N Engl J Med* 2006;355:549-59.

49 Lindsberg PJ, Soinne L, Tatlisumak T, Roine RO, Kallela M, Häppölä O, et al. Long-term outcome after intravenous thrombolysis of basilar artery occlusion. *JAMA* 2004;292:1862-6.

50 St George's, University of London. Vertebral artery ischaemia stenting trial (VIST). www.vist.sgul.ac.uk.

51 Compter A, van der Worp HB, Schonewille WJ, Vos JA, Algra A, Lo TH, et al. VAST: vertebral artery stenting trial. Protocol for a randomised safety and feasibility trial. *Trials* 2008;9:65.

52 Johnston SC, Rothwell PM, Nguyen-Huynh MN, Giles MF, Elkins JS, Bernstein AL, et al. Validation and refinement of scores to predict very early stroke after transient ischaemic attack. *Lancet* 2007;369:283-92.

53 Sheehan OC, Merwick A, Kelly LA, Hannon N, Marnane M, Kyne L, et al. Diagnostic usefulness of ABCD2 score to distinguish TIA and minor ischemic stroke from non-cerebrovascular events: the North Dublin TIA study. *Stroke* 2009;40:3449-54.

The management of spasticity in adults

Krishnan Padmakumari Sivaraman Nair, consultant[1], Jonathan Marsden, professor[2]

[1]Department of Neurology, Royal Hallamshire Hospital, Sheffield Teaching Hospitals NHS Foundation Trust, Sheffield, UK

[2]School of Health Professions, Faculty of Health and Human Sciences, University of Plymouth, Plymouth, UK

Correspondence to: K P S Nair siva.nair@sth.nhs.uk

Cite this as: *BMJ* 2014;349:g4737

DOI: 10.1136/bmj.g4737

http://www.bmj.com/content/349/bmj.g4737

Spasticity is a common disorder affecting people with long term neurological conditions such as stroke, multiple sclerosis, and traumatic brain and spinal cord injuries. A systematic review of 24 studies on the epidemiology of leg spasticity reported a prevalence of 28-38% in patients with stroke, 41-66% in patients with multiple sclerosis, and 13% in patients with traumatic brain injury.[1]

Spasticity varies from a subtle neurological sign to a gross increase in tone causing immobility of joints. The disorder is associated with several complications, including falls, pain, pressure ulcers, infections, and contractures,[2] although it is not clear whether these complications are caused by spasticity or co-exist independently.[1] Spasticity increases care needs and utilisation of healthcare resources,[3] and carers of patients with spasticity are more likely to experience anxiety and depression.[4] Some patients may make use of their spasticity to sit, stand, walk, or transfer. Management of spasticity requires a balanced approach, weighing the benefits of treatment against the usefulness of the spasticity. Current interventions to treat spasticity lack a robust evidence base, and guidelines often depend on expert recommendations. This review discusses the assessment and treatment of spasticity in adults.

What is spasticity?

Spasticity has been defined as "disordered sensorimotor control resulting from an upper motor neuron (UMN) lesion, presenting as intermittent or sustained involuntary activation of muscles."[5] Upper motor neurone syndrome may be associated with other clinical signs: positive features include exaggerated tendon reflexes, released reflexes, and upgoing plantars; negative features include motor weakness, slowness of movement, loss of dexterity, and loss of selective motor control. Lesions affecting the frontal motor cortex and its connections lead to increased excitation of spinal motor neurones[6] and a lower threshold to respond to stimuli such as stretch.[7] Overactivity of spinal motor neurones results in spasticity.

What are the clinical features of spasticity?

High muscle tone in spasticity characteristically affects the antigravity muscle groups. In the arms, the tone is usually high in adductors of the shoulders; flexors of elbows, wrist, and fingers; and pronators of forearm (figure). Excessive flexion of fingers and adduction of the thumb results in the characteristic clenched fist with "thumb in palm" deformity. In the legs, the high tone due to spasticity is particularly prominent in adductors of the hips, flexors of the knees, and plantar flexors and invertors of the ankle. Hyperextension of the big toe as a result of persistent high tone of extensor hallucis longus is another feature of spasticity, and patients may report difficulty in using footwear.

The high muscle tone associated with spasticity varies with the speed of the movement—that is, the faster the stretch, the greater the resistance. The resistance is felt as a catch after an initial few degrees of movement. This resistance then builds up; as the movement continues the resistance suddenly gives way. This "clasp-knife phenomenon" is evident during the initial stages of spasticity. Other clinical features of spasticity are clonus, spasms, spastic dystonia, and spastic co-contractions (box 1).

What is the differential diagnosis of spasticity?

The differential diagnosis of spasticity includes contractures, rigidity, and catatonia.

Contracture is a shortening and reduction in elasticity of muscles, tendons, ligaments, joint capsules, and skin, which is accompanied by an increase in the resistance to passive stretch.[6 8] After immobilisation, sarcomeres shorten and muscle and elastic tissue are replaced with connective tissue and fat.[6] Left unchecked, this process can result in permanent loss of motion in joints. Unlike spasticity, contractures do not show dynamic changes such as clasp knife phenomenon, catch and variation of tone with speed of movement, and position of limb. Sometimes stretching under sedation may be required to differentiate spasticity from contractures.

Rigidity is associated with disorders of the basal ganglia. Unlike spasticity, the high tone in rigidity is non-selective and affects all muscles acting on a joint equally. The resistance to passive movements due to rigidity is felt throughout the range of movement and does not change with speed of movement. In Parkinson's disease, rigidity associated tremors give a "cog wheel" feel on passive movement.

Catatonia is a neuropsychiatric syndrome characterised by abnormal posturing, gegenhalten, and "waxy flexibility." Gegenhalten or counterhold is an increase in muscle tone proportional to the force applied. In waxy flexibility, patients maintain their limbs in positions placed by others for a long time. When the limb is moved passively, the muscles stiffen in proportion to the force applied, as if the patient is actively opposing movement. Catatonia is caused by several psychiatric, neurological, and medical conditions. Presence of signs such as excitement, impulsivity, perseveration, combativeness, automatic obedience, stupor, mutism, staring, grimacing, stereotypical movements, echolalia, echopraxia, and withdrawal should raise a suspicion of catatonia.[9]

How is spasticity assessed?

Clinicians encounter patients with spasticity either as the initial symptom of a neurological illness or the worsening of existing spasticity due to a known long term neurological condition.

SUMMARY POINTS

- Spasticity is a frequent and debilitating feature of common neurological conditions such as stroke, multiple sclerosis, and traumatic brain and spinal cord injuries
- The disorder is often associated with pain and discomfort and increased care needs
- Spasticity is difficult to manage and requires a collaborative approach involving multiple disciplines
- The evidence for both drug and non-drug treatments of spasticity is limited
- More research is required to determine the effectiveness of various treatments of spasticity

Approach to adults presenting with new onset spasticity

Spasticity could be the initial manifestation of several neurological conditions (table 1). An assessment includes history of onset and progression of symptoms such as weakness, abnormal sensations, pain, and bladder, bowel, and sexual dysfunction. An inquiry into family history, history of overseas travel, dietary preferences, and compromised immunity may be warranted. These patients require a neurological examination of muscle tone, motor power, and reflexes, and a careful search for a sensory level.

Approach to adults presenting with worsening of spasticity

Spasticity is a common feature of several long term neurological conditions such as stroke, traumatic brain and spinal cord injury, and multiple sclerosis. A long term neurological condition may be a more common reason for consultations involving spasticity compared with new onset spasticity in general practice. When spasticity worsens, these patients may experience a variety of symptoms, such as pain, stiffness, involuntary movements, deterioration of mobility, increase in care needs, and sexual dysfunction.

The worsening of spasticity could be due to:

Triggers—spasticity can be aggravated by visceral or somatic stimuli below the level of injury (box 2)[10]

Disease progression—worsening of spasticity could also be a sign of the progression of the primary neurological disease, as in progressive forms of multiple sclerosis. In people with spinal cord injury, worsening spasticity may indicate development of post-traumatic syringomyelia.

New disease—worsening of spasticity could indicate a coincidental new disease (table 1).

The first step in the assessment of patients with worsening spasticity is to look for triggers (box 2). The education of patients and carers in recognising these triggers is an important part of management. If no underlying triggers are identified or if the spasticity continues to worsen, coincidental new disease should be excluded (table 1).

When should a patient with spasticity be referred?

Consider patients for referral to neurology services if they have new onset spasticity, spasticity that worsens rapidly without any triggers, or new neurological signs.

Referral to a rehabilitation specialist needs to be considered if patients fail to tolerate or respond to adequate doses of oral antispasticity drugs; spasticity affects

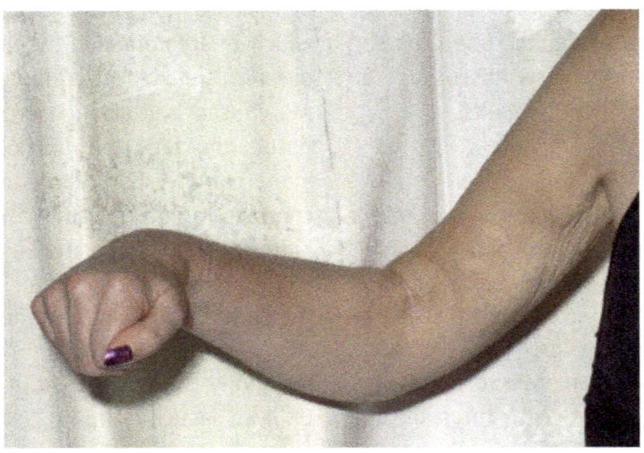

Spasticity of arm showing excessive flexion of elbow, wrist, and fingers

BOX 1 CLINICAL FEATURES OF SPASTICITY

Clonus

- Involuntary rhythmic contractions triggered by stretch; these can interfere with walking, transfers, sitting, and care

Spasms

- Sudden involuntary movements that often involve multiple muscle groups and joints in response to somatic or visceral stimuli

Spastic dystonia

- Tonic muscle overactivity without any triggers owing to the inability of motor units to cease firing after a voluntary or reflex activity[6]; results in characteristic limb postures and contractures

Spastic co-contraction

- Inappropriate activation of antagonistic muscles during voluntary activity due to lack of reciprocal inhibition causing a loss of dexterity and slowness in movements[6]

Table 1 Neurological conditions that may present initially with spasticity

Causes	Clinical features	Investigations
Spinal cord compression:		
Spinal canal stenosis, tumours affecting spinal cord	Sensory level: bladder, bowel, and sexual dysfunction	Magnetic resonance imaging
Autoimmune disorders:		
Primary progressive multiple sclerosis	Slowly progressive course without remissions and relapses	Magnetic resonance imaging, cerebrospinal fluid for oligoclonal bands
Neurodegenerative conditions:		
Motor neurone disease	Presence of lower motor neurone signs such as wasting and fasciculation	Electromyography
Infections:		
Tuberculosis of spine, Human T lymphotropic virus (HTLV1) myelopathy	Compromised immunity; contact with tuberculosis	Magnetic resonance imaging, HTLV serology
Inherited conditions:		
Hereditary spastic paraparesis, leucodystrophy	Family history of neurodegenerative conditions	Magnetic resonance imaging, genetic testing, very long chain fatty acids, white cell enzymes
Nutritional:		
Subacute combined degeneration of the cord, (vitamin B12 deficiency), copper deficiency	Nutritional history, eating disorders, use of zinc supplements	Vitamin B12, serum copper
Vascular:		
Spinal vascular malformations	Slowly progressive symptoms, combination of upper and lower motor neurone signs with sensory signs	Magnetic resonance imaging, spinal angiography

posture, mobility, and care; or spasticity is associated with considerable pain and discomfort.

What is the impact of spasticity?

The impact of spasticity extends beyond the physical effects to psychological and social aspects of life.[11] Poor posture makes transfers and changes in position difficult and can contribute to pressure ulcers. Severe spasticity makes hygiene tasks, such as the cleaning of hands, axillae, elbows, and genital areas particularly difficult. Spasticity can also interfere with bowel and bladder care and sexual relationships.

Spasticity can be potentially useful for some patients. Stiffness of the weak muscles helps with tasks such as sitting, transfers, standing, and walking. Spasticity of long finger flexor muscles enables people to hold implements such as cutlery or a toothbrush. An individualised assessment looking at whether patients are making use of spasticity as a strategy to compensate for weakness is required before embarking on treatment.

People with spasticity also have additional neurological symptoms such as weakness, poor postural reactions, and sensory loss. The contribution of these symptoms to loss of function should be assessed.

What is the aim of the management of spasticity?

The aim of management is to reduce the impact of spasticity on patients and to prevent secondary complications. This requires a multidisciplinary team including doctors, physiotherapists, occupational therapists, orthotists, nurses, and wheel chair engineers. The first step is to agree on the aims of treatment with patients and carers (box 3). Interventions also need to be tailored according to the patient's activity, care needs, and access to physiotherapy.

Differentiating between spasticity and contracture is important, as this guides treatment options. Broadly, drug interventions will be effective at targeting spasticity, whereas non-drug interventions have a greater impact on contracture. Guidelines on multiple sclerosis from the National Institute for Health and Care Excellence recommend physiotherapy for the management of all patients with spasticity, and drug interventions for spasticity causing pain, discomfort, loss of independence, and limitation of activities.[12]

BOX 2 TRIGGERS FOR WORSENING OF SPASTICITY

- Skin—ulcers, ingrown toenails, boils, and skin infections
- Visceral—constipation, urinary tract infections, urinary tract calculi, pain during menstruation
- Devices—improper seating, ill fitting orthotics, failure of intrathecal baclofen pump
- Drugs—rapid withdrawal of antispasticity drugs
- Others—infections, injuries, deep vein thrombosis, stress

What are the non-drug interventions for spasticity?

Stretching and splinting

Manual stretching, often as part of a home management programme, has long been a cornerstone of the management of spasticity. However, the effect of stretching on spasticity and contractures is still largely an evidence-free zone. A meta-analysis of four trials with a total of 161 participants found no significant effect of stretching on spasticity.[13] Splinting has the advantage of providing a stretch over a more prolonged period compared with manual stretching. A before and after design study on 10 patients and a controlled trial of 15 patients showed that splinting reduced the spasticity of the fingers and wrists, measured using the modified Ashworth scale.[14] [15] The modified Ashworth scale is an ordinal scale and measures the resistance of the limb to passive movements by the assessor.

The disadvantage is that splinting often holds the joint in a fixed position rather than applying a constant torque. The use of lycra based garments (dynamic fabricated orthoses) is another way of applying a stretch over longer periods

SOURCES AND SELECTION CRITERIA

We searched the databases PubMed, AMED, Embase, Medline, British Nursing Index, and CINAHL using the keywords "spasticity", "contracture", "upper motor neurone", and "muscle tone" from 2004 to 2014. We based this review on evidence from systematic reviews, guidelines by national and international organisations, and clinical trials published in English.

BOX 3 AIMS OF TREATMENT FOR SPASTICITY

- Relief of pain and discomfort
- Improvement of posture
- Facilitation of sitting, standing, and walking
- Reduction in burden of care
- Improvement of hygiene in areas such as palm, axilla, and groin
- Improvement in body image and self esteem
- Prevention of complications such as pressure ulcers

Table 2 Details of oral antispasticity drugs

Drug	Indication	Dose	Side effects
Baclofen	Preferred oral antispasticity drug	Starting dose 5 mg three times daily; titration 5-10 mg weekly; maximum dose 90-120 mg/day divided into 3 doses; lower doses in renal failure; taper by up to 15 mg/week	Weakness, drowsiness, dizziness, sexual dysfunction, urinary incontinence. Sudden withdrawal may cause rebound spasticity, seizures, and hallucinations. Should be used with caution during pregnancy
Tizanidine	Second line treatment if baclofen is not tolerated or not effective	Starting dose 2 mg at bedtime; titration, increased by 2 mg weekly; maximum dose 36 mg/day divided into 3 or 4 doses; taper by 4 mg/week	Dry mouth, gastrointestinal disturbance, hypotension, and acute hepatitis. Monitor liver enzymes
Dantrolene	Second line treatment if baclofen is not tolerated or not effective	Starting dose 25 mg/day; titration, increase in steps of 25 mg/week; maximum dose 100 mg 3 or 4 times daily, taper by 25 mg/week	Hepatotoxicity, weakness, dizziness, and diarrhoea. Monitor liver enzyme levels
Gabapentin	Spasticity associated with pain	300 mg once daily on day 1, then 300 mg twice daily on day 2, then 300 mg 3 times daily on day 3, then increased according to response in steps of 300 mg every 2 or 3 days, up to maximum of 3600 mg daily	Weight gain, gastrointestinal disturbance, confusion, depression, hostility, and sleep disturbances. Need electrocardiography to monitor for QT interval prolongation

while not rigidly fixing a joint. Customised, reinforced panels can direct the stretch appropriately, although they need adjustment for this to be maintained throughout the day. An open labelled crossover trial of 16 patients and a case series of six patients with chronic stroke suggest that these garments increase the range of movements at the wrist and fingers.[16 17] However, an open labelled trial of 13 patients showed no significant benefit with this intervention.[18]

Postural management and standing

Postural management involves managing postural alignment to prevent or reduce contracture and spasticity in people with severe symptoms. Management includes systems to maintain alignment when sitting, standing, and in bed. Standing frames allow people to remain upright for prolonged periods by providing the required support at the ankle, knee, or hip.

A crossover study on six patients with multiple sclerosis noted an increase in the range of movement at the ankle after the use of a standing frame for 30 minutes daily for three weeks.[19] Another small trial on eight patients with spinal cord injury showed that standing reduced spasticity, measured using the modified Ashworth scale.[20]

Exercises

Strengthening exercises improve motor control and function and, contrary to conventional beliefs, do not worsen spasticity. A meta-analysis of 15 randomised controlled trials showed that strengthening exercises improved strength and activity after stroke and did not worsen spasticity. The evidence of the effect on spasticity was based on three studies with a total of 61 participants.[21] Strong trunk, pelvic, and shoulder girdle muscles provide the stability required for accurate control of the distal movements. Exercises may be avoided in patients who are otherwise not fit, are in the immediate postoperative period, have osteoporosis, or are severely limited in their passive range of movement.

Constraint induced therapy is a technique of training the affected arm while restraining the unaffected arm. A trial of this technique on 10 patients showed a reduction in spasticity, measured using the modified Ashworth scale.[22] In a small trial of seven patients with chronic spinal cord injury, treadmill training of walking with body weight support showed a reduction in spasticity, measured using the same scale.[23]

Other physical modalities

Several physical modalities have been tried to reduce spasticity, such as extracorporeal shock wave therapy, whole body vibration, transcutaneous electrical stimulation, repetitive transcranial magnetic stimulation, transcranial direct current stimulation, and electromagnetic therapy. A Cochrane review of nine randomised controlled trials with 341 participants using these non-drug modalities for the treatment of spasticity in multiple sclerosis found "low level" evidence only for repetitive transcranial magnetic stimulation.[24] All these techniques require further evidence before they can be recommended for the treatment of spasticity.

What are the drug interventions for spasticity?

Oral antispasticity drugs

Commonly used oral antispasticity drugs (table 2) are those acting on the γ-aminobutyric acid (GABA)ergic system (baclofen, gabapentin, and benzodiazepines) and $\alpha 2$ adrenergic system (tizanidine) and those that block calcium release into the muscles (dantrolene). Although these drugs have been used for several decades, evidence for their efficacy is poor. A systematic review of 101 studies on oral antispasticity drugs noted a "dearth" of good quality trials and found limited evidence for efficacy of baclofen, tizanidine, and dantrolene in spasticity.[25] A Cochrane review on the management of spasticity after spinal cord injury found nine trials with a total of 218 participants,[26] Only tizanidine resulted in a significant reduction in the Ashworth score. Patients taking tizanidine also had significantly more adverse events than those taking placebo (81% v 53%). None of the oral antispasticity drugs resulted in improvement of function.[26] In a systematic review of 12 randomised control trials of 469 patients with non-progressive neurological disorders, the evidence on the efficacy of oral antispasticity drugs was "scarce and weak." Among all oral antispasticity drugs, tizanidine resulted in a reduction in the Ashworth score but did not improve function.[27]

Baclofen is the most preferred oral antispasticity drug. NICE guidelines recommend baclofen as a first line drug for the treatment of spasticity in multiple sclerosis and in children and young adults.[12 28] The second line options are tizanidine and dantrolene. Benzodiazepines have a similar efficacy to antispasticity drugs but more troublesome side effects. Drowsiness and behavioural side effects limit the use of benzodiazepines during the day time. Clonazepam is particularly useful for the treatment of nocturnal spasms. The usual starting dose is 250 µg at night, and the maximum dose is 1 mg.

Patients who do not respond to one type of oral antispasticity drug may respond to another. Evidence on the use of a combination of oral antispasticity agents is lacking. A combination of two drugs may be tried only in special circumstances: when spasticity is not responding to any single agent and in patients who could tolerate only small doses of antispasticity drugs.

Only around 50% of adults comply with treatment with oral antispasticity drugs.[29] Reduction of spasticity often unmasks underlying weakness due to the upper motor neurone syndrome or reliance on spasticity for postural stability and function, or both. It is important to mention this undesirable effect of treatment to patients. They should be advised to report any increase in weakness or falls after starting treatment. These drugs should be started at a small dose and increased in small increments.[30] It is also important to review the effects of oral antispasticity drugs periodically and to taper and stop them if they are not effective.[30] Even if drugs are apparently ineffective, it is better to taper the dose before stopping to avoid a rebound increase in spasticity from sudden discontinuation.

The timing of administering oral spasticity drugs and the dose should be tailored to the patient's lifestyle. Patients who are walking often require lower doses of antispasticity drugs during the day time as spasticity frequently facilitates standing and walking. A dose may be required before going to bed as spasticity often increases with change in posture. Furthermore, a dose immediately after awakening to reduce high tone may facilitate care in the morning.

Spasticity can worsen during pregnancy.[31] No data are available about the effects of antispasticity drugs during pregnancy in humans. Neonatal baclofen withdrawal syndrome has been reported in babies born to mothers taking the drug during pregnancy.[32] Antispasticity drugs are also secreted in human milk. During pregnancy these drugs should be prescribed judiciously and only if clearly indicated.

Cannabinoids

Cannabinoids are the pharmacologically active compounds in marijuana.[33] They act on cannabinoid receptors (CB-1 and CB-2), which are widely distributed in brain and spinal cord. Tetrahydrocannabinol, an agonist of both receptors, reduces spasticity but causes sedation and psychotropic side effects. Cannabidiol has lower affinity to both receptors and reduces the psychotropic and sedative effects of tetrahydrocannabinol. A systematic review for the American Academy of Neurology concluded that oral cannabis extracts containing both these compounds are effective in improving patient reported outcomes in those with multiple sclerosis but not in changing objective measures of spasticity.[33] Nabiximols (Sativex; oromucosal spray, a 1:1 mixture of 9-δ-tetrahydrocannabinol and cannabidiol) is licensed for use to treat spasticity in people with multiple sclerosis in the United Kingdom. A meta-analysis of the original data pooled from 666 patients from three trials on nabiximols reported that it is well tolerated; 35% of the participants in the treatment arm showed a reduction of spasticity only on the patient reported outcome measures.[34] A further systematic review of six trials using a combination of tetrahydrocannabinol and cannabidiol reported no significant change in objective outcome measures but noted an improvement in patient reported outcome measures.[35] Side effects include taste disturbance, dry mouth, oral ulcers, dizziness, depression, mood changes, cognitive impairment, drowsiness, dysarthria, and blurred vision. As only 30-40% of people show a response to treatment, the use of cannabinoids should be reviewed and discontinued if there is no improvement after 4-6 weeks. The long term effects on cognition, behaviour, and mental health are unclear.

Botulinum toxin

When injected into skeletal muscle, botulinum toxin causes selective weakness of the target muscle by blocking the release of acetylcholine at the neuromuscular junction. It results in a focal reduction in spasticity without side effects of global weakness or sedation. Two randomised controlled trials, one on 96 and another on 333 adults with arm spasticity after stroke, showed a reduction in the modified Ashworth score but no significant improvement in function.[36 37] Currently, botulinum toxin is recommended for the treatment of patients with focal spasticity of the arms after stroke in the United Kingdom, United States, and Europe.[38 39 40] The botulinum toxins licensed for this purpose are onabotulinum toxin A (Botox; Allergan), abobotulinum toxin A (Dysport; Ipsen, Biopharm), and incobotulinum toxin A (Xeomin; Merz Pharma).

Therapeutic effects are seen in 7-10 days, peak in 4-6 weeks, and wane by 12 weeks. Patients should be reassessed in about four weeks after the initial injections to determine their efficacy and whether treatment goals have been attained. If required, further injections should be planned once every 12 weeks.[39]

Adverse events of botulinum toxin include dry mouth, injection site pain, respiratory tract infections, muscle weakness, urinary incontinence, falls, fever, and pain. Rarely, the toxin can cause transient dysphagia, which can sometimes result in the need for nasogastric feeding. Patients should be counselled about these adverse events and advised to seek medical help if they develop signs and symptoms of toxin spread.

Botulinum toxin injections for spasticity should be considered as part of a neurorehabilitation programme. Adjunctive interventions such as serial casting may help to maximise the outcome.[41]

ADDITIONAL EDUCATIONAL RESOURCES

Resources for healthcare professionals

- Spasticity in adults: management using botulinum toxin (www.rcplondon.ac.uk/spasticity-in-adults-management-botulinum-tox)—gives evidence based guidance on patient selection, assessment, setting of treatment goals, and follow-up for use of botulinum toxin injections for the management of arm spasticity
- Spasticity in children and young people with non-progressive brain disorders (http://publications.nice.org.uk/spasticity-in-children-and-young-people-with-non-progressive-brain-disorders-cg145)—provides advice on management of spasticity and associated motor disorders in children and young adults up to age 19 years
- Management of spasticity and associated features (www.ebrainjnc.com/learning/course/view.php?id=530)—this e-learning module describes the mechanism, assessment, and management of spasticity (free but requires registration)

Resources for patients

- Resources for people living with spasticity (www.spinalcord.org/resources-for-people-living-with-spasticity)—a compilation of resources on spasticity for patients and care givers
- A to Z of MS: spasticity (www.mstrust.org.uk/atoz/spasticity.jsp)—information on spasticity for patients with multiple sclerosis (site has links to webcast and fact sheets on spasticity)
- Spasms and stiffness (www.mssociety.org.uk/what-is-ms/signs-and-symptoms/spasms-and-stiffness)—describes causes, effects, and treatment options for spasticity affecting people with multiple sclerosis

TIPS FOR NON-SPECIALISTS

- Spasticity is often associated with other signs and symptoms such as weakness, poor postural reactions, and sensory loss; these should also be looked for and addressed
- Look for triggers or independent neurological causes, or both, in people presenting with worsening of pre-existing spasticity
- Involve patients and carers while formulating aims of management of spasticity
- Consider non-pharmacological interventions such as exercises, stretching, splinting, and posture management in all patients with spasticity
- Oral antispasticity drugs should be started at a low dose and gradually titrated up; they should be withdrawn in small decrements
- All antispasticity drugs cause muscle weakness
- Consider referral for botulinum toxin injections for focal spasticity
- Consider referral for intrathecal baclofen pump or chemical neurolysis for severe, treatment resistant spasticity

Intrathecal baclofen

A relatively small dose of baclofen administered intrathecally achieves a high concentration of the drug within the spinal cord resulting in good muscle relaxation without systemic side effects. The intrathecal baclofen pump both stores and delivers programmable doses of baclofen through a catheter into the spinal subarachnoid space. The pump can be programmed to administer a selected dose of baclofen. The drug is effective in the treatment of spasticity secondary to spinal cord disorders, stroke, and multiple sclerosis.[42 43 44] A systematic review of eight non-randomised controlled trials on intrathecal baclofen in 162 people with spinal cord injury found a significant reduction in spasticity measured using the Ashworth scale. The reviewers could not identify any randomised controlled trial that met their inclusion criteria.[45] The intrathecal baclofen pump is indicated for carefully selected patients with significant limb spasticity despite adequate treatment with oral antispasticity drugs.

The frequency of complications from using the intrathecal baclofen pump varies from zero to 2.24 per implant.[46] Procedure related complications include infection, skin erosions, and cerebrospinal fluid leak and seroma formation around the pump. Abrupt withdrawal of intrathecal baclofen due to pump failure, battery failure, catheter block, or patient non-compliance to treatment can cause a clinical emergency, with features similar to the neuroleptic malignant syndrome.[47] Signs of acute baclofen withdrawal include high fever, confusion, rebound spasticity, and muscle rigidity. Therefore patients need to comply with treatment and attend the hospital regularly for monitoring and pump refills. The treatment of acute intrathecal baclofen withdrawal is intrathecal baclofen through a temporary external catheter. Pending this, patients should be started on oral baclofen 90-120 mg/day.

Chemical neurolysis

Chemical neurolysis involves an intraneural injection of phenol, or alcohol destruction of peripheral nerves by protein coagulation. Chemical neurolysis is effective in treating spasticity in large, powerful muscle groups close to the trunk, such as adductors of the thighs. A randomised controlled trial of 20 patients found that an intraneural injection of either 5% phenol or 50% alcohol resulted in a significant reduction in the spasticity of plantar flexors at the ankle.[48] A retrospective case review of 20 patients with spasticity due to spinal cord injuries showed that chemical neurolysis of obturator nerve with phenol resulted in a significant reduction in the adductor spasticity.[49] Side effects include skin sloughing, wound infection, necrosis of muscle near the injection site, and pain. Injecting phenol into the lumbar intrathecal space results in chemical neurolysis of cauda equina. This is an option for people with severe spasticity of the legs who have lost bladder and bowel functions and have no functional movement and no sensation in their legs. A retrospective review of 40 patients who received intrathecal phenol showed that 31 had good improvement and seven experienced side effects.[50]

Contributors: Both authors did the literature search, reviewed the evidence, and drafted, reviewed, and edited the article. KPSN is the guarantor.

Competing interests: We have read and understood the BMJ Group policy on declaration of interests and declare the following interest: in 2009 KPSN was a site investigator for a clinical trial of Sativex for spasticity funded by GW Pharmaceuticals, United Kingdom.

Provenance and peer review: Not commissioned; externally peer reviewed.

Patient consent: Obtained.

1 Martin A, Abogunrin S, Kurth H, Dinet J. Epidemiological, humanistic and economic burden of illness of lower limb spasticity in adults: a systematic review. *Neuropsychiatr Dis Treat* 2014:10;111-22.
2 Kheder A, Nair KPS. Spasticity: pathophysiology, evaluation and management. *Pract Neurol* 2012;12:289-98.
3 Tyry T, Salter A, Largent J, Ann Marrie R. The impact of spasticity severity on healthcare utilization among MS patients: a large-scale six-year follow-up study. *J Neurol Sci* 2013;333:376-7.
4 Denno MS, Gillard PJ, Graham GD, Dibonaventura MD, Goren A, Varon SF, et al. Anxiety and depression associated with caregiver burden in caregivers of stroke survivors with spasticity. *Arch Phys Med Rehabil* 2013;94:1731-6.
5 Pandyan AD, Gregoric M, Barnes MP, Wood D, Van Wijck F, Burridge J, et al. Spasticity: clinical perceptions, neurological realities and meaningful measurement. *Disabil Rehabil* 2005;27:2-6.
6 Yelnik AP, Simon O, Parratte B, Gracies JM. How to clinically assess and treat muscle overactivity in spastic paresis. *J Rehabil Med* 2010;42:801-7.
7 Nielsen JB, Crone C, Hultborn H. The spinal pathophysiology of spasticity from a basic science point of view. *Acta Physiol Scand* 2007;189:171-80.
8 O'Dwyer NJ, Ada L, Neilson PD. Spasticity and muscle contracture following stroke. *Brain* 1996:119;1737-49.
9 Daniels J. Catatonia: clinical aspects and neurobiological correlates. *J Neuropsychiatry Clin Neurosci* 2009;21:371-80.
10 Phadke CP, Balasubramanian CK, Ismail F, Boulias C. Revisiting physiologic and psychological triggers that increase spasticity. *Am J Phys Med Rehabil* 2013;92:357-69.
11 Morley A, Tod A, Cramp M, Mawson S. The meaning of spasticity to people with multiple sclerosis: what can health professionals learn? *Disabil Rehabil* 2013;35:1284-92.
12 National Collaborating Centre for Chronic Conditions. Multiple sclerosis: national clinical guideline for diagnosis and management in primary and secondary care. Royal College of Physicians, 2004.
13 Katalinic OM, Harvey LA, Herbert RD, Moseley AM, Lannin NA, Schurr K. Stretch for the treatment and prevention of contractures. *Cochrane Database Syst Rev* 2010;9:CD007455.
14 Jo HM, Song JC, Jang SH. Improvements in spasticity and motor function using a static stretching device for people with chronic hemiparesis following stroke. *Neurorehabilitation* 2013;32:369-75.
15 Kim EH, Chang MC, Seo JP, Jang SH, Song JC, Jo HM. The effect of a hand stretching device during the management of spasticity in chronic hemiparetic stroke patients. *Ann Rehabil Med* 2013;37:235-40.
16 Gracies JM, Marosszeky JE, Renton R, Sandanam J, Gandevia SC, Burke D. Short-term effects of dynamic lycra splints on upper limb in hemiplegic patients. *Arch Phys Med Rehabil* 2000;81:1547-55.
17 Doucet BM, Mettler JA. Effects of a dynamic progressive orthotic intervention for chronic hemiplegia: a case series. *J Hand Ther* 2013;26:139-46.
18 Ibuki A, Bach T, Rogers D, Bernhardt J. The effect of tone-reducing orthotic devices on soleus muscle reflex excitability while standing in patients with spasticity following stroke. *Prosthet Orthot Int* 2010;34:46-57.
19 Baker K, Cassidy E, Rone-Adams S. Therapeutic standing for people with multiple sclerosis: efficacy and feasibility. *Int J Ther Rehabil* 2007;14:104-9.
20 Manella KJ, Field-Fote EC. Modulatory effects of locomotor training on extensor spasticity in individuals with motor-incomplete spinal cord injury. *Restor Neurol Neurosci* 2013;31:633-46.
21 Ada L, Dorsch S, Canning CG. Strengthening interventions increase strength and improve activity after stroke: a systematic review. *Aust J Physiother* 2006;52:241-8.
22 Kagawa S, Koyama T, Hosomi M, Takebayashi T, Hanada K, Hashimoto F, et al. Effects of constraint-induced movement therapy on spasticity in patients with hemiparesis after stroke. *J Stroke Cerebrovasc Dis* 2013;22:364-70.
23 Manella KJ, Field-Fote EC. Modulatory effects of locomotor training on extensor spasticity in individuals with motor-incomplete spinal cord injury. *Restor Neurol Neurosci* 2013;31:633-46.
24 Amatya B, Khan F, La Mantia L, Demetrios M, Wade DT. Non pharmacological interventions for spasticity in multiple sclerosis. *Cochrane Database Syst Rev* 2013;2:CD009974.
25 Chou R, Peterson K, Helfand M. Comparative efficacy and safety of skeletal muscle relaxants for spasticity and musculoskeletal conditions: a systematic review. *J Pain Symptom Manage* 2004;28:140-75.
26 Taricco M, Pagliacci MC, Telaro E, Adone R. Pharmacological interventions for spasticity following spinal cord injury: results of a Cochrane systematic review. *Eura Medicophys* 2006;42:5-15.
27 Montane E, Vallano A, Laporte JR. Oral antispastic drugs in nonprogressive neurologic diseases: a systematic review. *Neurology* 2004;63:1357-63.
28 National Institute for Health and Care Excellence. Spasticity in children and young people with non- progressive brain disorders. (Clinical Guideline 145.) 2012. http://guidance.nice.org.uk/CG145.
29 Halpern R, Gillard P, Graham GD, Varon SF, Zorowitz RD. Adherence associated with oral medications in the treatment of spasticity. *PM R* 2013;5:747-56.
30 Simon O, Yelnik AP. Managing spasticity with drugs. *Eur J Phys Rehabil Med* 2010;46:401-10.

31 Ghidini A, Healey A, Andreani M, Simonson MR. Pregnancy and women with spinal cord injuries. *Acta Obstet Gynecol Scand* 2008;87:1006-10.

32 Moran LR, Almeida PG, Worden S, Huttner KM. Intrauterine baclofen exposure: a multidisciplinary approach. *Paediatrics* 2004;114:267-9.

33 Koppel BS, Brust JCM, Fife T, Bronstein J, Youssof S, Gronseth G, et al. Systematic review: efficacy and safety of medical marijuana in selected neurological disorders: Report of the guideline development subcommittee of the American Academy of neurology. *Neurology* 2014;82:1556-63.

34 Wade DT, Collin C, Stott C, Duncombe P. Meta-analysis of the efficacy and safety of Sativex (nabiximols), on spasticity in people with multiple sclerosis. *Mult Scler* 2010;16:707-14.

35 Lakhan SE, Rowland M. Whole plant cannabis extracts in the treatment of spasticity in multiple sclerosis: a systematic review. *BMC Neurol* 2009;9:59.

36 McCrory P, Turner-Stokes L, Baguley IJ, De Graff S, Katrak P, Sandanam J et al. Botulinum toxin for treatment of upper limb spasticity following stroke: a multi-centre randomized placebo-controlled study of effects on quality of life and other person centred outcomes. *J Rehabil Med* 2009;41:536-44.

37 Shaw L, Rodgers H, Price C, van Wijck F, Shackley P, Steen N, et al. BoTULS: a multicentre randomised controlled trial to evaluate the clinical effectiveness and cost-effectiveness of treating upper limb spasticity due to stroke with botulinum toxin type A. *Health Technol Assess* 2010;14(6).

38 Royal College of Physicians, British Society of Rehabilitation Medicine, Chartered Society of Physiotherapy, Association of Chartered Physiotherapists Interested in Neurology. Spasticity in adults: management using botulinum toxin. National guidelines. RCP, 2009.

39 Wissel J, Ward AB, Erztgaard P, Bensmail D, Hecht MJ, Lejune TM, et al. European consensus table on the use of botulinum toxin type A in adult spasticity. *J Rehabil Med* 2009;41:13-25.

40 Simpson DM, Gracies JM, Graham HK, Miyasaki JM, Naumann M, Russmann B, et al. Assessment: botulinum neurotoxin for the treatment of spasticity (an evidence based review): report of the therapeutics and technology assessment subcommittee of the American Academy of Neurology. *Neurology* 2008;70:1691-8.

41 Lee SJ Sung IY, Jang DH, Yi JH, Lee JH, Ryu JS. The effect and complication of botulinum toxin type A injection with serial casting. *Ann Rehabil Med* 2011;35:344-53.

42 Zahavi A, Geertzen JH, Middel B, Staal M, Rietman JS. Long term effect of intrathecal baclofen on impairment, disability and quality of life in patients with severe spasticity of spinal origin *J Neurol Neurosurg Psychiatry* 2004;75:1553-7.

43 Schiess MC, Oh IJ, Stimming EF, Lucke J, Acosta F, Fisher S, et al. Prospective 12-month study of intrathecal baclofen therapy for post stroke spastic upper and lower extremity motor control and functional improvement. *Neuromodulation* 2011;14:38-45.

44 Bensmail D, Peskine A, Roche N, Mailhan L, Thiebaut JB, Bussel B. Intrathecal baclofen for treatment of spasticity of multiple sclerosis patients. *Mult Scler* 2006;12:101-3.

45 McIntyre A, Mays R, Mehta R, Janzen S, Townson A, Hsieh J, et al. Examining the effectiveness of intrathecal baclofen on spasticity in individuals with chronic spinal cord injury: a systematic review. *J Spinal Cord Med* 2014;37:11-8.

46 Stetkarova I, Yabion SA, Kofler M, Stokic DS. Procedure and device related complications of intrathecal baclofen administration for management of adult muscle hypertonia: a review. *Neurorehabil Neural Repair* 2010:24; 609-19.

47 Ross JC, Cook AM, Stewart GL, Fahy BG. Acute intrathecal baclofen withdrawal: a brief review of treatment options. *Neurocrit Care* 2011;14:103-8.

48 Kocabas H, Salli A, Demir AH, Ozerbil OM. Comparison of phenol and alcohol neurolysis of tibial nerve motor branches to the gastrocnemius muscle for treatment of spastic foot after stroke: a randomized controlled pilot study. *Eur J Phys Rehabil Med* 2010;46:5-10.

49 Yasar E, Tok F, Taskaynatan MA, Yilmaz B, Balaban B, Alaca R. The effects of phenol neurolysis of the obturator nerve on distribution of buttock seat interface pressure in spinal cord injury patients with hip adductor spasticity. *Spinal Cord* 2010;48:828-31.

50 Pinder C, Bhakta B, Kodavali K. Intrathecal phenol: an old treatment revisited. *Disabil Rehabil* 2008;30:381-6.

First seizures in adults

Heather Angus-Leppan, consultant neurologist and epilepsy lead[1], honorary senior lecturer[2]

[1]Clinical Neurosciences, Royal Free London NHS Foundation Trust and Barnet Chase Farm Hospitals NHS Trust, London, UK

[2]Institute of Neurology, University College London and Centre for Restorative Neuroscience, Imperial College London

Correspondence to: H Angus-Leppan, Royal Free Hospital, Pond Street, London NW3 2QG heather.angus-leppan@nhs.net

Cite this as: BMJ 2014;348:g2470

DOI: 10.1136/bmj.g2470

http://www.bmj.com/content/348/bmj.g2470

A seizure is a clinical manifestation of presumed or proved abnormal electrical activity in the brain. A first seizure can range from a fleeting subjective experience such as déjà vu or a twitch (myoclonic jerk) through to a tonic-clonic convulsion. Some seizure manifestations overlap with normal phenomena. A single seizure may be provoked (with an acute precipitant that may or may not recur) or unprovoked (idiopathic or of unknown cause). Epilepsy is defined as more than one seizure.

This article focuses on the diagnosis of first seizures and differentiation from their "mimics" in adults. The diagnosis is correct in only two thirds of cases or less and relies almost exclusively on the clinical history.[1 2 3 4 5 6 7 8 9] Information for patients, particularly regarding risks of recurrence, investigation and treatment, driving, and mortality, will be discussed.

This review uses older seizure terminology,[10 11] as this is better understood by most readers and succinctly conveys important clinical concepts. Where the revised terminology differs, this is noted in the text and the supplementary table.[12]

How common are first seizures?

Few data about the frequency of minor (non-convulsive) first seizures exist. Many minor first seizures are unrecognised. The recorded incidence of first seizure (provoked and unprovoked) in Europe is approximately 70 per 100 000 per year,[13 14] with twice that incidence in poorer countries.[15 16 17] Febrile seizures are the "first seizure" with the highest worldwide incidence (50 per 100 000 per year), usually occurring in the first three years of life.[18]

The cumulative lifetime incidence of single seizures and recurrent epileptic seizures (including febrile seizures) is estimated as 5-10%.[19 20] The prevalence of epilepsy is between 0.5% and 1% of the population.[20] Epileptic seizures are responsible for 1% of hospital admissions and 3% of emergency department attendances.[21]

First seizures are not always declared in epidemiological questionnaires,[22 23] because of social stigma, fears about losing the driving licence, and concerns about employment.[24 25] Few epidemiological studies of provoked seizures have been done, as episodes are often indexed under their provocation (for example, alcohol withdrawal or head injury) rather than seizure and may not reach neurological attention.[26]

Transient loss of consciousness is the most commonly recorded and studied presentation of "first seizure." In 2005-06 100 000 hospital attendances in the United Kingdom were for transient loss of consciousness.[27] The table summarises the causes of transient loss of consciousness from several descriptive studies. These include epileptic seizure, syncope, and non-epileptic attack disorder.

Diagnosing a first seizure: how do people present?

In addition to the patient's history, an eyewitness account is very important and should be sought whenever possible. The patient's and eyewitness's histories are not only critical for diagnosis of the event. The "first seizure" may be a major event after other missed minor epileptic events, so that the diagnosis is epilepsy rather than a single seizure.[8 9] Clinically, clarifying whether the first seizure occurred with or without loss of awareness or consciousness is useful.

Seizures without loss of consciousness

The brief duration and a clear description of the experience define these seizures, which patients often do not recognise as important. If patients present, it is often to primary care. Early recognition allows for correct management and may change the diagnosis from a single seizure to epilepsy.

Myoclonus

Myoclonus is a sudden irregular jerk caused by involuntary muscle activity, involving the trunk or one or more limbs. Many causes of myoclonus exist—it may be physiological or pathological. In primary care, it is important to be aware of hypnic myoclonus (physiological) and acute causes related to drugs and to refer other patients with myoclonus (including seizures). Myoclonus in the awake state usually requires specialist assessment. Hypnic (night time) myoclonus is the most common form of myoclonus, experienced as a jolt, which may be dramatic and awaken the person, on drifting into sleep. Most of us have experienced this at least once, and patients can be reassured that this is a normal phenomenon.

Drugs (including some narcotics, antidepressants, and antipsychotics) cause myoclonus, as can drug toxicity or withdrawal. Secondary causes include epileptic seizure. A myoclonic seizure varies from a subtle unrecognised jerk, presenting as "clumsiness" or dropping of an object, to a violent jolt causing a fall. It may be the first feature of juvenile myoclonic epilepsy, the most common form of myoclonic epilepsy, classically with myoclonic jerks or clumsiness occurring in the first hours after awakening, especially after sleep deprivation. Recognition, referral, and treatment of these may prevent a full tonic-clonic seizure. Other causes include post-hypoxic brain damage (such as

SUMMARY POINTS

- First seizures range from a brief subjective experience (aura) to a major tonic-clonic seizure
- Up to 10% of people living to 80 years of age have one or more seizures; half of these are febrile convulsions
- In 85% of patients, the diagnosis comes from the history; blood tests, electrocardiography, electroencephalography, and sometimes magnetic resonance imaging are important for classification and risk prediction
- 50% of patients with an apparent "first seizure" have had other minor seizures, so their diagnosis is epilepsy
- Low risk patients with first seizures have no neurological deficits, normal magnetic resonance imaging and electroencephalography, and a 35% risk of recurrence at five years; they are not usually offered treatment
- High risk patients with first seizures have neurological deficit, magnetic resonance imaging and/or electroencephalography abnormalities, and a 70% risk of recurrence at five years; they are offered treatment

after cardiac arrest), encephalopathy, encephalitis, and neurodegeneration (which will present with other clinical features such as cognitive change) and spinal myoclonus due to injury or disease.[28]

Aura (simple partial subjective seizure)
Epileptic auras are brief (seconds only) and should be distinguished from migraine auras, which usually last several minutes. They can be autonomic, usually a rising epigastric sensation, lasting seconds. Psychic epileptic auras such as déjà vu are often unpleasant and out of the realm of any normal experience, sometimes intensely so; they may involve distortions of time or a feeling of separation or depersonalisation. Déjà vu (already seen) and jamais vu (never seen) refer to a false impression that a present experience is familiar. They refer to something heard, experienced, or seen. These are common auras of a temporal lobe seizure. They need to be distinguished from normal experience (such as occasional bland déjà vu), psychiatric illness (usually prolonged and with persistent behavioural or personality change), and migrainous auras (lasting many minutes in the setting of other features of migraine). Sensory epileptic auras are often simple, unformed elementary hallucinations (such as metallic taste, coloured spots, tinnitus, tingling), are usually positive (as opposed to the loss of function seen in stroke), and last seconds (as opposed to migraine and stroke). Complex hallucinations, such as formed objects or scenes or formed words or sentences, are very unlikely to be epileptic.[29] An aura is designated as a "focal seizure without impairment of consciousness or awareness involving subjective sensory or psychic phenomena only" in the revised classification.[12]

Simple partial motor seizure
These are clonic (regular shaking), tonic (stiffening), or dystonic (spasm), usually in a distal limb, and are usually brief (lasting seconds). They must be distinguished from spasticity due to cortical or spinal disease (such as occurs in about 30% of patients with multiple sclerosis or stroke, in which other clinical features and characteristic disabilities will indicate the diagnosis) or focal dystonia (such as writer's cramp, which is situation specific). Rigors can be mistaken for a first seizure, particularly in children.[30] A simple partial motor seizure is designated as a "focal motor seizure without impairment of consciousness or awareness" in the revised classification.[12]

Seizures with loss of consciousness

Absences
Previously referred to as "petit mal," these last seconds or less, with disruption of awareness, activity, and sometimes learning. They may happen many times a day. A motionless stare, sometimes with eyelid fluttering, may be observed. They start in childhood but continue into adulthood in 7-80% of cases. They are more likely to persist to adulthood if onset is in later childhood or in adolescence, if they are difficult to treat, and if they are associated with other types of seizures.[31] Absences may present late, with the person being unaware of them or having tolerated them for decades.[32] They must be distinguished from daydreaming, cognitive difficulties, hearing or visual loss, autism, and psychological difficulties, as well as from complex partial seizures (see below). A decline in academic performance at school should alert family, teachers, and healthcare professionals to the possibility of absence seizures. The electroencephalogram is diagnostic in more than 90% of cases.[9] If electroencephalography is unavailable, hyperventilation may induce a typical event.

Complex partial seizure
Some impairment of awareness, consciousness, and/or memory of the event occurs during a complex partial seizure.[10] These sometimes evolve from an aura (simple partial seizure). They may be a motionless stare or automatisms (automatic involuntary movements) such as lip smacking, fiddling, and rubbing or pseudo-purposeful movements. Objects in the immediate vicinity may be used; movements may include dressing and undressing, hitting out, or vocalisations. Tasks involving detailed cognition, such as loading a gun, finding a key and unlocking a cabinet, or typing in a password, would not be expected. Episodes last for seconds to minutes, and communication is usually impaired. These are designated as "focal seizures with impairment of consciousness or awareness" in the revised terminology.[12]

Tonic-clonic seizure (convulsion)
Tonic-clonic seizures may have no warning (if generalised from onset) or may start with an aura (if focal with secondary generalisation) before consciousness is lost. Often an initial cry is followed by a loss of tone and a fall, then a phase of tonic rigidity followed by regular rhythmic shaking in all limbs, trunk, and face, lateral tongue biting, and cyanosis. Eyes are usually open.[33 34] The usual duration is 1-2 minutes, and postictal confusion (a period usually longer than 10 minutes characterised by disorientation, poor concentration, poor short term memory, and decreased verbal and interactive skills) occurs.[10]

Differential diagnosis of transient loss of consciousness
Up to 35% of people will experience at least one episode of transient loss of consciousness by the age of 60 years.[35] The differentiation of tonic-clonic seizures from syncope and non-epileptic attack disorder is discussed below. This may be difficult, particularly if no eyewitness account is available. No single clinical feature or investigation is pathognomonic.

Postictal confusion,[7 34 36] cyanosis,[36] lateral tongue biting,[36] preceding déjà vu or jamais vu,[36] confirmed unresponsiveness,[36] head or eye turning to one side,[7 36] and rhythmic limb shaking or unusual (dystonic) posturing are strong seizure markers.[34 36] Seizure is five times more likely than syncope if the patient has postictal confusion characterised by disorientation ($P<0.001$).[7] Patients themselves are poor judges of their own postictal confusion, and the eyewitness account is crucial for this information.[7] Incontinence and injury do not discriminate between seizure, syncope, and non-epileptic attack disorder.[7]

Syncope
Transient loss of consciousness is much more commonly caused by syncope, particularly reflex (vasovagal) syncope, than by seizure. Many cases will not reach medical attention. Prodromal blurred vision, sweating, dizziness, dyspnoea, nausea, or palpitations,[7 36 37] precipitation by prolonged sitting or standing,[36] and pallor during the episode are common.[34] If movements occur, they are usually brief, often myoclonic jerks. However, syncope can sometimes be convulsive with tonic-clonic movements, owing to cerebral

hypoxia, particularly if the patient is not able to assume the horizontal position.[38] Eyes are usually open in both syncope and epileptic seizures but not in non-epileptic attacks.[33 38 39] Nausea or sweating before the event make seizure much less likely than syncope.[7] Cardiac syncope may be an apparently bland event, with no prodrome, brief loss of consciousness, and pallor, sweatiness, or clamminess, followed by rapid recovery. Cyanosis strongly suggests cardiac rather than reflex syncope.[7] Cardiac syncope due to arrhythmia or structural abnormality of the heart doubles the standardised mortality ratio and needs urgent investigation.[37]

Non-epileptic attack disorder

These are episodes resembling seizures but caused by psychological or psychiatric illness. They are also called non-epileptic seizures, dissociative seizures, or psychogenic non-epileptic seizures and were previously called pseudo-seizures or hysterical seizures (but they are not seizures). Sometimes the term "non-epileptic attack" is misused for any event that is not epilepsy (including syncope, psychiatric or psychological events, and migraine)

Non-epileptic attack disorder occurs in about 12-18% of people with transient loss of consciousness,[40] can be difficult to diagnose and manage, and presents in many forms. A successful outcome is more likely when the diagnosis is made early.[41] Key features are prolonged apparent loss of consciousness with normal colour or oxygen saturation on room air, fluctuating motor activity, asynchronous movements, pelvic thrusting, side to side head or body movements, ictal crying, some responsiveness such as resistance to eye opening, memory recall, and rapid post-event recovery. If the event is one of prolonged shaking and apparent loss of consciousness (more than 10 minutes) and the patient retains normal colour, the event is almost never an epileptic seizure.

Should first status epilepticus and seizure clusters be considered first seizure or epilepsy?

A cluster of seizures or status epilepticus within 24 hours is defined as a form of first seizure,[42] but this is controversial and not solidly supported by data.[43] Strong grounds exist for revising the inclusion of seizure clusters and first status epilepticus in the definition of first seizure.

In children, the risk of recurrence for multiple seizures in one day is double that for a single seizure, strongly supporting the argument for calling this epilepsy.[44] In adults, the recurrence rate after discharge from hospital is unclear. Some series suggest no increased risk of subsequent seizures if the patient presented with multiple seizures in the first 24 hours.[45] However, 16% of first status epilepticus patients die during their inpatient stay, whereas the immediate mortality from a single seizure is negligible.[46] Of those surviving the first 30 days, the long term standardised mortality rate for first seizure status epilepticus is more than double that for a brief single first seizure.[47] Management of first status epilepticus and seizure clusters is very different from that of a single seizure. Early management of "first status epilepticus" will be the same as for status epilepticus in patients with known epilepsy.

Who is most at risk?

Worldwide, social deprivation is closely associated with first seizures and epilepsy.[48] Young people and older people are at the highest risk for first seizure (as well as for epilepsy).[18 49] The frequency and cause of first seizures also vary in different economic and geographical settings.

> **SOURCES AND SELECTION CRITERIA**
>
> I consulted my personal archive of references and searched Medline and the Cochrane Collaboration and Clinical Evidence databases, using "seizure", "first seizure", and specific topics. I also consulted the National Institute for Health and Care Excellence's guidelines. I carefully examined randomised controlled trials, systematic reviews, and meta-analyses. Ranges of results are used in preference to averages, because pooling results from methodologically diverse studies is not accurate

Provoked seizures in early life are usually febrile convulsions,[50] caused by viral infection in 80%, with 8% due to meningitis (viral or bacterial).[51] Unprovoked remote symptomatic seizures in children are more commonly due to prenatal than postnatal factors.[13] An unprovoked idiopathic (presumed genetic) first seizure occurs in childhood or teenage years, commonly with a family history of idiopathic epilepsy.[52]

Worldwide, in adults, infections such as acute meningitis, encephalitis, malaria, HIV related disease, and cysticercosis are common causes of first seizures.[53] Provoked seizures due to intoxication and withdrawal from alcohol are also frequent.[13 54] In later life, vascular disease becomes the most common cause.[55] Brain tumours, including metastases, are responsible for about 4% of first seizures.[13] Paradoxically, lower grade primary tumours are more likely to present with a seizure than are higher grade ones.[56]

How should first seizure be managed?

Following a first seizure of any kind, all patients should be referred to a specialist for investigation. In the UK, patients with a first seizure see a wide range of health professionals including paramedical officers, emergency department nurses and doctors, primary care doctors, neurologists, other physicians, and specialist nurses, or none at all in at least 25% of cases.[48] If a tonic-clonic seizure is witnessed then stabilisation, removal of surrounding dangers, and examination for acute factors (including blood glucose, metabolic disturbance, sepsis, toxins and withdrawal states, acute stroke, and brain injury) are the starting points. If the tonic-clonic seizure lasts longer than two minutes, benzodiazepines (such as rectal diazepam, buccal midazolam, or intravenous lorazepam) are usually given as rescue medication. Admission is needed if the seizure recurs or continues, an underlying cause requiring acute treatment exists, level of consciousness is reduced, a neurological deficit is present, or social support for discharge is inadequate.[57] A provoked (acute symptomatic) first seizure with a trigger may need urgent treatment (such as for infection, encephalitis, metabolic disturbance, toxicity, haemorrhage). Remote or progressive symptomatic causes (such as chronic cerebrovascular disease or brain tumour) may also need treatment. A single seizure without loss of consciousness does not usually need any first aid.

Why is investigation after first seizure important?

When the history has not clarified whether the event was a seizure, the investigations are unlikely to do so. Retaking the history from the patient and from eyewitnesses is often more useful. Clinical assessment contributes more than 85% of the diagnostic yield in transient loss of consciousness.[1 4] Warning patients that investigations are unlikely to change the clinical diagnosis and may all be normal, even with a firm diagnosis of an epileptic seizure, is important.[4]

After a first seizure, further seizures (that is, epilepsy) occur in between 6% and 82% of patients.[18 58] Averaging these figures does not allow prediction of the risk for an individual. Thorough clinical assessment and investigations help to establish the type of seizure, cause, and recurrence risk. Provoked seizures are more common in people with an underlying genetic or other tendency to epilepsy,[52] and a single trigger (such as alcohol) should not be assumed to be the only cause.

What investigations are needed after first seizure in acute setting?

The most important initial tests in the acute setting are blood glucose measurement (for hypoglycaemia or hyperglycaemia) and electrocardiography. Electrocardiography is mandatory in anyone with loss of consciousness, as syncope of any cardiac cause may present as a secondary hypoxic seizure, and potentially fatal arrhythmias, particularly long QT syndromes (Brugada syndrome), will otherwise be missed.[59] Cardiac disease is the most common cause of non-traumatic sudden death in young people, sometimes preceded by potentially treatable cardiac syncope.[60]

Other blood tests will exclude hyponatraemia or hypernatremia, hypocalcaemia or hypercalcaemia, hypothyroidism, uraemia, liver failure, anaemia (which can trigger syncope), leucocytosis (suggesting infection, although mild leucocytosis can occur after a seizure), and eosinophilia (a clue to parasitosis, an important cause of a first seizure in many parts of the world).[48] Although the yield of blood tests is low,[1 4 59] they are needed to determine whether the seizure is provoked.[50]

What investigations will be done at early specialist follow-up?

Early specialist assessment by a neurologist can reduce investigations, improve diagnostic accuracy, and save time for the patient.[4 61] If, for example, the neurologist revises the diagnosis from seizure to reflex syncope, no further investigations are needed beyond the blood tests and electrocardiography.

Electroencephalography is useful in suspected first seizure for predicting recurrence and in classification of the seizure (idiopathic generalised or focal). Yield is highest in the first 24 hours after the seizure.[9] Relevant abnormalities (spikes and/or slow waves)[59 62] are found in 8-50% of cases.[59] The yield is increased by activation procedures (hyperventilation and photic stimulation)[63] and with electroencephalography after sleep deprivation (up to 80% yield, but also an increase to 4% in false positives).[9] An electroencephalogram is unhelpful when the diagnosis is syncope, as it does not "rule out" epilepsy and has a false positive rate of 4%.[64]

Is brain imaging needed in all first seizure patients?

Many guidelines advocate magnetic resonance imaging in all first seizure patients.[59] However, no sound justification exists in idiopathic epilepsy presenting at a young age. For example, in an 18 year old with a single convulsion, previous early morning myoclonic jerks, normal neurological examination, and an electroencephalogram with 3/second spike and wave discharges, the diagnosis of juvenile myoclonic epilepsy (idiopathic) is clear cut. Relevant lesions on magnetic resonance imaging are not found in patients with electroencephalogram proved idiopathic epilepsy. Magnetic resonance imaging can be safely restricted to first seizure patients without clinical or electroencephalographic evidence of idiopathic epilepsy.[65] Overall, magnetic resonance imaging has a yield of 10% in first seizures and is superior in resolution to computed tomography scanning, especially for temporal lobe epilepsy.[59]

Computed tomography scanning is useful for first seizure patients with acute head injury or patients with reduced level of consciousness. It is safer and faster than magnetic resonance imaging for acutely unwell patients,[65] and it may influence acute management in 9-17% of patients.[66]

Is this a first seizure and will it recur?

This is a critical question. The first step is to go back to the history. Up to half of people with a "first seizure" have historical evidence of non-convulsive seizures or nocturnal seizures (bed wetting, tongue biting, blood on the pillow, early morning headache, or "hangover" without alcohol), which suggests that the diagnosis is epilepsy.[8 9 13 67]

Studies with varying methods and follow-up from two to 26 years estimate the risk of recurrence after a first seizure to be between 6% and 82%.[68 69] Maximum recurrence risk is within the first 3-6 months.[8 18] For the individual patient, predictive factors need to be examined. For example, after a febrile convulsion, the risk of developing epilepsy is 6%, reducing over time.[68] Neurological deficits (prenatal injury,

Causes of transient loss of consciousness. Values are numbers (percentages)

Cause	Eagle, 1985—?syncope; emergency department*	Day et al, 1982—first episode (LOC); emergency department†	Angus-Leppan, 2008—first and recurrent episode (LOC); neurology clinic‡	Angus-Leppan, 2013; emergency department§
Syncope—all	—	—	40 (25)	—
Syncope—vasovagal	64 (35)	57 (29)	—	30 (35)
Syncope—orthostatic	16 (10)	7 (3)	—	—
Syncope—cardiac	15 (9)	17 (9)	—	10 (12)
Epilepsy	2 (1)	58 (29)	68 (43)	20 (23)
Non-epileptic attack disorder	3 (1)	14 (7)	19 (12)	10 (11)
Other	7 (5)	20 (10)	11 (7)	—
Unknown	69 (39)	25 (13)	20 (13)	16 (19)
Total	176	198	158	86

LOC=loss of consciousness.
**Patients with first and recurrent events.[90]*
†Patients with first events only.[1]
‡Patients with first and recurrent events.[4]
§Patients with first events only (unpublished).

neurological deficit, intellectual disability) or relevant magnetic resonance imaging or electroencephalographic abnormalities (spikes, slow waves, or both) are the strongest predictors of recurrence across many studies.[70] For patients with one or both of these factors, the risk of recurrence is 70% over five years.[71] For patients without these factors, recurrence is estimated at 35%.[70 71]

To treat or not to treat?

After a first seizure, the default position is not to give antiepileptic drug treatment. We offer treatment to first seizure patients with a high risk of recurrence, because of known neurological deficit, a magnetic resonance imaging or electroencephalographic abnormality, or individual factors.[72] These include risk of fracture or injury, social isolation, and the need to return to driving as soon as possible.

Does early treatment improve long term prognosis and prevent death?

Early treatment reduces the risk of recurrence but does not improve the long term prognosis.[71 73] It has not been shown to reduce mortality due to epilepsy. These findings apply predominantly to low risk patients, as randomisation to early or delayed treatment occurs only when both doctor and patient are uncertain about whether to treat.

Should we treat if provocation is ongoing?

We have no solid evidence regarding treatment if the provocation continues (for example, ongoing alcohol or drug intake, brittle diabetes, or hypothyroidism or hypercalcaemia that is taking months to correct). The natural history of alcohol use and seizures suggests an increasing risk of further events with each recurrence, directly due to alcohol,[74] head injuries, or alcoholic brain damage. Hypoglycaemia causes neuronal damage, which predisposes to further seizures.[75] Although treatment is not proved, it may protect from further seizures and can be justified while the chronic provoking factors remain.

What follow-up is recommended after first seizure?

Specialist review and investigations are recommended for first seizure patients within four weeks.[65] Unless the diagnosis is revised to syncope, follow-up with results will usually occur after about three months, earlier if abnormalities are found. Further specialist follow-up depends on the estimated risk of recurrence, whether drug treatment has been started, and other individual factors. Many patients with a first seizure and normal investigations will be discharged to primary care, with specialist review if a further event occurs. Patients may remain concerned, even after explanation, when told that they have had a seizure and they cannot drive but their tests are normal and they do not need further specific treatment or specialist follow-up. Primary care physicians have an important role in further explanation, particularly in the significant minority of first seizure patients in whom the diagnosis may trigger depression and anxiety.[76]

What should we advise with regards to driving?

Driving is often a great concern to patients with a first seizure.[77] People with epilepsy have 40% more serious road traffic accidents than do other people.[78] Initial advice to the first seizure patient should be not to drive until medically advised otherwise, whether or not the diagnosis is certain. First seizures should be reported to the Driver and Vehicle Licensing Agency (DVLA) in the UK or the equivalent body internationally.

Driving regulations vary considerably between, and sometimes within, countries. In the UK, decision making is centralised.[79] The regulatory body, the DVLA, gathers information from treating doctors, with the advantage of separating the therapeutic relationship and decision making about driving. New regulations allow some patients with only simple partial seizures to drive. If the first seizure is unprovoked, investigations are normal, and no neurological deficit is present, driving will usually be permitted after six months. Otherwise, driving is usually permitted after 12 months seizure free. Commercial licences are subject to more stringent regulation.[79]

TIPS FOR FIRST CONTACT DOCTOR

- After stabilisation of a patient with a first seizure, take a careful history from the patient and eyewitness(es)
- Blood tests and electrocardiography are important, especially for hypoglycaemia and arrhythmias
- Advise the patient not to drive and not to bath alone; give details of educational resources (see box)
- Refer to a specialist for early review (further assessment, tests, and antiepileptic drugs if indicated)

QUESTIONS FOR FUTURE RESEARCH

- What are the recurrence rates of defined seizure types analysed by their cause?
- What is the optimal management strategy for first seizure patients, particularly regarding antiepileptic drugs?
- When should we treat provoked seizures with antiepileptic drugs?
- Are first status epilepticus and multiple seizures a "first seizure" or epilepsy?
- What causes sudden unexpected death in epilepsy and what prevents it for first seizure patients?
- How can we improve the way we advise first seizure patients on lifestyle and safety?

ADDITIONAL EDUCATIONAL RESOURCES

Resources for healthcare professionals

- National Institute for Health and Care Excellence, UK (guidance.nice.org.uk/Topic)—Free guidelines, no registration needed; recommendations and references on initial assessment
- Scottish Intercollegiate Guidelines Network (sign.ac.uk/guidelines/published/index.html)—Free guidelines, no registration needed; recommendations and references on initial assessment
- Epilepsy.com (www.epilepsy.com)—Links and information pages, including links to videos with examples of different seizure types

Resources for patients and healthcare professionals

- Epilepsy Action (epilepsy.org.uk)—Free site with information for patients; no registration needed; explanations, descriptions, useful links, literature
- Epilepsy Society (epilepsysociety.org.uk; 01494 601 400)—Free site and helpline; no registration needed; information on important topics, links, brochure, helpline
- International League Against Epilepsy (ilae-epilepsy.org)—No registration needed; information and links to other sites; information pages on important topics

What advice should be given about safety at home and at leisure?

Patients should be advised to have showers rather than baths, ideally with a heat controlled system.[80] If this is not possible, an informed relative or carer should be present and available during bathing. Ideally, household members should be trained in first aid.

Swimming can be safe, with an informed lifeguard or another person trained in first aid. For some patients with intellectual disability or other medical needs, swimming guidelines are advisable and can be individually tailored to the need.[81] The UK Sport Diving Medical Committee recommends that the person is off medication and seizure free for five years before scuba diving.[82] For this and other potentially hazardous activities such as downhill skiing, abseiling, bungee jumping, cycling, parachuting, and gliding, no clear evidence base exists for our advice.

What advice should be given regarding sex following first seizure?

Little evidence exists on epilepsy and sexuality, particularly in women. No data are available on the risks of injury with a seizure during sexual activity. One study in patients with severe epilepsy estimated that 8% of seizures occurred during intercourse or masturbation and that 25% feared a seizure during sexual activity, but these figures cannot be extrapolated to patients with first seizures.[83] Hyposexuality and sexual concerns are common, but doctors, nurses, and patients are often uneasy about discussing them.[84 85] In the absence of any firm evidence, we should tell patients to continue with their normal level of sexual activity and answer any specific questions.

Should we warn all patients about sudden unexpected death in epilepsy?

In the UK, specialists are mandated to discuss sudden unexpected death in epilepsy with all patients with epilepsy,[65] but not for first seizure patients. Only 5% of neurologists discussed sudden unexpected death in epilepsy with all patients; 60% discussed it with some, usually high risk, patients or those who specifically asked about it.[86] The standardised mortality rate after a first seizure is about 2.3,[87] which overlaps with the 2-4 described for epilepsy.[88] If we discuss sudden death with patients with epilepsy, we should also do so with patients with first seizures and those with cardiac syncope. Discussing sudden unexpected death in epilepsy at the first visit is not always appropriate, as there is much to discuss and sometimes a risk of information overload. Content and timing of this discussion must be individualised to prevent a negative psychological effect.[89]

I greatly appreciate the support of S Powis and the Royal Free Hospital research scheme, C Burghes and the Royal Free Charity, and my colleagues. I thank R J Guiloff for suggestions.

Contributors: HAL planned the organisation, content, and structure of the paper on the basis of the BMJ's guidelines for writing a clinical review.

Competing interests: I have read and understood the BMJ Group policy on declaration of interests and declare the following interests: none.

Provenance and peer review: Commissioned: externally peer reviewed.

1 Day SC, Cook EF, Funkenstein H, Goldman L. Evaluation and outcome of emergency room patients with transient loss of consciousness. *Am J Med* 1982;73:15-23.

2 Leach JP, Lauder R, Nicolson A, Smith DF. Epilepsy in the UK: misdiagnosis, mistreatment, and undertreatment? The Wrexham area epilepsy project. *Seizure* 2005;14:514-20.

3 Smith D, Defalla BA, Chadwick DW. The misdiagnosis of epilepsy and the management of refractory epilepsy in a specialist clinic. *QJM* 1999;92:15-23.

4 Angus-Leppan H. Diagnosing epilepsy in neurology clinics: a prospective study. *Seizure* 2008;17:431-6.

5 Forsgren L. Prospective incidence study and clinical characterization of seizures in newly referred adults. *Epilepsia* 1990;31:292-301.

6 Zaidi A, Clough P, Cooper P, Scheepers B, Fitzpatrick AP. Misdiagnosis of epilepsy: many seizure-like attacks have a cardiovascular cause. *J Am Coll Cardiol* 2000;36:181-4.

7 Hoefnagels W, Padberg G, Overweg J, Van der Velde E, Roos R. Transient loss of consciousness: the value of the history for distinguishing seizure from syncope. *J Neurol* 1991;238:39-43.

8 Hauser WA, Rich SS, Annegers JF, Anderson VE. Seizure recurrence after a 1st unprovoked seizure: an extended follow-up. *Neurology* 1990;40:1163-70.

9 King MA, Newton MR, Jackson GD, Fitt GJ, Mitchell LA, Silvapulle MJ, et al. Epileptology of the first-seizure presentation: a clinical, electroencephalographic, and magnetic resonance imaging study of 300 consecutive patients. *Lancet* 1998;352:1007-11.

10 Angeles DK. Proposal for revised clinical and electroencephalographic classification of epileptic seizures. *Epilepsia* 1981;22:489-501.

11 Commission on Classification and Terminology of the International League Against Epilepsy. Proposal for revised classification of epilepsies and epileptic syndromes. *Epilepsia* 1989;30:389-99.

12 Berg AT, Berkovic SF, Brodie MJ, Buchhalter J, Cross JH, van Emde Boas W, et al. Revised terminology and concepts for organization of seizures and epilepsies: report of the ILAE Commission on Classification and Terminology, 2005-2009. *Epilepsia* 2010;51:676-85.

13 Jallon P, Goumaz M, Haenggeli C, Morabia A. Incidence of first epileptic seizures in the canton of Geneva, Switzerland. *Epilepsia* 1997;38:547-52.

14 Loiseau J, Loiseau P, Guyot M, Duche B, Dartigues JF, Aublet B. Survey of seizure disorders in the French southwest: I. Incidence of epileptic syndromes. *Epilepsia* 1990;31:391-6.

15 Placencia M, Suarez J, Crespo F, Sander JW, Shorvon SD, Ellison RH, et al. A large-scale study of epilepsy in Ecuador: methodological aspects. *Neuroepidemiology* 1992;11:74-84.

16 Meinardi H, Scott RA, Reis R, Sander JW, for the ILAE Commission on the Developing World. The treatment gap in epilepsy: the current situation and ways forward. *Epilepsia* 2001;42:136-49.

17 Lavados J, Germain L, Morales A, Campero M, Lavados P. A descriptive study of epilepsy in the district of El Salvador, Chile, 1984-1988. *Acta Neurol Scand* 1992;85:249-56.

18 Hart Y, Sander J, Shorvon S, Johnson A. National general practice study of epilepsy: recurrence after a first seizure. *Lancet* 1990;336:1271-4.

19 Hauser WA, Annegers JF, Kurland LT. Incidence of epilepsy and unprovoked seizures in Rochester, Minnesota: 1935-1984. *Epilepsia* 1993;34:453-68.

20 Hauser WA, Annegers JF, Rocca WA. Descriptive epidemiology of epilepsy: contributions of population-based studies from Rochester, Minnesota. *Mayo Clin Proc* 1996;71:576-86.

21 All Party Parliamentary Group on Epilepsy. Wasted money, wasted lives: the human and economic cost of epilepsy in England. Stationery Office, 2007.

22 Zielinski JJ. Epidemiology and medicosocial problems of epilepsy in Warsaw: final report on research program. Psychoneurological Institute, 1974.

23 Beran RG, Michelazzi J, Hall L, Tsimnadis P, Loh S. False-negative response rate in epidemiologic studies to define prevalence ratios of epilepsy. *Neuroepidemiology* 1985;4:82-5.

24 Jacoby A, Baker G, Smith D, Dewey M, Chadwick D. Measuring the impact of epilepsy: the development of a novel scale. *Epilepsy Res* 1993;16:83-8.

25 Bellon M, Walker C, Peterson C, Cookson P. The "E" word: epilepsy and perceptions of unfair treatment from the 2010 Australian Epilepsy Longitudinal Survey. *Epilepsy Behav* 2013;27:251-6.

26 Bellon M, Walker C, Peterson C. Seizure-related injuries and hospitalizations: self-report data from the 2010 Australian Epilepsy Longitudinal Survey. *Epilepsy Behav* 2013;26:7-10.

27 National Institute for Health and Clinical Excellence. Transient loss of consciousness ('blackouts') management in adults and young people. NICE, 2010.

28 Caviness JN, Brown P. Myoclonus: current concepts and recent advances. *Lancet Neurol* 2004;3:598-607.

29 Angus-Leppan H. Migraine: mimics, borderlands and chameleons. *Pract Neurol* 2013;13:308-18.

30 Cross JH. Pitfalls in the diagnosis and differential diagnosis of epilepsy. *Paediatr Child Health* 2009;19:199-202.

31 Panayiotopoulos C, Chroni E, Daskalopoulos C, Baker A, Rowlinson S, Walsh P. Typical absence seizures in adults: clinical, EEG, video-EEG findings and diagnostic/syndromic considerations. *J Neurol Neurosurg Psychiatry* 1992;55:1002-8.

32 Marini C, King M, Archer J, Newton M, Berkovic S. Idiopathic generalised epilepsy of adult onset: clinical syndromes and genetics. *J Neurol Neurosurg Psychiatry* 2003;74:192-6.

33 Chung SS, Gerber P, Kirlin KA. Ictal eye closure is a reliable indicator for psychogenic nonepileptic seizures. *Neurology* 2006;66:1730-1.

34 Thijs RD, Wagenaar WA, Middelkoop HA, Wieling W, van Dijk JG. Transient loss of consciousness through the eyes of a witness. *Neurology* 2008;71:1713-8.

35 Ganzeboom KS, Mairuhu G, Reitsma JB, Linzer M, Wieling W, Van Dijk N. Lifetime cumulative incidence of syncope in the general population: a study of 549 Dutch subjects aged 35-60 years. *J Cardiovasc Electrophysiol* 2006;17:1172-6.
36 Sheldon R, Rose S, Ritchie D, Connolly SJ, Koshman M-L, Lee MA, et al. Historical criteria that distinguish syncope from seizures. *J Am Coll Cardiol* 2002;40:142-8.
37 Soteriades ES, Evans JC, Larson MG, Chen MH, Chen L, Benjamin EJ, et al. Incidence and prognosis of syncope. *N Engl J Med* 2002;347:878-85.
38 Lempert T, Bauer M, Schmidt D. Syncope: a videometric analysis of 56 episodes of transient cerebral hypoxia. *Ann Neurol* 1994;36:233-7.
39 Lempert T. [Syncope: phenomenology and differentiation from epileptic seizures] [German]. *Nervenarzt* 1997;68:620-4.
40 Reuber M, Jamnadas-Khoda J, Broadhurst M, Grunewald R, Howell S, Koepp M, et al. Psychogenic nonepileptic seizure manifestations reported by patients and witnesses. *Epilepsia* 2011;52:2028-35.
41 Reuber M, Pukrop R, Bauer J, Helmstaedter C, Tessendorf N, Elger CE. Outcome in psychogenic nonepileptic seizures: 1 to 10-year follow-up in 164 patients. *Ann Neurol* 2003;53:305-11.
42 Commission on Epidemiology and Prognosis, International League Against Epilepsy. Guidelines for epidemiologic studies on epilepsy. *Epilepsia* 1993;34:592-6.
43 Haut SR, Shinnar S. Considerations in the treatment of a first unprovoked seizure. *Semin Neurol* 2008;28:289-96.
44 Camfield P, Camfield C. Epilepsy can be diagnosed when the first two seizures occur on the same day. *Epilepsia* 2000;41:1230-3.
45 Kho LK, Lawn ND, Dunne JW, Linto J. First seizure presentation: do multiple seizures within 24 hours predict recurrence? *Neurology* 2006;67:1047-9.
46 Rossetti A, Hurwitz S, Logroscino G, Bromfield E. Prognosis of status epilepticus: role of aetiology, age, and consciousness impairment at presentation. *J Neurol Neurosurg Psychiatry* 2006;77:611-5.
47 Logroscino G, Hesdorffer DC, Cascino GD, Annegers JF, Bagiella E, Hauser WA. Long-term mortality after a first episode of status epilepticus. *Neurology* 2002;58:537-41.
48 Crombie D. A survey of the epilepsies in general practice: a report by the Research Committee of the College of General Practitioners. *Br Med J* 1960;2:416-22.
49 Loiseau J, Loiseau P, Duche B, Guyot M, Dartigues JF, Aublet B. A survey of epileptic disorders in southwest France: seizures in elderly patients. *Ann Neurol* 1990;27:232-7.
50 Beghi E, Carpio A, Forsgren L, Hesdorffer DC, Malmgren K, Sander JW, et al. Recommendation for a definition of acute symptomatic seizure. *Epilepsia* 2010;51:671-5.
51 Lewis HM, Parry JV, Parry RP, Davies HA, Sanderson P, Tyrrell D, et al. Role of viruses in febrile convulsions. *Arch Dis Child* 1979;54:869-76.
52 Panayiotopoulos CP. A clinical guide to epileptic syndromes and their treatment. Bladon Medical Publishing, 2002.
53 Carpio A, Hauser WA. Epilepsy in the developing world. *Curr Neurol Neurosci Rep* 2009;9:319-26.
54 Leone M, Tonini C, Bogliun G, Monaco F, Mutani R, Bottacchi E, et al. Chronic alcohol use and first symptomatic epileptic seizures. *J Neurol Neurosurg Psychiatry* 2002;73:495-9.
55 Szaflarski JP, Rackley AY, Kleindorfer DO, Khoury J, Woo D, Miller R, et al. Incidence of seizures in the acute phase of stroke: a population-based study. *Epilepsia* 2008;49:974-81.
56 Van Breemen MS, Wilms EB, Vecht CJ. Epilepsy in patients with brain tumours: epidemiology, mechanisms, and management. *Lancet Neurol* 2007;6:421-30.
57 Dunn M, Breen D, Davenport R, Gray A. Early management of adults with an uncomplicated first generalised seizure. *Emerg Med J* 2005;22:237-42.
58 Hauser WA, Anderson VE, Loewenson RB, McRoberts SM. Seizure recurrence after a first unprovoked seizure. *N Engl J Med* 1982;307:522-8.
59 Krumholz A, Wiebe S, Gronseth G, Shinnar S, Levisohn P, Ting T, et al. Practice parameter: evaluating an apparent unprovoked first seizure in adults (an evidence-based review): report of the Quality Standards Subcommittee of the American Academy of Neurology and the American Epilepsy Society. *Neurology* 2007;69:1996-2007.
60 Eckart RE, Scoville SL, Campbell CL, Shry EA, Stajduhar KC, Potter RN, et al. Sudden death in young adults: a 25-year review of autopsies in military recruits. *Ann Intern Med* 2004;141:829-34.
61 Angus-Leppan H, Leach JP. A new era in acute neurological consultations. *Eur J Neurol* 2010;17(4):e26-7.
62 Smith SJ. EEG in the diagnosis, classification, and management of patients with epilepsy. *J Neurol Neurosurg Psychiatry* 2005;76(suppl 2):ii2-7.
63 Angus-Leppan H. Seizures and adverse events during routine scalp electroencephalography: a clinical and EEG analysis of 1000 records. *Clin Neurophysiol* 2007;118:22-30.
64 Zivin L Marsan CA. Incidence and prognostic significance of "epileptiform" activity in the EEG of non-epileptic subjects. *Brain* 1968;91:751-78.
65 National Institute for Health and Clinical Excellence. The epilepsies: the diagnosis and management of the epilepsies in adults and children in primary and secondary care. NICE, 2012.
66 Harden CL, Huff JS, Schwartz TH, Dubinsky RM, Zimmerman RD, Weinstein S, et al. Reassessment: neuroimaging in the emergency patient presenting with seizure (an evidence-based review): report of the Therapeutics and Technology Assessment Subcommittee of the American Academy of Neurology. *Neurology* 2007;69:1772-80.
67 Shinnar S, Berg AT, Moshe SL, Petix M, Maytal J, Kang H, et al. Risk of seizure recurrence following a first unprovoked seizure in childhood: a prospective study. *Pediatrics* 1990;85:1076-85.
68 Neligan A, Bell GS, Giavasi C, Johnson AL, Goodridge DM, Shorvon SD, et al. Long-term risk of developing epilepsy after febrile seizures: a prospective cohort study. *Neurology* 2012;78:1166-70.
69 Berg AT, Shinnar S. The risk of seizure recurrence following a first unprovoked seizure: a quantitative review. *Neurology* 1991;41:965-72.
70 Kim LG, Johnson TL, Marson AG, Chadwick DW, for the MRC MESS Study Group. Prediction of risk of seizure recurrence after a single seizure and early epilepsy: further results from the MESS trial. *Lancet Neurol* 2006;5:317-22.
71 Marson A, Jacoby A, Johnson A, Kim L, Gamble C, Chadwick D, et al. Immediate versus deferred antiepileptic drug treatment for early epilepsy and single seizures: a randomised controlled trial. *Lancet* 2005;365:2007-13.
72 Cole C, Pointu A, Wellsted DM, Angus-Leppan H. A pilot study of the epilepsy risk awareness checklist (ERAC) in people with epilepsy and learning disabilities. *Seizure* 2010;19:592-6.
73 Leone MA, Solari A, Beghi E. Treatment of the first tonic-clonic seizure does not affect long-term remission of epilepsy. *Neurology* 2006;67:2227-9.
74 Ng SK, Hauser WA, Brust JC, Susser M. Alcohol consumption and withdrawal in new-onset seizures. *N Engl J Med* 1988;319:666-73.
75 Burns CM, Rutherford MA, Boardman JP, Cowan FM. Patterns of cerebral injury and neurodevelopmental outcomes after symptomatic neonatal hypoglycemia. *Pediatrics* 2008;122:65-74.
76 Velissaris SL, Saling MM, Newton MR, Berkovic SF, Wilson SJ. Psychological trajectories in the year after a newly diagnosed seizure. *Epilepsia* 2012;53:1774-81.
77 Sander JW. Ultimate success in epilepsy—the patient's perspective. *Eur J Neurol* 2005;12(suppl 4):3-11.
78 Taylor J, Chadwick D, Johnson T. Risk of accidents in drivers with epilepsy. *J Neurol Neurosurg Psychiatry* 1996;60:621-7.
79 Driver and Vehicle Licensing Agency. 2014. www.dvla.gov.uk/medical/ataglance.
80 Seneviratne U. Management of the first seizure: an evidence based approach. *Postgrad Med J* 2009;85:667-73.
81 Burt J, Cole C. Swimming guidelines for adults with epilepsy: Jennifer Burt and Christine Cole describe how guidelines designed to ensure the safety of swimmers with epilepsy were researched, consulted on and distributed. *Learning Disability Practice* 2008;11(10):12-6.
82 Almeida Mdo R, Bell GS, Sander JW. Epilepsy and recreational scuba diving: an absolute contraindication or can there be exceptions? A call for discussion. *Epilepsia* 2007;48:851-8.
83 Fenwick PB, Toone BK, Wheeler MJ, Nanjee MN, Grant R, Brown D. Sexual behaviour in a centre for epilepsy. *Acta Neurolog Scand* 1985;71:428-35.
84 Lambert MV. Seizures, hormones and sexuality. *Seizure* 2001;10:319-40.
85 Duncan S, Blacklaw J, Beastall G, Brodie M. Antiepileptic drug therapy and sexual function in men with epilepsy. *Epilepsia* 1999;40:197-204.
86 Morton B, Richardson A, Duncan S. Sudden unexpected death in epilepsy (SUDEP): don't ask, don't tell? *J Neurol Neurosurg Psychiatry* 2006;77:199-202.
87 Hauser WA, Beghi E. First seizure definitions and worldwide incidence and mortality. *Epilepsia* 2008;49(suppl 1):8-12.
88 Sander JW. Comorbidity and premature mortality in epilepsy. *Lancet* 2013;382:1618-9.
89 Ng YS, Davenport R, Duncan S, Derry C. Complications of the SUDEP (sudden unexpected death in epilepsy) discussion. *J Neurol Neurosurg Psychiatry* 2013;84(11):e2-e.
90 Eagle KA, Black HR, Cook EF, Goldman L. Evaluation of prognostic classifications for patients with syncope. *Am J Med* 1985;79:455-60.

Drug treatment of epilepsy in adults

Dieter Schmidt, head, Epilepsy Research Group[1],
Steven C Schachter, chief academic officer, Consortia for Improving Medicine with Innovation and Technology[2]

[1]Epilepsy Research Group, Goethestr. 5, 14163 Berlin, Germany

[2]Departments of Neurology, Beth Israel Deaconess Medical Center, Massachusetts General Hospital and Harvard Medical School, Boston, MA, USA

Correspondence to: D Schmidt dbschmidt@t-online.de

Cite this as: *BMJ* 2014;348:g2546

DOI: 10.1136/bmj.g254

http://www.bmj.com/content/348/bmj.g254

ABSTRACT

Epilepsy is a serious, potentially life shortening brain disorder, the symptoms of which can be successfully treated in most patients with one or more antiepileptic drug. About two in three adults with new onset epilepsy will achieve lasting seizure remission on or off these drugs, although around half will experience mild to moderately severe adverse effects. Patients with epilepsy, especially the 20-30% whose seizures are not fully controlled with available drugs (drug resistant epilepsy), have a significantly increased risk of death, as well as psychiatric and somatic comorbidities, and adverse effects from antiepileptic drugs. Newer drugs have brought more treatment options, and some such as levetiracetam cause fewer drug interactions and less hypersensitivity than older ones. However, they do not reduce the prevalence of drug resistant epilepsy or prevent the development of epilepsy in patients at high risk, such as those with a traumatic brain injury. The development of antiepileptic drugs urgently needs to be revitalized so that we can discover more effective antiseizure drugs for the treatment of drug resistant epilepsy, including catastrophic forms. Antiepileptogenic agents to prevent epilepsy before the first seizure in at risk patients and disease modifying agents to control ongoing severe epilepsy associated with progressive underlying disease are also needed.

Introduction

Epilepsy is a heterogeneous and serious brain disorder with multifactorial origins and manifestations. It comprises many seizure types and epilepsy syndromes,[1] some of which are life shortening.[2] Although 70-80% of patients with new onset epilepsy have complete seizure control with current antiepileptic drugs,[3 4] unmet treatment needs remain. About half of patients report at least one adverse effect during treatment with first line antiepileptic drugs.[5 6] Drug resistant epilepsy occurs in 20-30% of patients newly diagnosed with epilepsy, depending on the definition used.[7] Long term observations have shown that 14% of patients with new onset childhood epilepsy who remain in remission for many years will develop refractory epilepsy while still being treated with antiepileptic drugs.[4] Treatment is empirical and often based on trial and error. Seizures are widely recognized as the clinical hallmark of epilepsy, but epileptogenesis—the disease process by which epilepsy develops after brain insults or as a result of gene mutations—begins before the first seizure and probably continues after the onset of seizures.[8 9] Although current antiepileptic drugs achieve symptomatic seizure relief, which is why they are more appropriately called antiseizure drugs, they do not prevent or reverse the pathological process that underlies human epilepsy or other clinical manifestations of epilepsy, such as the comorbidity of epilepsy. They therefore do not prevent the development of epilepsy, even in patients at high risk (for example, after brain injury or craniotomy),[10] and nor do they exert disease modifying effects that prevent or reverse drug resistant epilepsy. Also, they do not prevent or eliminate the substantial behavioral, cognitive, and somatic comorbidities seen in many patients with epilepsy.[11]

These life limiting currently unmet needs provide a roadmap for the development of more effective antiseizure drugs, as well as for disease modifying and antiepileptogenic drugs.[9 12 13] In this review, we critically assess the current drug treatment of epilepsy in adults and briefly examine prospects for tackling current unmet needs. Drug treatment in children with epilepsy is covered elsewhere.[14] Non-drug based treatments for epilepsy, such as epilepsy surgery, diets, and brain stimulation, are beyond the scope of this review.

SUMMARY POINTS

- Roughly 70-80% of adults with new onset epilepsy will become seizure free with current antiepileptic drugs, although around half will experience adverse effects
- About 20-30% continue to have drug resistant epilepsy with seizures, adverse effects, increased mortality, and substantial psychiatric and somatic comorbidities
- Newer antiepileptic drugs have brought more treatment options and increased ease of use but do not reduce the frequency of drug resistant epilepsy or prevent epilepsy in those at risk
- There is an urgent need to revitalize the development of antiepileptic drugs to discover more effective drugs for the treatment of drug resistant epilepsy
- Antiepileptogenic compounds that prevent epilepsy before the first seizure in at risk patients are needed, as well as disease modifying drugs to control ongoing severe epilepsy and its comorbidities

Epidemiology

Worldwide about 65 million people have epilepsy,[15] making it the most common neurological disorder after stroke and a major burden for public health systems.[16 17] The prevalence of epilepsy varies by population. In developed countries, the annual incidence of epilepsy is nearly 50 per 100 000 population and prevalence is around 700 per 100 000.[18] In low and middle income countries, such estimates are generally higher. For example, in Ethiopia, a developing country, the prevalence of epilepsy is as high as 29.5/1000 (95% confidence interval 20.5/1000 to 40.9).[15 17]

When to start treatment

The Multicentre Study of Early Epilepsy and Single Seizures trial shows that starting antiepileptic drugs after a first seizure reduces the risk of a second seizure compared with no treatment or delayed treatment.[20] Immediate treatment increased the time to second seizure (hazard ratio 1.3, 95% confidence interval 1.1 to 1.6) and first occurrence of a tonic-clonic seizure (1.5, 1.2 to 1.8). It also reduced the time to achieve two year remission of seizures (P=0.023).[20] Table 1 details factors that place patients at high risk for recurrence. It is justifiable to recommend treatment after the first seizure in patients at higher risk of recurrence because such patients have a slightly better long term outcome with early versus delayed treatment (table 2).

Accordingly, the new practical clinical definition of epilepsy proposed by the International League Against Epilepsy (ILAE) includes certain patients after their first seizure. Such patients are those with a probability of further seizures "similar to the general recurrence risk (≥60%) after two unprovoked seizures, occurring over the next 10 years," or, as in the previous definition, those patients who have had two unprovoked seizures more than 24 hours apart.[21] One important consequence of the revised definition of epilepsy is that all clinicians who encounter patients after a first seizure need to be familiar with the varied clinical presentations of seizures, especially those that are non-convulsive, as well as the appropriate investigations to determine the underlying cause.[22]

For patients diagnosed as having epilepsy,[22] treatment with an antiepileptic drug is usually recommended, especially if further seizures might cause serious morbidity or mortality. Underlying this standard recommendation is a 73% risk of seizure recurrence (95% confidence interval 59% to 87%) within four years of two unprovoked seizures.[23] The risk of a third seizure is nearly twice as high in patients whose seizures have a known cause as in those with idiopathic or cryptogenic seizures,[23] as defined by the ILAE.[24] Nevertheless, no randomized controlled trials have been performed in unselected patients who have had two or more seizures, and the size of the treatment effect of antiepileptic drugs is currently unknown.[25] If the diagnosis of epilepsy is uncertain, it may be best not to start antiepileptic drugs but to undertake further evaluations, such as electroencephalography monitoring, or adopt a watch and wait approach.[26]

Table 1 Prognostic index from the Multicentre Study of Early Epilepsy and Single Seizures trial* [20]

Prognostic index	Summary score†
Single seizure before presentation	0
Two or three seizures before presentation	1
Four or more seizures before presentation	2
Add if present:	
Neurologic disorder or deficit	1
Abnormal electroencephalogram	1

**Reproduced, with permission, from Lancet Neurology.*[20]
†Low risk of recurrence=0; medium risk=1; high risk=2-4. Antiepileptic drugs should generally be considered for patients in the medium or high recurrence risk groups.

Selecting the first antiepileptic drug

Ideally, antiepileptic drugs should fully control seizures, be well tolerated with no long term safety problems (such as teratogenicity, hypersensitivity reactions, or organ toxicity), and be easy for clinicians to prescribe and patients to take (once or twice daily, no drug interactions, and no need for serum monitoring).[26] The introduction of more than 15 antiepileptic drugs since the 1980s has provided more choice but has made it more difficult, even for epilepsy specialists, to select the optimum drug for individual patients because each drug has its advantages and limitations (figs 1-4).

Effectiveness in new onset epilepsy

Most patients with newly diagnosed epilepsy have a constant course that can be predicted early on.[31] [32] About 50% of patients with new onset focal or generalized seizures, as internationally defined,[24] become seizure free while taking the first appropriately selected and dosed first line antiepileptic drug (assuming that patients have access to healthcare resources; box 1).[4 7 33 34]

The current evidence base of comparative efficacy among first line antiepileptic drugs is limited to a surprisingly few class I trials (box 2).

Class I evidence for the comparative efficacy and effectiveness of drugs for new onset epilepsy is limited.[19] The SANAD trial, a large randomized unblinded pragmatic study of antiepileptic drug monotherapy in new onset epilepsy, showed similar efficacy of carbamazepine, lamotrigine, and oxcarbazepine, but a lower comparative efficacy of gabapentin and topiramate, for treating focal seizures.[44] Time to 12 month remission was the primary efficacy parameter. Compared with carbamazepine, the hazard ratios (95% confidence interval) were 0.72 (0.58 to 0.89; P<0.05) for gabapentin, 0.81 (0.66 to 1.00; P<0.05) for topiramate, 1.01 (0.83 to 1.22; P>0.05) for lamotrigine, and 0.92 (0.73 to 1.18; P>0.05) for oxcarbazepine. A hazard ratio greater than one indicates that 12 month remission occurs more rapidly on that drug than with carbamazepine.[44]

In another unblinded randomized study, levetiracetam monotherapy was as effective as controlled release carbamazepine for focal seizures or extended release valproic acid/valproate for generalized seizures in patients with new onset epilepsy.[45] The hazard ratio for time to treatment withdrawal was 1.02 (0.74 to 1.41) for levetiracetam versus

Drug*	Presumed main mechanism of action	Approved use (FDA, EMA)	Main uses	Main limitations
Potassium bromide (1857)	GABA potentiation?	Generalized tonic-clonic seizures, myoclonic seizures	Focal and generalized seizures	Currently for adjunctive use only, not in wide use anymore, sedative
Phenobarbital (1912)	GABA potentiation	Partial and generalized convulsive seizures, sedation, anxiety disorders, sleep disorders	Focal and generalized seizures (intravenous); most cost effective treatment for epilepsy, particularly in low resource countries	Enzyme inducer, not useful in absence seizures, skin hypersensitivity. Less effective than carbamazepine or phenytoin for focal seizures in mostly new onset epilepsy
Phenytoin (1938)	Na^+ channel blocker	Partial and generalized convulsive seizures	First line drug (intravenous) for focal and generalized seizures with focal onset; similar efficacy to carbamazepine[47]	Enzyme inducer, non-linear pharmacokinetics. Not useful for absence or myoclonic seizures; skin hypersensitivity
Primidone (1954)	GABA potentiation	Partial and generalized convulsive seizures	Focal and generalized seizures	Enzyme inducer, not useful in absence seizures, sedative, skin hypersensitivity. Less effective than carbamazepine or phenytoin for focal seizures in new onset epilepsy
Ethosuximide (1958)	T-type Ca^{2+} channel blocker	Absence seizures	First line antiepileptic drug, no skin hypersensitivity. Use for absence seizures only. As effective as valproate for new onset absence seizures	Gastrointestinal adverse effects, insomnia, psychotic episodes

*Year in which the drug was first approved or marketed in the US or Europe.
EMA=European Medicines Agency; FDA= US Food and Drug Administration; GABA=γ-aminobutyric acid.

Fig 1 Characteristics of widely used first generation antiepileptic drugs for the treatment of epilepsy[9 27 28 29]

extended release valproic acid and 0.84 (0.66 to 1.07) for levetiracetam versus controlled release carbamazepine.[45]

For treatment of refractory partial epilepsy, taking into account baseline risk, random effects meta-analysis was used to derive pooled estimates of odds ratios and number needed to treat or number needed to harm (NNT/NNH).[46]

Sixty two placebo controlled trials (12 902 patients) and eight head to head randomized controlled trials (1370

Drug*	Presumed main mechanism of action	Approved use (FDA, EMA)	Main uses	Main limitations
Diazepam (1963)	GABA potentiation	Convulsive disorders, status epilepticus, anxiety, alcohol withdrawal	Intravenous use, no clinical hepatotoxicity, no skin hypersensitivity, use for focal and generalized seizures	Currently for adjunctive use and emergency use only, sedative, substantial tolerance (loss of efficacy)
Carbamazepine (1964)	Na^+ channel blockade	Partial and generalized convulsive seizures, trigeminal pain, bipolar disorder	First line drug for focal and generalized seizures with focal onset; none of the newer drugs has currently been shown to be more efficacious than carbamazepine	Enzyme inducer, not useful for absence or myoclonic seizures, skin hypersensitivity
Valproate (1967)	Multiple (for example, GABA potentiation, glutamate (NMDA) inhibition, sodium channel and T-type calcium channel blockade)	Partial and generalized convulsive seizures, absence seizures, migraine prophylaxis, bipolar disorder	First line drug (used intravenously) for focal and generalized seizures; none of the newer drugs has cuurently been shown to be more efficacious than valproate; no skin hypersensitivity	Enzyme inhibitor, substantial teratogenicity, weight gain
Clonazepam (1968)	GABA potentiation	Lennox-Gastaut syndrome, myoclonic seizures, panic disorders	No clinical hepatotoxicity, use for focal and generalized seizures	Currently for adjunctive use only, sedative, substantial tolerance (loss of efficacy)
Clobazam (1975)	GABA potentiation	Lennox-Gastaut syndrome, anxiety disorders	No clinical hepatotoxicity. Use for focal and generalized seizures	Currently for adjunctive use only, sedative, substantial tolerance (loss of efficacy)

*Year in which the drug was first approved or marketed in the US or Europe.
EMA=European Medicines Agency; FDA=US Food and Drug Administration; GABA=γ-aminobutyric acid; NMDA=N-methyl-D-aspartate subtype of glutamate receptors.

Fig 2 Characteristics of widely used second generation antiepileptic drugs for the treatment of epilepsy[9 27 28 29]

Drug*	Presumed main mechanism of action	Approved use (FDA, EMA)	Main uses	Main limitations
Vigabatrin (1989)	GABA potentiation	Infantile spasms, complex partial seizures (currently for adjunctive use only)	No clinical hepatotoxicity. Use for infantile spasms, focal and generalized seizures with focal onset	Not useful for absence or myoclonic seizures. Causes a visual field defect and weight gain. Not as efficacious as carbamazepine for focal seizures
Lamotrigine (1990)	Na^+ channel blocker	Partial and generalized convulsive seizures, Lennox-Gastaut syndrome, bipolar disorder	First line drug for focal and generalized seizures	Enzyme inducer, skin hypersensitivity. Not as effective as valproate for new onset absence seizures
Oxcarbazepine (1990)	Na^+ channel blocker	Partial seizures	First line drug for focal and generalized seizures with focal onset	Enzyme inducer, hyponatremia, skin hypersensitivity. Not useful for absence or myoclonic seizures
Gabapentin (1993)	Ca^{2+} blocker ($\alpha 2\delta$ subunit)	Partial and generalized convulsive seizures, postherpetic and diabetic neuralgia, restless leg syndrome	No clinical hepatotoxicity. Use for focal and generalized seizures with focal onset	Currently for adjunctive use only. Not useful for absence or myoclonic seizures and can cause weight gain. Not as effective as carbamazepine for new onset focal seizures
Topiramate (1995)	Multiple (GABA potentiation, glutamate (AMPA) inhibition, sodium and calcium channel blockade)	Partial and generalized convulsive seizures, Lennox-Gastaut syndrome, migraine prophylaxis	First line drug for focal and generalized seizures. No clinical hepatotoxicity	Cognitive side effects, kidney stones, speech problems, weight loss. Not as effective as carbamazepine for new onset focal seizures
Levetiracetam (2000)	SV2A modulation	Partial and generalized convulsive seizures, partial seizures, GTCS, juvenile myoclonic epilepsy	First line drug (intravenous) for focal and generalized seizures with focal onset and myoclonic seizures. No clinical hepatotoxicity. As efficacious as carbamazepine for new onset focal seizures	Not useful for absence or myoclonic seizures. Psychiatric side effects
Zonisamide (2000)	Na^+ channel blocker	Partial seizures	First line drug for focal and generalized seizures. No clinical hepatotoxicity. Non-inferior to carbamazepine for new onset focal seizures	Cognitive side effects, kidney stones, sedative, weight loss
Stiripentol (2002)	GABA potentiation, Na^+ channel blocker	Dravet syndrome	Use for seizures in Dravet syndrome. No clinical hepatotoxicity	Currently for adjunctive use only
Pregabalin (2004)	Ca^{2+} blocker ($\alpha 2\delta$ subunit)	Partial seizures, neuropathic pain, generalized anxiety disorder, fibromyalgia	Use for focal and generalized seizures with focal onset. No clinical hepatotoxicity	Currently for adjunctive use only, not useful for absence or myoclonic seizures, weight gain
Rufinamide (2004)	Na^+ channel blockade	Lennox-Gastaut syndrome	Use for seizures in Lennox-Gastaut syndrome. No clinical hepatotoxicity	Currently for adjunctive use only
Lacosamide (2008)	Enhanced slow inactivation of voltage gated Na^+ channels	Partial seizures	Use (intravenous) for focal and generalized seizures with focal onset. No clinical hepatotoxicity	Currently for adjunctive use only
Eslicarbazepine acetate (2009)	Na^+ channel blocker	Partial seizures	Use for focal and generalized seizures with focal onset	Currently for adjunctive use only, enzyme inducer, hyponatremia
Perampanel (2012)	Glutamate (AMPA) antagonist	Partial seizures	Use for focal and generalized seizures with focal onset	Currently for adjunctive use only. Not useful for absence or myoclonic seizures

*Year in which the drug was first approved or marketed in the US or Europe.
AMPA=α-amino-3-hydroxy-5-methyl-4-isoxazolepropionic acid subtype of glutamate receptors; EMA=European Medicines Agency; FDA=US Food and Drug Administration; GABA=γ-aminobutyric acid; GTCS=generalized tonic clonic seizures on awakening; SV2A=synaptic vesicle protein.

Fig 3 Characteristics of widely used third generation antiepileptic drugs for the treatment of epilepsy[9 27 28 29]

RESPONSE TO ANTIEPILEPTIC DRUGS

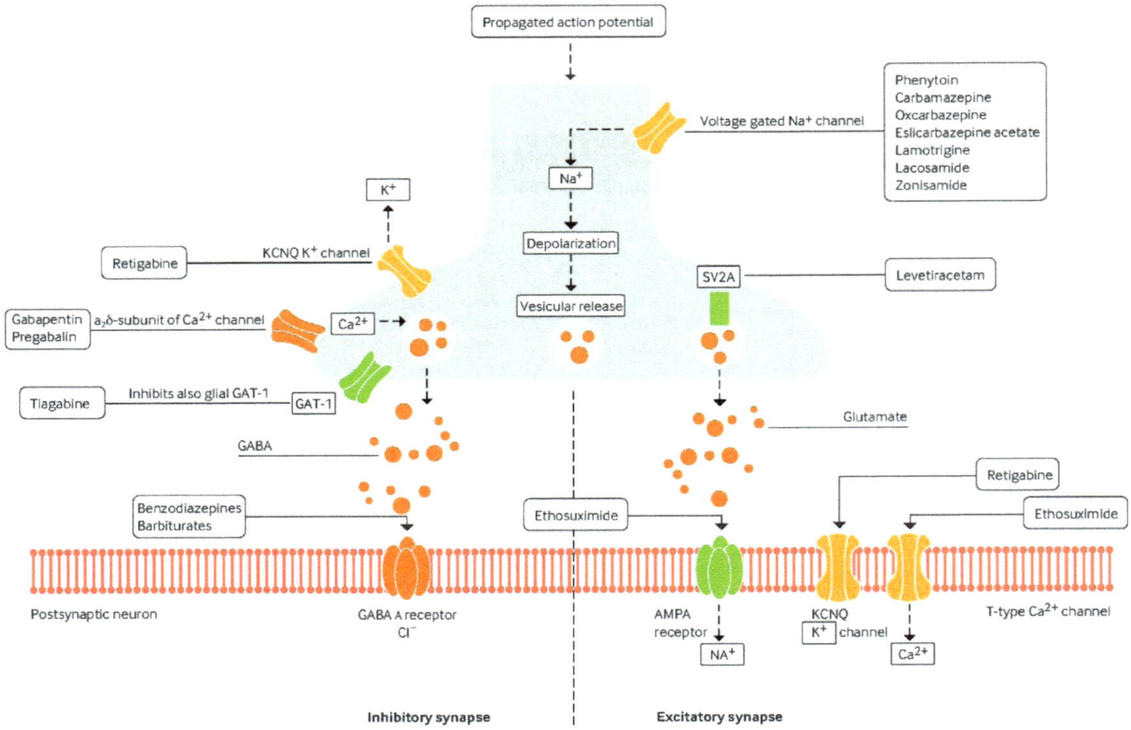

Fig 4 Mechanisms of action of antiepileptic drugs, which act by diverse mechanisms, mainly involving modulation of voltage activated ion channels, potentiation of GABA, and inhibition of glutamate.[27 30] Approved antiepileptic drugs have effects on inhibitory (left hand side) and excitatory (right hand side) nerve terminals. The antiepileptic efficacy in trials of most of these drugs as initial add-on does not differ greatly, indicating that seemingly similar antiseizure activity can be obtained by mechanisms aimed at diverse targets. However, putative mechanisms of action were determined only after discovering the antiseizure effects; mechanism driven drug discovery has been largely ignored.[9] Abbreviations: AMPA, α-amino-3-hydroxy-5-methyl-4-isoxazole propionic acid; GABA, γ-aminobutyric acid; GAT-1, sodium dependent and chloride dependent GABA transporter 1; SV2A, synaptic vesicle glycoprotein 2A. Modified, with permission, from *Nature Reviews Neurology*.[28]

Drug	Suggested titration of daily dose	Suggested range of average target dose (total mg/day; frequency of dosing)	Target plasma concentration (mg/L)
Carbamazepine	200-400 mg every 7 days	600-1200 bid or tid	3-12
Clobazam	10 mg/day	10-60 mg bid or qd	NA
Eslicarbazepine	400 mg every 3-7 days	800-1200 qd	NA
Felbamate	300 mg every 7 days	2400-3600 bid, tid	20-45
Gabapentin	300 mg every 1-3 days	900-3600 bid, tid	NA
Lacosamide	100 mg every 3-7 days	400-600 bid	NA
Lamotrigine	Monotherapy: 25 mg for 2 weeks, 50 mg for the next 2 weeks, then increases of 50-100 mg/week; add-on in the presence of valproate: 25 mg every other day for 2 weeks, 25 mg/day for the next 2 weeks, then increases of 25-50 mg/week; add-on in the presence of enzyme inducing drugs: 50 mg for 2 weeks, 100 mg for the next 2 weeks, then increases of 50-100 mg/week	100-400 qd, bid	2-15
Levetiracetam	500 mg every 1-3 days	1000-3000 bid	NA
Oxcarbazepine	150 mg every 3-7 days	800-1800 bid, tid	7.5-20 (MHD)
Phenobarbital	50 mg every 7 days	50-200 qd, bid	10-40
Phenytoin	50-100 mg every 3-5 days; beyond 200 mg in 25-30 mg steps	200-300 bid, tid, qd for extended release availability	5-25
Perampanel	2 mg every 3-7 days	8-12 qd	NA
Pregabalin	75-150 mg every 3-7 days	150-600 bid, tid	NA
Primidone	62.5-250 mg every 7 days	500-750 bid, tid	10-40 (PHB)
Retigabine	100 mg/day increased by 150 mg/day	900-1200 bid, tid	NA
Tiagabine	6 mg every 5-7 days	36-60 bid, tid	NA
Topiramate	25 mg for 1-2 weeks; beyond 100 mg, 25-50 mg/week	100-400 bid, tid	NA
Vigabatrin	500 mg every 7 days	500-3000 bid	NA
Valproate	500 mg every 3-7 days	600-1500 bid slow release	40-120
Zonisamide	100 mg every 3-7 days	200-600 bid, tid	NA

MHD=monohydroxy metabolite; NA=not applicable; PHB=phenobarbital; qd=once a day; bid=twice a day; tid=three times a day.

Fig 5 Dosages and effective plasma concentrations of antiepileptic drugs for the treatment of epilepsy in adults[26 47]

BOX 1 DISEASE BURDEN AND TREATMENT GAP

The global burden from epilepsy as measured by disability adjusted life years increased by 30% between 1990 and 2010.[35] In 2010, the disease burden from epilepsy was higher than that for Alzheimer's disease and other dementias, multiple sclerosis, and Parkinson's disease combined.[35]

The often substantial comorbidity of epilepsy includes injury and drowning, depression and anxiety associated with high suicide rates, and mortality three times the rate expected in the general population, including sudden unexplained death in epilepsy (SUDEP).[36] Estimates indicate that most people with epilepsy in developing countries live in rural and remote areas and have no easy access to skilled medical care.[37 38] The difference between the number of people with active epilepsy and the number who are being appropriately treated in a given population at a given point in time is known as the treatment gap.[37]

Epilepsy imposes a large economic burden on patients and their families, particularly in rural and remote regions and the developing world.[37] Throughout the world, epilepsy imposes an additional hidden burden associated with stigmatization and discrimination against patients and their families in the community, workplace, school, and home. Social isolation, emotional distress, dependence on family, poor employment opportunities, and personal injury add to the suffering of people with epilepsy.[38] Because of the seriousness of the disorder and its psychosocial dimensions, it is worrying that epilepsy is often suboptimally diagnosed and managed, even in developed countries, and especially among certain socioeconomic groups.[11 39]

How to close the treatment gap

The Global Campaign Against Epilepsy, which is jointly sponsored by the World Health Organization, ILAE, and International Bureau for Epilepsy, advocates using phenobarbital to close the high treatment gap in low income countries.[40] The suggested first step is for all patients with epilepsy to be given phenobarbital, which will control seizures in most of them. In resource poor countries, phenobarbital can cost as little as $5 (£3; €3.7) to $10 a year. Phenobarbital has an extremely low potential for misuse.[41] Its use in developed countries has been limited by a comparative trial that showed that phenobarbital and primidone (which is metabolized to phenobarbital) were less well tolerated than phenytoin or carbamazepine.[42] This finding is less relevant for resource poor countries when the only choice is between phenobarbital or no treatment at all. The side effects of phenobarbital—mainly sedation, possible mild cognitive impairment, and depression—can be minimized by using the lowest possible effective dose.[41] Thus, phenobarbital is the current drug of choice for large scale, community based programs, particularly in rural and remote areas of developing countries.[41] Despite the availability of phenobarbital for more than 90 years and its modest cost, the treatment gap for epilepsy still exceeds 90% in many developing countries.[41]

Table 2 Estimates of seizure recurrence risk from the Multicentre Study of Early Epilepsy and Single Seizures trial*

Treatment	1 year probability of recurrence (%)	3 year probability of recurrence (%)	5 year probability of recurrence (%)
Low risk:			
Early start	26	35	39
Delayed start	19	28	30
Medium risk:			
Early start	24	35	39
Delayed start	35	50	56
High risk:			
Early start	36	46	50
Delayed start	59	67	73

**Modified, with permission, from Lancet Neurology.[20] All results were significantly different.*

patients) were included. Pooled odds ratios for responder and withdrawal rates (versus placebo) were 3.00 (95% confidence interval 2.63 to 3.41) and 1.48 (1.30 to 1.68), respectively. Indirect comparisons of responder rate based on relative measurements of treatment effect favored topiramate (1.52, 1.06 to 2.20) over all other antiepileptic drugs, whereas gabapentin (0.67, 0.46 to 0.97) and lacosamide (0.66, 0.48 to 0.92) were less efficacious, without significant heterogeneity. When analyses were based on absolute estimates (NNTs), topiramate and levetiracetam were more efficacious, with gabapentin and tiagabine being less efficacious. Withdrawal rates were higher with oxcarbazepine (1.60, 1.12 to 2.29) and topiramate (1.68, 1.07 to 2.63), and lower with gabapentin (0.65, 0.42 to 1.00) and levetiracetam (0.62, 0.43 to 0.89). However, differences were too small to make any conclusions about which new drugs had superior effectiveness. The choice of drug for refractory partial epilepsy should therefore be guided more by other aspects, such as patient characteristics and pharmacoeconomics, than only by evidence from randomized trials.[46]

Figure 5 lists dosages and effective plasma concentrations of antiepileptic drugs for the treatment of epilepsy in adults. The incidence of many adverse events can be reduced by slow titration and avoiding high dosages.

Tolerability and safety of drugs in new onset epilepsy

Given the similar efficacy of many first line antiepileptic drugs in new onset epilepsy, comparative tolerability and safety become important considerations when selecting treatment.

Figure 6 provides an overview of the main tolerability and safety considerations for currently available antiepileptic drugs. The evidence base for the comparative tolerability of individual drugs given as monotherapy is limited to short term

BOX 2 PREFERRED FIRST LINE ANTIEPILEPTIC DRUGS FOR NEW ONSET AND REFRACTORY EPILEPSY IN ADULTS[26 43]

All drugs that are regarded as first line for new onset cases are also considered for patients with refractory epilepsy because they differ from one another in their pharmacological profile.

New onset partial epilepsies

- Carbamazepine
- Gabapentin
- Lamotrigine
- Levetiracetam
- Oxcarbazepine
- Topiramate
- Valproate

New onset idiopathic generalized epilepsies

- Lamotrigine
- Topiramate
- Valproate

Refractory partial epilepsy

- Lacosamide
- Pregabalin
- Zonisamide
- Perampanel
- Clobazam

Refractory idiopathic generalized epilepsies

- Clobazam
- Levetiracetam

Adverse effect	CBZ	CLB	ESL	ETS	FBM	GBP	LCM	LEV	LTG	OXC	PGN	PER	PHB	PHT	TGB	RTG	TPM	VPA	VGB	ZNS
EARLY ONSET ADVERSE EVENTS																				
Somnolence	–	High	Medium	Medium	–	Medium	Medium	Medium	Medium	–	Medium	–	High	–	High	Medium	High	–	Medium	High
Dizziness	–	High	–	Medium	–	Medium	Medium	Medium	Medium	High	–	–	–	High	High	–	High	–	Medium	Medium
Seizure aggravation	Medium	Medium	Medium	–	–	Medium	–	–	–	–	Medium	–	–	Medium	Medium	–	–	–	High	
Gastrointestinal	Medium	–	–	High	Medium	Low	–	Low	–	Medium	–	–	–	–	–	–	–	Medium	–	Medium
Hypersensitivity (SJS/TEN)	Medium	–	Medium	Medium	Medium	–	–	–	Medium	Medium	–	–	Medium	Medium	–	–	Medium	–	–	Medium
Rash	Medium	–	–	–	–	–	–	–	Medium	Medium	–	–	–	Medium	–	–	–	–	–	–
LATE ONSET ADVERSE EVENTS																				
Encephalopathy														Medium				Medium	High	
Depression				Medium									Medium	Medium	Medium				Medium	
Behavioral problems								Medium				Medium	High	Medium	Medium		High		High	Medium
Psychotic episodes	Low			High	Low	Medium		Low					Low	Low	Low		Low	Low	High	
Leukopenia	High			Medium	Medium					Low			Medium	Medium						
Aplastic anemia	Medium			Medium	High								Medium	Medium						
Thrombocytopenia					Medium													High		
Megaloblastic anemia	Low												Medium	Medium						
Pancreatitis						Low												Medium		
Liver failure					Medium													Medium		
Nephrolithiasis																	Low			Medium
Osteoporosis	Low												Medium	Medium				Low		
Hyponatremia	Low		Medium							Medium										
Weight gain	Medium					Medium					High							Medium	Medium	
Weight loss					High												Medium			Medium
Cognition impaired	Medium	Medium	Medium										High	Medium			Medium			Medium
Teratogenicity																	Medium	High		
Retinal dysfunction																High		High		

CLB=clobazam; CBZ=carbamazepine; ESL=eslicarbazepine; ETS=ethosuximide; FBM=felbamate; GBP=gabapentin; LEV=levetiracetam; LCM=lacosamide; LTG=lamotrigine; OXC=oxcarbazepine; PER=perampanel; PGB=pregabalin; PHB=phenobarbital; PHT=phenytoin; PRM=primidone; RTG=retigabine; ; TPM=topiramate; VPA=valproate; VGB=vigabatrin; ZNS=zonisamide; SJS/TEN=Stevens-Johnson syndrome or toxic epidermal necrolysis. Key: – no increase, low risk, medium risk, high risk

Fig 6 Overview of adverse effects of individual antiepileptic drugs.[9 26 29]

randomized controlled trials, which typically show a similar proportion of patients with adverse effects when comparing newer drugs such as levetiracetam and zonisamide with carbamazepine.[33 48] In the SANAD trial, about 50% of patients reported at least one adverse effect from carbamazepine or valproic acid/valproate as well as from newer drugs, such as lamotrigine, gabapentin, oxcarbazepine, and topiramate.[5 6] There is thus no compelling evidence that these recently approved drugs are better tolerated than older ones.[5 6 49 50] With regard to safety, valproic acid/valproate seems to be the most teratogenic antiepileptic drug on the market,[51 52] and newer drugs, such as gabapentin and levetiracetam, cause fewer or no dermatological hypersensitivity reactions and do not induce or inhibit hepatic enzyme function.

Pharmacogenomics may be helpful in selecting specific antiepileptic drugs.[53] People of Asian descent who take carbamazepine, lamotrigine, or phenytoin and carry the *HLA-B*15:02* allele have a significantly increased risk of developing Stevens-Johnson syndrome or toxic epidermal necrolysis.[54] In drug specific analysis, the carrier rate of *HLA-B*15:02* was significantly higher in patients with carbamazepine related Stevens-Johnson syndrome or toxic epidermal necrolysis than in carbamazepine tolerant controls (92.3% *v* 11.9%, $P<0.005$; odds ratio 89.2, 19.2 to 413.8). This was also true in patients with phenytoin related Stevens-Johnson syndrome or toxic epidermal necrolysis compared with phenytoin tolerant controls (46.7% *v* 20.0%, $P=0.045$; 3.50, 1.10 to 11.18.[55] Screening is therefore recommended before starting these drugs in patients with Han Chinese and South East Asian ancestry.[56]

With older antiepileptic drugs, drug interactions can greatly lower the efficacy of other drugs, including other antiepileptic drugs when taken in combination; this is not a problem with newer non-enzyme inducing agents, such as gabapentin, lamotrigine, and levetiracetam (fig 7).

The evidence on the potential adverse effects of long term enzyme induction with antiepileptic drugs has been recently reviewed.[60] Clinical problems can occur as a result of pharmacokinetic interactions altering the serum concentration and, possibly, the efficacy or the adverse effects of concurrently taken antiepileptic drugs and other drugs when the inducer is introduced or withdrawn.[60] Enzyme induction will continue for as long as the patient takes the inducer and will affect future drugs that are prescribed. The enzyme inducing effects of antiepileptic drugs therefore have implications for the general health of people with epilepsy.

Whether enzyme inducing antiepileptic drugs should still be used as first line treatment for newly diagnosed epilepsy when many non-inducing, equally effective, alternatives are available is a point for discussion and further research. Several clinical scenarios require patients to be switched to a non-enzyme inducing antiepileptic drug. Examples include patients who need pharmacotherapy for cancer or those

Drug	Clinically relevant interactions when added to other drugs including antiepileptic drugs	Clinically relevant interactions when other drugs are added
Carbamazepine	Lowers plasma concentrations of lamotrigine, tiagabine, and valproate; lowers efficacy of drugs for other disorders*	Plasma concentration increased by a variety of drugs, including erythromycin, propoxyphene, isoniazid, cimetidine, verapamil, diltiazem, and fluoxetine
Clobazam	No relevant change	No relevant change
Eslicarbazepine	Lowers plasma concentrations and lower efficacy of other drugs*	Plasma concentration reduced by enzyme inducers
Ethosuximide	Uncertain	Plasma concentration reduced by enzyme inducers
Felbamate	Increases plasma concentrations of valproate, phenytoin, phenobarbital, carbamazepine epoxide	Plasma concentration reduced by enzyme inducers
Gabapentin	No relevant change	No relevant change
Lacosamide	No relevant change	Plasma concentration reduced by enzyme inducers
Lamotrigine	No relevant change	Plasma concentration increased by valproate and reduced by enzyme inducers
Levetiracetam	No relevant change	No relevant change
Oxcarbazepine	Lowers plasma concentrations of lamotrigine, phenytoin, tiagabine, and valproate; lowers efficacy of drugs for other disorders* at doses of >900 mg oxcarbazepine	Plasma concentration reduced by enzyme inducers
Perampanel	No relevant change	Plasma concentration reduced by enzyme inducers
Phenobarbital	Lower plasma concentrations of lamotrigine, oxcarbazepine, phenytoin, tiagabine, and valproate; lowers efficacy of drugs for other disorders*	Plasma concentration increased by valproate and felbamate
Phenytoin†	Lower plasma concentrations of lamotrigine, tiagabine, and valproate; lowers efficacy of drugs for other disorders*	Valproate competes for protein binding
Pregabalin	No relevant change	No relevant change
Primidone	Lower plasma concentrations of lamotrigine, oxcarbazepine, phenytoin, tiagabine, valproate, and others; lowers efficacy of drugs for other disorders*	Plasma concentration reduced by enzyme inducers
Retigabine	No relevant change	No relevant change
Topiramate	No relevant change	Plasma concentration reduced by enzyme inducers
Valproate	Higher toxicity of phenytoin, phenobarbital, and primidone (which is mainly metabolized to phenobarbital)	Plasma concentration reduced by enzyme inducers
Vigabatrin	No relevant change	No relevant change
Zonisamide	No relevant change	Plasma concentration reduced by enzyme inducers

*Inducers of cytochrome P450 system. †Need to monitor serum concentrations.

Fig 7 Summary of drug interaction properties of common antiepileptic drugs.[56,57,58,59] *Inducers of cytochrome P 450 enzyme system. †Need to monitor serum concentrations

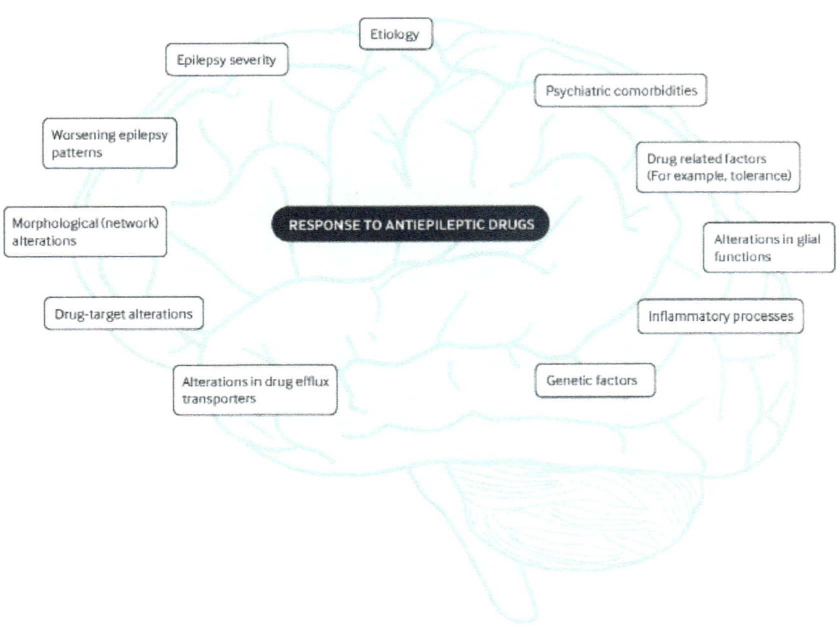

Fig 8 Possible determinants of antiepileptic drug resistance in human and experimental epilepsies.[67] Modified, with permission, from *Nature Reviews*[9]

BOX 3 STOPPING ANTIEPILEPTIC DRUGS IN PATIENTS IN REMISSION

High risk profile for seizure recurrence off antiepileptic drugs[106]

- Being 16 years or older
- Taking more than one antiepileptic drug
- Having seizures after starting drug treatment
- History of generalized tonic-clonic seizures
- History of myoclonic seizures
- Having an abnormal electroencephalogram in previous year

When it may be safe to discontinue[114,115]

- Freedom from seizures for more than two years implies a 60% chance of persistent remission in certain epilepsy syndromes
- Favorable factors:
  - Control easily achieved on a low dose of one drug
  - No previous unsuccessful attempts at withdrawal
  - Normal neurological examination and electroencephalogram
  - Primary generalized epilepsy except juvenile myoclonic epilepsy
  - Benign syndromes

SOURCES AND SELECTION CRITERIA

References for this review were identified through searches of publications listed by PubMed and ScienceDirect from 1 January 1980 to 1 September 2013. We used the search terms "epilepsy", "treatment", "antiepileptic drugs", "efficacy", "effectiveness", "antiepileptogenesis", "antiepileptogenic drugs", "disease modification", "adverse effects", "antiepileptic drugs discovery", "antiepileptic drugs preclinical development", "antiepileptic drugs clinical development", and "humans". References were also identified from relevant review articles and through searches of the authors' files. Only articles published in English were reviewed. We excluded articles published in non-peer reviewed journals. The final reference list was based on relevance to the topics covered in the review. We included publications published between 1983 and 2013, including meta-analyses. Publications of evidence classes I-IV were included because of the limited evidence base on the drug treatment of epilepsy.[19]

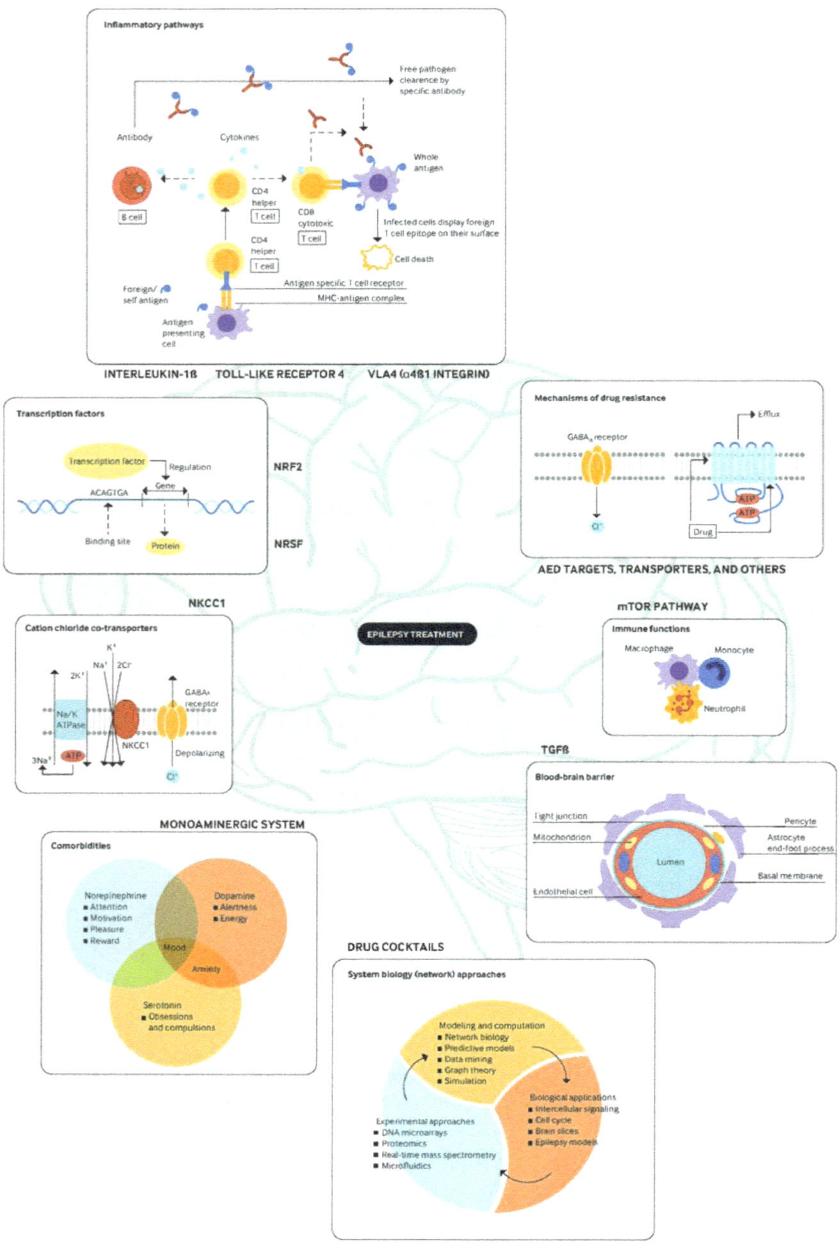

Fig 9 Examples of novel targets that are particularly interesting for development of antiseizure or antiepileptogenic drugs. Modified, with permission, from *Nature Reviews*.[9] GABAA=γ-aminobutyric acid type A; NKCC1=bumetanide sensitive sodium-(potassium)-chloride cotransporter 1; MHC=major histocompatibility complex; NRF2=nuclear factor erythroid 2 related factor 2; NRSF=neurone restrictive silencer factor; TGFβ=transforming growth factor β; VLA4=very late antigen 4 (α4β1 integrin)

with other life threatening diseases treated with drugs that are inducible by concurrent antiepileptic drug treatment.

People with epilepsy who are established on enzyme inducing antiepileptic drugs should be screened regularly for associated long term problems, such as osteoporosis and sexual dysfunction. The patient's other care providers should be advised about the potential for harmful pharmacokinetic interactions. Switching patients to non-enzyme inducing drugs to avoid these interactions should be done with caution, particularly if seizures are not fully controlled. For seizure-free patients, the risks and benefits of switching need to be carefully weighed given the paucity of data on comparative likelihood of seizure control. In all such situations, the benefits and risks of both courses of action should be discussed with patients and their families.[60]

Finally, patients may be using over-the-counter dietary supplements or herbal preparations, some of which may interact with antiepileptic drugs—for example, *Gingko biloba* or St John's wort can interact with hepatically metabolized antiepileptic drugs.[61]

Optimizing drug regimens

Iatrogenic overtreatment is a leading cause of poor tolerability to antiepileptic drugs. This can occur by unnecessarily exceeding the recommended dosage for a particular drug (fig 5) or through pharmacokinetic or pharmacodynamic effects of other, including inappropriately prescribed, drugs.[62] Adverse effects and the patient's perceived risk of adverse effects or safety risks may compromise adherence to the prescribed dose. Poor adherence, in turn, may lower treatment efficacy, with potentially fatal results,[63] and paradoxically cause heightened or prolonged adverse effects by not allowing tolerance of adverse effects to develop.[64]

Target plasma concentrations are available for several antiepileptic drugs (fig 5) but are less useful for optimizing dosages and dosing schedules than for monitoring the patient's clinical course and adherence to therapy.[26] Except for phenytoin, for which monitoring is strongly recommended, particularly at concentrations above 20 mg/L because of the non-linear saturation dose kinetics, monitoring of plasma concentrations of other drugs is needed only to confirm suspected non-adherence or to evaluate unexplained toxicity or uncontrolled seizures in individual cases.[26 65] Even so, although therapeutic drug monitoring may improve the benefit to risk ratio of treatment, there are many practical limitations,[65] including latency in the occurrence of adverse effects or seizures and constraints in when the blood can be sampled, owing to travel time to phlebotomy services. In addition, further work is needed to clarify the role of drug monitoring in improving seizure control during pregnancy and identifying serum drug concentrations that may be considered safe for fetal exposure.[66]

Drug resistant epilepsy

Drug resistant epilepsy is one of the most important unmet needs in the daily management of epilepsy,[11] and it provides a challenge to our understanding of the mechanisms underlying drug resistance and how it can be overcome or avoided (fig 8).

Any patient in whom at least two trials of adequately selected and dosed antiepileptic drugs have not brought sustained remission fulfils the ILAE criteria for drug resistant epilepsy.[68] Many other definitions exist for different purposes.[7 26 69] Epilepsy may also be considered drug resistant if treatment does not stop seizures for 12 months, for whatever reason. By this wide definition, which is based on an influential hospital based observational study,[7] and which is increasingly being used in the US, 36% of newly treated patients have drug resistant seizures.[7] However, if the definition of frequent and severe seizures despite optimal treatment is used, with alternative treatments such as surgery being included, only 5-10% of newly diagnosed patients are estimated to have drug resistant seizures.[70] A diagnosis of absolute drug resistance may require failure of at least six antiepileptic drugs, because about 17% of patients become seizure free when additional antiepileptic drugs are given, even when two to five drugs have previously failed to control seizures.[32 71 72] These data suggest that there is no room for complacency among physicians treating patients who have had persistent seizures over many years despite taking multiple antiepileptic drugs.

The mechanisms underlying drug resistant epilepsy are still not fully understood (fig 9).[8 73 74] Current theories include the transporter hypothesis, the target hypothesis, the network hypothesis, the gene variant hypothesis, and the intrinsic severity hypothesis.[8 75] However, none of these hypotheses can convincingly explain how drug resistance arises in human epilepsy,[67] and a new synthesis or breakthrough in understanding is needed. Interestingly, a history of depression and a high frequency of seizures before treatment onset have been associated with drug resistance.[76 77] These and other observations suggest that common neurobiological factors may underlie disease severity, psychiatric comorbidity, and drug resistant epilepsy, although more work is clearly needed.[67]

Recent progress in our understanding of mechanisms involved in ictogenesis and epileptogenesis now permits a shift towards target based validation studies in animal models of refractory epilepsy or epileptogenesis. Systems biology approaches are a promising source for targets. Such approaches take advantage of newer high throughput technologies to profile large numbers and types of molecules by using functional genomics, transcriptomics, epigenomics, proteomics, and metabolomics, enabling identification of causal pathways from the myriad of competing hypotheses, and thus assisting in defining candidate targets.[78] Molecular profiling of epileptic brain tissues from animal models and humans also holds promise to identify new ictogenic and epileptogenic drug targets, and it might be possible to discover a final common pathway of genes consistently induced at human epileptic foci.[78] This is supported by the recent identification of several promising pathways and potential drug targets, with particularly interesting examples illustrated in fig 10. More extensive discussion of individual targets is available elsewhere.[9]

No class I evidence has shown superior efficacy for any particular antiepileptic drug with market authorization for treating drug resistant epilepsy.[11] In addition, there is no evidence that modern antiepileptic drugs have substantially lowered the proportion of patients with drug resistance.[11] New add-on antiepileptic drugs are only moderately more effective than placebo. In a recent meta-analysis of 54 randomized controlled add-on trials in 11 106 patients with refractory epilepsy, the benefit in efficacy between adding a new antiepileptic drug and adding placebo was only 6% for freedom from seizures and 21% for a 50% reduction in seizure frequency.[79] This suggests that better strategies for finding more effective antiseizure drugs are needed for refractory epilepsy.

Failure of the first drug to induce sustained seizure remission and drug resistant epilepsy

There are two options for patients who continue to have seizures despite taking the first antiepileptic drug: an alternative monotherapy (substitution) or combination therapy (add-on), which usually means adding a second drug to the current monotherapy.[26 80] Randomized trials have not provided evidence of which strategy is best.[81 82] Although substitution is preferable for patients with serious idiosyncratic side effects from the first drug, many physicians prefer add-on treatment with small increments in dose, mainly because it avoids the possibility of breakthrough seizures after discontinuation of the baseline

Drug	Dose
FIRST STAGE: EARLY STATUS EPILEPTICUS	
Diazepam, intravenous bolus (not exceeding 2-5 mg/min)	10-20 mg
Diazepam, rectal administration	10-30 mg
Clonazepam, intravenous bolus (not exceeding 2 mg/min)	1-2 mg at 2 mg/min*
Lorazepam, intravenous bolus	0.007 mg/kg (usually 4 mg)*
Midazolam, buccal or intranasal	5-10 mg* intravenous
SECOND STAGE: ESTABLISHED STATUS EPILEPTICUS	
Fosphenytoin, intravenous bolus (not exceeding 100 mg phenytoin	Loading dose: 15-20 mg phenytoin equivalents/kg, no faster than 100-150 mg phenytoin equivalents/min
Levetiracetam, intravenous bolus	Optimal dose not known, most often used: 2000-4000 mg
Phenytoin, intravenous bolus/infusion (not exceeding 50 mg/min)	15-20 mg/kg at 25 mg/min
Phenobarbital, intravenous bolus (not exceeding 100 mg/min)	10-20 mg/kg
Valproate, intravenous bolus	15-30 mg/kg
THIRD STAGE: REFRACTORY STATUS EPILEPTICUS	
Midazolam	0.1-0.3 mg/kg at 4 mg/min bolus followed by infusion of 0.05-0.4 mg/kg/h
Thiopentone	100-250 mg bolus over 20 s then further 50 mg boluses every 2-3 min until seizures are controlled. Then an infusion of 3-5 mg/kg/h to maintain burst suppression on electroencephalography
Propofol	2 mg/kg bolus followed by an infusion of 5–10 mg/kg/h to maintain burst suppression on electroencephalography

*May be repeated.

Fig 10 Doses and routes of administration of drugs used to treat different stages of tonic-clonic status epilepticus. From the consensus document of the workshop of European epileptologists[106]

drug.[26] In addition, add-treatment has become easier to implement and maintain with modern non-enzyme inducing drugs.[60]

For patients whose clinical course meets the study specific definition of drug resistant epilepsy,[68] relatively short term randomized controlled trials show that the chance of freedom from seizures declines with successive drug regimens, most markedly from the first to the third antiepileptic drug, especially in patients with localization related epilepsies.[32] In one representative observational study from an epilepsy clinic, seizure-free rates decreased from 61.8% for the first antiepileptic drug to 41.7% after one drug proved ineffective.[71] In patients who had no response to the first drug, the proportion who subsequently became seizure free was much smaller (11%) when treatment failed because of lack of efficacy rather than intolerable side effects (41%) or an idiosyncratic reaction (55%).[7] Encouragingly, a longitudinal observational study encompassing almost 40 years of follow-up found that nearly four of five patients whose seizures were not initially controlled after two trials of suitable antiepileptic drugs eventually entered remission for at least one year, and half had at least a five year remission.[83] Idiopathic or cryptogenic causes were the only significant predictor of entering remission in this study.

Treatment of special patient groups

One of the standards of good clinical care is to tailor the treatment of epilepsy on the basis of the patient's individual needs.[26]

Women

People with epilepsy, and particularly women, have a higher risk of bone fracture than the general population.[84] This increased risk is secondary to epilepsy (that is, breaking a bone during a seizure) and use of antiepileptic drugs, especially enzyme inducing ones.[60 85] These drugs independently increased the risk of fracture in the Women's Health Initiative study,[86] as well as in a Danish population based case-control study and a Korean study.[85 87] The Women's Health Initiative determined the associations between the use of antiepileptic drugs and falls, fractures, and bone mineral density over an average of 7.7 years of follow-up in women aged 50-79 years in a longitudinal cohort analysis. After adjustment for covariates, use of antiepileptic drugs was positively associated with total fractures (hazard ratio 1.44, 1.30 to 1.61), all site specific fractures including the hip (1.51, 1.05 to 2.17), clinical vertebral fractures (1.60, 1.20 to 2.12), lower arm or wrist fractures (1.40, 1.11 to 1.76), other clinical fractures (1.46, 1.29 to 1.65), and two or more falls (1.62, 1.50 to 1.74), and was not associated with baseline bone mineral density or changes in bone mineral density ($P \geq 0.064$ for all sites). Use of more than one antiepileptic drug and use of enzyme inducing antiepileptic drugs were significantly associated with total fractures (1.55, 1.15 to 2.09 and 1.36, 1.09 to 1.69, respectively). The Women's Health Initiative concluded that in clinical practice, postmenopausal women who use antiepileptic drugs should be considered at increased risk for fracture and attention to fall prevention may be particularly important in these women. Antiepileptic drugs, especially enzyme inducing ones, have been shown to decrease bone mineral density and alter bone metabolism. Induction of cytochrome P can accelerate the metabolism of vitamin D to polar inactive metabolites.[60] The use of risedronate plus calcium and vitamin D has been shown to prevent the occurrence of new fractures in male patients with a high risk of fractures.[88] Further studies are needed to clarify the mechanisms by which enzyme inducing antiepileptic drugs have these effects on bone and whether newer non-enzyme inducing drugs have advantages over enzyme inducing ones.

Pregnant women and neonates

Although two of three women with epilepsy who become pregnant remain seizure free throughout pregnancy, antiepileptic drug dosages may need to be adjusted, particularly when seizures occur in the first trimester. Women prescribed lamotrigine and possibly levetiracetam, topiramate, and oxcarbazepine may also need dose adjustment to compensate for the increased clearance of these drugs during pregnancy and to reduce the risk of breakthrough seizures.[89 90 91]

Offspring of women with epilepsy who took an antiepileptic drug during pregnancy seem to have an increased risk of being small for gestational age and having a one minute Apgar score of less than 7.[91] Many antiepileptic drugs are associated with major congenital malformations, and prescribers should routinely consult an updated package insert or patient information leaflet for the latest recommendations of regulatory agencies. For example, the use of valproic acid monotherapy in the first trimester is associated with significantly increased risks for six of the 14 malformations under consideration. The adjusted odds ratios were as follows: spina bifida, 12.7 (7.7 to 20.7); atrial septal defect, 2.5 (1.4 to 4.4); cleft palate, 5.2 (2.8 to 9.9); hypospadias, 4.8 (2.9 to 8.1); polydactyly, 2.2 (1.0 to 4.5); and craniosynostosis, 6.8 (1.8 to 18.8).[92 93]

A recent guideline for treatment of women with epilepsy also suggested that intrauterine exposure to valproate monotherapy reduces cognitive outcomes for offspring, as has also been suggested for phenytoin and phenobarbital.[94] If clinically possible, antiepileptic drugs known to be associated with congenital malformations, including valproate, as well as combinations of antiepileptic drugs, should be avoided during pregnancy, especially during the first trimester. Similarly, valproate, phenytoin, phenobarbital, and antiepileptic drug polytherapy should be avoided throughout pregnancy if clinically possible to prevent unfavorable cognitive outcomes in offspring.[94]

The risk of major congenital malformations seems to be influenced not only by the specific antiepileptic drug but also by dose and other variables.[95 96] The lowest malformation rate was seen in the International Registry of Antiepileptic Drugs and Pregnancy (EURAP) with less than 300 mg per day of lamotrigine and less than 400 mg per day of carbamazepine compared with valproic acid and phenobarbital at all studied doses, and with carbamazepine at doses greater than 400 mg per day.[95] Folate supplementation ($\geq$0.4 mg folic acid/day) is recommended during pregnancy because this lowers the risk of cognitive teratogenicity in babies born to women with epilepsy.[96] Primidone and levetiracetam pass into breast milk in amounts that may be clinically important, unlike valproate, phenobarbital, phenytoin, and carbamazepine.[96]

Older people

The change in pharmacokinetics and higher sensitivity to adverse events of many antiepileptic drugs associated with aging usually require more cautious selection of drugs and dosing in older people. Lower glomerular filtration rates should prompt reduced doses of renally excreted drugs. Changes in body fat, albumin, and cytochrome P450 also occur, and oxcarbazepine related hyponatremia may be more common.[26 97] In addition, concomitant diseases, such as hypertension, are common in this age group and often require medication, increasing the possibility of drug interactions with antiepileptic drugs. Therefore, monotherapy with a well tolerated antiepileptic drug that is not associated with drug interactions, such as gabapentin and lamotrigine,[98] low dose topiramate,[99] and levetiracetam (no class I evidence available), is preferable. Providers should be aware that adherence to antiepileptic drug regimens may be more difficult in older people with cognitive decline.

Patients with comorbidities

Many disorders are more common in people with epilepsy than in the general population, including cardiac, gastrointestinal, and respiratory disorders; stroke; dementia; and migraine.[100] Alzheimer's disease and migraine are not only more common in patients with epilepsy but are also risk factors for the development of seizures, suggesting a bidirectional association and shared disease mechanisms.[100]

The lifetime community based prevalence of depression, suicidal ideation, and generalized anxiety disorder is twice as high in patients with epilepsy than in the general population.[101] Depression and anxiety substantially affect quality of life and are associated with an increased suicide rate.[102] The psychiatric comorbidities of epilepsy may also manifest as psychogenic non-epileptic seizures or panic attacks.[103] Psychiatric comorbidities are associated with a worse response to the treatment of the epilepsy, whether by drugs or surgery. Comorbid mood and anxiety disorders have also been associated with more adverse effects when taking antiepileptic drugs.[77]

Before starting antidepressants in patients with epilepsy, it is important to look for possible iatrogenic causes of depression. Antiepileptic drugs such as phenobarbital, vigabatrin, topiramate, tiagabine, levetiracetam, and clobazam can induce depressive symptoms in patients with epilepsy. Several second generation (carbamazepine and valproate) and third generation (lamotrigine and pregabalin) drugs are associated with mood stabilizing properties, so discontinuation of one of these could precipitate depression.[77 103] Patients with both epileptic seizures and psychogenic non-epileptic seizures may benefit from reducing high doses of antiepileptic drugs or the number of drugs given, if possible.[103]

Treatments for psychiatric disorders in patients with epilepsy are severely lacking. Current clinical experience suggests that carbamazepine, valproate, and lamotrigine cannot counteract established depression in patients with epilepsy. Although pregabalin is approved for both epilepsy and generalized anxiety disorder, it is has not been comprehensively studied as treatment for patients with epilepsy and comorbid psychiatric disorders.

The ability of antidepressants to counteract depression in patients with epilepsy has not been properly studied.[77 103] Only two double blind controlled trials have been reported. One small study showed that high dose amitriptyline was superior to placebo against major depressive episodes.[104] Reassuringly, the other trial found that sertraline did not increase seizure frequency or severity.[105] Selective serotonin reuptake inhibitors (SSRIs) and selective noradrenaline reuptake inhibitors (SNRIs) have been assessed in patients with intractable epilepsy in open label trials, and fewer seizures were seen during treatment with the SSRIs fluoxetine or citalopram.[103] The only exception among antidepressant drugs was bupropion, which caused more seizures in patients with epilepsy.[103] Taken together, these studies suggest that SSRIs and SNRIs may reduce seizures and depressive symptoms in patients with epilepsy and depression, although further controlled trials are needed. Work is also needed to evaluate anecdotal observations that SSRIs and SNRIs increase the number of seizures in patients with slow hepatic metabolism or when taken in overdose.[103] Until then, SSRIs with minor pharmacokinetic interactions, such as escitalopram and citalopram, should be considered as first line drugs, followed by sertraline. Fluoxetine and paroxetine interfere with cytochrome P450, so their use may require antiepileptic drug dosages to be adjusted.[10]

AREAS FOR FUTURE RESEARCH

To identify:

- Molecular targets that may lead to the discovery of novel drugs to treat drug resistant epilepsy
- The cellular mechanisms that trigger epileptogenesis after brain insults
- The cellular mechanisms that lead to seizure remission without relapse on or off antiepileptic drugs (cure)
- Molecular targets that may lead to the discovery of novel drugs to prevent epilepsy before the first seizure
- Molecular targets that may lead to the discovery of novel drugs to prevent psychiatric and cognitive comorbidity

ADDITIONAL EDUCATIONAL RESOURCES—GUIDELINES

- American Academy of Neurology and American Epilepsy Society. Efficacy and tolerability of the new antiepileptic drugs I: treatment of new onset epilepsy. 2004. www.neurology.org/content/62/8/1252.full.pdf+html
- American Academy of Neurology and American Epilepsy Society. Efficacy and tolerability of the new antiepileptic drugs II: treatment of refractory epilepsy. 2004. www.neurology.org/content/62/8/1261.full.pdf
- American Academy of Neurology and American Epilepsy Society. Management issues for women with epilepsy—focus on pregnancy: teratogenesis and perinatal outcomes. 2009. www.neurology.org/content/73/2/133.full.pdf
- American Academy of Neurology and American Epilepsy Society. Management issues for women with epilepsy—focus on pregnancy: obstetrical complications and change in seizure frequency. 2009. www.neurology.org/content/73/2/126.full.pdf
- National Institute for Health and Care Excellence. The epilepsies: the diagnosis and management of the epilepsies in adults and children in primary and secondary care. 2012. http://guidance.nice.org.uk/CG137
- Guidelines for Management of Epilepsy in India (GEMIND). www.epilepsyindia.org/ies/GUIDELINES/Gemind_Combine.pdf
- Glauser T, Ben-Menachem E, Bourgeois B, Cnaan A, Guerreiro C, Kälviäinen R, et al; ILAE Subcommission on AED Guidelines. Updated ILAE evidence review of antiepileptic drug efficacy and effectiveness as initial monotherapy for epileptic seizures and syndromes. *Epilepsia* 2013;54:551-63

Patients with status epilepticus and prolonged acute convulsive seizures

Tonic-clonic status epilepticus is associated with serious morbidity and mortality, and treatment depends on seizure stage (fig 10).[106] Unfortunately, this is a therapeutic area in which there are few randomized trials, and their absence has impeded definitive assessment of alternative therapeutic options, particularly in treatment of stage 2 and stage 3 seizures. The regulatory agencies have not licensed drugs for status epilepticus because of the lack of randomized studies.[106]

In the first stage (early status epilepticus), buccal midazolam has become an important out-of-hospital treatment option. A randomized controlled trial showed that buccal midazolam achieved seizure cessation in 8 min compared with 15 min for rectal diazepam ($P<0.01$). The rate of respiratory depression did not differ between groups.[107] In UK community practice, rectal diazepam and unlicensed buccal midazolam are the two treatment options used for acute epileptic seizures. In practice, outside the US rectal diazepam is rarely used, with unlicensed buccal midazolam being widely recommended and prescribed by physicians. More recently a licensed preparation of buccal midazolam has become available.[108] In a double blind study of children and adults with convulsions that had lasted for more than five minutes, and who were still seizing when paramedics arrived, midazolam given by intramuscular autoinjector had equal efficacy to intravenous lorazepam, with comparable safety. The primary efficacy outcome in this study was absence of seizures on arrival at the emergency department, without emergency medical system rescue therapy.[109] Patients treated with intramuscular midazolam were more likely to have stopped seizing on arrival at the emergency department and were less likely to be admitted to the hospital or an intensive care unit.[109]

In the second stage (established status epilepticus), preferred treatment choices include intravenous valproate, levetiracetam, and lacosamide among the newer antiepileptic drugs, as well as the older agents fosphenytoin, phenytoin, and phenobarbital (fig 8). In the third stage (refractory status epilepticus), midazolam, thiopentone, and propofol are available choices (fig 10). Further treatments such as various anesthetics and non-pharmacological treatments may be considered as well, including immunotherapy for cryptogenic refractory status epilepticus.[110] None of the drugs for the second or third stage has been studied in sufficiently powered randomized controlled trials, and multicenter randomized controlled comparative trials are needed.[111] Treatment in individual cases should include consideration of any underlying causes of status epilepticus.[111]

Stopping antiepileptic drugs

Patients who become seizure free and remain so for a prolonged time often wish to discontinue treatment. The decision to discontinue antiepileptic drugs should be based on the patient's risks of seizure recurrence after discontinuation, which overall is twice as high in the two years after discontinuing drugs compared with continuing to take them (box 3). Other studies suggest that the risk of seizure recurrence when patients stop taking antiepileptic drugs is as high as 34% (27% to 43%), with a wide range of 12-66%.[112] Adults seem to have a higher risk of recurrence than children (39% *v* 31%).[113] The revised ILAE definition of epilepsy states that "epilepsy is considered to be resolved for individuals who either had an age dependent epilepsy syndrome but are now past the applicable age or those who have remained seizure free for the last 10 years and off anti-seizure medicines for at least the last five years."[21]

Considerations for counseling patients include driving, pregnancy, work, and family. Other considerations are that a recurrent seizure may be embarrassing and stigmatizing for the patient. It could also result in loss of a driver's license or, rarely, accidental or seizure related death. Furthermore, restarting antiepileptic drugs after seizure recurrence does not guarantee immediate and sustained resumption of seizure control.[116] However, the impact of ongoing drug related side effects and drug interactions may argue in favor of discontinuing treatment. It may be advisable to offer discontinuation using a slow taper schedule in suitable patients after a thorough and documented discussion of the pros and cons.

This recommendation also applies to stopping antiepileptic drugs for patients in seizure remission after epilepsy surgery.[117 118] Epilepsy surgery improves the prognosis of surgical candidates, with rates of freedom from seizures of 50-80%, depending on the cause of epilepsy, type and site of surgery, age group, and duration of follow-up.[118] Unfortunately, in many series, outcomes are given without reference to whether patients are seizure free on or off antiepileptic drugs, the latter often being referred to as an indicator of cure.[119] It has long been recommended that antiepileptic drugs are continued for at least one or two years after surgery, largely on the basis of antiepileptic drug withdrawal policies in non-surgical cohorts. Furthermore, it was suggested that after successful epilepsy surgery, duotherapy is preferable to monotherapy to maintain seizure control.[120] This raises the question of whether it is justifiable to discontinue antiepileptic drugs after surgical remission in all patients.

After temporal lobe surgery, the average proportion of adults who were cured (at least five years seizure free and off drugs) was only 25%.[119] A systematic review found that cure was more common in children (27%) than in adults (19%).[121] This was confirmed in a recent Swedish study—twice as many children were seizure free and had stopped antiepileptic drugs than adults 10 years after surgery.[122]

Why are postoperative cure rates so much lower than the overall surgical seizure freedom rates reported in the literature? Firstly, the follow-up periods of observation may have been too short. It takes time to achieve complete discontinuation of antiepileptic drugs and at least an additional five years of remission off these drugs to establish cure.[117] Most published studies had shorter postoperative follow-up intervals. Secondly, postoperative seizure freedom rates are not stable but decline over time,[123] and the extent of this decline probably depends on underlying disease.[124] Median long term (>5 years) seizure freedom rates ranged from only 27% to 66%,[121 122] closer to the reported cure rates of 19-45% in a recent review.[117]

How can seizures relapse after antiepileptic drug withdrawal in patients who have had complete resection of the presumed cause of epilepsy? One possible explanation is that most epilepsies do not develop from alterations in a single localized target; rather, they arise from complex alterations that result in a wide epileptic network in the brains of individual patients.[125] Variability of network properties and the extent of these networks may explain why even complete resection does not guarantee cure, because only part of the potentially epileptogenic network may have been removed.[126] The development of antiepileptogenic drugs in the future may improve cure rates for medical treatment, and the discovery of biomarkers to assess the extent of the epileptogenic network in an individual patient may offer a chance to improve surgical cure rates.

There is no proof that antiepileptic drug withdrawal itself negatively affects long term seizure outcomes in patients who have become seizure free under drug treatment or after epilepsy surgery. Discontinuation of drugs merely unveils the natural course of the epileptic disorder in medically treated patients and unmasks true postoperative outcome. Given the available evidence, the risk of relapse is probably determined more by the clinical characteristics of the epilepsy syndrome or failure of the surgical procedure to eliminate relevant epileptogenic brain networks than by antiepileptic drug withdrawal and its timing.

Emerging treatments

Novel approaches to the development of new drugs are emerging.[9] These offer hope of finding more effective antiseizure drugs to treat ongoing drug resistant epilepsy, antiepileptogenic agents to prevent symptomatic or genetic epilepsy before the first seizure, and disease modifying agents to mitigate established epilepsy. Our understanding of the mechanisms mediating the development of epilepsy, the causes of drug resistance, and the emerging role of pharmacogenetics for drug discovery have grown substantially over the past decade.[9,127] Finally, new strategies are being explored, such as joint endeavors between academia and industry, identification and application of tools for new target driven and systems biology based approaches, and comparative preclinical proof-of-concept studies and innovative clinical trials designs.[9]

Barriers to the development of new drugs for drug resistant epilepsy

Reliance on established animal models that were used to bring previous antiepileptic drugs to the market as the preferred method to test experimental compounds as well as clinically inadequate trial designs in humans are roadblocks in the development of more effective antiepileptic drugs for drug resistant epilepsy.[11] Novel preclinical and clinical approaches for the discovery and development of drugs with more effective antiseizure activity have recently been suggested.[9,28,128] Potential targets for future drug discovery and development have been proposed (fig 10).

The currently accepted minimum measure for efficacy in randomized controlled trials is a statistical difference between the placebo arm and the treatment arm in the proportion of patients showing at least a 50% reduction in seizure frequency versus the baseline period.[11,129,130,131] This bar is disappointingly low from a clinical perspective because 50% seizure reduction has not been shown to be beneficial for overall health or quality of life of patients,[132] and nor does it satisfy the requirements for a driver's license.[133] This policy has led to the approval of several new antiepileptic drugs without demonstrated superiority over older ones, and which have entered the market at higher prices. A concern with placebo controlled trials is the increasingly unpredictable and unexpectedly high placebo response rates, which have been held responsible, at least in part, for the failure of new antiepileptic drugs to show efficacy in placebo controlled add-on trials.[128,134] Another concern is that placebo use seems to be associated with an increased rate of sudden unexplained death in clinical trials.[125]

Clinical features such as a history of epilepsy surgery or lifetime exposure to seven or more antiepileptic drugs are associated with a low placebo response,[135,136] which may maximize the treatment effect of the experimental antiepileptic drug versus placebo. However, limiting clinical trials to patients with these clinical features may restrict the generalizability of the findings. If variations of placebo mechanisms are left uncontrolled, it will be more difficult to document any specific effects of a drug. Novel clinical trial designs for the development of antiepileptic drugs that de-emphasize the use of placebo controls have recently been proposed.[9,131] A further concern is that current trial designs do not take into account the heterogeneity of the causes and severity of disease in trial participants with drug resistant epilepsy. Although clinical features such as lifetime exposure to an increasing number of antiepileptic drugs seem to be associated with a decreased likelihood of eventual remission in patients with new onset epilepsy,[7,32,71,83] current trial designs do not stratify patients on the basis of the severity of disease as measured by the total number of antiepileptic drugs they have taken, for example. This needs more attention and, if confirmed, may render a comparison of efficacy results between trials with individual antiepileptic drugs more difficult.

Conclusions

Most patients will achieve lasting remission of seizures on generally well tolerated antiseizure drug treatment, and the availability of many new antiepileptic drugs over the past three decades has brought more treatment options. Yet about 20-30% of patients continue to experience seizures despite all available drug options, and even more are at high risk of neuropsychiatric comorbidities.

New drugs with fewer side effects and better efficacy than the currently available ones are urgently needed. Antiepileptogenic and disease modifying agents are also needed. Because many large drug companies have stopped innovating in this therapeutic area, it is becoming increasingly important for foundations and government agencies to fund the discovery of new antiepileptic drugs, and to do so at a level commensurate with the substantial prevalence and costs of drug resistant epilepsy.

Contributors: DS wrote an early version of most sections of the manuscript and revised the manuscript. SCS edited early and revised versions of the manuscript, contributed as author to sections of the manuscript, and is guarantor.

Competing interests: We have read and understood the BMJ Group policy on declaration of interests and declare the following interests: DS has received hospitality and consulting fees in the past two years from Eisai, Sun, UCB, and Viropharma. None of the companies has had any input to the manuscript. SCS: none declared.

Provenance and peer review: Commissioned; externally peer reviewed.

1 Tejada J, Costa KM, Bertti P, Garcia-Cairasco N. The epilepsies: complex challenges needing complex solutions. *Epilepsy Behav* 2013;26:212-28.
2 Berg AT, Berkovic SF, Brodie MJ, Buchhalter J, Cross JH, van Emde Boas W, et al. Revised terminology and concepts for organization of seizures and epilepsies: report of the ILAE Commission on Classification and Terminology, 2005-2009. *Epilepsia* 2010;51:676-85.
3 Cockerell OC, Johnson AL, Sander JW, Shorvon SD. Prognosis of epilepsy: a review and further analysis of the first nine years of the British National General Practice Study of Epilepsy, a prospective population-based study. *Epilepsia* 1997;38:31-46.
4 Sillanpää M, Schmidt D. Natural history of treated childhood-onset epilepsy: prospective, long-term population-based study. *Brain* 2006;129:617-24.
5 Marson AG, Al-Kharusi AM, Alwaidh M, Appleton R, Baker GA, Chadwick DW, et al. The SANAD study of effectiveness of valproate, lamotrigine, or topiramate for generalised and unclassifiable epilepsy: an unblinded randomised controlled trial. *Lancet* 2007;369:1016-26.

6 Marson AG, Al-Kharusi AM, Alwaidh M, Appleton R, Baker GA, Chadwick DW, et al. The SANAD study of effectiveness of carbamazepine, gabapentin, lamotrigine, oxcarbazepine, or topiramate for treatment of partial epilepsy: an unblinded randomised controlled trial. *Lancet* 2007;369:1000-15.
7 Kwan P, Brodie MJ. Early identification of refractory epilepsy. *N Engl J Med* 2000;342:314-9.
8 Löscher W, Brandt C. Prevention or modification of epileptogenesis after brain insults: experimental approaches and translational research. *Pharmacol Rev* 2010;62:668-700.
9 Löscher W, Klitgaard H, Twyman RE, Schmidt D. New avenues for anti-epileptic drug discovery and development. *Nat Rev Drug Discov* 2013;12:757-76.
10 Temkin NR. Preventing and treating posttraumatic seizures: the human experience. *Epilepsia* 2009;50(suppl 2):10-3.
11 Löscher W, Schmidt D. Modern antiepileptic drug development has failed to deliver: ways out of the current dilemma. *Epilepsia* 2011;52:657-78.
12 French JA, White HS, Klitgaard H, Holmes GL, Privitera MD, Cole AJ, et al. Development of new treatment approaches for epilepsy: Unmet needs and opportunities. *Epilepsia* 2013;54(suppl 4):3-12.
13 Pitkänen A, Nehlig A, Brooks-Kayal AR, Dudek FE, Friedman D, Galanopoulou AS, et al. Issues related to development of antiepileptogenic therapies. *Epilepsia* 2013;54(suppl 4):35-43.
14 Hirtz D, Berg A, Bettis D, Camfield C, Camfield P, Crumrine P, et al. Practice parameter: treatment of the child with a first unprovoked seizure: report of the quality standards subcommittee of the American Academy of Neurology and the Practice Committee of the Child Neurology Society. *Neurology* 2003;60:166-75.
15 Ngugi AK, Bottomley C, Kleinschmidt I, Sander JW, Newton CR. Estimation of the burden of active and life-time epilepsy: a meta-analytic approach. *Epilepsia* 2010;51:883-90.
16 Schachter SC. Seizure disorders. In: Heggenhougen K, ed. International encyclopedia of public health, first edition. Elsevier, 2008;5:674-80.
17 Thurman DJ, Beghi E, Begley CE, Berg AT, Buchhalter JR, Ding D, et al. Standards for epidemiologic studies and surveillance of epilepsy. *Epilepsia* 2011;52(suppl 7):2-26.
18 Hirtz D, Thurman DJ, Gwinn-Hardy K, Mohamed M, Chaudhuri AR, Zalutsky R. How common are the "common" neurologic disorders? *Neurology* 2007;68:326-37.
19 Glauser T, Ben-Menachem E, Bourgeois B, Cnaan A, Guerreiro C, Kälviäinen R, et al. Updated ILAE evidence review of antiepileptic drug efficacy and effectiveness as initial monotherapy for epileptic seizures and syndromes. *Epilepsia* 2013;54:551-63.
20 Kim LG, Johnson TL, Marson AG, Chadwick DW; MRC MESS Study group. Prediction of risk of seizure recurrence after a single seizure and early epilepsy: further results from the mess trial. *Lancet Neurol* 2006;5:317-22.
21 Fisher RS, Acevedo C, Arzimanoglou A, Bogacz A, Cross JH, Elger C, et al. An operational clinical definition of epilepsy. *Epilepsia* www.ilae.org/Visitors/Centre/Documents/DefinitionofEpilepsy.pdf.
22 Schachter SC. An important step forward: commentary on "A practical clinical definition of epilepsy". *Epilepsia* [forthcoming].
23 Hauser WA, Rich SS, Lee JR, Annegers JF, Anderson VE. Risk of recurrent seizures after two unprovoked seizures. *N Engl J Med* 1998;338:429-34.
24 Commission on Classification and Terminology of the International League Against Epilepsy. Proposal for revised clinical and electroencephalographic classification of epileptic seizures. *Epilepsia* 1981;22:489-501.
25 Marson AG. When to start antiepileptic drug treatment and with what evidence? *Epilepsia* 2008;49(suppl 9):3-6.
26 Schmidt D. Drug treatment of epilepsy: options and limitations. *Epilepsy Behav* 2009;15:56-65.
27 Rogawski MA, Löscher W. The neurobiology of antiepileptic drugs. *Nat Rev Neurosci* 2004;5:553-64.
28 Bialer M, White HS. Key factors in the discovery and development of new antiepileptic drugs. *Nat Rev Drug Disc* 2010;9:68-82.
29 Abou-Khalil B, Schmidt D. Antiepileptic drugs: advantages and disadvantages. In: Stefan H, Theodore WH, eds. Handbook of clinical neurology. Vol 108. Epilepsy part II: treatment. Elsevier 2012:723-39.
30 Löscher W, Schmidt D. Epilepsy: perampanel—new promise for refractory epilepsy? *Nat Rev Neurol* 2012;8:661-2.
31 Sillanpää M, Schmidt D. Early seizure frequency and aetiology predict long-term medical outcome in childhood-onset epilepsy. *Brain* 2009;132:989-98.
32 Brodie MJ, Barry SJ, Bamagous GA, Norrie JD, Kwan P. Patterns of treatment response in newly diagnosed epilepsy. *Neurology* 2012;78:1548-54.
33 Brodie MJ, Perucca E, Ryvlin P, Ben-Menachem E, Meencke HJ; Levetiracetam Monotherapy Study Group. Comparison of levetiracetam and controlled-release carbamazepine in newly diagnosed epilepsy. *Neurology* 2007;68:402-8.
34 Privitera MD, Brodie MJ, Mattson RH, Chadwick DW, Neto W, Wang S, et al. Topiramate, carbamazepine and valproate monotherapy: double-blind comparison in newly diagnosed epilepsy. *Acta Neurol Scand* 2003;107:165-75.
35 Murray CJ, Vos T, Lozano R, Naghavi M, Flaxman AD, Michaud C, et al. Disability-adjusted life years (DALYs) for 291 diseases and injuries in 21 regions, 1990-2010: a systematic analysis for the Global Burden of Disease Study 2010. *Lancet* 2012;380:2197-223.
36 Sillanpää M, Shinnar S. Long-term mortality in childhood-onset epilepsy. *N Engl J Med* 2010;363:2522-9.
37 Meyer AC, Dua T, Ma J, Saxena S, Birbeck G. Global disparities in the epilepsy treatment gap: a systematic review. *Bull World Health Organ* 2010;88:260-6.
38 WHO. Disease control priorities related to mental, neurological, developmental and substance abuse disorders. 2006. www.who.int/mental_health/publications/financing/disease_control_priorities_mental_neurological_disorders/en/index.html.
39 Editorial. Epilepsy must become a higher priority in Europe. *Lancet Neurol* 2010;9:941.
40 De Boer HM, Moshe SL, Korey SR, Purpura DP. ILAE/IBE/WHO Global Campaign Against Epilepsy: a partnership that works. *Curr Opin Neurol* 2013;26:219-25.
41 Brodie MJ, Kwan P. Current position of phenobarbital in epilepsy and its future. *Epilepsia* 2012;53(suppl 8):40-6.
42 Mattson RH, Cramer JA, Collins JF, Smith DB, Delgado-Escueta AV, Browne TR, et al. Comparison of carbamazepine, phenobarbital, phenytoin, and primidone in partial and secondarily generalized tonic-clonic seizures. *N Engl J Med* 1985;313:145-51.
43 Perucca E, Tomson T. The pharmacological treatment of epilepsy in adults. *Lancet Neurol* 2011;10:446-56.
44 Marson AG, Appleton R, Baker GA, Chadwick DW, Doughty J, Eaton B, et al. A randomised controlled trial examining the longer-term outcomes of standard versus new antiepileptic drugs. The SANAD trial. *Health Technol Assess* 2007;11:1-149.
45 Trinka E, Marson AG, Van Paesschen W, Kälviäinen R, Marovac J, Duncan B, et al. KOMET: an unblinded, randomised, two parallel-group, stratified trial comparing the effectiveness of levetiracetam with controlled-release carbamazepine and extended-release sodium valproate as monotherapy in patients with newly diagnosed epilepsy. *J Neurol Neurosurg Psychiatry* 2013;84:1138-47.
46 Costa J, Fareleira F, Ascencao R, Borges M, Sampaio C, Vaz-Carneiro A. Clinical comparability of the new antiepileptic drugs in refractory partial epilepsy: a systematic review and meta-analysis. *Epilepsia* 2011;52:1280-91.
47 Faught E. Ezogabine: a new angle on potassium gates. *Epilepsy Curr* 2011;11:75-8.
48 Baulac M, Brodie MJ, Patten A, Segieth J, Giorgi L. Efficacy and tolerability of zonisamide versus controlled-release carbamazepine for newly diagnosed partial epilepsy: a phase 3, randomised, double-blind, non-inferiority trial. *Lancet Neurol* 2012;17:579-88.
49 Gaitatzis A, Sander JW. The long-term safety of antiepileptic drugs. *CNS Drugs* 2013;27:435-55.
50 Guerrini R, Zaccara G, la Marca G, Rosati A. Safety and tolerability of antiepileptic drug treatment in children with epilepsy. *Drug Saf* 2012;35:519-33.
51 Tomson T, Battino D. Teratogenic effects of antiepileptic drugs. *Lancet Neurol* 2012;11:803-13.
52 Meador KJ, Baker GA, Browning N, Cohen MJ, Bromley RL, Clayton-Smith J, et al. Fetal antiepileptic drug exposure and cognitive outcomes at age 6 years (NEAD study): a prospective observational study. *Lancet Neurol* 2013;12:244-52.
53 Löscher W, Klotz U, Zimprich F, Schmidt D. The clinical impact of pharmacogenetics on the treatment of epilepsy. *Epilepsia* 2009;50:1-23.
54 Illing PT, Vivian JP, Purcell AW, Rossjohn J, McCluskey J. Human leukocyte antigen-associated drug hypersensitivity. *Curr Opin Immunol* 2013;25:81-9.
55 Cheung YK, Cheng SH, Chan EJ, Lo SV, Ng MH, Kwan P. HLA-B alleles associated with severe cutaneous reactions to antiepileptic drugs in Han Chinese. *Epilepsia* 2013;54:1307-14.
56 Benedetti MS. Enzyme induction and inhibition by new antiepileptic drugs: a review of human studies. *Fundam Clin Pharmacol* 2000;14:301-19.
57 Strolin-Benedetti M. Enzyme induction and inhibition by new antiepileptic drugs: a review of human studies. *Fundam Clin Pharmacol* 2000;14:301-9.
58 Patsalos PN, Perucca E. Clinically important drug interactions in epilepsy: general features and interactions between antiepileptic drugs. *Lancet Neurol* 2003;2:347-56.
59 Patsalos PN, Berry DJ, Bourgeois BF, Cloyd JC, Glauser TA, Johannessen SI, et al. Antiepileptic drugs—best practice guidelines for therapeutic drug monitoring: a position paper by the subcommission on therapeutic drug monitoring, ILAE Commission on Therapeutic Strategies. *Epilepsia* 2008;49:1239-76.
60 Brodie MJ, Mintzer S, Pack AM, Gidal BE, Vecht CJ, Schmidt D. Enzyme induction with antiepileptic drugs: cause for concern? *Epilepsia* 2013;54:11-27.
61 Ekstein D, Schachter SC. Natural products in epilepsy—the present situation and perspectives for the future. *Pharmaceuticals* 2010;3:1426-45.
62 Schmidt D. Strategies to prevent overtreatment with antiepileptic drugs in patients with epilepsy. *Epilepsy Res* 2002;52:61-9.
63 Faught E, Duh MS, Weiner JR, Guérin A, Cunnington MC. Nonadherence to antiepileptic drugs and increased mortality: findings from the RANSOM Study. *Neurology* 2008;71:1572-8.
64 Löscher W, Schmidt D. Experimental and clinical evidence for loss of effect (tolerance) during prolonged treatment with antiepileptic drugs. *Epilepsia* 2006;47:1253-84.

65 Pirie DA, Wattar BH, Pirie AM, Houston V, Siddiqua A, Doug M, et al. Effects of monitoring strategies on seizures in pregnant women on lamotrigine: a meta-analysis. *Eur J Obstet Gynecol Reprod Biol* 2013; published online 24 Oct.

66 Adab N. Therapeutic monitoring of antiepileptic drugs during pregnancy and in the postpartum period: is it useful? *CNS Drugs* 2006;20:791-800.

67 Schmidt D, Löscher W. New developments in antiepileptic drug resistance: an integrative view. *Epilepsy Curr* 2009;9:47-52.

68 Kwan P, Arzimanoglou A, Berg AT, Brodie MJ, Hauser WA, Mathern G, et al. Definition of drug resistant epilepsy: consensus proposal by the ad hoc Task Force of the ILAE Commission on Therapeutic Strategies. *Epilepsia* 2010;51:1069-77.

69 Picot MC, Baldy-Moulinier M, Daurès JP, Dujols P, Crespel A. The prevalence of epilepsy and pharmacoresistant epilepsy in adults: a population-based study in a western European country. *Epilepsia* 2008;49:1230-8.

70 Hauser WA. The natural history of drug resistant epilepsy: epidemiologic considerations. *Epilepsy Res Suppl* 1992;5:25-8.

71 Schiller Y, Najjar Y. Quantifying the response to antiepileptic drugs: effect of past treatment history. *Neurology* 2008;70:54-65.

72 Sillanpää M, Schmidt D. Is incident drug-resistance of childhood-onset epilepsy reversible? A long-term follow-up study. *Brain* 2012;135:2256-62.

73 Margineanu DG. Systems biology, complexity, and the impact on antiepileptic drug discovery. *Epilepsy Behav* 2013; published online 30 Sep.

74 Schmidt D, Löscher W. Drug resistance in epilepsy: putative neurobiologic and clinical mechanisms. *Epilepsia* 2005;46:858-77.

75 Kwan P, Schachter SC, Brodie MJ. Drug-resistant epilepsy. *N Engl J Med* 2011;365:919-26.

76 Hitiris N, Mohanraj R, Norrie J, Sills GJ, Brodie MJ. Predictors of pharmacoresistant epilepsy. *Epilepsy Res* 2007;75:192-6.

77 Kanner AM. Do psychiatric comorbidities have a negative impact on the course and treatment of seizure disorders? *Curr Opin Neurol* 2013;26:208-13.

78 Loeb JA. Identifying targets for preventing epilepsy using systems biology. *Neurosci Lett* 2011;497:205-12.

79 Beyenburg S, Stavem K, Schmidt D. Placebo-corrected efficacy of modern antiepileptic drugs for refractory epilepsy: systematic review and meta-analysis. *Epilepsia* 2010;51:7-26.

80 Karceski S, Morrell MJ, Carpenter D. Treatment of epilepsy in adults: expert opinion, 2005. *Epilepsy Behav* 2005;7:S1-64.

81 Deckers CLP, Hekster YA, Keyser A, van Lier HJJ, Meinardi H, Renier WO. Monotherapy versus polytherapy for epilepsy: a multicenter double-blind randomized study. *Epilepsia* 2001;42:1387-94.

82 Beghi E, Gatti G, Tonini C, Ben-Menachem E, Chadwick DW, Nikanorova M, et al. Adjunctive therapy versus alternative monotherapy in patients with partial epilepsy failing on a single drug: a multicentre, randomized, pragmatic controlled trial. *Epilepsy Res* 2003;57:1-13.

83 Marson A, Jacoby A, Johnson A, Kim L, Gamble C, Chadwick D. Immediate versus deferred antiepileptic drug treatment for early epilepsy and single seizures: a randomised controlled trial. *Lancet* 2005;365:2007-13.

84 Pack A. Bone health in people with epilepsy: is it impaired and what are the risk factors? *Seizure* 2008;17:181-6.

85 Vestergaard P, Rejnmark L, Mosekilde L. Fracture risk associated with use of antiepileptic drugs. *Epilepsia* 2004;45:1330-7.

86 Carbone LD, Johnson KC, Robbins J, Larson JC, Curb JD, Watson K, et al. Antiepileptic drug use, falls, fractures, and BMD in postmenopausal women: findings from the women's health initiative (WHI). *J Bone Miner Res* 2010;25:873-81.

87 Kim SH, Lee JW, Choi KG, Chung HW, Lee HW. A 6-month longitudinal study of bone mineral density with antiepileptic drug monotherapy. *Epilepsy Behav* 2007;10:291-5.

88 Lazzari AA, Dussault PM, Thakore-James M, Gagnon D, Baker E, Davis SA, et al. Prevention of bone loss and vertebral fractures in patients with chronic epilepsy—antiepileptic drug and osteoporosis prevention trial. *Epilepsia* 2013; published online 6 Sep.

89 Battino D, Tomson T, Bonizzoni E, Craig J, Lindhout D, Sabers A, et al; EURAP Study Group. Seizure control and treatment changes in pregnancy: Observations from the EURAP epilepsy pregnancy registry. *Epilepsia* 2013;54:1621-7.

90 Reisinger TL, Newman M, Loring DW, Pennell PB, Meador KJ. Antiepileptic drug clearance and seizure frequency during pregnancy in women with epilepsy. *Epilepsy Behav* 2013;29:13-8.

91 Harden CL, Meador KJ, Pennell PB, Koppel BS, Hovinga CA, Gidal B, et al. Management issues for women with epilepsy—focus on pregnancy (an evidence-based review): II. Teratogenesis and perinatal outcomes: report of the quality standards subcommittee and therapeutics and technology subcommittee of the American Academy of Neurology and the American Epilepsy Society. *Epilepsia* 2009;50:1237-46.

92 Wyszynski DF, Nambisan M, Surve T, Alsdorf RM, Smith CR, Holmes LB; Antiepileptic Drug Pregnancy Registry. Increased rate of major malformations in offspring exposed to valproate during pregnancy. *Neurology* 2005;64:961-5.

93 Jentink J, Loane MA, Dolk H, Barisic I, Garne E, Morris JK, et al; EUROCAT Antiepileptic Study Working Group. Valproic acid monotherapy in pregnancy and major congenital malformations. *N Engl J Med* 2010;362:2185-9.

94 Harden CL, Pennell PB, Koppel BS, Hovinga CA, Gidal B, Meador KJ, et al. Management issues for women with epilepsy—focus on pregnancy (an evidence-based review): III. Vitamin K, folic acid, blood levels, and breast-feeding: report of the quality standards subcommittee and therapeutics and technology assessment subcommittee of the American Academy of Neurology and the American Epilepsy Society. *Epilepsia* 2009;50:1247-55.

95 Tomson T, Battino D, Bonizzoni E, Craig J, Lindhout D, Sabers A, et al. Dose-dependent risk of malformations with antiepileptic drugs: an analysis of data from the EURAP epilepsy and pregnancy registry. *Lancet Neurol* 2011;10:609-17.

96 Meador KJ, Loring DW. Risks of in utero exposure to valproate. *JAMA* 2013;309:1730-1

97 Robertson MM, Trimble MR. The treatment of depression in patients with epilepsy. A double-blind trial. *J Affect Disord* 1985;9:127-36.

98 Rowan AJ, Ramsay RE, Collins JF, Pryor F, Boardman KD, Uthman BM, et al. New onset geriatric epilepsy: a randomized study of gabapentin, lamotrigine, and carbamazepine. *Neurology* 2005;64:1868-73.

99 Ramsay RE, Uthman B, Pryor FM, Rowan AJ, Bainbridge J, Spitz M, et al. Topiramate in older patients with partial-onset seizures: a pilot double-blind, dose-comparison study. *Epilepsia* 2008;49:1180-5.

100 Gaitatzis A, Sisodiya SM, Sander JW. The somatic comorbidity of epilepsy: a weighty but often unrecognized burden. *Epilepsia* 2012;53:1282-93.

101 Tellez-Zenteno JF, Patten SB, Jette N, Williams J, Wiebe S. Psychiatric comorbidity in epilepsy: a population-based analysis. *Epilepsia* 2007;48:2336-44.

102 Fazel S, Wolf A, Långström N, Newton CR, Lichtenstein P. Premature mortality in epilepsy and the role of psychiatric comorbidity: a total population study. *Lancet* 2013;382:1646-54.

103 Kanner AM. The treatment of depressive disorders in epilepsy: what all neurologists should know. *Epilepsia* 2013;54(suppl 1):3-12.

104 Robertson MM, Trimble MR. The treatment of depression in patients with epilepsy. A double-blind trial. *J Affect Disord* 1985;9:127-36.

105 Noe KH, Locke DE, Sirven JI. Treatment of depression in patients with epilepsy. *Curr Treat Options Neurol* 2011;13:371-9.

106 Shorvon SD, Baulac TM, Cross H, Trinka E, Walker M; for the Task Force on Status Epilepticus of the ILAE. The drug treatment of status epilepticus in Europe: consensus document from a workshop at the first London colloquium on status epilepticus. *Epilepsia* 2008;49:2177-84.

107 McIntyre J, Robertson S, Norris E, Appleton R, Whitehouse WP, Phillips B, et al. Safety and efficacy of buccal midazolam versus rectal diazepam for emergency treatment of seizures in children: a randomised controlled trial. *Lancet* 2005;366:205-10.

108 European Medicines Agency. Buccolam 2.5 mg oromucosal solution: summary of product characteristics. www.ema.europa.eu/docs/en_GB/document_library/EPAR_-_Product_Information/human/002267/WC500112310.pdf.

109 Silbergleit R, Lowenstein D, Durkalski V, Conwit R; Neurological Emergency Treatment Trials (NETT) Investigators. RAMPART (Rapid Anticonvulsant Medication Prior to Arrival Trial): a double-blind randomized clinical trial of the efficacy of intramuscular midazolam versus intravenous lorazepam in the prehospital treatment of status epilepticus by paramedics. *Epilepsia* 2011;52(suppl 8):45-7.

110 Shorvon S. The treatment of status epilepticus. *Curr Opin Neurol* 2011;24:165-70.

111 Ferlisi M, Shorvon S. The outcome of therapies in refractory and super-refractory convulsive status epilepticus and recommendations for therapy. *Brain* 2012;135:2314-28.

112 Schmidt D, Löscher W. Uncontrolled epilepsy following discontinuation of antiepileptic drugs in seizure-free patients: a review of current clinical experience. *Acta Neurol Scand* 2005;111:291-300.

113 Berg AT, Shinnar S. Relapse following discontinuation of antiepileptic drugs: a meta-analysis. *Neurology* 1994;44:601-8.

114 Medical Research Council Antiepileptic Drug Withdrawal Study Group. Randomised study of antiepileptic drug withdrawal in patients in remission. *Lancet* 1991;337:1175-80.

115 American Academy of Neurology Practice parameter: a guideline for discontinuing antiepileptic drugs in seizure-free patients—summary statement. *Neurology* 1996;47:600-2.

116 Bonnett LJ, Shukralla A, Tudur-Smith C, Williamson PR, Marson AG. Seizure recurrence after antiepileptic drug withdrawal and the implications for driving: further results from the MRC Antiepileptic Drug Withdrawal Study and a systematic review. *J Neurol Neurosurg Psychiatry* 2011;82:1328-33.

117 Schmidt D, Baumgartner C, Löscher W. Seizure recurrence after planned discontinuation of antiepileptic drugs in seizure-free patients after epilepsy surgery: a review of current clinical experience. *Epilepsia* 2004;45:179-86.

118 Braun KPJ, Schmidt D. Stopping antiepileptic drugs in seizure-free patients. *Curr Opin Neurol* [forthcoming].

119 Schmidt D, Baumgartner C, Löscher W. The chance of cure following surgery for drug-resistant temporal lobe epilepsy. What do we know and do we need to revise our expectations? *Epilepsy Res* 2004;187-201.

120 Zeng TF, An DM, Li JM, Li YH, Chen L, Hong Z, et al. Evaluation of different antiepileptic drug strategies in medically refractory epilepsy patients following epilepsy surgery. Epilepsy Res 2012;101:14-21.

121 Tellez-Zenteno JF, Dhar R, Hernandez-Ronquillo L Wiebe S. Long-term outcomes in epilepsy surgery: antiepileptic drugs, mortality, cognitive and psychosocial aspects. *Brain* 2007;130:334-45.
122 Edelvik A, Rydenhag B, Olsson I, Flink R, Kumlien E, Källän K, et al. Long-term outcomes of epilepsy surgery in Sweden: a national prospective and longitudinal study. *Neurology* 2013;81:1244-51.
123 Najm I, Jehi L, Palmini A, Gonzalez-Martinez J, Paglioli E, Bingaman W. Temporal patterns and mechanisms of epilepsy surgery failure. *Epilepsia* 2013;54:772-82.
124 Bulacio JC, Jehi L, Wong C, Gonzalez-Martinez J, Kotagal P, Nair D, et al. Long-term seizure outcome after resective surgery in patients evaluated with intracranial electrodes. *Epilepsia* 2012;53:1722-30.
125 Engel J Jr, Thompson PM, Stern JM, Staba RJ, Bragin A, Mody I. Connectomics and epilepsy. *Curr Opin Neurol* 2013;26:186-94.
126 Wiebe W, Jette N. Pharmacoresistance and the role of surgery in difficult to treat epilepsy. *Nat Rev Neurol* 2012;8:669-77.
127 Schmidt D. Is antiepileptogenesis a realistic goal in clinical trials? Concerns and new horizons. *Epilept Disord* 2012;14:105-13.
128 Halford JJ, Ben-Menachem E, Kwan P, Ness S, Schmitt J, Eerdekens M, et al. A randomized, double-blind, placebo-controlled study of the efficacy, safety, and tolerability of adjunctive carisbamate treatment in patients with partial-onset seizures. *Epilepsia* 2011;52:816-25.
129 Perucca E. What clinical trial designs have been used to test antiepileptic drugs and do we need to change them? *Epilept Disord* 2012;14:124-31.
130 Perucca E, French J, Bialer M. Development of new antiepileptic drugs: challenges, incentives, and recent advances. *Lancet Neurol* 2007;6:793-804.
131 Friedman D, French JA. Clinical trials for therapeutic assessment of antiepileptic drugs in the 21st century: obstacles and solutions. *Lancet Neurol* 2012;11:827-34.
132 Birbeck GL, Hays RD, Cui X, Vickrey BG. Seizure reduction and quality of life improvements in people with epilepsy. *Epilepsia* 2002;43:535-8.
133 Lossius R, Kinge E, Nakken KO. Epilepsy and driving: considerations on how eligibility should be decided. *Acta Neurol Scand Suppl* 2010;190:67-71.
134 Baulac M, Leon T, O'Brien TJ, Whalen E, Barrett J. A comparison of pregabalin, lamotrigine, and placebo as adjunctive therapy in patients with refractory partial-onset seizures. *Epilepsy Res* 2010;91:10-9.
135 Ryvlin P, Cucherat M, Rheims S. Risk of sudden unexpected death in epilepsy in patients given adjunctive antiepileptic treatment for refractory seizures: a meta-analysis of placebo-controlled randomised trials. *Lancet Neurol* 2011;10:961-8.
136 Schmidt D, Beyenburg S, D'Souza J, Stavem K. Clinical features associated with placebo response in refractory focal epilepsy. *Epilepsy Behav* 2013;27:393-8.

Management of chronic epilepsy

Fergus J Rugg-Gunn, consultant neurologist[1 2],
Josemir W Sander, professor of neurology[1 2 3]

[1]Department of Clinical and Experimental Epilepsy, UCL Institute of Neurology, Queen Square, London, UK

[2]Epilepsy Society, Chalfont St Peter, UK

[3]SEIN-Epilepsy Institute in the Netherlands Foundation, Heemstede, Netherlands

Correspondence to: L Sander, Box 29, UCL Institute of Neurology, London WC1N 3BG, UK l.sander@ucl.ac.uk

Cite this as: BMJ 2012;345:e4576

DOI: 10.1136/bmj.e4576

http://www.bmj.com/content/345/bmj.e4576

Epilepsy can be defined pragmatically as the occurrence of at least two unprovoked epileptic seizures. It is the commonest serious neurological condition in adults, directly affecting over 400 000 people in the United Kingdom and up to 60 million people worldwide.[1] Prevalence of epilepsy in developed countries is about 0.5%; however, the lifetime risk of a person having a non-febrile epileptic seizure is much higher at 2-5%, implying, for most patients, remittance of the condition or premature death.

Risk of a second seizure occurring within two years of the first event is about 50%. Early treatment with antiepileptic drugs after the first seizure does not affect the long term prognosis, with 75-80% achieving remission at five years, irrespective of whether treatment began after the first seizure or only after a recurrence.[2 3] Treatment is therefore typically reserved for people who have had at least two seizures; the risk of a third seizure in these patients is over 70%. A tailored approach to treatment should always be adopted, since there could be circumstances in which treatment after a first seizure is appropriate (for example, presence of a structural lesion on neuroimaging) or deferred (for example, in those with very infrequent seizures).

Most people with epilepsy eventually become free of seizures on antiepileptic drugs. Nevertheless, about 20-30% of patients continue to have seizures despite treatment.[4] By extrapolating this proportion to the UK, an estimated 100 000 people with epilepsy need continuing, hospital based medical treatment. Of this group, over 35 000 will have more than one seizure a month. Epilepsy carries an increased risk of morbidity and premature mortality with standardised mortality rates two to threefold higher than the general population.[5 6] This raised risk is partly due to the underlying cause of the epilepsy but is also a direct result of seizures, such as an increased risk of accidents (including drowning) and sudden unexpected death in epilepsy (a condition that affects at least 500 people with epilepsy in the UK annually). On this basis, seizure remission, wherever possible, is a major goal.

SUMMARY POINTS

- Epilepsy is common, affecting over 400 000 people in the United Kingdom
- Epileptic seizures are associated with an increased risk of morbidity and premature mortality
- Quality of life depends on seizure freedom and lack of adverse effects from drug treatment
- Comorbidities and the effects on lifestyle, mood, and relationships are also important
- Up to 75% of people with epilepsy become seizure-free on treatment
- Choice of drug treatment should be tailored to each person, as determined by their characteristics, the epilepsy syndrome, seizure types, lifestyle issues, and cotreatments
- Combination treatment could be needed for patients who do not respond to monotherapy
- Review diagnosis and treatment compliance for patients who do not respond to treatment
- Consider other treatment options, such as surgery, in people with chronic focal epilepsy

The implications of chronic epilepsy extend beyond continued seizures, and encompass cognitive difficulties, mood disturbance, and lifestyle issues, the effective treatment of which involves a coordinated response from both primary and secondary care.

The purpose of this review was to examine the literature on how to manage adults with chronic epilepsy.

Who gets epilepsy?

The incidence of epilepsy is increased in childhood, at least partly because of brain malformations, perinatal cerebral insults, and genetic disorders, and in later life, usually as a result of cerebrovascular disease. Nevertheless, seizures could start at any age and may follow a cerebral insult, such as head injury, intracranial infections, or tumours. The risk of developing epilepsy increases in the presence of learning disability or after a prolonged or lateralised febrile convulsion in childhood. Genetic factors contribute either directly (for example, in the autosomal dominantly inherited condition tuberous sclerosis) or in a more complex pattern of polygenic inheritance. Overall, genetic factors are thought to contribute to about 40% of people with epilepsy.

What is the goal of epilepsy treatment?

In all people with epilepsy, the goal should be to achieve seizure freedom. Reducing a person's seizures by 50%, for example, from six seizures to three seizures a month might have a minimal effect on quality of life.[7] This is largely because of the restrictions to a person's lifestyle that remain until seizure freedom, such as the inability to drive, difficulties obtaining work, and maintaining a relationship. Nevertheless, antiepileptic drugs have both idiosyncratic and often more predictable chronic side effects, and seizure freedom should not be relentlessly pursued at the expense of quality of life; intrusive side effects also have a negative effect on quality of life.[7] Common side effects that lead to withdrawal of drug treatment include drowsiness, dizziness, lethargy, and cognitive slowing. These side effects are a particular concern for combination antiepileptic drug treatment.

How is epilepsy managed?

The diagnosis of epilepsy is clinical—that is, it is made on the basis of a description of the seizure by both a patient and a witness. It is mandatory to try to obtain a witness description, which is often more informative than the person's account of the event, which may be confounded by loss of awareness, confusion, and amnesia. Investigations such as a brain scan by magnetic resonance imaging or an electroencephalography recording should be used to corroborate clinical suspicion and not as screening tests, owing to the presence of both false positive and false negative information. Patients should be referred to a specialist for evaluation if a seizure is suspected, but drug treatment is typically started only after a second seizure.

The choice of initial monotherapy has been guided by several important studies (including, most recently, SANAD[8][9]) and advice from the National Institute for Health and Clinical Excellence (NICE).[10] The antiepileptic drug strategy should be tailored to each patient's seizure type, epilepsy syndrome, cotreatment, comorbidity, lifestyle issues, and preferences (box 1).

Specialists should adjust the dose of the selected drug to achieve optimal seizure control, making increments if seizures continue in the absence of side effects and, for some drugs such as phenytoin, being guided by assays of serum drug concentrations. Zealous adherence to quoted therapeutic ranges of serum antiepileptic concentrations is, however, not appropriate. These data should always be secondary to the clinical picture of whether the person continues to have seizures or dose related side effects from antiepileptic drugs. Blood levels of antiepileptic drugs should also be monitored to detect non-adherence to the prescription, suspected toxicity, and in the management of specific clinical conditions such as status epilepticus, organ failure and pregnancy, in which serum levels may fall resulting in the re-emergence of seizures.

Treatment should be initiated and continuing therapy should be planned by the specialist. If management is straightforward, continuing drug treatment can be prescribed in primary care if local circumstances or licensing allow. The duration of each treatment trial before deciding on continuing or changing to an alternative drug depends on the occurrence of side effects and seizure frequency. For example, it will take longer to establish whether a drug has been effective in a patient with very infrequent seizures than in a patient with daily or weekly seizures.

What affects seizure control and prognosis in chronic epilepsy?

Several factors influence prognosis, and specifically, the chance of patients becoming seizure-free. Perinatal neurological insult and learning disability are associated with an increased risk of developing chronic epilepsy. Only about 10% of people with an epileptic structural lesion on magnetic resonance imaging, such as hippocampal sclerosis, achieve seizure freedom with drug treatment alone. For some of these, epilepsy surgery offers the best chance of becoming seizure-free and improving quality of life.[11]

An important factor in the probability of subsequent remission is the frequency of seizures within the first six months after seizure onset; 95% of patients with two seizures in the first six months achieve a five year remission, compared with only 24% of those with more than ten seizures.[12] The probability of seizure remission decreases significantly with each successive treatment failure. About 50% of people become seizure-free with their first antiepileptic drug, whereas only 11% who discontinued the first appropriate drug owing to a lack of efficacy become seizure-free on a second drug, and only 4% become seizure-free on a third drug or beyond.[13] A recent series of studies has suggested, however, that this view is overly pessimistic. For example, in a review of the effect of 265 drug changes in 155 people with chronic epilepsy, 16% were rendered seizure-free after introduction of one drug, whereas a further 21% had a considerable reduction in seizure frequency. Overall, 28% of the cohort was rendered seizure-free by one or more changes to their drug treatment.[14]

BOX 1 INFORMATION NEEDS

General epilepsy information
- Explanation of what the condition is
- Classification
- Investigations
- Syndrome
- Epidemiology
- Prognosis
- Genetics
- Sudden unexpected death in epilepsy

Antiepileptic drugs
- Choice of drug
- Efficacy
- Side effects
- Adherence
- Drug interactions
- Free prescriptions

Seizure triggers
- Lack of sleep
- Alcohol and recreational drugs
- Stress
- Photosensitivity

First aid
- General guidelines

Issues for women
- Contraception
- Preconception
- Pregnancy and breastfeeding
- Menopause

Lifestyle
- Driving regulations
- Employment
- Education
- Leisure
- Relationships
- Safety at home

Possible psychosocial consequences
- Perceived stigma
- Memory loss
- Depression
- Anxiety
- Maintain mental wellbeing
- Self esteem
- Sexual difficulties
- Support organisations
- Address and telephone numbers

BOX 2 TRIGGERS FOR REFERRAL TO SECONDARY CARE
- All patients with a suspected epileptic seizure
- All patients who continue to have epileptic seizures (that is, active epilepsy)
- Patients who have possible side effects, both acute and chronic, from drug treatment
- Patients with stable epilepsy but a change of circumstances, such as pregnancy
- Consideration of treatment withdrawal
- Patients needing additional specialist information, such as preconception counselling

What are the factors to consider if seizure control is suboptimal?

Is the diagnosis correct?

A patient's failure to respond to adequate trials of antiepileptic drugs should prompt specialists to review the diagnosis. One study showed that up to 20-30% of people attending tertiary referral centres with presumed chronic epilepsy did not in fact have the condition, with the most common differential diagnoses being dissociative seizures and neurocardiogenic or cardiac syncope.[15]

Is the drug treatment appropriate?

Some antiepileptic drugs could exacerbate seizure disorders if used injudiciously. The most common examples are the use of carbamazepine, oxcarbazepine, phenytoin, pregabalin, and gabapentin in primary generalised epilepsy, all of which can exacerbate not only absences and myoclonic jerks but also convulsive seizures.[16] Therefore, a patient's seizure disorder must be classified accurately, although this is not possible in some instances and drugs with a broad spectrum of activity should be used (table).

What other medications and illnesses need to be considered?

Other non-epilepsy drugs may lower the seizure threshold, including antimalarial compounds (such as chloroquine, mefloquine), smoking cessation drugs (such as bupropion), antidepressants, and antipsychotics (such as amitriptyline and clozapine). Use of these drugs should be questioned if seizure control is suboptimal. Systemic illnesses, such as sepsis, renal or hepatic disease, or an endocrine disturbance, may cause treatment failure and should be investigated.

Is adherence to treatment adequate?

If there are doubts about adherence to treatment, the patient and carer should be questioned sensitively about this. Serum concentrations of antiepileptic drugs can also be obtained. Inspecting the packaging and drugs themselves may rarely yield prescribing or dispensing errors. If adherence is a problem, consider using dossett boxes, prepackaged treatment packs, and reminder services (such as alarms or regular, timed text messages).

Has the patient had a good trial with a maximally tolerated dose of all major antiepileptic drugs?

People with poorly controlled epilepsy are usually under the care of a specialist neurology team. If seizures continue despite a maximally tolerated dose of individual first line drugs, specialists should trial a combination of two first line drugs for that seizure type. The chance of dual therapy controlling seizures, if monotherapy has been unsuccessful, is 10-15%. If dual therapy does not help, the drug which seems to have the most effect and fewest side effects should be continued, and the second drug should be gradually replaced with an adjunctive drug. NICE guidelines may help in selecting an alternative, second line antiepileptic drug (table).[10] The chance of a 50% reduction in seizures from the addition of a second line drug is 20-50%, with the chance of the patient becoming seizure-free less than 10%.

If the second line drug is effective, consider withdrawing the initial drug. Prescription of an unhelpful second line drug should not be continued. If adjunctive treatment is ineffective or not tolerated, discuss this with the person, and possibly refer them to a tertiary epilepsy specialist. Current NICE guidelines recommend other antiepileptic drugs to consider at this point for focal epilepsy, such as lacosamide, eslicarbazepine acetate, pregabalin, zonisamide, retigabine, and tiagabine, as well as the older substances phenobarbitone and phenytoin.[10]

Over the past 20 years, the number of antiepileptic drugs available has increased markedly (see figure and table). Similarities exist between drugs in terms of efficacy and indications, but there is a wide range of dosing strategies,

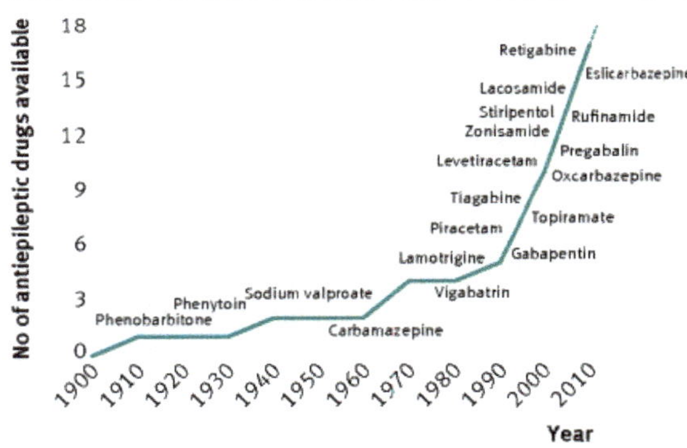

Antiepileptic drugs available in the UK over the past 20 years, in addition to acetazolamide, clobazam, clonazepam, and ethosuximide

NICE guidelines on antiepileptic drug treatment[10]

Epileptic seizure type	First line treatment	Adjunctive treatment	Other drugs to consider on referral to tertiary care	Do not consider (may worsen seizures)
Generalised tonic-clonic	Carbamazepine, lamotrigine, oxcarbazepine,* sodium valproate	Clobazam, lamotrigine, levetiracetam, sodium valproate, topiramate	–	Carbamazepine, gabapentin, oxcarbazepine, phenytoin, pregabalin, tiagabine, vigabatrin
Tonic or atonic	Sodium valproate	Lamotrigine*	Rufinamide*, topiramate*	Carbamazepine, gabapentin, oxcarbazepine, pregabalin, tiagabine, vigabatrin
Absence	Ethosuximide, lamotrigine,* sodium valproate	Ethosuximide, lamotrigine,* sodium valproate	Clobazam, clonazepam, levetiracetam,* topiramate,* zonisamide*	Carbamazepine, gabapentin, oxcarbazepine, phenytoin, pregabalin, tiagabine, vigabatrin
Myoclonic	Levetiracetam,* sodium valproate, topiramate*	Levetiracetam, sodium valproate, topiramate*	Clobazam, clonazepam, piracetam, zonisamide*	Carbamazepine, gabapentin, oxcarbazepine, phenytoin, pregabalin, tiagabine, vigabatrin
Focal	Carbamazepine, lamotrigine, levetiracetam, oxcarbazepine, sodium valproate	Carbamazepine, clobazam, gabapentin, lamotrigine, levetiracetam, oxcarbazepine, sodium valproate, topiramate	Eslicarbazepine acetate, lacosamide, phenobarbital, phenytoin, pregabalin, retigabine, tiagabine, vigabatrin, zonisamide	–

**At the time of publication of NICE guidelines in January 2012, this drug did not have UK marketing authorisation for this indication or population.*

pharmacokinetic and pharmacodynamic interactions, and side effect profiles. This complexity has led to a degree of "prescribing paralysis" among non-specialists, and clinicians will often retreat to established and trusted drugs, rather than considering more contemporary and newly licensed drugs.

Which drug should the patient try next?
With a large number of drugs to choose from, how do specialists choose drugs rationally—that is, tailor the choice of treatment to an individual? Many placebo controlled trials of adjunctive antiepileptic drugs have formed the bases on which individual drugs have been licensed. Establishing which drug is the most effective and well tolerated by comparing these trials is difficult because of different trial designs, patient selection, and outcome measures. Nevertheless, detailed analysis shows no clear statistical difference between the drugs in terms of efficacy and tolerability,[17 18] and therefore one drug cannot be stated as conclusively better than another.

Head to head trials of adjunctive and combination treatments offer greater potential for establishing a drug hierarchy. Few such studies exist, and those that have been undertaken frequently evaluate outcome measures other than seizure frequency, such as mood changes and aggression.[19] These goals are laudable but do little to inform which drug or combination to recommend next for people with refractory epilepsy to improve seizure control.

In reality, the choice of the third or fourth antiepileptic drug or beyond is complex and involves looking at the evidence, clinical experience, and individual characteristics and concerns. For example, in people with comorbidities such as migraine, choosing a drug with adjunctive preventative properties for migraines may be beneficial (such as topiramate, sodium valproate, pregabalin, or gabapentin). In people with anxiety or depression, compounds that are also indicated for generalised anxiety disorder (such as pregabalin) or other drugs with mood stabilising properties (such as valproate and lamotrigine) may be worth considering earlier than other substances. In people with an elevated body mass index, consider avoiding pregabalin, sodium valproate, and gabapentin, and consider instead topiramate and zonisamide, which are commonly associated with weight loss.

The presence of cotreatments, particularly those affected by enzyme inducing drugs, may influence the choice of drug. Oral anticoagulants may need an increased dose to maintain appropriate anticoagulation levels, and hormonal contraceptives are rendered less effective, even with a dose adjustment, in the presence of drugs such as carbamazepine, phenytoin, and higher dose topiramate. Other drugs with favourable pharmacokinetics, such as levetiracetam, may be better choices. Teratogenicity is a clear concern with all drugs, and particularly in combinations including sodium valproate.[20]

How can the total drug load be minimised?
It is important to reduce and discontinue antiepileptic drugs if their prescription has not aided seizure control and they are suspected of giving rise to adverse effects. Reduction of the number of antiepileptic drugs frequently results in patients feeling better and improved seizure control.[21] The rate at which these drugs should be withdrawn in this situation is controversial and should be planned and supervised by specialist services. Some drugs can be safely withdrawn fairly rapidly, but conventional withdrawal occurs over a period of weeks. This period is particularly important in the withdrawal of benzodiazepines and barbiturates, which could precipitate status epilepticus if withdrawn too rapidly.[22] Making only one drug change at a time is recommended, to determine cause and effect if there is any improvement or deterioration.

SOURCES AND SELECTION CRITERIA

This clinical review is based on personal experience, reference archives, and a wide literature search of PubMed using the search terms "adult epilepsy", "management of epilepsy", and "antiepileptic drugs". We also consulted guidelines from the International League against Epilepsy, American Academy of Neurology, PubMed search for adult epilepsy, and antiepileptic drug and clinical management guidelines from the National Institute for Health and Clinical Excellence (clinical guideline 137, 2012).

What about epilepsy surgery?
In focal epilepsy, if satisfactory seizure control cannot be achieved by antiepileptic drugs, consider an evaluation for epilepsy surgery. This treatment is especially indicated if a lesion with concordant clinical features has been detected on magnetic resonance imaging, but should be considered in patients with a focal onset epilepsy and ongoing seizures despite optimal doses of two to three antiepileptic drugs (as monotherapy or in combination).

How often should people with epilepsy be reviewed?
Current NICE guidelines recommend that all people with epilepsy should have a yearly structured review. In adults, this review may be undertaken by a general practitioner or specialist, depending on how well the epilepsy is controlled and the presence of specific lifestyle issues, such as consideration of pregnancy, driving regulations, or drug cessation (box 2). At this review, people should have access to written and visual information, counselling services, timely and appropriate investigations, and tertiary services (box 1). In particular, if seizures are not controlled or diagnosis is uncertain, patients should be referred to tertiary services for further assessment.[10]

What should an epilepsy review include?

Pharmacological aspects
At the annual epilepsy review, the person's treatment should be discussed. This discussion will include an evaluation of the effectiveness of the prescribed drugs and presence of adverse effects. Common side effects to almost all drugs include drowsiness, dizziness, and lethargy; these effects, in addition to specific side effects for each drug, should be actively sought. The effect of comorbidities and use of cotreatments should be reviewed, such as the oral contraceptive pill or anticoagulants. Routine monitoring of antiepileptic drugs is not indicated because it is unlikely to alter drug management in isolation.

Non-pharmacological aspects
The implications and consequences of chronic epilepsy should be considered, which often are more devastating than the seizures themselves. Patients should be given general safety advice about cooking with a microwave oven, safe bathing, and recreational activities. The driving regulations should be discussed if appropriate, and patients

should be reminded that a one year period of seizure freedom is required before being eligible to drive. Issues regarding epilepsy, antiepileptic drugs, contraception, and pregnancy should be considered in women of childbearing age and further advice sought from a specialist if relevant. A discussion of reasonable expectations and limitations with regard to the prognosis and the prospects for independent living, leisure and social life, and employment is also important. For patients and their families, the support of an epilepsy specialist nurse[23] and of voluntary organisations, such as the Epilepsy Society (www.epilepsysociety.org.uk) or Epilepsy Action (www.epilepsy.org.uk), are invaluable.

Contributors: Both authors conceptualised, drafted, and reviewed the paper. JWS is the guarantor.

Competing interests: All authors have completed the Unified Competing Interest form at www.icmje.org/coi_disclosure.pdf (available on request from the corresponding author) and declare: no support from any organisation for the submitted work; FRG has received honorariums and travel expenses from UCB, GlaxoSmithKline, and Eisai; JWS has received research support, honorariums, and travel expenses from UCB, Janssen-Cilag, GlaxoSmithKline, Viropharma, and Eisai; JWS and FRG are based at University College London Hospitals/University College London, which received a proportion of funding from the Department of Health's National Institute for Health Research Biomedical Research Centres funding scheme.

Provenance and peer review: Commissioned; externally peer reviewed.

1 Ngugi AK, Kariuki SM, Bottomley C, Kleinschmidt I, Sander JW, Newton CR. Incidence of epilepsy: a systematic review and meta-analysis. *Neurology* 2011;77:1005-12.
2 Leone MA, Solari A, Beghi E. Treatment of the first tonic-clonic seizure does not affect long-term remission of epilepsy. *Neurology* 2006;67:2227-9.
3 Marson A, Jacoby A, Johnson A, Kim L, Gamble C, Chadwick D. Immediate versus deferred antiepileptic drug treatment for early epilepsy and single seizures: a randomised controlled trial. *Lancet* 2005;365:2007-13.
4 Annegers JF, Hauser WA, Elveback LR. Remission of seizures and relapse in patients with epilepsy. *Epilepsia* 1979;20:729-37.
5 Cockerell OC, Johnson AL, Sander JW, Hart YM, Goodridge DM, Shorvon SD. Mortality from epilepsy: results from a prospective population-based study. *Lancet* 1994;344:918-21.
6 Lhatoo SD, Johnson AL, Goodridge DM, MacDonald BK, Sander JW, Shorvon SD. Mortality in epilepsy in the first 11 to 14 years after diagnosis: multivariate analysis of a long-term, prospective, population-based cohort. *Ann Neurol* 2001;49:336-44.
7 Gilliam F. Optimizing health outcomes in active epilepsy. *Neurology* 2002;58(suppl 5):S9-20.
8 Marson AG, Al-Kharusi AM, Alwaidh M, Appleton R, Baker GA, Chadwick DW, et al. The SANAD study of effectiveness of valproate, lamotrigine, or topiramate for generalised and unclassifiable epilepsy: an unblinded randomised controlled trial. *Lancet* 2007;369:1016-26.
9 Marson AG, Al-Kharusi AM, Alwaidh M, Appleton R, Baker GA, Chadwick DW, et al. The SANAD study of effectiveness of carbamazepine, gabapentin, lamotrigine, oxcarbazepine, or topiramate for treatment of partial epilepsy: an unblinded randomised controlled trial. *Lancet* 2007;369:1000-15.
10 National Institute for Health and Clinical Excellence. Clinical guideline 137. NICE, 2012.
11 Wiebe S, Blume WT, Girvin JP, Eliasziw M. A randomized, controlled trial of surgery for temporal-lobe epilepsy. *N Engl J Med* 2001;345:311-8.
12 MacDonald BK, Johnson AL, Goodridge DM, Cockerell OC, Sander JW, Shorvon SD. Factors predicting prognosis of epilepsy after presentation with seizures. *Ann Neurol* 2000;48:833-41.
13 Kwan P, Brodie MJ. Early identification of refractory epilepsy. *N Engl J Med* 2000;342:314-9.
14 Luciano AL, Shorvon SD. Results of treatment changes in patients with apparently drug-resistant chronic epilepsy. *Ann Neurol* 2007;62:375-81.
15 Smith D, Defalla BA, Chadwick DW. The misdiagnosis of epilepsy and the management of refractory epilepsy in a specialist clinic. *QJM* 1999;92:15-23.
16 Chaves J, Sander JW. Seizure aggravation in idiopathic generalized epilepsies. *Epilepsia* 2005;46(suppl 9):133-9.
17 Marson AG, Kadir ZA, Hutton JL, Chadwick DW. The new antiepileptic drugs: a systematic review of their efficacy and tolerability. *Epilepsia* 1997;38:859-80.
18 Marson AG, Hutton JL, Leach JP, Castillo S, Schmidt D, White S, et al. Levetiracetam, oxcarbazepine, remacemide and zonisamide for drug resistant localization-related epilepsy: a systematic review. *Epilepsy Res* 2001;46:259-70.
19 Meador KJ, Loring DW, Hulihan JF, Kamin M, Karim R. Differential cognitive and behavioral effects of topiramate and valproate. *Neurology* 2003;60:1483-8.
20 Meador KJ, Baker GA, Browning N, Clayton-Smith J, Combs-Cantrell DT, Cohen M, et al. Cognitive function at 3 years of age after fetal exposure to antiepileptic drugs. *N Engl J Med* 2009;360:1597-605.
21 Albright P, Bruni J. Reduction of polypharmacy in epileptic patients. *Arch Neurol* 1985;42:797-9.
22 Duncan JS, Shorvon SD, Trimble MR. Discontinuation of phenytoin, carbamazepine, and valproate in patients with active epilepsy. *Epilepsia* 1990;31:324-33.
23 Hosking PG, Duncan JS, Sander JW. The epilepsy nurse specialist at a tertiary care hospital-improving the interface between primary and tertiary care. *Seizure* 2002;11:494-9.

Chronic migraine

Todd J Schwedt, associate professor of neurology

Mayo Clinic, Phoenix, AZ 85054, USA

Correspondence to: T J Schwedt schwedt.todd@mayo.edu

Cite this as: *BMJ* 2014;348:g1416

DOI: 10.1136/bmj.g1416

http://www.bmj.com/content/348/bmj.g1416

ABSTRACT

Chronic migraine is a disabling neurologic condition that affects 2% of the general population. Patients with chronic migraine have headaches on at least 15 days a month, with at least eight days a month on which their headaches and associated symptoms meet diagnostic criteria for migraine. Chronic migraine places an enormous burden on patients owing to frequent headaches; hypersensitivity to visual, auditory, and olfactory stimuli; nausea; and vomiting. It also affects society through direct and indirect medical costs. Chronic migraine typically develops after a slow increase in headache frequency over months to years. Several factors are associated with an increased risk of transforming to chronic migraine. The diagnosis requires a carefully performed patient interview and neurologic examination, sometimes combined with additional diagnostic tests, to differentiate chronic migraine from secondary headache disorders and other primary chronic headaches of long duration. Treatment takes a multifaceted approach that may include risk factor modification, avoidance of migraine triggers, drug and non-drug based prophylaxis, and abortive migraine treatment, the frequency of which is limited to avoid drug overuse. This article provides an overview of current knowledge regarding chronic migraine, including epidemiology, risk factors for its development, pathophysiology, diagnosis, management, and guidelines. The future of chronic migraine treatment and research is also discussed.

Introduction

Migraine is a neurologic condition characterized by attacks of headache; hypersensitivity to visual, auditory, olfactory, and cutaneous stimuli; nausea; and vomiting. Most people with migraine have "episodic migraine"—fewer than 15 days of headache each month. However, a subgroup of people with migraine has "chronic migraine," defined as at least 15 days of headache each month, including at least eight days a month on which the headache and associated symptoms are consistent with fully developed migraine attacks. Typically, chronic migraine develops after a slow increase in headache frequency over months to years, a process termed "migraine transformation." Chronic migraine is common, often affects people during their most productive years of life, exerts substantial individual and societal costs, and is associated with numerous comorbid disorders. Treatment includes avoidance of migraine triggers and risk factor modification, as well as drug and non-drug based treatments to prevent and abort migraine attacks.

This article uses the latest data to review the frequency of chronic migraine, risk factors associated with transformation to chronic migraine and reversion back to episodic migraine, the individual and societal burdens from chronic migraine, the pathophysiology of chronic migraine, and its diagnosis. Although few treatments have been adequately investigated specifically for chronic migraine, evidence based and experience based recommendations for treatment are discussed. This review concludes with recommended topics to discuss with patients, thoughts about the future of research and treatment, a summary of published guidelines on the diagnosis and treatment of chronic migraine, and a discussion of the design of chronic migraine clinical trials.

Epidemiology

Estimates of the prevalence of chronic migraine throughout the world range from 0% to 5.1%, with most general population studies reporting a prevalence of 1.4-2.2%.[1] The variation probably reflects true differences among populations and the use of different definitions. Data from the United States show that the prevalence of chronic migraine increases throughout adolescence, peaks in midlife, and then declines after age 50 years (fig 1).[2] The highest prevalence is in women aged 18-49 years.[2] In population based samples, chronic migraine accounts for about 8% of all migraine cases.[2] The proportion of migraineurs with a chronic migraine pattern increases slightly with age.

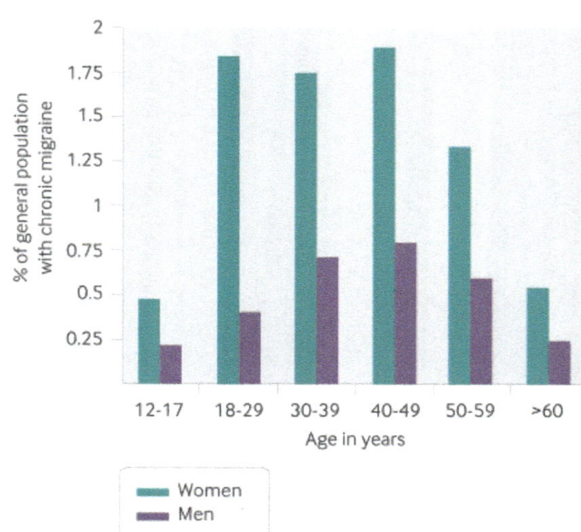

Fig 1 Prevalence of chronic migraine in the United States according to age[2]

SUMMARY POINTS

- Chronic migraine describes the migraine pattern in which a person has at least 15 headache days a month, including at least eight days a month with fully developed migraines
- Chronic migraine is a common and disabling neurologic disorder
- Patients with less frequent migraines (episodic migraine) should be counseled on avoiding risk factors associated with transformation to chronic migraine
- The treatment of chronic migraine includes avoidance of risk factors for chronic migraine, avoidance of migraine attack triggers, use of prophylactic and abortive drugs, and non-drug treatment
- The recognition and management of disorders that are comorbid with chronic migraine optimizes patient outcomes

Transformation and reversion factors

Each year, about 2.5% of people with episodic migraine transform to chronic migraine.[3] Factors associated with an increased risk of transformation include obesity, snoring, sleep disorders, excessive caffeine intake, psychiatric disease, high frequency of headaches at baseline, frequent use of abortive migraine drugs, female sex, lower socioeconomic status, comorbid pain disorders, history of head or neck injury, and presence of cutaneous allodynia.[4 5 6] Major life changes, such as divorce, marriage, or change of employment status, also increase the risk of transformation to chronic migraine.[7]

Clinicians must be aware of modifiable risk factors associated with the development of chronic migraine so that they can counsel their patients to avoid these risk factors. Patients and clinicians must be especially aware of too frequent use of migraine abortive drugs ("medication overuse") as a risk factor because it is common in this clinical population. The prevalence of chronic migraine with medication overuse is 0.3-1.1% in the general population.[1] About half of people with chronic migraine who present to specialty headache clinics have medication overuse.[8] Estimates of medication overuse among people with chronic migraine in the general population vary widely—from one third to two thirds.[1]

The risk of developing chronic migraine depends on the frequency with which abortive drugs are used and the type of drug used. The highest risks are associated with barbiturates (odds ratio 1.7; critical frequency of five usage days/month) and opioids (odds ratio 1.4; critical frequency of eight usage days/month).[3] Overuse of migraine specific agents such as triptans is also associated with an increased risk of transformation, albeit a lower risk than that associated with overuse of butalbital and opiates.[9 10 11] Non-steroidal anti-inflammatory drugs (NSAIDs) might reduce the risk of transformation in patients with up to nine headache days a month but increase the risk in patients with 10-14 headache days a month.[3 12]

Fortunately, patients with chronic migraine often revert to episodic migraine. A general population study of 383 people with chronic migraine found that 33.9% had persistent chronic migraine during the two years after enrollment, 26.1% reverted to fewer than 10 headache days a month (low frequency episodic migraine), and 40% transitioned in and out of chronic migraine.[13] These data are consistent with results from other studies suggesting that chronic migraine is a "fluid" state, with many patients flowing in and out of a chronic migraine pattern over time.[6] Factors that may be associated with reversion of chronic migraine include lower baseline frequency of headaches (15-19 *v* 25-31 headache days/month), absence of allodynia, adherence to prophylactic drugs, withdrawal of overused abortive drugs, and physical exercise.[6 13]

Box 1 lists the risk factors associated with chronic migraine transformation and reversion.

Individual and societal effects

Individual and societal costs related to migraine are enormous. According to the Global Burden of Disease 2010 study, migraine accounts for about 1% of global disability adjusted life years and is the 30th leading cause of disability adjusted life years.[14] Annual direct and indirect costs from headache are estimated at $20bn (£12.2bn; €14.7bn) in the United States and annual costs from migraine are €27bn in Europe.[15 16]

As expected, chronic migraine results in substantially greater disability than episodic migraine. Compared with episodic migraine, people with chronic migraine have lower income, are less likely to be employed full time, and are more likely to be occupationally disabled.[17] A large population based study found that over a three month period, 57% of people with chronic migraine missed at least five days of work or school compared with 24% of those with episodic migraine. In addition, 58% of those with chronic migraine and 18% with episodic migraine reported reduced productivity with household chores for at least five days over the three months.[18] About 25% of people with chronic migraine have very severe headache related disability according to scores on the migraine disability assessment scale, and about 90% have at least moderate levels of migraine related disability.[19 20] Compared with people with episodic migraine, those with chronic migraine are significantly more likely to have headaches of severe intensity and longer duration, whether treated or not; they are also more likely to have comorbid disorders.[20]

The use of healthcare resources is greater for patients with chronic migraine than for those with episodic migraine. People with chronic migraine visit primary care providers, specialists, and emergency departments more often. They are also admitted to hospital more often and require diagnostic tests and migraine drugs more often.[20 21] Annual

BOX 1 FACTORS ASSOCIATED WITH AN INCREASED RISK FOR TRANSFORMATION AND REVERSION OF CHRONIC MIGRAINE[3 4 5 6 7 13]

Transformation to chronic migraine
- Obesity
- Snoring
- Sleep disorders
- Excessive caffeine intake
- Psychiatric disease
- High baseline headache frequency
- Overuse of migraine abortive drugs
- Major life changes
- Head or neck injury
- Cutaneous allodynia
- Female sex
- Comorbid pain disorders
- Lower socioeconomic status

Reversion to episodic migraine
- Adherence to migraine prophylactic drugs
- Lower baseline headache frequency
- Absence of cutaneous allodynia
- Physical exercise
- Withdrawal of overused migraine abortive drugs

BOX 2 CHRONIC MIGRAINE DIAGNOSTIC CRITERIA[40]
- A: Headache (tension-type like or migraine like) on ≥15 days/month for >3 months and fulfilling criteria B and C
- B: Occurring in a patient who has had ≥5 attacks of migraine with or without aura
- C: On ≥8 days/month for >3 months, fulfilling any of the following:
  - Migraine without aura diagnostic criteria
  - Migraine with aura diagnostic criteria
  - Believed by the patient to be migraine at onset and relieved by a triptan or ergot derivative
- D: Not better accounted for by another headache diagnosis

total medical costs (direct and indirect) are 4.4 times greater in patients with chronic migraine ($7750) than in those with episodic migraine ($1757), with about 70% of the cost associated with chronic migraine being attributable to lost productive time.[22] In people with chronic migraine, an average of 4.6 hours of lost productive time per week is attributed to headache—0.8 hours of work absenteeism and 3.8 hours of presenteeism.[23]

Pathophysiology

The pathophysiology of chronic migraine and the mechanisms that result in transformation are not fully understood. However, the roles of atypical pain processing, central sensitization, cortical hyperexcitability, and neurogenic inflammation have been studied.

Atypical modulation of pain might play a role in transformation. Reduced inhibition of pain by regions of the descending pain modulatory pathway has been identified in chronic migraine.[24] In migraineurs, pain induced functional activation of pain inhibiting brainstem regions and the functional connectivity of brainstem pain modulatory regions are atypical.[25 26] Furthermore, the extent of these abnormalities correlates with the presence of cutaneous allodynia, a symptom of central sensitization.[25 26] It is postulated that recurrent migraine attacks lead to sensitization of the trigeminal system, which results in a reduced threshold for activation of this system, more frequent migraine attacks, and transformation to chronic migraine.[5] Cortical hyperexcitability might also contribute to transformation.[27 28 29] Transcranial magnetic stimulation studies of patients with chronic migraine suggest that the occipital cortex of these patients is hyperexcitable, even more so than in patients with episodic migraine.[30] The extent to which lack of cortical inhibition versus intrinsic cortical excitability contributes to this state is not clear.[31]

There is evidence that the structure and function of other pain processing regions in the brains of patients with migraine—for example, regions that participate in sensory discriminative, affective, and cognitive pain processing—are also atypical. Several studies have found positive correlations between the extent of these abnormalities and increasing frequency of headaches, suggesting that they are precursors to or biomarkers of transformation to chronic migraine.[32 33 34 35] Neuroimaging studies that have specifically studied patients with chronic migraine have found atypical pain processing and atypical structure of pain processing brain regions in this condition.[36 37 38]

Exuberant release of vasoactive neuropeptides such as calcitonin gene related peptide (CGRP) and the resultant neurogenic inflammation might also contribute to the pathophysiology of chronic migraine. A recent study found raised plasma concentrations of CGRP in migraineurs during the interictal phase of migraine compared with participants without migraine.[39] Furthermore, CGRP concentrations were higher in patients with chronic migraine than in those with episodic migraine. It is not clear whether high CGRP concentrations are the result of more frequent migraine attacks, thus serving as a potential biomarker of chronic migraine, or whether they are part of the process that leads to more frequent migraine attacks.

SOURCES AND SELECTION CRITERIA

PubMed was searched for manuscripts published between 1950 and October 2013 using the following search terms: "chronic migraine" or "transformed migraine" or "refractory chronic migraine" or "chronic migraine" and "prevalence" or "chronic migraine" and "incidence" or "chronic migraine" and "treatment" or "chronic migraine" and "disability" or "chronic migraine" and "diagnosis" or "chronic migraine" and "pathophysiology" or "chronic migraine" and "comorbidity" or "chronic migraine" and "guidelines." The search was limited to the English language. In addition, the reference lists of identified manuscripts and the author's own files were searched for relevant publications. Manuscripts were selected for inclusion on the basis of the author's assessment of the paper's originality, as well as its importance and relevance to the topics included in this review.

Diagnosis

History and examination

Diagnosis is made on the basis of the patient's symptoms and exclusion of other causes of frequent headache (box 2). The diagnostic process begins with a carefully obtained headache history, to collect the information needed to determine the level of suspicion for a primary versus a secondary headache disorder and to assign a specific headache diagnosis. While collecting information about medical history and headache characteristics, the clinician is searching for "red flag" features that increase the likelihood of a secondary headache disorder and may thus lead to further diagnostic testing. Box 3 lists common red flags.

General physical and neurologic examinations are performed, with any potentially relevant abnormalities increasing the suspicion for a secondary headache disorder. In addition to the typical neurologic examination, the examination should include attention to the patient's neck and shoulders, temporal artery pulses, and temporomandibular joint. A funduscopic examination should be performed and the examiner should palpate over the occipital and supraorbital nerves in search of tenderness. Abnormal neurologic findings cannot be attributed to migraine without first considering other causes. Most patients will present with typical features of chronic migraine and normal examination findings, so will not need additional diagnostic testing. However, further diagnostic evaluation is warranted when the history and examination leave the clinician with concerns that a secondary headache disorder exists.

Discussion of the indications for individual diagnostic tests is beyond the scope of this article. Tests that may be needed depend on the clinician's specific suspicions; they include blood tests, cervical spine imaging, sinus imaging, brain imaging, imaging of the brain arteries and venous sinuses, imaging of the cervical arteries, polysomnography, and lumbar puncture for cerebrospinal fluid analysis and measurement of opening pressure.

BOX 3 RED FLAGS FOR A SECONDARY HEADACHE DISORDER[41]

- Abnormal findings on neurologic examination
- Focal neurologic symptoms that are not consistent with typical migraine aura symptoms
- Systemic symptoms such as fevers, chills, and weight loss
- Rapid increase in headache frequency
- Orthostatic worsening of symptoms
- Exertional worsening of symptoms
- New onset headaches
- Thunderclap headaches (very severe headache that reaches maximum intensity in <1 min)
- Headaches in a patient with existing risk factors for a secondary headache (such as cancer or hypercoagulable state)
- Overuse of headache abortive drugs

Differentiating chronic migraine from other primary headaches

Once it is known that the patient has a primary headache disorder, the specific headache type must be determined. Chronic migraine is one of several primary headaches that manifests with at least 15 headache days a month for at least three consecutive months. Chronic migraine can be differentiated from these other primary chronic headaches with a similar pattern by first considering the duration of individual headaches. Headaches that are shorter than four hours are considered "short" and ones that are longer than four hours are "long."[42] Chronic headaches of long duration are attributed to one of four diagnoses: chronic migraine, new daily persistent headache, hemicrania continua, or chronic tension-type headache. These four headache types are usually easy to differentiate from one another (fig 2).

New daily persistent headache is differentiated according to the manner in which the headache condition began. Unlike patients with chronic migraine, who typically develop the disease after a slow progression in headache frequency, patients with new daily persistent headache have continuous headache within the first 24 hours of headache onset. Although new daily persistent headache can have similar features to those seen in chronic migraine, the timing of onset differentiates it from chronic migraine.

Hemicrania continua is a continuous side locked headache of mild to moderate severity, with superimposed exacerbations of pain associated with ipsilateral cranial autonomic features (such as lacrimation, conjunctival injection, or rhinorrhea). Although mild to moderate cranial autonomic features can be present with migraine, the autonomic features of hemicrania continua are more common and more prominent. Occasionally it can be difficult to differentiate chronic migraine from hemicrania continua on the basis of symptoms alone. However, hemicrania continua is an "indometacin responsive" headache syndrome, meaning it is completely responsive to adequate doses of indometacin. Thus, a trial of indometacin is necessary for the formal diagnosis of hemicrania continua and helps to differentiate this condition from chronic migraine.[40]

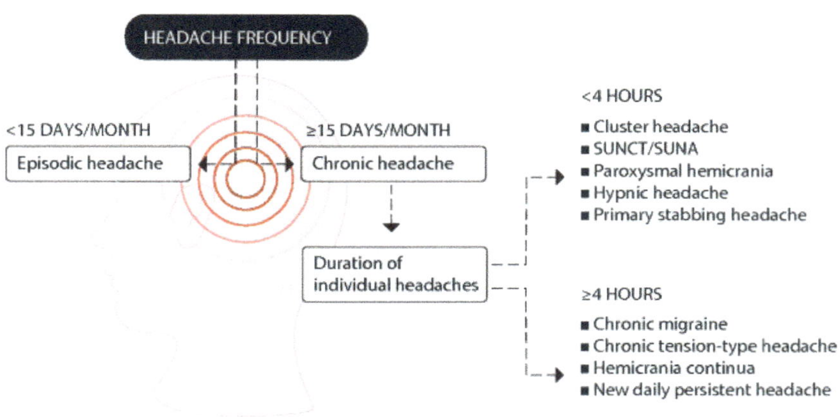

Fig 2 Differentiating chronic migraine from other primary headaches. The differentiation of primary headaches is first made according to headache frequency. Headaches occurring on fewer than 15 days a month are considered "episodic," whereas those occurring on at least 15 days a month are considered "chronic." Chronic headaches can be subdivided according to the duration of individual headaches. Headaches shorter than four hours are considered "short duration," whereas those lasting at least four hours are "long duration." Chronic migraine is a chronic headache of long duration. SUNCT=short lasting unilateral neuralgiform headache attacks with conjunctival injection and tearing; SUNA=short lasting unilateral neuralgiform headache attacks with cranial autonomic symptoms

Chronic tension-type headache is a "featureless" headache—it is not accompanied by migraine symptoms such as hypersensitivity to light and sound, nausea, or vomiting. In addition, the pain of tension-type headache is mild to moderate, whereas the pain of full-blown migraine attacks is moderate to severe. Notably, patients with chronic migraine often have days on which headaches resemble tension-type headache. They must, however, have at least eight days a month during which they experience full-blown migraine symptoms or are successfully treated with a triptan or ergot derivative for a presumed migraine before full expression of migraine features.[40]

Comorbid conditions

The identification and management of disorders that are comorbid with chronic migraine improve treatment outcomes. Chronic migraine is comorbid with sleep disorders, fatigue, other pain disorders, other neurologic disorders, psychiatric illness, cerebrovascular disease, cardiovascular disease, and gastrointestinal problems.[43 44 45 46 47 48 49] Compared with people with episodic migraine, patients with chronic migraine are twice as likely to have depression, anxiety, and other chronic pain. They are also significantly more likely to have bipolar disorder, respiratory illness (such as asthma and chronic obstructive pulmonary disease), heart disease, and vascular risk factors (such as hypertension and high cholesterol).[17]

Treatment

The main goals of treatment are to reduce the frequency of migraine attacks and to reduce migraine related disability while avoiding the overuse of migraine abortive

BOX 4 MEDICATION OVERUSE HEADACHE

- Headache occurs on at least 15 days/month in a patient with a pre-existing headache disorder
- Regular overuse* for longer than 3 months of one or more drugs that can be used for acute or symptomatic headache treatment
- Not better accounted for by another headache diagnosis

**Intake of ergotamine, triptans, opioids, combination analgesics (such as tablets that combine simple analgesics with opioids, butalbital, or caffeine), or drugs from multiple drug classes on at least 10 days/month. Intake of simple analgesics for at least 15 days/month.*

BOX 5 DRUG PROPHYLAXIS OF CHRONIC MIGRAINE*

Highest level evidence (≥2 randomized placebo controlled trials)

- Topiramate
- OnabotulinumtoxinA

Lower quality evidence (1 randomized study)

- Sodium valproate
- Gabapentin
- Tizanidine
- Amitriptyline

Lowest quality evidence (open label study)

- Atenolol
- Memantine
- Pregabalin
- Zonisamide

**The drugs listed have been studied specifically for prophylaxis in chronic migraine. However, drugs used for prophylaxis of episodic migraine are often used in chronic migraine, even in the absence of data supporting their use in this context.*

drugs. These goals are achieved through a combination of avoiding migraine triggers, dealing with modifiable risk factors, and using pharmacologic and non-pharmacologic prophylaxis. Migraine abortive drugs are also needed, but their frequency of use must be limited to avoid overuse and medication overuse headache. Medication overuse is diagnosed if abortive drugs are used regularly for more than three months on 10 or more, or 15 or more, days a month, depending on the drug (box 4).[40]

Risk factor modification and trigger avoidance

As discussed above, several risk factors for the development of chronic migraine and for the reversion to episodic migraine have been identified. On the basis of clinical experience and emerging data, it is recommended that the management of chronic migraine includes providing the patient with advice regarding exposure to modifiable risk factors.[50 51 52 53 54] Depending on the individual patient, advice might include losing weight, participating in a regular exercise routine, avoiding caffeine, avoiding alcohol, avoiding stress or modifying the response to stressors, getting sufficient sleep, and avoiding overuse of migraine abortive drugs. Patients should be instructed to maintain a daily headache diary, an activity that helps patients track their migraine patterns and identify their migraine triggers. Once triggers are identified, measures should be taken to avoid exposure to them.

Prophylaxis

Drug with high quality evidence (≥2 randomized placebo controlled trials)

Data from relatively large randomized placebo controlled studies provide support for the use of topiramate and onabotulinumtoxinA (botulinum toxin type A) for prophylaxis in chronic migraine (box 5). Although many drugs used for prophylaxis in episodic migraine and chronic migraine are prescribed off label, onabotulinumtoxinA is the only one that is approved by the Food and Drug Administration for chronic migraine.

Topiramate has been studied for prophylaxis in three randomized placebo controlled clinical trials.[55 56 57] In the Silberstein study, 306 patients with a baseline of 17 migraine/migrainous days a month received topiramate at a mean dose of 86 mg/day (maximum dose 100 mg/day) or placebo. At 90 days, topiramate was superior to placebo for the primary efficacy endpoint of change from baseline in the mean number of monthly migraine/migrainous days (topiramate −6.4 days *v* placebo −4.7 days, P=0.01). A high dropout rate limits the quality of study results, with only 55.8% of the patients treated with topiramate and 55.2% of those treated with placebo completing the trial.

In the other two trials of topiramate, most patients overused migraine abortive drugs and sample sizes were relatively small.[55 57] Nonetheless, both found topiramate to be superior to placebo. In Diener and colleagues' study, after about three months of follow-up, 100 mg of topiramate reduced the mean number of monthly migraine days when compared with placebo. The treatment group (n=32) had 3.5 (standard deviation 6.3) fewer days with migraine a month (baseline headache frequency 15.5 (4.6) migraine days a month) compared with 0.2 (4.7) fewer days with migraine a month (baseline headache frequency 16.4 (4.4) migraine days a month; P<0.05 for comparison between treatment groups) in the placebo group (n=27). In Silvestrini and colleagues' study, 28 patients with an average baseline headache frequency of 21 days a month were randomized 1:1 to low dose topiramate at 50 mg daily or placebo. During month two of treatment, participants receiving topiramate had fewer headache days than those receiving placebo (8.1 (8.1) *v* 20.6 (3.4); P<0.001). More common topiramate related side effects in these studies included weight loss, paresthesias, fatigue, difficulty concentrating, dry mouth, and nausea.

Two large randomized placebo controlled studies with identical study designs have investigated onabotulinumtoxinA for prophylaxis in chronic migraine.[58 59 60 61] In total, 1384 participants were randomized 1:1 to injections of onabotulinumtoxinA or placebo. Two thirds of subjects met criteria for overuse of abortive migraine drugs. Baseline headache frequency averaged nearly 20 days with headache per 28 days. A pooled analysis of the two trials found reductions in the mean change from baseline in number of headache days in participants treated with onabotulinumtoxinA and in those receiving placebo injections. However, onabotulinumtoxinA was significantly more effective than placebo at all time points from four weeks until 24 weeks after the first treatment. At the primary endpoint of 24 weeks, the mean reduction in headache days was 8.4 days per 28 days in the onabotulinumtoxinA group and 6.6 days per 28 days in the placebo group (P<0.001). More common onabotulinumtoxinA related side effects in these studies included neck pain, other musculoskeletal pain, injection site pain, eyelid ptosis, muscular weakness, and headache.

Drugs with lower quality evidence (1 randomized trial)

Sodium valproate was studied in a small randomized placebo controlled clinical trial in which 17 patients with chronic migraine received 500 mg sodium valproate twice daily, whereas 12 received placebo.[62] After three months, patients taking sodium valproate had significantly fewer headaches (5.2 *v* 22 headache days a month), whereas those receiving placebo had no change from baseline (22.3 headache days a month; P<0.05 for comparison between the two cohorts). Reported treatment related side effects included somnolence, tremor, impotence, and hair loss.

Gabapentin 2400 mg was investigated for prophylaxis in a study of 95 participants—22 with chronic migraine and 58 with "combination migraine and tension-type headache"—some of whom were "analgesic overusers."[63] Gabapentin was significantly better than placebo for the proportion of days free of headache (10% of days headache free at baseline *v* 26.6% of days headache free with gabapentin *v* 17.5% of days headache free with placebo; P<0.001 for comparison of gabapentin and placebo). Treatment outcomes for patients with migraine were not reported separately from those for patients with tension-type headache. Adverse events experienced by more than 5% of patients taking gabapentin included dizziness, somnolence, ataxia, and nausea.

Tizanidine (mean dose of 18 mg/day) was compared with placebo in a 1:1 randomized clinical trial of prophylaxis for frequent headaches in 92 participants who met criteria for efficacy analyses (at least eight weeks of double blind treatment without major protocol violations).[64] About 75% of participants had chronic migraine. Tizanidine was significantly superior to placebo for the primary endpoint of headache index (headache index = sum (headache days ×

average intensity × duration in hours)/28 days; P=0.0025). Post hoc analysis showed no differences in outcomes between patients with chronic migraine and those with migrainous or tension-type headaches. Tizanidine associated side effects included somnolence, dizziness, dry mouth, and asthenia.

Amitriptyline was compared with onabotulinumtoxinA for prophylaxis in a 1:1 randomized but non-blinded non-placebo controlled trial of 72 patients with chronic migraine.[65] Amitriptyline, at doses of 25-50 mg daily, had similar benefits to onabotulinumtoxinA. The number of days with pain was reduced by at least 50% in 72% of participants receiving amitriptyline and 67.8% of those taking onabotulinumtoxinA. Pain intensity was reduced by at least 3 points on a visual analog scale in 55.6% of patients receiving amitriptyline and 50% of those taking onabotulinumtoxinA. Lastly, the number of doses of analgesic given was reduced by least 50% in 71% of patients receiving amitriptyline and 77% of those taking onabotulinumtoxinA. Common side effects of amitriptyline included weight gain, dry mouth, somnolence, and constipation.

Open label studies provide lower quality but promising evidence for effective treatment of chronic migraine with atenolol, memantine, zonisamide, and pregabalin.[66 67 68 69]

Prophylaxis with a combination of drugs might be considered if the response to monotherapy is poor.[70] Published data in support of combining migraine prophylactic drugs are limited, and one study suggests that a combination of topiramate and propranolol is no more effective than topiramate alone for treating chronic migraine.[71] However, combination therapy is often used in clinical practice. The efficacy of this treatment approach requires further investigation. If combination therapy is used, drugs with differing mechanisms of action should be considered.

Drugs used for both episodic migraine and chronic migraine

Many drugs commonly used for treating episodic migraine are used for treating chronic migraine, despite the lack of evidence supporting their utility in this form of migraine. It is generally assumed that these drugs are effective in chronic migraine, but future investigations should test this assumption.

Non-drug treatments

Non-drug treatments such as physical therapy, behavioral therapy (for example, relaxation techniques, biofeedback, and cognitive behavioral therapy), massage, acupuncture, and physical exercise may be considered as adjuncts for the treatment of chronic migraine.[54 72 73 74 75] The choice of treatment should be guided by the needs of individual patients. For example, a patient with muscle tension in the neck and shoulders might benefit from physical therapy and massage, whereas someone with migraine related anxiety might be a good candidate for relaxation therapy.

Refractory chronic migraine

Despite use of best treatments, some patients with chronic migraine are refractory to conventional treatments. The prevalence of refractory chronic migraine in the general population is unknown, but about 5% of patents seen in specialty headache clinics are estimated to have refractory migraine, mostly refractory chronic migraine.[76] Before labeling a patient as having refractory migraine, it is important to assess the details of previous trials of treatment, including adherence to treatment, the maximum dose of drug used, and the duration for which the treatment was trialed. It is not uncommon for patients to consider themselves to have "failed" numerous drug treatments, when in reality they were not given adequate trials owing to the use of sub-therapeutic doses or insufficient trial durations (or both).

Topics to discuss with patients

Active participation in treatment

The high frequency of symptoms in chronic migraine and the often unpredictable timing of severe migraine attacks can result in patients feeling that they have no control over their illness.[77 78] This can translate into patients taking a passive role in their treatment. It must be stressed to patients that treatment outcomes will be optimized only if they take an active role in their treatment. Active participation can include:

- Maintaining a headache and migraine trigger diary to identify migraine triggers and assess changes in migraine patterns over time
- Modifying lifestyle to minimize exposure to migraine triggers and risk factors
- Adhering to drug and non-drug based treatments.

Avoid drug overuse

Patients must be counseled about the negative effects of overusing abortive drugs. Until educated about drug overuse, most patients do not recognize that the frequent use of abortive migraine drugs can lead to headaches becoming more frequent and less responsive to other treatments for migraine. Clinicians should set limits on the average number of days a week that abortive migraine drugs can be used. On the basis of expert opinion, drug overuse is diagnosed in patients who have regularly used ergotamines, triptans, opioids, combination analgesics, or drugs from multiple classes on at least 10 days a month or simple analgesics on at least 15 days a month for at least three months (box 4).[40] For the successful avoidance of drug overuse, it is essential that the clinician works with the patient to find effective prophylactic treatments that reduce headache frequency. If drug overuse is present, treatment typically consists of patient education and counseling, withdrawal of the overused drug, and migraine prophylactic treatment.[79 80]

Be patient with prophylactic treatments

Patients with migraine often expect immediate results from new drugs. To improve adherence to treatment and reduce patient frustration, clinicians should make patients aware of the expected interval between starting a new drug and obtaining relief. Once the target dose is reached, six to eight weeks of treatment might be needed before maximum benefits are realized.

The goal is control

Patients should be advised that a realistic goal of treatment is to reduce the frequency and severity of their migraine symptoms and their migraine related disability. Unfortunately, the goal is not complete remission or cure of migraine.

Looking ahead

Research

An improved understanding of the pathophysiologic mechanisms involved in the transformation from episodic migraine to chronic migraine and reversion to episodic migraine is needed to develop methods of inhibiting transformation and supporting reversion. Several laboratories have developed animal models that reflect physiologic components of chronic migraine. It is hoped that such models will yield insights into mechanisms of chronic migraine transformation and reversion.[81 82 83 84]

A recent study in humans suggests that plasma concentrations of CGRP measured between migraine attacks might serve as a biomarker for chronic migraine.[39] Future studies should evaluate the utility of measuring concentrations of CGRP and other vasoactive neuropeptides to predict transformation, predict treatment responses, and assess early responses to migraine prophylaxis. Structural and functional neuroimaging biomarkers for predicting transformation and reversion and for predicting treatment response are also being sought. Structural measures (such as cortical thickness and volumetrics) and functional measures (such as regional activation and resting state functional connectivity) might help to advance our understanding of mechanisms involved in chronic migraine and help to identify chronic migraine biomarkers. Studies investigating genetic profiles that predispose people to developing chronic migraine are needed. Large, longitudinal, multicenter studies that collect detailed phenotypic, biologic, and neuroimaging data would greatly enhance the efficiency of chronic migraine research.

Further work is needed to delineate the diagnostic criteria for chronic migraine more accurately. The current diagnostic requirement of at least 15 headache days a month was set arbitrarily on the basis of expert consensus. Future studies should explore associations between the frequency of headache and physiologic, imaging, and phenotypic characteristics with the goal of refining criteria that differentiate episodic migraine from chronic migraine. These studies should also explore further subgrouping of patients with chronic migraine, such as differentiating patients who have constant, unremitting headache from those who have periods of freedom from headache.

Future drug treatments

New drugs that are more effective, better tolerated, and have fewer contraindications are needed. Several new classes of drug are under investigation for the abortive or prophylactic treatment of migraine. These include: CGRP antagonists, anti-CGRP antibodies, anti-CGRP receptor antibodies, 5-hydroxytryptamine type 1F (5HT-1F) receptor agonists, nitric oxide synthetase inhibitors, pituitary adenylate activating peptide (PACAP) receptor antagonists, transient receptor potential subfamily V member 1 (TRPV1) antagonists, and glutamate receptor antagonists (clinicaltrials.gov).[85] New methods of delivering existing migraine abortive drug are under study, including transdermal delivery of sumatriptan, a bidirectional nasal delivery system for sumatriptan, and oral inhalation of dihydroergotamine (clinicaltrials.gov).[86] In addition, drugs commonly used for treating episodic migraine should be tested for efficacy in chronic migraine in well designed randomized placebo controlled clinical trials.

KEY RESEARCH QUESTIONS

- What mechanisms underlie transformation from episodic migraine to chronic migraine?
- What animal models are optimal for studying chronic migraine?
- How can transformation to chronic migraine be best predicted and prevented at the level of the individual patient?
- What are the safest and most effective treatments for chronic migraine?

Future non-drug treatments

Electrical stimulation of peripheral nerves and transcranial brain stimulation are of interest for the treatment of chronic migraine.

A supraorbital and supratrochlear percutaneous nerve stimulator is available over the counter. A small, sham controlled study of this device (active stimulation n=34; sham stimulation n=33) in people with episodic migraine showed that 20 minutes of daily stimulation for three months resulted in 38% of patients having at least a 50% reduction in monthly migraine days (*v* 12.1% in the sham stimulation group, P=0.023).[87] The effectiveness of this stimulator in chronic migraine has yet to be investigated.

Occipital nerve stimulation through implanted stimulators continues to be investigated for the treatment of refractory chronic migraine. Several open label case series and two sham controlled clinical trials suggest that occipital nerve stimulation might provide some benefit for these patients.[88 89 90 91 92] However, the larger of the two sham controlled trials (the only one powered to test an a priori defined primary outcome) failed to show superiority of occipital nerve stimulation over sham stimulation for the primary outcome of at least a 50% reduction in average pain intensity with no increase in average headache duration.[92] Furthermore, adverse event rates, mostly as a result of lead migration, infection, and persistent stimulator related pain, have consistently been high in published reports. Further occipital nerve stimulation trials are currently under way (clinicaltrials.gov). Dual occipital and supraorbital nerve stimulation is also of interest.[93 94]

Sphenopalatine ganglion stimulation, vagal nerve stimulation, transcranial magnetic stimulation, and transcranial direct current stimulation have each shown early evidence of possible benefit for migraine treatment but require additional investigations to determine their safety and efficacy.[95 96 97 98]

Surgical deactivation of migraine trigger sites has been investigated in observational studies and a small controlled trial.[99 100 101 102] However, results from randomized controlled multicenter trials with long term follow-up have not been published. Therefore, there is currently insufficient evidence to support the use of such surgery for the treatment of migraine and it should be considered only within the context of clinical research trials.[103 104]

Chronic migraine guidelines

Chronic migraine diagnostic criteria

The newest diagnostic criteria for chronic migraine are available in the latest International Classification of Headache Disorders guideline.[40] These criteria should be used for assigning the diagnosis in all research studies and can help clinicians make a diagnosis in their patients.

Defining refractory chronic migraine

Guidelines for considering a patient with chronic migraine as "refractory" to treatment are available.[105 106 107 108] Such a definition is important for determining when it might be appropriate to recommend less well proved treatments or treatments that are still being investigated and are associated with greater risk (such as implanted stimulators). On the basis of expert consensus, the American Headache Society proposed the following definition for refractory chronic migraine:

- Headaches seriously interfere with function or quality of life despite modification of triggers, lifestyle factors, and adequate trials of drugs with established efficacy
- The patient did not respond to adequate trials of preventive drugs, alone or in combination, from at least two of four drug classes including β blockers, anticonvulsants, tricyclics, and calcium channel blockers
- The patient did not respond to adequate trials of abortive drugs, including both a triptan and dihydroergotamine intranasal or injectable formulation and either non-steroidal anti-inflammatory drugs or combination analgesics, unless contraindicated.

Management

Management guidelines specifically for chronic migraine are available from the Latin American and Brazilian Headache Societies, the German Migraine and Headache Society/German Society for Neurology, and the Austrian Headache Society/Swiss Headache Society.[109 110] Guidelines for the management of episodic migraine are available from the American Headache Society and American Academy of Neurology, Canadian Headache Society, the European Federation of Neurological Societies (EFNS), the Taiwan Headache Society, the Italian Society for the Study of Headache, headache specialists in India, and the Croatian Society for Neurovascular Disorders.[111 112 113 114 115 116 117 118 119] Although a comparison of guidelines is beyond the scope of this review, Loder and colleagues have published a comparison of the 2012 American Headache Society/American Academy of Neurology guidelines with the Canadian guidelines and the EFNS guidelines.[120] The European Headache Federation recently published a position statement on the use of neuromodulation for the treatment of chronic headaches.[121]

Clinical trial design for studies of chronic migraine

The International Headache Society clinical trials guidelines (2012) include guidance on conducting migraine clinical trials.[122] Guidelines for trials of prophylactic drugs for chronic migraine were published in 2008.[123] A series of papers was recently published that discusses important statistical considerations when studying the transformation and reversion of chronic migraine.[124 125 126 127]

Conclusions

Chronic migraine is a common neurologic condition that causes substantial pain, migraine hypersensitivity, and disability. Typically, chronic migraine develops after a slow increase in headache frequency over months to years. Clinicians and patients must be aware of modifiable risk factors associated with transformation to chronic migraine and reversion to episodic migraine. In addition to risk factor modification, treatment includes the avoidance of migraine attack triggers and the use of drug and non-drug abortive and prophylactic treatments.

Substantial advances have been achieved in defining chronic migraine, describing its pathophysiology, identifying risk factors associated with transformation and reversion, and identifying effective treatments. However, further work is needed within each of these areas. Animal models of chronic migraine, careful endophenotyping of patients, and advanced neuroimaging are likely to yield important additional insights. Furthermore, existing and new treatments for episodic migraine need to be studied in well designed clinical trials for their utility in treating chronic migraine.

Competing interests: I have read and understood the BMJ Group policy on declaration of interests and declare the following: in the past three years I have received personal compensation for consulting from Allergan, Levadex, Pfizer, Supernus, and Zogenix; I have received personal compensation for speaking from Allergan; and I have received research support from Merck.

Provenance and peer review: Commissioned; externally peer reviewed.

1 Natoli JL, Manack A, Dean B, Butler Q, Turkel CC, Stovner L, et al. Global prevalence of chronic migraine: a systematic review. *Cephalalgia* 2010;30:599-609.

2 Buse DC, Manack AN, Fanning KM, Serrano D, Reed ML, Turkel CC, et al. Chronic migraine prevalence, disability, and sociodemographic factors: results from the American Migraine Prevalence and Prevention Study. *Headache* 2012;52:1456-70.

3 Bigal ME, Serrano D, Buse D, Scher A, Stewart WF, Lipton RB. Acute migraine medications and evolution from episodic to chronic migraine: a longitudinal population-based study. *Headache* 2008;48:1157-68.

4 Bigal ME, Lipton RB. Obesity is a risk factor for transformed migraine but not chronic tension-type headache. *Neurology* 2006;67:252-7.

5 Louter MA, Bosker JE, van Oosterhout WP, van Zwet EW, Zitman FG, Ferrari MD, et al. Cutaneous allodynia as a predictor of migraine chronification. *Brain* 2013;136:3489-96.

6 Scher AI, Midgette LA, Lipton RB. Risk factors for headache chronification. *Headache* 2008;48:16-25.

7 Scher AI, Stewart WF, Buse D, Krantz DS, Lipton RB. Major life changes before and after the onset of chronic daily headache: a population-based study. *Cephalalgia* 2008;28:868-76.

8 Davies P. Medication overuse headache: a silent pandemic. *Pain* 2012;153:7-8.

9 Evers S, Gralow I, Bauer B, Suhr B, Buchheister A, Husstedt IW, et al. Sumatriptan and ergotamine overuse and drug-induced headache: a clinicoepidemiologic study. *Clin Neuropharmacol* 1999;22:201-6.

10 Limmroth V, Katsarava Z, Fritsche G, Przywara S, Diener HC. Features of medication overuse headache following overuse of different acute headache drugs. *Neurology* 2002;59:1011-4.

11 Lipton RB, Serrano D, Nicholson RA, Buse DC, Runken MC, Reed ML. Impact of NSAID and triptan use on developing chronic migraine: results from the American Migraine Prevalence and Prevention (AMPP) study. *Headache* 2013;53:1548-63.

12 Starling AJ, Hoffman-Snyder C, Halker RB, Wellik KE, Vargas BB, Dodick DW, et al. Risk of development of medication overuse headache with nonsteroidal anti-inflammatory drug therapy for migraine: a critically appraised topic. *Neurologist* 2011;17:297-9.

13 Manack A, Buse DC, Serrano D, Turkel CC, Lipton RB. Rates, predictors, and consequences of remission from chronic migraine to episodic migraine. *Neurology* 2011;76:711-8.

14 Murray CJ, Vos T, Lozano R, Naghavi M, Flaxman AD, Michaud C, et al. Disability-adjusted life years (DALYs) for 291 diseases and injuries in 21 regions, 1990-2010: a systematic analysis for the Global Burden of Disease Study 2010. *Lancet* 2012;380:2197-223.

15 Stovner LJ, Andree C. Impact of headache in Europe: a review for the Eurolight project. *J Headache Pain* 2008;9:139-46.

16 Stewart WF, Ricci JA, Chee E, Morganstein D, Lipton R. Lost productive time and cost due to common pain conditions in the US workforce. *JAMA* 2003;290:2443-54.

17 Buse DC, Manack A, Serrano D, Turkel C, Lipton RB. Sociodemographic and comorbidity profiles of chronic migraine and episodic migraine sufferers. *J Neurol Neurosurg Psychiatry* 2010;81:428-32.

18 Bigal ME, Serrano D, Reed M, Lipton RB. Chronic migraine in the population: burden, diagnosis, and satisfaction with treatment. *Neurology* 2008;71:559-66.

19 Buse D, Manack A, Serrano D, Reed M, Varon S, Turkel C, et al. Headache impact of chronic and episodic migraine: results from the American Migraine Prevalence and Prevention study. *Headache* 2012;52:3-17.

20 Stokes M, Becker WJ, Lipton RB, Sullivan SD, Wilcox TK, Wells L, et al. Cost of health care among patients with chronic and episodic migraine in Canada and the USA: results from the International Burden of Migraine Study (IBMS). *Headache* 2011;51:1058-77.

21 Blumenfeld AM, Varon SF, Wilcox TK, Buse DC, Kawata AK, Manack A, et al. Disability, HRQoL and resource use among chronic and episodic

migraineurs: results from the International Burden of Migraine Study (IBMS). *Cephalalgia* 2011;31:301-15.
22 Munakata J, Hazard E, Serrano D, Klingman D, Rupnow MF, Tierce J, et al. Economic burden of transformed migraine: results from the American Migraine Prevalence and Prevention (AMPP) study. *Headache* 2009;49:498-508.
23 Stewart WF, Wood GC, Manack A, Varon SF, Buse DC, Lipton RB. Employment and work impact of chronic migraine and episodic migraine. *J Occup Environ Med* 2010;52:8-14.
24 Aurora SK, Barrodale PM, Tipton RL, Khodavirdi A. Brainstem dysfunction in chronic migraine as evidenced by neurophysiological and positron emission tomography studies. *Headache* 2007;47:996-1003; discussion 1004-7.
25 Moulton EA, Burstein R, Tully S, Hargreaves R, Becerra L, Borsook D. Interictal dysfunction of a brainstem descending modulatory center in migraine patients. *PLoS One* 2008;3:e3799.
26 Schwedt TJ, Larson-Prior L, Coalson RS, Nolan T, Mar S, Ances BM, et al. Allodynia and descending pain modulation in migraine: a resting state functional connectivity analysis. *Pain Med* 2014;15:154-65.
27 Aurora SK. Spectrum of illness: understanding biological patterns and relationships in chronic migraine. *Neurology* 2009;72(5 suppl):S8-13.
28 Aurora SK. Is chronic migraine one end of a spectrum of migraine or a separate entity? *Cephalalgia* 2009;29:597-605.
29 Aurora SK, Kulthia A, Barrodale PM. Mechanism of chronic migraine. *Curr Pain Headache Rep* 2011;15:57-63.
30 Aurora SK, Barrodale P, Chronicle EP, Mulleners WM. Cortical inhibition is reduced in chronic and episodic migraine and demonstrates a spectrum of illness. *Headache* 2005;45:546-52.
31 Diener HC, Dodick DW, Goadsby PJ, Lipton RB, Olesen J, Silberstein SD. Chronic migraine—classification, characteristics and treatment. *Nat Rev Neurol* 2011;8:162-71.
32 Kim JH, Suh SI, Seol HY, Oh K, Seo WK, Yu SW, et al. Regional grey matter changes in patients with migraine: a voxel-based morphometry study. *Cephalalgia* 2008;28:598-604.
33 Maleki N, Becerra L, Nutile L, Pendse G, Brawn J, Bigal M, et al. Migraine attacks the basal ganglia. *Mol Pain* 2011;7:71.
34 Schmitz N, Admiraal-Behloul F, Arkink EB, Kruit MC, Schoonman GG, Ferrari MD, et al. Attack frequency and disease duration as indicators for brain damage in migraine. *Headache* 2008;48:1044-55.
35 Valfre W, Rainero I, Bergui M, Pinessi L. Voxel-based morphometry reveals gray matter abnormalities in migraine. *Headache* 2008;48:109-17.
36 De Tommaso M, Losito L, Difruscolo O, Libro G, Guido M, Livrea P. Changes in cortical processing of pain in chronic migraine. *Headache* 2005;45:1208-18.
37 Mongini F, Keller R, Deregibus A, Barbalonga E, Mongini T. Frontal lobe dysfunction in patients with chronic migraine: a clinical-neuropsychological study. *Psychiatry Res* 2005;133:101-6.
38 Schwedt TJ, Schlaggar BL, Mar S, Nolan T, Coalson RS, Nardos B, et al. Atypical resting-state functional connectivity of affective pain regions in chronic migraine. *Headache* 2013;53:737-51.
39 Cernuda-Morollon E, Larrosa D, Ramon C, Vega J, Martinez-Camblor P, Pascual J. Interictal increase of CGRP levels in peripheral blood as a biomarker for chronic migraine. *Neurology* 2013;81:1191-6.
40 The International Classification of Headache Disorders, 3rd ed (beta version). *Cephalalgia* 2013;33:629-808.
41 Bigal ME, Lipton RB. The differential diagnosis of chronic daily headaches: an algorithm-based approach. *J Headache Pain* 2007;8:263-72.
42 Welch KM, Goadsby PJ. Chronic daily headache: nosology and pathophysiology. *Curr Opin Neurol* 2002;15:287-95.
43 Bigal ME, Kurth T, Santanello N, Buse D, Golden W, Robbins M, et al. Migraine and cardiovascular disease: a population-based study. *Neurology* 2010;74:628-35.
44 Chen YC, Tang CH, Ng K, Wang SJ. Comorbidity profiles of chronic migraine sufferers in a national database in Taiwan. *J Headache Pain* 2012;13:311-9.
45 De Tommaso M, Sardaro M, Serpino C, Costantini F, Vecchio E, Prudenzano MP, et al. Fibromyalgia comorbidity in primary headaches. *Cephalalgia* 2009;29:453-64.
46 Kruit MC, van Buchem MA, Launer LJ, Terwindt GM, Ferrari MD. Migraine is associated with an increased risk of deep white matter lesions, subclinical posterior circulation infarcts and brain iron accumulation: the population-based MRI CAMERA study. *Cephalalgia* 2010;30:129-36.
47 Riedl A, Schmidtmann M, Stengel A, Goebel M, Wisser AS, Klapp BF, et al. Somatic comorbidities of irritable bowel syndrome: a systematic analysis. *J Psychosom Res* 2008;64:573-82.
48 Spector JT, Kahn SR, Jones MR, Jayakumar M, Dalal D, Nazarian S. Migraine headache and ischemic stroke risk: an updated meta-analysis. *Am J Med* 2010;123:612-24.
49 Teixeira AL, Costa EA, da Silva AA Jr, dos Santos IA, Gomez RS, Kummer A, et al. Psychiatric comorbidities of chronic migraine in community and tertiary care clinic samples. *J Headache Pain* 2012;13:551-5.
50 Verrotti A, Agostinelli S, D'Egidio C, Di Fonzo A, Carotenuto M, Parisi P, et al. Impact of a weight loss program on migraine in obese adolescents. *Eur J Neurol* 2013;20:394-7.
51 Hershey AD, Powers SW, Nelson TD, Kabbouche MA, Winner P, Yonker M, et al. Obesity in the pediatric headache population: a multicentre study. *Headache* 2009;49:170-7.
52 Narin SO, Pinar L, Erbas D, Ozturk V, Idiman F. The effects of exercise and exercise-related changes in blood nitric oxide level on migraine headache. *Clin Rehabil* 2003;17:624-30.
53 Pryse-Phillips WE, Dodick DW, Edmeads JG, Gawel MJ, Nelson RF, Purdy RA, et al. Guidelines for the nonpharmacologic management of migraine in clinical practice. Canadian Headache Society. *CMAJ* 1998;159:47-54.
54 Varkey E, Cider A, Carlsson J, Linde M. Exercise as migraine prophylaxis: a randomized study using relaxation and topiramate as controls. *Cephalalgia* 2011;31:1428-38.
55 Diener HC, Bussone G, Van Oene JC, Lahaye M, Schwalen S, Goadsby PJ. Topiramate reduces headache days in chronic migraine: a randomized, double-blind, placebo-controlled study. *Cephalalgia* 2007;27:814-23.
56 Silberstein SD, Lipton RB, Dodick DW, Freitag FG, Ramadan N, Mathew N, et al. Efficacy and safety of topiramate for the treatment of chronic migraine: a randomized, double-blind, placebo-controlled trial. *Headache* 2007;47:170-80.
57 Silvestrini M, Bartolini M, Coccia M, Baruffaldi R, Taffi R, Provinciali L. Topiramate in the treatment of chronic migraine. *Cephalalgia* 2003;23:820-4.
58 Aurora SK, Dodick DW, Turkel CC, DeGryse RE, Silberstein SD, Lipton RB, et al. OnabotulinumtoxinA for treatment of chronic migraine: results from the double-blind, randomized, placebo-controlled phase of the PREEMPT 1 trial. *Cephalalgia* 2010;30:793-803.
59 Aurora SK, Winner P, Freeman MC, Spierings EL, Heiring JO, DeGryse RE, et al. OnabotulinumtoxinA for treatment of chronic migraine: pooled analyses of the 56-week PREEMPT clinical program. *Headache* 2011;51:1358-73.
60 Diener HC, Dodick DW, Aurora SK, Turkel CC, DeGryse RE, Lipton RB, et al. OnabotulinumtoxinA for treatment of chronic migraine: results from the double-blind, randomized, placebo-controlled phase of the PREEMPT 2 trial. *Cephalalgia* 2010;30:804-14.
61 Dodick DW, Turkel CC, DeGryse RE, Aurora SK, Silberstein SD, Lipton RB, et al. OnabotulinumtoxinA for treatment of chronic migraine: pooled results from the double-blind, randomized, placebo-controlled phases of the PREEMPT clinical program. *Headache* 2010;50:921-36.
62 Yurekli VA, Akhan G, Kutluhan S, Uzar E, Koyuncuoglu HR, Gultekin F. The effect of sodium valproate on chronic daily headache and its subgroups. *J Headache Pain* 2008;9:37-41.
63 Spira PJ, Beran RG. Gabapentin in the prophylaxis of chronic daily headache: a randomized, placebo-controlled study. *Neurology* 2003;61:1753-9.
64 Saper JR, Lake AE 3rd, Cantrell DT, Winner PK, White JR. Chronic daily headache prophylaxis with tizanidine: a double-blind, placebo-controlled, multicenter outcome study. *Headache* 2002;42:470-82.
65 Magalhaes E, Menezes C, Cardeal M, Melo A. Botulinum toxin type A versus amitriptyline for the treatment of chronic daily migraine. *Clin Neurol Neurosurg* 2010;112:463-6.
66 Calandre EP, Garcia-Leiva JM, Rico-Villademoros F, Vilchez JS, Rodriguez-Lopez CM. Pregabalin in the treatment of chronic migraine: an open-label study. *Clin Neuropharmacol* 2010;33:35-9.
67 Edvardsson B. Atenolol in the prophylaxis of chronic migraine: a 3-month open-label study. *Springerplus* 2013;2:479.
68 Pascual-Gomez J, Alana-Garcia M, Oterino A, Leira R, Lainez-Andres JM. [Preventive treatment of chronic migraine with zonisamide: a study in patients who are refractory or intolerant to topiramate]. *Rev Neurol* 2008;47:449-51.
69 Bigal M, Rapopot A, Sheftell F, Tepper D, Tepper S. Memantine in the preventive treatment of refractory migraine. *Headache* 2008;48:1337-42.
70 Peterlin BL, Calhoun AH, Siegel S, Mathew NT. Rational combination therapy in refractory migraine. *Headache* 2008;48:805-19.
71 Silberstein SD, Dodick DW, Lindblad AS, Holroyd K, Harrington M, Mathew NT, et al. Randomized, placebo-controlled trial of propranolol added to topiramate in chronic migraine. *Neurology* 2012;78:976-84.
72 Andrasik F. Behavioral treatment of migraine: current status and future directions. *Expert Rev Neurother* 2004;4:403-13.
73 Nestoriuc Y, Martin A. Efficacy of biofeedback for migraine: a meta-analysis. *Pain* 2007;128:111-27.
74 Pistoia F, Sacco S, Carolei A. Behavioral therapy for chronic migraine. *Curr Pain Headache Rep* 2013;17:304.
75 Yang CP, Chang MH, Liu PE, Li TC, Hsieh CL, Hwang KL, et al. Acupuncture versus topiramate in chronic migraine prophylaxis: a randomized clinical trial. *Cephalalgia* 2011;31:1510-21.
76 Irimia P, Palma JA, Fernandez-Torron R, Martinez-Vila E. Refractory migraine in a headache clinic population. *BMC Neurol* 2011;11:94.
77 Martin NJ, Holroyd KA, Penzien DB. The headache-specific locus of control scale: adaptation to recurrent headaches. *Headache* 1990;30:729-34.
78 Scharff L, Turk DC, Marcus DA. The relationship of locus of control and psychosocial-behavioral response in chronic headache. *Headache* 1995;35:527-33.
79 Hagen K, Albretsen C, Vilming ST, Salvesen R, Gronning M, Helde G, et al. Management of medication overuse headache: 1-year randomized multicentre open-label trial. *Cephalalgia* 2009;29:221-32.
80 Zeeberg P, Olesen J, Jensen R. Discontinuation of medication overuse in headache patients: recovery of therapeutic responsiveness. *Cephalalgia* 2006;26:1192-8.
81 Melo-Carrillo A, Lopez-Avila A. A chronic animal model of migraine, induced by repeated meningeal nociception, characterized

by a behavioral and pharmacological approach. *Cephalalgia* 2013;33:1096-105.
82 Oshinsky ML, Gomonchareonsiri S. Episodic dural stimulation in awake rats: a model for recurrent headache. *Headache* 2007;47:1026-36.
83 Pusic AD, Grinberg YY, Mitchell HM, Kraig RP. Modeling neural immune signaling of episodic and chronic migraine using spreading depression in vitro. *J Vis Exp* 2011;(52). pii: 2910.
84 Stucky NL, Gregory E, Winter MK, He YY, Hamilton ES, McCarson KE, et al. Sex differences in behavior and expression of CGRP-related genes in a rodent model of chronic migraine. *Headache* 2011;51:674-92.
85 Silberstein SD. Emerging target-based paradigms to prevent and treat migraine. *Clin Pharmacol Ther* 2013;93:78-85.
86 Rapoport AM. The therapeutic future in headache. *Neurol Sci* 2012;33(suppl 1):S119-25.
87 Schoenen J, Vandersmissen B, Jeangette S, Herroelen L, Vandenheede M, Gerard P, et al. Migraine prevention with a supraorbital transcutaneous stimulator: a randomized controlled trial. *Neurology* 2013;80:697-704.
88 Oh MY, Ortega J, Bellotte JB, Whiting DM, Alo K. Peripheral nerve stimulation for the treatment of occipital neuralgia and transformed migraine using a c1-2-3 subcutaneous paddle style electrode: a technical report. *Neuromodulation* 2004;7:103-12.
89 Popeney CA, Alo KM. Peripheral neurostimulation for the treatment of chronic, disabling transformed migraine. *Headache* 2003;43:369-75.
90 Saper JR, Dodick DW, Silberstein SD, McCarville S, Sun M, Goadsby PJ. Occipital nerve stimulation for the treatment of intractable chronic migraine headache: ONSTIM feasibility study. *Cephalalgia* 2011;31:271-85.
91 Schwedt TJ, Dodick DW, Hentz J, Trentman TL, Zimmerman RS. Occipital nerve stimulation for chronic headache--long-term safety and efficacy. *Cephalalgia* 2007;27:153-7.
92 Silberstein SD, Dodick DW, Saper J, Huh B, Slavin KV, Sharan A, et al. Safety and efficacy of peripheral nerve stimulation of the occipital nerves for the management of chronic migraine: results from a randomized, multicenter, double-blinded, controlled study. *Cephalalgia* 2012;32:1165-79.
93 Hann S, Sharan A. Dual occipital and supraorbital nerve stimulation for chronic migraine: a single-center experience, review of literature, and surgical considerations. *Neurosurg Focus* 2013;35:E9.
94 Reed KL, Black SB, Banta CJ 2nd, Will KR. Combined occipital and supraorbital neurostimulation for the treatment of chronic migraine headaches: initial experience. *Cephalalgia* 2010;30:260-71.
95 Cecchini AP, Mea E, Tullo V, Curone M, Franzini A, Broggi G, et al. Vagus nerve stimulation in drug-resistant daily chronic migraine with depression: preliminary data. *Neurol Sci* 2009;30(suppl 1):S101-4.
96 Lipton RB, Pearlman SH. Transcranial magnetic simulation in the treatment of migraine. *Neurotherapeutics* 2010;7:204-12.
97 Teepker M, Hotzel J, Timmesfeld N, Reis J, Mylius V, Haag A, et al. Low-frequency rTMS of the vertex in the prophylactic treatment of migraine. *Cephalalgia* 2010;30:137-44.
98 Tepper SJ, Rezai A, Narouze S, Steiner C, Mohajer P, Ansarinia M. Acute treatment of intractable migraine with sphenopalatine ganglion electrical stimulation. *Headache* 2009;49:983-9.
99 Chepla KJ, Oh E, Guyuron B. Clinical outcomes following supraorbital foraminotomy for treatment of frontal migraine headache. *Plast Reconstr Surg* 2012;129:656e-62e.
100 Guyuron B, Kriegler JS, Davis J, Amini SB. Comprehensive surgical treatment of migraine headaches. *Plast Reconstr Surg* 2005;115:1-9.
101 Guyuron B, Kriegler JS, Davis J, Amini SB. Five-year outcome of surgical treatment of migraine headaches. *Plast Reconstr Surg* 2011;127:603-8.
102 Guyuron B, Reed D, Kriegler JS, Davis J, Pashmini N, Amini S. A placebo-controlled surgical trial of the treatment of migraine headaches. *Plast Reconstr Surg* 2009;124:461-8.
103 Loder E, Weizenbaum E, Frishberg B, Silberstein S. Choosing wisely in headache medicine: the American Headache Society's list of five things physicians and patients should question. *Headache* 2013;53:1651-9.
104 Mathew PG. A critical evaluation of migraine trigger site deactivation surgery. *Headache* 2014;54:142-52.
105 Bussone G. Clinical considerations on chronic migraine, pharmacoresistance and refractoriness. *Neurol Sci* 2010;31(suppl 1):S83-5.
106 D'Amico D, Leone M, Grazzi L, Bussone G. When should "chronic migraine" patients be considered "refractory" to pharmacological prophylaxis? *Neurol Sci* 2008;29(suppl 1):S55-8.
107 Schulman EA, Lake AE 3rd, Goadsby PJ, Peterlin BL, Siegel SE, Markley HG, et al. Defining refractory migraine and refractory chronic migraine: proposed criteria from the refractory headache special interest section of the American Headache Society. *Headache* 2008;48:778-82.
108 Schulman EA, Peterlin BL, Lake AE 3rd, Lipton RB, Hanlon A, Siegel S, et al. Defining refractory migraine: results of the RHSIS survey of American Headache Society members. *Headache* 2009;49:509-18.
109 Giacomozzi AR, Vindas AP, da Silva AA Jr, Bordini CA, Buonanotte CF, Roesler CA, et al. Latin American consensus on guidelines for chronic migraine treatment. *Arq Neuropsiquiatr* 2013;71:478-86.
110 Straube A, Gaul C, Forderreuther S, Kropp P, Marziniak M, Evers S, et al. [Therapy and care of patients with chronic migraine: expert recommendations of the German Migraine and Headache Society/ German Society for Neurology as well as the Austrian Headache Society/Swiss Headache Society]. *Nervenarzt* 2012;83:1600-8.
111 Treatment Guideline Subcommittee of the Taiwan Headache Society. [Treatment guidelines for preventive treatment of migraine]. *Acta Neurol Taiwan* 2008;17:132-48.
112 Evers S, Afra J, Frese A, Goadsby PJ, Linde M, May A, et al. EFNS guideline on the drug treatment of migraine—revised report of an EFNS task force. *Eur J Neurol* 2009;16:968-81.
113 Holland S, Silberstein SD, Freitag F, Dodick DW, Argoff C, Ashman E. Evidence-based guideline update: NSAIDs and other complementary treatments for episodic migraine prevention in adults: report of the Quality Standards Subcommittee of the American Academy of Neurology and the American Headache Society. *Neurology* 2012;78:1346-53.
114 Pringsheim T, Davenport W, Mackie G, Worthington I, Aube M, Christie SN, et al. Canadian Headache Society guideline for migraine prophylaxis. *Can J Neurol Sci* 2012;39(2 suppl 2):S1-59.
115 Ravishankar K, Chakravarty A, Chowdhury D, Shukla R, Singh S. Guidelines on the diagnosis and the current management of headache and related disorders. *Ann Indian Acad Neurol* 2011;14(suppl 1):S40-59.
116 Sarchielli P, Granella F, Prudenzano MP, Pini LA, Guidetti V, Bono G, et al. Italian guidelines for primary headaches: 2012 revised version. *J Headache Pain* 2012;13(suppl 2):S31-70.
117 Silberstein SD. Practice parameter: evidence-based guidelines for migraine headache (an evidence-based review): report of the quality standards subcommittee of the American Academy of Neurology. *Neurology* 2000;55:754-62.
118 Silberstein SD, Holland S, Freitag F, Dodick DW, Argoff C, Ashman E. Evidence-based guideline update: pharmacologic treatment for episodic migraine prevention in adults: report of the quality standards subcommittee of the American Academy of Neurology and the American Headache Society. *Neurology* 2012;78:1337-45.
119 Vukovic Cvetkovic V, Kes VB, Seric V, Solter VV, Demarin V, Janculjak D, et al. Report of the Croatian Society for Neurovascular Disorders, Croatian Medical Association. Evidence based guidelines for treatment of primary headaches—2012 update. *Acta Clin Croat* 2012;51:323-78.
120 Loder E, Burch R, Rizzoli P. The 2012 AHS/AAN guidelines for prevention of episodic migraine: a summary and comparison with other recent clinical practice guidelines. *Headache* 2012;52:930-45.
121 Martelletti P, Jensen RH, Antal A, Arcioni R, Brighina F, de Tommaso M, et al. Neuromodulation of chronic headaches: position statement from the European Headache Federation. *J Headache Pain* 2013;14:86.
122 Tfelt-Hansen P, Pascual J, Ramadan N, Dahlof C, D'Amico D, Diener HC, et al. Guidelines for controlled trials of drugs in migraine: third edition. A guide for investigators. *Cephalalgia* 2012;32:6-38.
123 Silberstein S, Tfelt-Hansen P, Dodick DW, Limmroth V, Lipton RB, Pascual J, et al. Guidelines for controlled trials of prophylactic treatment of chronic migraine in adults. *Cephalalgia* 2008;28:484-95.
124 Houle TT, Turner DP, Houle TA, Smitherman TA, Martin V, Penzien DB, et al. Rounding behavior in the reporting of headache frequency complicates headache chronification research. *Headache* 2013;53:908-19.
125 Houle TT, Turner DP, Smitherman TA, Penzien DB, Lipton RB. Influence of random measurement error on estimated rates of headache chronification and remission. *Headache* 2013;53:920-9.
126 Lipton RB, Penzien DB, Turner DP, Smitherman TA, Houle TT. Methodological issues in studying rates and predictors of migraine progression and remission. *Headache* 2013;53:930-4.
127 Turner DP, Smitherman TA, Penzien DB, Lipton RB, Houle TT. Rethinking headache chronification. *Headache* 2013;53:901-7.

Pharmacological prevention of migraine

Nathan Fenstermacher, physician assistant, Morris Levin, co-director, Thomas Ward, co-director

Dartmouth Headache Centre, Dartmouth Hitchcock Medical Centre, Lebanon, NH 03756, USA

Correspondence to: N Fenstermacher nathan.p.fenstermacher@hitchcock.org

Cite this as: BMJ 2011;342:d583

DOI: 10.1136/bmj.d583

http://www.bmj.com/content/342/bmj.d583

People who have migraine experience intermittent attacks of unilateral, pulsating, and moderate to severe headache with associated nausea or photophobia and phonophobia (or all these symptoms). These attacks typically start before the age of 40, often in childhood or teenage years, and occur most commonly from the second to the fourth decade of life.[1] Attacks may be infrequent or frequent. Chronic migraine is diagnosed when attacks regularly occur on more than 15 days a month. Box 1 shows the International Headache Society's classification criteria for migraine without aura.

Recent population studies have shown the worldwide prevalence of migraine to be greater than 10%. The prevalence of migraine in the United States has been estimated at 18% for women, 6% for men, and 12% overall.[2 3] Migraine clearly affects women more than men, and its aetiology also seems to have a hereditary component. The World Health Organization ranks migraine 19th on the list of diseases worldwide that cause disability.[w1] In spite of recent advances in treatment options for migraine, both acute and preventive, these treatments continue to be underused,[3 4] which leaves patients with unnecessary suffering and increases the burden on the healthcare system. We review the different types of preventive treatment and discuss how they should be used to treat migraine effectively.

When to consider prevention for migraine

Specific clinical guidelines on when it is clinically appropriate to start preventive treatment vary between different countries and organisations. A high frequency of migraine, inadequate responsiveness to drugs used to treat migraine acutely, and migraines that greatly interfere with activities of daily life are accepted criteria for starting preventive treatment.[5 6 7] Box 2 lists the European Federation of Neurological Societies and American Academy of Neurology guidelines for starting preventive treatment. It is important to consider coexisting medical conditions and psychological diagnoses when deciding on a preventive treatment. A single drug may effectively treat the coexisting condition and prevent migraines in some circumstances. The importance of the discussion between practitioner and patient about preventive drugs and the reasons for considering their use is often overlooked. Shared decision making, which ensures that the patient understands the reasons for starting preventive treatment and feels comfortable with the drug chosen, increases the likelihood of adherence to the preventive treatment plan. Because overuse of analgesics and other acute drugs may make preventive drugs less effective, the patient should also be instructed to limit their use.[8] Simple analgesics should ideally be used on fewer than 15 days a month and combination analgesics and other acute drugs be limited to 10 days a month.[w2]

SUMMARY POINTS

- Accurate diagnosis of migraine is crucial to establishing an effective treatment plan
- Migraine cannot be cured, just prevented
- A preventive management plan must take into account coexisting conditions and the patient's preferences
- Preventive treatment should aim to decrease the frequency and severity of acute attacks, make acute treatments more efficacious, and minimise adverse drug reactions

What are the goals of preventive treatment?

The goals of preventive treatment mirror the criteria for starting these drugs. The major targets of preventive treatment are reduced frequency and severity of migraine headaches, and it is helpful to communicate this to the patient.[5 6 7] An important point to stress early on is that migraine has no cure, and the goal is to manage and reduce the burden of the disease. The patient's disability is reduced if these main goals are achieved. Other goals of preventive treatment include reduced use of acute drugs and fewer visits to the emergency room or doctor's surgery. Patients also need to understand that it may take time for a drug to become effective, most often two to three months at an adequate dose. Asking patients to keep a headache calendar or diary is an effective way to monitor progress.

What do the treatments prevent?

The pathogenesis of migraine is not completely understood. Studies of patients prescribed commonly used drugs for preventing migraine have shown that that these drugs suppress cortical spreading depression.[w3] However the complex mechanisms of action of migraine preventive drugs are unclear.

What drugs are available for the prevention of migraine?

Although preventive options for migraine may be either pharmacological or non-pharmacological, we will discuss the pharmacological option only. Certain β blockers, calcium channel blockers, tricyclic antidepressants, and antiepileptic drug are considered first line preventive treatments, and many other drugs are considered second and third line options.[5] Only five drugs are currently approved by the Food and Drug Administration (FDA) for prevention of episodic migraine. These are propranolol, timolol, valproate, topiramate, and methysergide. OnabotulinumtoxinA (Botox) is now FDA approved for the treatment of chronic migraine. European and US treatment recommendations have only a few minor differences (table).[5 6] The evidence for the recommendations is derived from clinical trials where available.

β blockers

Propranolol and metoprolol have been evaluated in randomised placebo controlled trials for their efficacy in migraine prevention. A Cochrane review of available studies in 2004 concluded that propranolol is effective in preventing migraines in the short term, with insufficient data to make a conclusion regarding long term treatment.[9] Sustained release options offer the benefits of once daily dosing and improved compliance. β blockers are a good choice of preventive drug for patients with coexistent hypertension, but they should not be used for patients with asthma and must be used with caution in patients with depression.

BOX 1 INTERNATIONAL HEADACHE SOCIETY'S CLASSIFICATION CRITERIA FOR MIGRAINE WITHOUT AURA[1]

At least five attacks fulfilling criteria A-C

- A: Headache attacks lasting 4-72 hours (untreated or unsuccessfully treated)
- B: Headache has at least two of the following characteristics:
  - Unilateral location
  - Pulsating quality
  - Moderate or severe pain intensity
  - Aggravation by, or causes avoidance of, routine physical activity
- C: During headache at least one of the following occurs:
  - Nausea or vomiting
  - Photophobia and phonophobia
- D Not attributed to another disorder

BOX 2 CRITERIA FOR STARTING PREVENTIVE TREATMENT[6 7]

- Quality of life, business duties, or school attendance is severely impaired
- Two or more attacks a month
- Migraine attacks do not respond to acute drug treatment
- Frequent, very long, or uncomfortable auras occur

Drugs for the prevention of migraine

Drug	Target dose	Common adverse drug reactions	Strength of evidence (US)†	Strength of evidence (Europe)‡
β blockers				
Propranolol	80-160 mg once daily	Hypotension	A	A
Metoprolol	25-100 mg once-twice daily	Hypotension	B	A
Atenolol	25-100mg once daily	Hypotension	B	NA
Calcium channel blockers				
Flunarizine	5-15 mg once daily	Weight gain, tardive dyskinesia	NA	A
Verapamil	80-120 mg once-three times daily	Bradycardia, hypotension	B	NA
Amlodipine	5-10 mg once daily	Oedema	NA	NA
Other antihypertensives				
Lisinopril	20 mg once daily	Cough	NA	C
Candesartan	16 mg once daily		NA	C
Antidepressants				
Amitriptyline	25-75 mg once daily	Anticholinergic side effects	A	B
Nortriptyline	10-100 mg once daily	Anticholinergic side effects	C	NA
Fluoxetine	10-40 mg once daily		B	NA
Venlafaxine	75-150 mg twice daily	Drowsiness, urinary retention	NA	B
Anticonvulsants				
Valproate	250-500 mg twice daily	Weight gain, tremor, hair loss	A	A
Topiramate	50-100 mg twice daily	Nephrolithiasis, acute glaucoma	A	A
Gabapentin	300-1200 mg three times daily	Drowsiness, dizziness	B	C
Lamotrigine	50-300 mg once daily	Stevens-Johnson syndrome	NA	NA
Zonisamide	25-400 mg once daily	Nephrolithiasis, sulfonamide allergy	NA	NA
Supplements and herbs				
Riboflavin	200 mg twice daily		B	C
Coenzyme Q10	100 mg three times daily	Gastrointestinal upset	NA	C
Magnesium	400-600 mg once daily	Diarrhoea	B	C
Others				
Methysergide	2 mg once daily	Retroperitoneal fibrosis	A	
OnabotulinumtoxinA	155 U		A	

†Taken from American Academy of Neurology practice parameter.
‡Taken from European Federation of Neurological Societies guidelines.

Calcium channel blockers

Flunarazine—a calcium channel blocker not available in all countries—causes a mild reduction in the frequency of migraine attacks.[10] Calcium channel blockers that are more widely available, such as amlodipine and verapamil, are effective options for some patients.[w4] As with most other antihypertensive drugs, hypotension and pedal oedema are side effects to watch out for, but otherwise these drugs are well tolerated.

Other antihypertensive drugs

Several drugs belonging to the angiotensin converting enzyme inhibitor class and the angiotensin receptor blocker class have been studied as potential treatments for preventing migraine, although because of a lack of definitive data for migraine prevention, these drugs are second or third tier options. A randomised, placebo controlled, crossover study showed that lisinopril, an angiotensin converting enzyme inhibitor, decreased both the number of days with migraine and headache severity by 20%.[11] One randomised controlled trial found that candesartan, an angiotensin receptor blocker, reduced the number of days of migraine a month by nearly five days compared with placebo.[12] Both these classes of drugs may be alternative choices for patients with or without hypertension who do not tolerate, or do not respond to, β blockers or calcium channel blockers.

Antidepressants

Amitriptyline, a tricyclic antidepressant, has been shown to be effective in preventing migraine in several randomised controlled trials and is considered a first line option in the US.[13] The dose of amitriptyline used to prevent migraine is lower than the recommended dose to treat depression, and benefits in migraine are independent of improvement in depression. The effective use of other tricyclics, such as protriptyline and nortriptyline, has been reported, but high level evidence to support their use is lacking. Patients may experience anticholinergic side effects such as dry mouth and constipation when taking tricyclic drugs. Selective serotonin reuptake inhibitors have proved to be no more effective than placebo for preventing migraine attacks.[14] The serotonin and noradrenaline reuptake inhibitor venlafaxine has been shown to be effective in prevention of migraine compared with placebo and selective serotonin reuptake inhibitors. One randomised controlled trial found that venlafaxine decreased the number of days with migraine compared with placebo.[15] Serotonin and noradrenaline reuptake inhibitors may be appropriate for patients with chronic pain from other conditions, such as fibromyalgia.

Antiepileptic drugs

Several antiepileptic drugs have been shown to be effective in preventing migraine in randomised controlled trials, and valproate and topiramate are generally considered first line treatment choices since a Cochrane review in 2008 found them to be effective.[16 17 18 19] The same Cochrane review also concluded that the class as a whole is generally well tolerated and can help reduce the frequency of migraine attacks.[17] Valproate must be used with caution in women of childbearing age because of its association with neural tube defects in offspring. Warn patients about weight gain, hair loss, and tremor when prescribing valproate. Topiramate has been associated with weight loss.[18] A history of renal stones is a relative contraindication for using topiramate.

Topiramate may be effective in treating chronic migraine and may be useful in patients whose headaches are complicated by overuse of acute drugs.[w5] The evidence that gabapentin is effective in preventing migraine is variable, and it is not considered a first line treatment choice. Gabapentin is helpful for patients with other pain conditions, but it has to be taken three times a day. Lamotrigine may be useful for patients who have migraine with aura.[w6]

Supplements and herbs

Several vitamins, minerals, and herbal remedies can be used to prevent migraine and may appeal to patients who wish to avoid taking daily prescription drugs. These treatments offer the benefits of few adverse drug reactions and drug interactions. Butterbur, or *Petasites hybridus*, is effective but warn patients to use only properly processed plant extracts because the leaves of the plant are potentially carcinogenic. Petasites decreases the frequency of migraine attack, and one study found a statistically significant decrease (≥50%) in the frequency of migraine.[19] Coenzyme Q10 can decrease the frequency of attacks, but it has little effect on the severity of migraine and does not reduce the use of acute drugs.[20] Magnesium oxide and riboflavin (vitamin B-2) have also been shown to reduce the frequency of attacks.[21 22] A negative Cochrane systematic review and meta-analysis of studies that examined the effectiveness of feverfew, derived from the *Tanacetum parthenium* plant, has limited its use.[23]

Other drugs

Methysergide, an ergot derivative, is an effective preventive option. Its use is limited to six month periods with recommended drug holidays because of the potential development of retroperitoneal, pleural, and cardiac valve fibrosis. Although it was approved by the FDA for prevention of migraine, methysergide is no longer available in the US. Its major metabolite, methylergonovine, is however used by some practitioners.

Botulinum toxin A

The use of botulinum toxin A has gained a great deal of attention in recent years. The results of trials to date have not proved clear efficacy over placebo in episodic migraine, and it is known to be ineffective for tension-type headache.[24 w7] However, the FDA has approved botulinum toxin A for the treatment of patients with chronic migraine, and it is licensed in the United Kingdom for the same indication.[25] It is administered every three months as 155 units distributed over 31 injection sites, which include the forehead, temporalis muscles, suboccipital areas, upper posterior cervical musculature, and trapezius muscles.

Combination treatment

For patients who fail to respond to single preventive drugs, the use of more than one drug may prove effective—for example, a combination of propranolol and amitriptyline.

When should preventive treatment be discontinued?

The frequency of follow-up visits is tailored to the patient's individual needs and response to treatment. Guidelines for discontinuing preventive drugs are arbitrary, and treatment decisions should be made on a case by case basis. For example, if coexisting conditions are being treated, the clinician might decide not to discontinue drugs. Drugs might need to be discontinued slowly in patients who react to quick changes in medication. Drugs are usually discontinued in patients who have shown no clear benefit after an adequate trial duration.

TIPS FOR NON-SPECIALISTS

- When choosing a preventive drug, carefully consider treating coexisting conditions with the same drug, if appropriate
- To improve treatment adherence, take the time to explain the rationale for starting preventive drugs to the patient and answer any questions
- Limit polypharmacy if possible; however, multiple drugs may be needed
- Limit the use of analgesic drugs because current evidence suggests that when analgesic use is high, preventive drugs are less effective

SOURCES AND SELECTION CRITERIA

The content of this article is based in part on guidelines from the United States Headache Consortium, which use an evidence based medicine format but include data up to 1997 only.[5] These guidelines are available at the American Academy of Neurology website (www.aan.com). We also included guidelines on the management of migraine from the European Federation of Neurological Societies.[6 7] In addition, we used Cochrane reviews as well as peer reviewed publications in headache and neurological journals obtained from Medline searches.

ADDITIONAL EDUCATIONAL RESOURCES

All the resources below provide more information on classification and treatment options in a clear and concise manner as well as links to other resources

Resources for clinician

- International Headache Society (www.ihs-headache.org)
- American Headache Society (www.americanheadachesociety.org)
- European Headache Federation (www.ehf-org.org)
- British Association for the Study of Headache (www.bash.org.uk)
- European Federation of Neurological Societies (www.efns.org)

Resources for patients

- American Headache Society (www.achenet.org)
- Migraine Action Association (www.migraine.org.uk)
- World Headache Alliance (www.w-h-a.org/)
- More on migraine: This film presents some of the latest research into the causes of this debilitating condition. It also highlight the current best practice for drug therapy, and discusses whether complementary therapies can play a role in treating migraine.media-1v110.1136/bmj.d583v1

Contributors: NF did most of the writing. The article was revised and edited several times before submission by all three authors.

Competing interests: All authors have completed the Unified Competing Interest form at www.icmje.org/coi_disclosure.pdf (available on request from the corresponding author) and declare: no support from any organisation for the submitted work; ML has received honorariums for lectures from NuPathe, Merck, and Allergan and has served as a consultant for NuPathe in the past year. He has been on the Speaker's Bureau with Merck and Astellas; TW has consulted with NuPathe, MAP Pharma, and Pfizer in the past year; he has been on the Speaker's Bureau with Merck, Zogenix/Astrellen,

Allergan, and Valeant; he has received research support from Merck, Allergan, GSK, NMT Medical, and Solstice within the past three years; no other relationships or activities that could appear to have influenced the submitted work.

Provenance and peer review: Commissioned; externally peer reviewed.

1 Headache Classification Committee of the International Headache Society. The international classification of headache disorders. 2nd ed. *Cephalalgia* 2004;24(suppl 1):1-160.
2 Silberstein SD, Lipton RB, Dodick DW. Wolff's headache and other head pain. 8th ed. Oxford University Press, 2008.
3 Stovner LJ, Hagen K, Jensen R, Katsarava Z, Lipton RB, Scher AI, et al. The global burden of headache: a documentation of headache prevalence and disability worldwide. *Cephalalgia* 2007;27:193-210.
4 Lipton RB, Bigal M, Diamond M, Freitag F, Reed ML, Stewart WF, et al. Migraine prevalence, disease burden, and the need for preventive therapy. *Neurology* 2007;68:343-9.
5 Silberstein SD. Practice parameter: evidence-based guidelines for migraine headache (an evidence-based review): report of the quality standards subcommittee of the American Academy of Neurology. *Neurology* 2000;55:754-62.
6 Evers S, Afra J, Frese A, Goadsby PJ, Linde M, May A, et al. EFNS guideline on the drug treatment of migraine- revised report of an EFNS task force. *Eur J Neurol* 2009;16:968-81.
7 Antonaci F, Dumitrache C, De Cillis I, Allena M. A review of current European guidelines for migraine. *J Headache Pain* 2010;11:13-9.
8 Mathew N, Kurman R, Perez F. Drug induced refractory headache—clinical features and management. *Headache* 1990;30:634-8.
9 Linde K, Rossnagel K. propranolol for migraine prophylaxis. *Cochrane Database Syst Rev* 2004;2:CD003225.
10 Reveix Herault L, Cardona A, Ospina E, Carrillo P. Effectiveness of flunazarine in the prophylaxis of migraine: a meta-analytical review of the literature. *Revista de Neurol* 2003;36:907-12.
11 Schrader H, Stovner L, Helde G, Sand T, Bovim G. Prophylactic treatment of migraine with angiotensin converting enzyme inhibitor (lisinopril): randomized, placebo controlled, crossover study. *BMJ* 2001;322:19.
12 Trovnik E, Stovner L, Helde G, Sand T, Bovim G. Prophylactic treatment of migraine with an angiotensin II receptor blocker: a randomized controlled trial. *JAMA* 2003;289:65-9.
13 Couch JR, Hassanein RS. Amitriptyline in migraine prophylaxis. *Arch Neurol* 1979;36:695-9.
14 Moja L, Cusi C, Sterzi R, Canepari C. Selective serotonin re-uptake inhibitors (SSRI) for preventing migraine and tension-type headaches. *Cochrane Database Syst Rev* 2005;3:CD002919.
15 Ozyalcin S, Talu G, Kiziltan E, Yucel B, Ertas M, Disci R. The efficacy and safety of venlafaxine in the prophylaxis of migraine. *Headache* 2005;45:144-52.
16 Jensen R, Brinck T, Olesen J. Sodium valproate has a prophylactic effect in migraine without aura: a triple-blind, placebo-controlled crossover study. *Neurology* 1994;44:647-51.
17 Mulleners WM, Chronicle EP. Anticonvulsants in migraine prophylaxis: a Cochrane review. *Cephalalgia* 2008;28:585-97.
18 Silberstein SD, Neto W, Schmitt J, Jacobs D. Topiramate in migraine prevention: results of a large controlled trial. *Arch Neurol* 2004;61:490-5.
19 Lipton RB, Gobel H, Einhaupl, Wilks K, Mauskop A. Petasites hybridus root (butterbur) is an effective preventive treatment for migraine. *Neurology* 2004;63:2240-4.
20 Sandor PS, Di Clemente L, Coppola G, Saenger U, Fumal A, Magis D, et al. Efficacy of coenzyme Q10 in migraine prophylaxis: a randomized controlled trial. *Neurology* 2005;64:713-5.
21 Schoener J, Jacquy J, Lenaerts M. Effectiveness of high-dose riboflavin in migraine prophylaxis—a randomized controlled trial. *Neurology* 1998;50:65-9.
22 Peikert A, Wilimzig C, Kohne-Volland R. Prophylaxis of migraine with oral magnesium: results from a prospective, multi-center, placebo-controlled and double-blind randomized study. *Cephalalgia* 1996;16:257-63.
23 Pittler MH, Ernst E. Feverfew for preventing migraine. *Cochrane Database Syst Rev* 2004;1:CD002286.
24 Evers S, Vollmer-Haase J, Schwaag S, Rahmann A, Husstedt IW, Frese A. Botulinum toxin A in the prophylactic treatment of migraine—a randomized double-blind, placebo-controlled study. *Cephalalgia* 2004;24:838-43.
25 Diener HC, Dodick DW, Aurora SK, Turkel CC, DeGryse RE, Lipton RB, et al. Onabotulinumtoxin A for treatment of chronic migraine: results from the double-blind, randomized, placebo-controlled phase of the PREEMPT 2 trial. *Cephalalgia* 2010;30:804-14.

Cluster headache

Alexander D Nesbitt, research fellow[1,2], Peter J Goadsby, professor of clinical neurology[2]

[1]Surrey Sleep Research Centre, University of Surrey, Guildford GU2 7XP, UK

[2]Department of Neurology, University of California, San Francisco, CA 94115, USA

Correspondence to: P J Goadsby pgoadsby@headache.ucsf.edu

Cite this as: *BMJ* 2012;344:e2407

DOI: 10.1136/bmj.e2407

http://www.bmj.com/content/344/bmj.e2407

Few, if any, medical disorders are more painful than cluster headache. Previously termed migrainous neuralgia, it was last reviewed in the *BMJ* nearly 50 years ago.[1] At that time, the authors stressed the importance of covering the topic in a general medical journal to aid recognition. Despite this remarkably prescient view, and the extreme and stereotyped nature of its presentation, cluster headache is still commonly misdiagnosed. Without a clear diagnosis, affected patients can wait many years before receiving adequate help, and they often endure unnecessary and unhelpful attempts at treatment before gaining any relief.[2]

Patients describe the pain of a single attack as being worse than anything else they have experienced, including childbirth. Many endure repeated attacks, lasting up to three hours, every single day. The severity of the pain has earned it the sobriquet "suicide headache," although in our experience this is a rare occurrence in this exceptional patient group.

The management of this condition differs from that of other headache disorders. This article will review the clinical entity of cluster headache by highlighting its unique and defining characteristics as an aid to correct diagnosis, before critically appraising current treatment methods. In doing so, we outline an up to date streamlined management strategy aimed at limiting the considerable burden that this condition places on patients.

What is cluster headache?

Cluster headache is a primary headache disorder classified with similar conditions known as trigeminal autonomic cephalalgias (table).[3] These conditions are typified by recurrent attacks of unilateral pain, which are very severe and usually involve the orbital or periorbital region innervated by the first (ophthalmic) division of the trigeminal nerve. Characteristic signs and symptoms of activation of the cranial autonomic pathways accompany the pain on the same side: lacrimation, conjunctival injection, nasal congestion or rhinorrhoea (or both), ptosis or miosis (or both), and periorbital oedema (box 1; fig 1).

The term cluster headache originates from the tendency of attacks to cluster together into bouts that last several weeks. In the episodic form of the disorder, the bouts can occur at certain times of year, often with a seasonal predilection.[4] They are separated by periods of remission, which last at least a month (box 2).[3] However, about 10% of patients have the chronic form of the disorder and have continuous attacks with no respite.

A well described physiological reflex arc, the trigeminovascular reflex, potentiates the trigeminal pain and cranial autonomic features of cluster headache by positive feedback mechanisms (fig 2).[8]

Functional imaging studies have detected activation ipsilateral to the pain in the region of the posterior hypothalamus (fig 2), which may have a pivotal role in integrating the pain, cranial autonomic features, and unique timing of cluster headache.[11]

Who gets it?

Pooled data from epidemiological studies give cluster headache a lifetime prevalence of 0.12%, with data from a door to door study in Norway showing a one year prevalence of 0.3%.[12] The condition has a heritable tendency in some families, and first degree relatives of affected people have an estimated 14-48-fold increased risk of developing it.[13]

The male to female ratio varies between 2.5:1 and 3.5:1.[4,14] Patients typically start to develop the attacks in their third to fifth decade, although patients as young as 4 years and as old as 96 years can be affected. There seems to be an association with smoking, with around 65% of patients being active smokers or reporting a history of smoking.[14] However, a causative link to smoking seems unlikely, because smoking cessation does not seem to alter the clinical course of the disorder and cannot easily account for the disorder in children.

The natural course of cluster headache can be difficult to predict, with some people showing a bidirectional transition between the episodic and chronic form of the condition. Less frequent bouts of attacks and more prolonged, and sometimes permanent, periods of remission can occur with advancing age.

How is cluster headache diagnosed?

The diagnosis of cluster headache is made by a careful history that elicits the clinical features of short lasting unilateral pain with cranial autonomic disturbances (box 2), and the cyclical nature of the bouts in which the attacks occur. Descriptions of the disorder are supported by three large prospective case series that use similar methods.[4,5,14]

SUMMARY POINTS

- Cluster headache is an excruciatingly painful primary headache disorder, which places an exceptional burden on those affected
- Attacks are one sided, generally last 15 minutes to three hours, and have a characteristic set of cranial autonomic features, which are accompanied by agitation
- Attacks occur from once every other day to eight times daily, in bouts that last several weeks, usually with complete remission between bouts
- Treat acute attacks with high flow oxygen (12 L/min for at least 15 minutes) or parenteral triptans (or both), such as subcutaneous sumatriptan 6 mg, unless contraindicated
- High doses of verapamil are often necessary as preventive treatment; electrocardiographic monitoring is mandatory when escalating doses

Where is the pain and what is it like?

The pain of cluster headache is unilateral in at least 97% of people with episodic disease and mainly focused behind the eye (88-92%), over the temple (69-70%), or over the maxilla (50-53%), although it may extend to other areas of the head and neck.[4,5,14] Between 14% and 18% of patients report that the pain shifts sides between bouts of attacks and less commonly during a bout, but never during the attack itself.[4,14] Patients often describe the pain as a sharp, piercing, burning, or pulsating sensation like "having a red hot poker forced through my eye," and they report that the intensity is so extreme it is unlike anything they have ever experienced ("11 out of 10").

How long does an attack last?

The diagnostic criteria (box 2) state that attacks should last between 15 and 180 minutes, although on rare occasions they can last longer. In the British series, a mean untreated minimum duration of 72 minutes and maximum duration of 159 minutes was reported.[4]

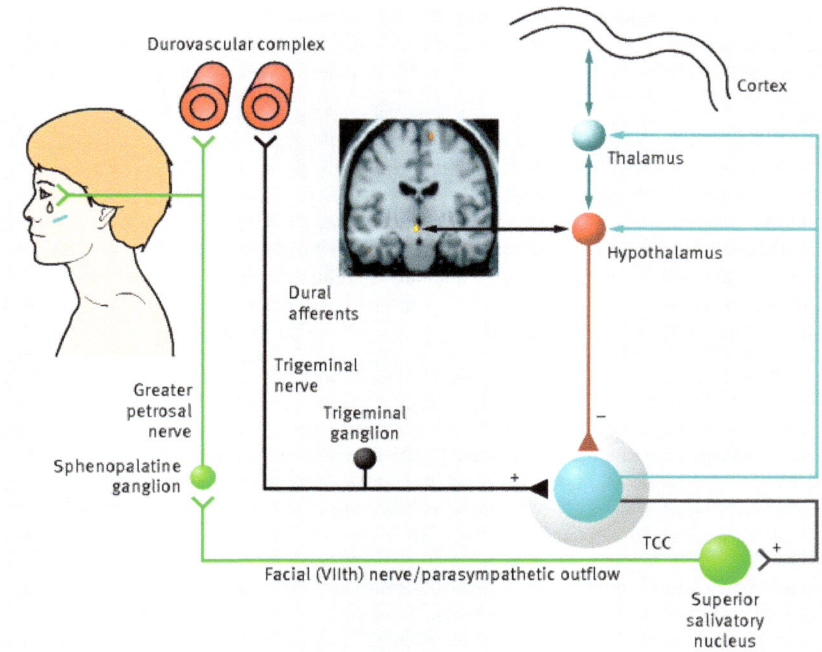

Fig 2 The trigeminovascular reflex. Nerve endings containing pain receptors innervate structures of the face and cranial vault, particularly the pain producing dura mater and cerebral blood vessels (the durovascular complex). This nociceptive information is carried to the brainstem in the trigeminal nerve, via the trigeminal ganglion. Within the brainstem, trigeminal fibres synapse in an area known as the trigeminocervical complex (TCC). From here, information ascends to the hypothalamus, thalamus, and cortex via pain processing pathways. In addition, the afferent trigeminal signals arriving at the TCC also stimulate the cranial parasympathetic system via the superior salivatory nucleus. This results in increased firing of parasympathetic fibres carried from the brainstem in the facial nerve and then greater superficial petrosal nerve, which synapse at the sphenopalatine ganglion. These fibres innervate facial structures (including the lacrimal gland and nasal mucosa, thus causing the lacrimation and rhinorrhoea seen with attacks) and the durovascular complex. Neurotransmitter release at these parasympathetic terminals (vasoactive intestinal polypeptide) causes further irritation of trigeminal sensory nerve endings and release of calcitonin gene related peptide, which potentiates the trigeminovascular reflex arc. It is this reflex that is responsible for the pain and facial parasympathetic signs of cluster headache attacks.[9] The ptosis and miosis seen with attacks arise from interruption of the oculosympathetic fibres that run with the internal carotid artery and through the cavernous sinus, where they are thought to be affected by local vascular distension.[10] The posterior hypothalamus, which shows a strong activation signal in functional imaging studies during attacks (insert), may modulate signalling through the TCC, perhaps providing a breaking mechanism to regulate the trigeminovascular reflex[9]

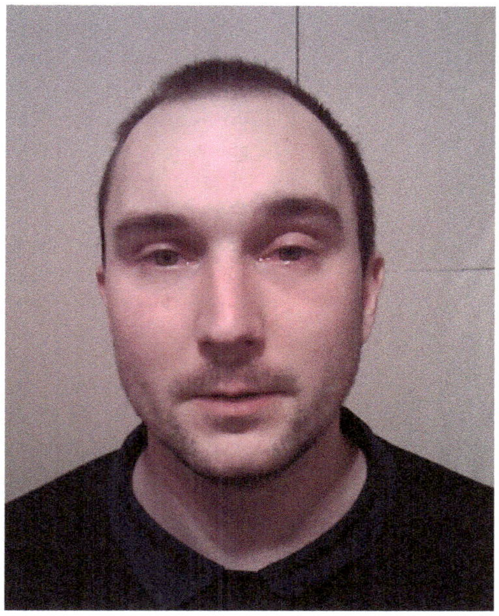

Fig 1 Cranial autonomic features during a cluster headache attack. This photograph was taken during an attack and clearly shows characteristic left periorbital oedema and left partial ptosis, with left conjunctival injection and tear formation. These signs reverted to normal when the attack stopped

BOX 1 CRANIAL AUTONOMIC FEATURES OF CLUSTER HEADACHE ATTACKS[4,5]*

- Ipsilateral lacrimation (91%)
- Ipsilateral conjunctival injection (77%)
- Ipsilateral nasal congestion or rhinorrhoea (75%/72%)
- Ipsilateral ptosis† (74%)
- Ipsilateral oedema of the eyelid or the face (or both) (74%)
- Ipsilateral sweating of the forehead or the face (or both) (38%)
- Ipsilateral miosis† (29%)

**Features are ipsilateral to the side of pain; not all features need to be present*

†A partial Horner's syndrome may persist to a lesser degree between attacks.

BOX 2 DIAGNOSTIC CRITERIA FOR CLUSTER HEADACHE[3]

A) At least five attacks fulfilling criteria B-D

B) Severe or very severe unilateral orbital, supraorbital, or temporal pain that lasts for 15-180 minutes if untreated

C) Headache accompanied by at least one of the following:

- Ipsilateral conjunctival injection or lacrimation (or both)
- Ipsilateral nasal congestion or rhinorrhoea (or both)
- Ipsilateral eyelid oedema
- Ipsilateral forehead and facial sweating
- Ipsilateral miosis or ptosis (or both)
- Restlessness or agitation

D) Attacks have a frequency of one every other day to eight each day

E) Not attributed to another disorder

- *Episodic cluster headache*: Attacks occurring in periods that last seven days to one year separated by pain-free periods that last one month or longer
- *Chronic cluster headache*: Attacks that occur for more than one year without remission or with remissions that last less than one month

The onset of pain is rapid, and the sensation increases from serious discomfort to excruciating pain over the course of a few minutes. The pain usually stays at maximal intensity for the duration of the attack, although it may wax and wane slightly, or be punctuated by super-intense stabs of pain. The attack will often end as abruptly as it started.

How often do individual attacks occur?

The frequency of attacks is also a feature of the diagnostic criteria (box 2), and it varies from one attack every 48 hours to eight separate attacks in 24 hours, although less frequent attacks may occur at the beginning and end of bouts.

The British study found the mean maximum number of attacks each day to be 4.6, with 37% of patients reporting a predictable time of onset during the day and 72% reporting attacks occurring at predictable times during the night, waking them from sleep.[4]

Which other symptoms occur with the attack?

Each attack is accompanied by one or more cranial autonomic symptom or sign on the same side as the pain (box 1; figs 1 and 2). All of these signs and symptoms are transient and resolve with the cessation of pain, although a partial Horner's syndrome or isolated ptosis may persist between attacks or even bouts as a result of local damage to oculosympathetic fibres during repeated attacks (fig 2).[10] The persistence of these signs in the context of the disorder need not cause undue alarm, unless they progressively worsen, in which case secondary causes should be considered and investigations or referral initiated.

Between 70% and 93% of patients describe a sense of restlessness and agitation during an attack and will often pace, rock back and forth, and bang their heads.[4 14] Most patients wish to isolate themselves and seek a cold environment. Between 28% and 50% report nausea,[4 5 14] and a further 23% may vomit during an attack.[4] More than half (54-64%) of patients have photophobia, often limited to the same side as the pain, with slightly fewer reporting an aversion to loud noise (43%) or strong smells (26%) during the attack.[4 14 15]

Aura phenomena, similar to those experienced during migraine, including visual phenomena and paraesthesia, precede attacks by up to 60 minutes in 14% of patients.[4]

Patients commonly have tenderness and cutaneous allodynia at and around the site of pain between attacks, including over the ipsilateral greater occipital nerve.[16]

Does anything trigger the attacks?

In over half of patients (53-63%), small quantities of alcohol, particularly red wine (70%), will precipitate an attack, usually within an hour of ingestion.[4 14 15] However, this is only the case during a bout rather than when in remission.

In most patients (72%), attacks are related to nocturnal sleep, with daytime naps also being triggers in some.[4] Small case series have reported a raised apnoea-hypopnoea index in some patients, suggesting a higher incidence of obstructive sleep apnoea, although no convincing mechanistic or therapeutic insights currently exist to explain this.[17]

Some patients report that odours from volatile organic compounds, such as perfume and paint, can also trigger attacks. Nitrates may trigger attacks,[18] and glyceryl trinitrate is used to provoke attacks experimentally.[11] Sildenafil has also been reported to induce attacks during a bout.[19]

How often do bouts of attacks occur?

Most people with cluster headache experience one bout a year, with a unimodal frequency distribution and mean bout duration of 8.6 weeks found in the British series. However, patients may go for several years without a bout (up to 20 in some cases), and others may have more frequent bouts each year.[4]

Comparison of the trigeminal autonomic cephalalgias based on cohorts studied,[4 6 7] the international classification of headache disorders,[3] and patients seen in practice*

Characteristic	Cluster headache	Paroxysmal hemicrania	SUNCT/SUNA
Sex (M:F)	3:1	1:1	1.5:1
Pain:			
Quality	Sharp/stabbing/throbbing	Sharp/stabbing/throbbing	Sharp/stabbing/throbbing
Severity	Very severe	Very severe	Severe
Distribution	V1>C2>V2>V3	V1>C2>V2>V3	V1>C2>V2>V3
Attacks:			
Frequency per day	1 every other day to 8/day	1-40 (>5/day for more than half the time)	3-200 (typically 100/day)
Length	15-180 min	2-30 min	5-240 s
Triggers			
Alcohol	+++	+	–
Nitroglycerin	+++	+	–
Cutaneous	–	–	+++
Agitation or restlessness	90%	80%	65%
Episodic *v* chronic	90:10	35:65	10:90
Circadian or circannual periodicity	Present	Absent	Absent
Treatment effects:			
Oxygen	80%	No effect	No effect
Sumatriptan 6 mg subcutaneously	75%	20%	<10%
Indomethacin	No effect	100%	No effect
Migrainous features with attacks:			
Nausea	50%	40%	25%
Photophobia or phonophobia	65%	65%	25%

**SUNCT/SUNA=short lasting unilateral neuralgiform headache attacks with conjunctival injection and tearing/short lasting unilateral neuralgiform headache attacks with cranial autonomic features; C=cervical; V=trigeminal.*

Which conditions resemble cluster headache?

The table highlights the main features of cluster headache and the other trigeminal autonomic cephalalgias, which although rare are the main differential diagnoses.

Secondary (or symptomatic) cluster headache may be caused by several structural lesions, particularly pituitary tumours, in addition to carotid dissections and cavernous sinus pathology, so magnetic resonance imaging of the brain and, potentially, carotid arteries is a useful part of the diagnostic investigation.[20]

Attacks of migraine tend to be less severe and to last longer; cranial autonomic features, if present, are less prominent and more likely to be bilateral.[21] Nausea, vomiting, and bilateral photophobia are common. Migraine lacks the striking timing patterns and clustering effects, and most patients prefer not to move during the episode, in contrast to the agitation and restlessness experienced during a cluster attack. Alcohol ingestion may also precipitate migraine, typically after a time delay of several hours.

Trigeminal neuralgia tends to affect people over the age of 50 years and consists of sudden short lasting stabs of lancinating pain, usually affecting the second and third divisions of the trigeminal nerve. It is not associated with cranial autonomic features and is often precipitated by touch, chewing, swallowing hot or cold liquids, and cold wind.[3]

How should patients with cluster headache be managed?

Effective management relies on shared responsibility between primary and secondary care, and all suspected cases should be initially referred for specialist neurological or headache assessment. Patients should be kept under long term follow-up and if possible be offered open appointments at times when bouts recur.

Treatment of individual attacks

Standard analgesia is ineffective, and there is no evidence to support the use of non-steroidal anti-inflammatory drugs, paracetamol (acetaminophen), codeine, or opioids in the treatment of individual attacks. Prescription of such agents should therefore be avoided. The mainstay of abortive treatment consists of inhaled oxygen and parenteral triptans.

Oxygen

A recent double blind randomised placebo controlled crossover trial found that 78% of subjects were pain free after inhalation of 100% oxygen at 12 L/min for 15 minutes ($P<0.001$).[22] Patients should continuously inhale oxygen at this rate for at least 15 minutes through a non-rebreathing facemask. Guidelines for oxygen use, including a prefilled home oxygen order form for doctors of patients in the United Kingdom, are provided on the website of the Organisation for the Understanding of Cluster Headache.

A PATIENT'S PERSPECTIVE

I am careful not to wake the children as I make my way downstairs. If they were to witness my nightly cluster ritual, they would never see me the same way again. Their father, fearless protector, diligent provider, crawling about in tears, beating his head on the hard wood floor. The pain is so intense I want to scream, but I never do. I go down three flights of stairs where I can't be heard, and drop to my knees. I place my hands on the back of my neck and lock my fingers together. I bind my head between my arms and squeeze as hard as I can in an attempt to crush my skull. I begin to roll around, banging my head on the floor, pressing my left eye with the full force of my palm. I search for the telephone that has always been my weapon of choice for creating a diversion, and I beat my left temple with the hand piece. I create a rhythm as I strike my skull, cursing the demon with each blow. With permission from www.clusterheadaches.com

Triptans

Parenteral triptans have been shown to be an effective treatment for individual attacks, whereas orally administered triptans have not. A randomised double blinded placebo controlled crossover study of sumatriptan 6 mg subcutaneous injections showed freedom from pain or a reduction to mild pain in 74% of attacks 15 minutes after administration ($P<0.001$).[23] The incidence of rebound and tachyphylaxis is lower in patients with cluster headache than in those with migraine when sumatriptan is injected up to twice daily on a long term basis. Good randomised placebo controlled evidence also supports the use of sumatriptan nasal spray 20 mg (57% of patients reported adequate relief ($P=0.002$) and 47% reported freedom from pain ($P=0.003$) at 30 minutes)[24] and zolmitriptan nasal spray 10 mg (61% ($P=0.002$) and 50% ($P=0.003$)).[25]

Preventive treatment

Preventive treatment aims to suppress the attacks for the duration of the bout, or over longer periods in those with chronic cluster headache, with the fewest possible side effects.

Consensus evidence, based on observation and one small randomised controlled trial,[26] suggests that a tapering course of corticosteroids—such as 1 mg/kg prednisolone (maximum 60 mg) for five days, which is then reduced by 10 mg every three days—may temporarily reduce the frequency of headaches. A preventive agent, with longer latency until onset of action, should be started at the same time.[27]

The preventive drug of choice is verapamil. This is based on consensus agreement and a small double blinded multicentre placebo controlled study.[28] Baseline

ONGOING AND FUTURE RESEARCH

- Imaging studies using functional and high resolution anatomical approaches aim to provide more detailed information on the activating mechanisms of attacks
- Future randomised controlled trials may assess the efficacy of the calcitonin gene related peptide inhibitors or receptor antagonists, a new class of headache abortive drugs
- Further investigation of the sleep and circadian physiology of patients is providing important mechanistic information designed to help develop new proof of concept treatments
- Randomised controlled trials of different methods of oxygen delivery will provide information that can help rapidly abort individual attacks
- Needleless triptan injections are currently being marketed
- New modes of neurostimulation, such as sphenopalatine ganglion stimulation, are being explored
- Patient databases will help enable longitudinal assessment of the natural course of the disorder

TIPS FOR NON-SPECIALISTS

- Consider cluster headache in anyone who presents with a regularly occurring severe unilateral headache that lasts for three hours or less
- A marked sense of agitation and need to move about can help differentiate cluster headache from migraine, which usually compels the patient to remain calm and still
- Conventional analgesia is ineffective and not worth trying
- Offer all patients short burst oxygen therapy and parenteral (injectable or nasal) triptans to treat attacks
- Prefilled, cluster specific home oxygen supply order forms and guidelines on use are available to download at www.ouchuk.org

electrocardiography should be performed before starting verapamil at a dose of 80 mg three times a day and increasing this by 80 mg each fortnight. Electrocardiography should be repeated 10 days after the dose change and reviewed before each dose increase, paying particular attention to the PR interval. This is essential because of the relatively high incidence of heart block associated with verapamil.[29] For adequate control, at least 480 mg daily is usually needed, and doses of up to 960 mg daily are sometimes needed.[28] At higher doses, other side effects of verapamil include constipation, dizziness, and peripheral oedema.

Verapamil can be slowly withdrawn and stopped once the bout is assumed to have ended and lower doses do not allow breakthrough attacks. The maximum efficacious dose achieved can then be given at the beginning of subsequent bouts, as long as a baseline electrocardiogram remains within normal limits.

Although evidence from controlled trials is limited, there is consensus that lithium may be a useful preventive treatment, even though it is generally of less use than verapamil and it is associated with more side effects and the need for regular plasma monitoring.[27]

Observational studies from the 1960s suggest that methysergide can be efficacious, particularly for short bouts, but its use is restricted by serious fibrotic side effects, and it should therefore be given for short periods only under specialist supervision.[27] Melatonin can be useful in doses of 9-15 mg at night, and this is supported by a small double blind pilot study.[30]

Other agents such as topiramate, sodium valproate, pizotifen, and gabapentin are occasionally used with some success, although data from clinical trials are limited.[27]

Nerve blocks and infusions

Data from a recent randomised controlled trial support the injection of a mixture of local anaesthetic and corticosteroid solution over the greater occipital nerve on the side of the pain.[31] This can be used as an effective bridging technique to allow an adequate dose of oral preventive drug to be achieved. Its use would normally be limited to once every eight to 12 weeks.

A repeated course of intravenous dihydroergotamine, when used according to established protocols in specialist centres only, was shown to break the cycle in a cohort study.[32]

Neuromodulation

The small proportion of people with chronic cluster headache who gain no meaningful benefit from preventive drugs should be considered for surgical intervention. Occipital nerve stimulation involves the extracranial implantation of stimulating electrodes around the greater occipital nerve, situated below the scalp and overlying the occipital bones.[33 34] Long term follow-up of a small cohort showed improvement in 71%, with 64% stating that they would recommend the procedure to others. This safe and effective technique should be considered part of routine care in selected patients with drug refractory chronic cluster headache.[35]

Because functional imaging studies show activation in the region of the posterior hypothalamus during attacks,[11] deep brain stimulation of this area is also being used to treat refractory cases. This technique offers good efficacy in about 60% of patients,[36] although a small controlled trial was negative, and death has been reported as a complication of this approach.[37] Its use should be restricted to patients who have failed peripheral stimulation techniques.

SOURCES AND SELECTION CRITERIA

We based this clinical review on personal reference archives, personal experience, and extensive literature searches of the PubMed and Cochrane databases using the search terms "cluster headache" and "trigeminal autonomic cephalalgia". We also consulted management guidelines from the European Federation of Neurological Sciences and the British Association for the Study of Headache.

ADDITIONAL EDUCATIONAL RESOURCES

Resources for healthcare professionals

- Organisation for the Understanding of Cluster Headache (OUCH UK; www.ouchuk.org/html/clusters_video5.asp)—Video of a patient enduring an attack, which shows the characteristic psychomotor agitation that accompanies an attack
- BMJ Learning (http://learning.bmj.com/learning/module-intro/.html?moduleId=5004479&searchTerm=%E2%80%9Ccluster%20headache%E2%80%9D&page=0)—A guide to diagnosis and management
- British Association for the Study of Headache (www.bash.org.uk)—Guidelines on the diagnosis and management of a range of primary headaches, including cluster headache; also gives details of regular meetings and teaching weekends for GPs, specialist registrars, and consultants throughout the UK
- International Headache Society (http://ihs-classification.org/en/)—Useful diagnostic criteria that cover all forms of primary and secondary headache disorders; registered members may take advantage of an online learning resource centre and access to the journal *Cephalalgia*

Resources for patients

Organisation for Understanding Cluster Headache (OUCH UK; www.ouchuk.org)—A unique patient support group that offers practical advice and information for patients and supporters plus an online support forum and regular meetings throughout the UK

Contributors: ADN initiated and planned the manuscript. ADN and PJG both contributed to the manuscript and provided figures. PJG critically revised drafts of the article and approved the content of the final version to be published. PJG is guarantor.

Competing interests: Both authors have completed the ICMJE uniform disclosure form at www.icmje.org/coi_disclosure.pdf (available on request from the corresponding author) and declare: ADN had financial support from the Patrick Berthoud Charitable Trust for the submitted work; no financial relationships with any organisations that might have an interest in the submitted work in the previous 3 years; no other relationships or activities that could appear to have influenced the submitted work. PJG has consulted for or lectured in sessions supported by Allergan, American Headache Society, Colucid, MAP Pharma, Merck, eNeura, Autonomic technologies, Boston Scientific, Eli-Lilly, Medtronic, Linde gases, Mennarini, BristolMyersSquibb, and Pfizer, and had grant support from GlaxoSmithKline, MAP Pharma, Merck, eNeura, and Amgen.

Provenance and peer review: Commissioned; externally peer reviewed.

Patient consent obtained.

1 Balla JI, Walton JN. Periodic migrainous neuralgia. *BMJ* 1964;1:219-21.
2 Bahra A, Goadsby PJ. Diagnostic delays and mis-management in cluster headache. *Acta Neurol Scand* 2004;109:175-9.
3 Headache Classification Committee of the International Headache Society. The international classification of headache disorders (second edition). *Cephalalgia* 2004;24(suppl 1):1-160.
4 Bahra A, May A, Goadsby PJ. Cluster headache: a prospective clinical study in 230 patients with diagnostic implications. *Neurology* 2002;58:354-61.

5 Donnet A, Lanteri-Minet M, Guegan-Massardier E, Mick G, Fabre N, Geraud G, et al. Chronic cluster headache: a French clinical descriptive study. *J Neurol Neurosurg Psychiatry* 2007;78:1354-8.
6 Cittadini E, Matharu MS, Goadsby PJ. Paroxysmal hemicrania: a prospective clinical study of thirty-one cases. *Brain* 2008;131:1142-55.
7 Cohen AS, Matharu MS, Goadsby PJ. Short-lasting unilateral neuralgiform headache attacks with conjunctival injection and tearing (SUNCT) or cranial autonomic features (SUNA). A prospective clinical study of SUNCT and SUNA. *Brain* 2006;129:2746-60.
8 Goadsby PJ. Pathophysiology of cluster headache: a trigeminal autonomic cephalgia. *Lancet Neurol* 2002;1:37-43.
9 Akerman S, Holland P, Goadsby PJ. Diencephalic and brainstem mechanisms in migraine. *Nat Rev Neurosci* 2011;12:570-84.
10 Drummond PD. Mechanisms of autonomic disturbance in the face during and between attacks of cluster headache. *Cephalalgia* 2006;26:633-41.
11 May A, Bahra A, Buchel C, Frackowiak RS, Goadsby PJ. Hypothalamic activation in cluster headache attacks. *Lancet* 1998;352:275-8.
12 Fischera M, Marziniak M, Gralow I, Evers S. The incidence and prevalence of cluster headache: a meta-analysis of population-based studies. *Cephalalgia* 2008;28:614-8.
13 Russell MB. Epidemiology and genetics of cluster headache. *Lancet Neurol* 2004;3:279-83.
14 Schurks M, Kurth T, de Jesus J, Jonjic M, Rosskopf D, Diener HC. Cluster headache: clinical presentation, lifestyle features, and medical treatment. *Headache* 2006;46:1246-54.
15 Irimia P, Cittadini E, Paemeleire K, Cohen AS, Goadsby PJ. Unilateral photophobia or phonophobia in migraine compared with trigeminal autonomic cephalalgias. *Cephalalgia* 2008;28:626-30.
16 Marmura MJ, Pello SJ, Young WB. Interictal pain in cluster headache. *Cephalalgia* 2010;30:1531-4.
17 Chervin RD, Zellek N, Lin X, Hall JM, Sharma N, Hedger KM. Sleep disordered breathing in patients with cluster headache. *Neurology* 2000;54:2302-6.
18 Ekbom K. Nitroglycerin as a provocative agent in cluster headache. *Arch Neurol* 1968;19:487-93.
19 Evans RW. Sildenafil can trigger cluster headaches. *Headache* 2006;46:173-4.
20 Wilbrink LA, Ferrari MD, Kruit MC, Haan J. Neuroimaging in trigeminal autonomic cephalgias: when, how, and of what? *Curr Opin Neurol* 2009;22:247-53.
21 Lai T-H, Fuh J-L, Wang S-J. Cranial autonomic symptoms in migraine: characteristics and comparison with cluster headache. *J Neurol Neurosurg Psychiatry* 2009;80:1116-9.
22 Cohen AS, Burns B, Goadsby PJ. High flow oxygen for treatment of cluster headache. A randomized trial. *JAMA* 2009;302:2451-7.
23 Ekbom K; the Sumatriptan Cluster Headache Study Group. Treatment of acute cluster headache with sumatriptan. *N Engl J Med* 1991;325:322-6.
24 Van Vliet JA, Bahra A, Martin V, Aurora SK, Mathew NT, Ferrari MD, et al. Intranasal sumatriptan in cluster headache—randomized placebo-controlled double-blind study. *Neurology* 2003;60:630-3.
25 Cittadini E, May A, Straube A, Evers S, Bussone G, Goadsby PJ. Effectiveness of intranasal zolmitriptan in acute cluster headache. A randomized, placebo-controlled, double-blind crossover study. *Arch Neurol* 2006;63:1537-42.
26 Jammes JL. The treatment of cluster headaches with prednisone. *Dis Nerv Syst* 1975;36:375-6.
27 May A, Leone M, Afra J, Linde M, Sandor PS, Evers S, et al. EFNS guidelines on the treatment of cluster headache and other trigeminal-autonomic cephalalgias. *Eur J Neurol* 2006;13:1066-77.
28 Leone M, D'Amico D, Frediani F, Moschiano P, Grazzi L, Attanasio A, et al. Verapamil in the prophylaxis of episodic cluster headache: a double-blind study versus placebo. *Neurology* 2000;54:1382-5.
29 Cohen AS, Matharu MS, Goadsby PJ. Electrocardiographic abnormalities in patients with cluster headache on verapamil therapy. *Neurology* 2007;69:668-75.
30 Leone M, D'Amico D, Moschiano F, Fraschini F, Bussone G. Melatonin versus placebo in the prophylaxis of cluster headache: a double-blind pilot study with parallel groups. *Cephalalgia* 1996;16:494-6.
31 Leroux E, Valade D, Taifas I, Vicaut E, Chagnon M, Roos C, et al. Suboccipital steroid injections for transitional treatment of patients with more than two cluster headache attacks per day: a randomised, double-blind, placebo-controlled trial. *Lancet Neurol* 2011;10:891-7.
32 Nagy AJ, Gandhi S, Bhola R, Goadsby PJ. Intravenous dihydroergotamine (DHE) for inpatient management of refractory primary headaches. *Neurology* 2011;77:1827-32.
33 Burns B, Watkins L, Goadsby PJ. Successful treatment of medically intractable cluster headache using occipital nerve stimulation (ONS). *Lancet* 2007;369:1099-106.
34 Magis D, Allena M, Bolla M, De Pasqua V, Remacle JM, Schoenen J. Occipital nerve stimulation for drug-resistant chronic cluster headache: a prospective pilot study. *Lancet Neurol* 2007;6:314-21.
35 Burns B, Watkins L, Goadsby PJ. Treatment of intractable chronic cluster headache by occipital nerve stimulation in 14 patients. *Neurology* 2009;72:341-5.
36 Leone M. Deep brain stimulation in headache. *Lancet Neurol* 2006;5:873-7.
37 Schoenen J, Di Clemente L, Vandenheede M, Fumal A, De Pasqua V, Mouchamps M, et al. Hypothalamic stimulation in chronic cluster headache: a pilot study of efficacy and mode of action. *Brain* 2005;128:940-7.

BPP UNIVERSITY SCHOOL OF HEALTH BMJ

Thunderclap headache

Anne Ducros, neurologist[1], Marie-Germaine Bousser, professor of neurology[2]

[1]Emergency Headache Centre, Head and Neck Clinic, Lariboisière Hospital, Assistance Publique Hôpitaux de Paris, 75010 Paris, France

[2]Neurology Department, Head and Neck Clinic, Lariboisière Hospital

Correspondence to: A Ducros anne.ducros@lrb.aphp.fr

Cite this as: *BMJ* 2012;345:e8557

DOI: 10.1136/bmj.e8557

http://www.bmj.com/content/346/bmj.e8557

Headache affects about 90% of the general population. The most common causes are migraine and episodic tension-type headache. A small proportion of patients present acutely to a primary care doctor, and the main objective is to identify those who require urgent investigations.

The term thunderclap headache is used to decribe a severe headache of instantaneous onset—one minute at the most.[1] Estimated incidence is about 43 per 100 000 adults per year in the developed world.[2] In our emergency headache centre, out of a total of 8000 patients each year, about 120 present with thunderclap headache. Any thunderclap headache, even in a patient with a history of recurrent headache, such as migraine, must be considered as secondary to a variety of causes, the foremost of which is subarachnoid haemorrhage.[3] [4] Making a diagnosis can be challenging. Even when brain computed tomography (CT) and lumbar puncture results are normal, the underlying cause can be serious—for example, cervical artery dissection, cerebral venous thrombosis, and reversible cerebral vasoconstriction syndrome (RCVS).[4] [5]

This review aims to describe the various causes of thunderclap headache and the role of investigations when CT and lumbar puncture investigations are normal.

What is a thunderclap headache?

This clinical form of headache is defined by its mode of onset and severity.[6] [7] A detailed history is needed to recognise a thunderclap headache. First ask the patient precisely how long the headache took to peak and then what the maximum severity was on an 11 point scale (0 no pain; 1-3 mild pain; 4-6 moderate pain; 7-9 severe pain; 10 worst pain ever). A headache that reaches 7 or more within less than one minute is a thunderclap headache. Headache that is present on awakening cannot by definition be called a thunderclap headache, although it may be one. Thunderclap headaches may last from minutes to several days. The location and type of pain are not specific. Thunderclap headaches may be single or recur over a few days. They may start spontaneously or during performance of the Valsalva manoeuvre, exertion, sexual activity, emotional stress, bathing, or showering. General practitioners should urgently refer a patient with thunderclap headache to the emergency department and, whenever possible, to a hospital with a neurology department.

How should a patient with thunderclap headache be assessed?

Circumstances preceding the onset, including exposure to vasoactive drugs, may provide clues to some diagnoses (box 1). Associated neurological symptoms and any abnormality in the neurological or physical examination increase the need for rapid evaluation. In particular, always check eyelids, pupils, visual field, and cerebellar function for subtle signs (box 2). The absence of any associated symptoms and a strictly normal examination do not exclude a serious cause—urgent diagnostic work-up is still needed.

What are the most common causes?

Subarachnoid haemorrhage

Systematic reviews and prospective observational studies have shown that about 70% of subarachnoid haemorrhages present primarily with headache, which has a thunderclap pattern in 50%.[8] [9] [10] [11] Subarachnoid haemorrhage is found in 11-25% of patients who present with thunderclap headache.[2] [9] Any thunderclap headache must raise suspicion of an underlying subarachnoid haemorrhage, even in an alert pain-free patient with a supple neck at the time of presentation.[10] The shortest duration of headache caused by a subarachnoid haemorrhage is unknown. Subarachnoid haemorrhage is initially misdiagnosed in about one of three patients, especially those who have a normal Glasgow coma scale score and present with isolated headache.[10]

First perform unenhanced brain CT, followed by lumbar puncture if the tomogram is normal,[3] [11] because a normal result does not exclude subarachnoid haemorrhage. CT results are normal in 2% of cases within 12 hours after headache onset, 10% after one day, and 50% after five days.[10] Systematic reviews show that magnetic resonance imaging (MRI) is as sensitive as CT for the detection of subarachnoid blood within the first few hours and becomes more sensitive after the first day.[11] However, like CT, the sensitivity of early MRI is not 100%.

A lumbar puncture is therefore needed in all cases of thunderclap headache after normal brain imaging.[10] If the cerebrospinal fluid (CSF) is bloodstained, it should immediately be centrifuged; yellow coloration (xanthochromia) of the supernatant indicates subarachnoid haemorrhage. This can be confirmed by spectrophotometry, which will show the presence of bilirubin formed in vivo. The sensitivity of spectrophotometry for bilirubin is close to 100% when lumbar puncture is performed 12 hours to two weeks after subarachnoid haemorrhage.[11]

In positive cases, search for a ruptured aneurysm using cerebral angiography. Non-traumatic subarachnoid haemorrhages are caused by a ruptured aneurysm in 85% of cases, whereas 10% are idiopathic perimesencephalic

SUMMARY POINTS

- Thunderclap headache is a severe headache that peaks within 60 seconds of onset
- Neurovascular disorders often present with thunderclap headache
- Infectious disorders, intracranial hypertension, and hypotension syndromes occasionally present with thunderclap headache
- Subarachnoid haemorrhage is the most common cause; diagnosis is based on plain brain computed tomography (CT) and, if normal, on lumbar puncture
- Suspect reversible cerebral vasoconstriction syndrome when thunderclap headaches recur over a few days
- Cervical artery dissection, cerebral venous thrombosis, reversible cerebral vasoconstriction syndrome, and pituitary apoplexy may present with isolated thunderclap headache and normal physical examination, CT, and cerebrospinal fluid
- When CT and cerebrospinal fluid are normal, other investigations are needed, including cervical and cerebral vascular imaging and brain magnetic resonance imaging

subarachnoid haemorrhages.[11] The remaining 5% are caused by rare conditions including intracranial arterial dissection, brain and spinal vascular malformations and tumours, angiitis, cerebral venous thrombosis,[11] and RCVS.[12]

Reversible cerebral vasoconstriction syndrome

In two prospective studies of patients with sudden onset headache investigated by plain brain CT and lumbar puncture if needed, 11-25% of cases had subarachnoid haemorrhage, 10-12% had other serious disorders (including strokes, tumours, and meningitis), and the remainder had "no underlying cause" and a good outcome on follow-up.[2 9] These studies led to the concept of "benign thunderclap headache" and to the suggestion that cerebral angiography was not necessary after normal results on CT and lumbar puncture.[9]

Systematic vessel imaging led to the recognition of RCVS as a common cause of thunderclap headache.[5] A systematic review, based on three large observational studies (two prospective and one retrospective) and numerous smaller case series and reports, showed that RCVS presents as isolated headaches in about 75% of cases.[13] On the basis of this review and our experience at the emergency headache centre, we believe that RCVS accounts for most "benign thunderclap headaches."

RCVS is characterised by severe headaches, with or without focal deficits and seizures, and diffuse segmental cerebral arterial vasoconstriction that resolves within three months.[12 13 14] Half of cases occur during the postpartum period or after exposure to serotoninergic agents, adrenergic substances, or cannabis.[5 14 15] Most patients have multiple thunderclap headaches that recur every day or so for a few days to four weeks.[5 13] The pain lasts from five minutes to

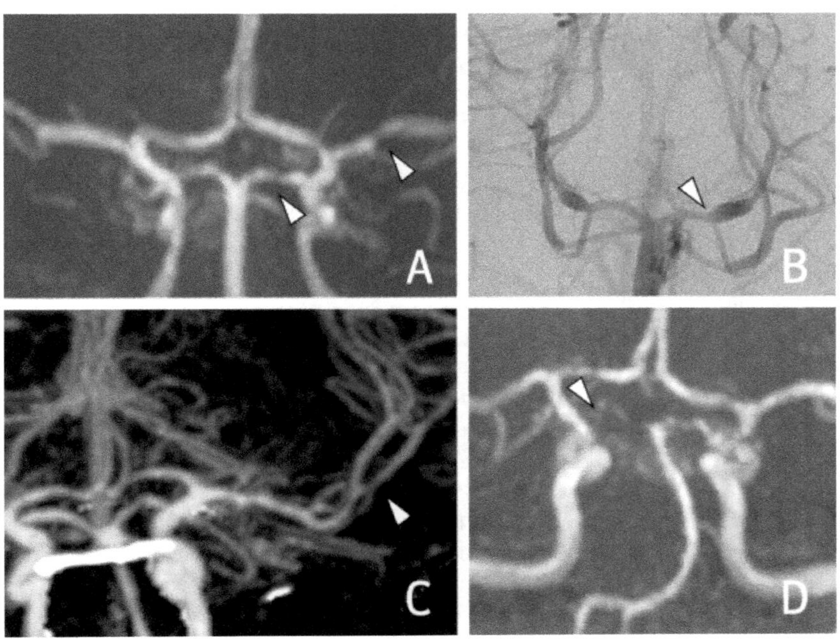

Cerebral angiography in cases with reversible cerebral vasoconstriction syndrome (RCVS). (A and D) Cerebral magnetic resonance angiography in two patients showing segmental constrictions (arrowheads); in (D) the right posterior cerebral artery is severely constricted. (B) Conventional catheter cerebral angiography in RCVS, showing segmental dilation of both posterior cerebral arteries (arrowhead). (C) Cerebral computed tomography angiography in RCVS showing a short stenosis of a branch of the left middle cerebral artery (arrowhead)

BOX 1 CIRCUMSTANCES PRECEDING THUNDERCLAP HEADACHE THAT POINT TO POSSIBLE CAUSES

- Mild trauma: Cervical arterial dissection, intracranial hypotension
- Intake of vasoactive substances: Illicit drugs (cannabis, cocaine, ecstasy, amphetamines, lysergide); antidepressants (selective serotonin reuptake inhibitors, mixed adrenaline (epinephrine) and serotonin reuptake inhibitors); α sympathomimetics (nasal decongestants, noradrenaline (norepinephrine)); migraine drugs (triptans and ergot alkaloid derivatives): reversible cerebral vasoconstriction syndrome (RCVS)
- Dural puncture: Intracranial hypotension
- Fever: Infectious disorders
- Postpartum: RCVS, cerebral venous thrombosis, eclampsia
- Ear, nose, and throat symptoms: Complicated sinusitis

BOX 2 OTHER SYMPTOMS AND SIGNS THAT CAN GIVE A CLUE TO THE DIAGNOSIS

- Neck stiffness: Subarachnoid haemorrhage or meningitis
- Transient loss of consciousness: Subarachnoid haemorrhage (around 50% of cases), colloid cyst of the third ventricle
- Epileptic seizure: Subarachnoid haemorrhage, other stroke, cerebral venous thrombosis, posterior reversible encephalopathy syndrome (PRES), reversible cerebral vasoconstriction syndrome (RCVS)
- Focal neurological symptoms: Subarachnoid haemorrhage, other stroke, cerebral venous thrombosis, PRES, RCVS
- Horner's sign or pulsatile tinnitus or tongue palsy: Dissection of the homolateral internal carotid artery
- Unilateral mydriasis with or without other signs of third cranial nerve paralysis: Aneurysm compressing the third nerve
- Patients avoid lying flat: Subarachnoid haemorrhage, intracranial hypertension syndrome, cerebral venous thrombosis, acute sinusitis
- Patients avoid standing up: Intracranial hypotension, cerebellar stroke
- Papilloedema: Intracranial hypertension
- Arterial hypertension: Subarachnoid haemorrhage, eclampsia, PRES, RCVS
- Electrocardiographic abnormalities: Subarachnoid haemorrhage, myocardial infarction with ectopic pain
- Asymmetrical blood pressure at upper limbs: Aortic arch dissection

TIPS FOR NON-SPECIALISTS

- Careful history taking is needed to identify a thunderclap headache because patients seldom mention how long their headache took to peak
- Obtain the time to peak and the precise intensity of the maximal pain on an 11 point scale (0 no pain; 1-3 mild pain; 4-6 moderate pain; 7-9 severe pain; 10 worst pain ever)
- Always refer a patient with thunderclap headache to the emergency department as soon as possible
- First line investigations always include plain brain computed tomography (CT) followed by a lumbar puncture if the tomogram is normal
- Patients with isolated thunderclap headache and normal physical examination, normal brain CT, and normal cerebrospinal fluid results can still have a serious underlying condition; refer to a multidisciplinary neurology team

a few hours. Sexual activity, emotion, exertion, coughing, straining, urination, bathing, and showering are common triggers. A prospective series showed that 60% of patients with isolated sexual headaches had RCVS.[16]

In RCVS presenting with isolated headaches, the results of plain brain CT are usually normal and cerebrospinal fluid is either normal or "near normal," with a mild increase in blood cell counts and protein concentrations.[5] RCVS is not always benign. Overall, one in four patients has a convexity subarachnoid haemorrhage—a non-aneurysmal, usually mild, subarachnoid haemorrhage in the sulcal spaces of the cerebral hemispheres, near the convexity.[13] Haemorrhagic and ischaemic stroke can occur, sometimes after a few days of isolated headaches in patients with initial normal brain imaging.[12 14] Diagnostic criteria for RCVS have been proposed (box 3).[13] Diagnosis requires the demonstration of diffuse arterial beading by cerebral angiography, usually magnetic resonance angiography (MRA) or CT angiography (CTA), even though these tests are less sensitive than catheter angiography (figure). MRA, CTA, and even catheter angiography may be normal up to six or seven days after headache onset in patients who are ultimately shown to have RCVS on repeat angiography.[12]

There is no evidence based treatment for RCVS. Patients should rest, with the duration and type of rest depending on initial severity. Some patients need bed rest in hospital for two weeks; in others, rest at home (avoiding exertion and sex but without bed rest) for a few days to two weeks is sufficient. All vasoactive substances should be removed and avoided even after vasoconstriction resolves (box 1).[13] Nimodipine—a smooth muscle relaxant that mainly affects cerebral arteries—is mostly used, despite scarce evidence of efficacy. Outcome is usually good, although a few patients are left with permanent deficits from strokes.[12 14] A few lethal cases—mostly postpartum—have been reported.[15]

What are the less common causes of thunderclap headache?

Causes detected by plain CT or lumbar puncture

Two large prospective studies found that other intracranial haemorrhages, easily seen on plain CT, accounted for 5-10% of cases of thunderclap headache (box 4).[2 9] Rarely, thunderclap headache is caused by ischaemic stroke, which can be diagnosed on plain CT, although diffusion weighted MRI is better.[17] Hydrocephalus and brain tumours such as colloid cysts of the third ventricle occasionally present as repeated thunderclap headaches with nausea and vomiting, because of acute intracranial hypertension provoked by movements, coughing, or straining.[4] Thunderclap headache may be followed by coma due to herniation, and the diagnosis can usually be made on plain CT. Acute sinusitis can also cause thunderclap headache but must be regarded as a diagnosis of exclusion.[18]

BOX 3 PROPOSED DIAGNOSTIC CRITERIA FOR REVERSIBLE CEREBRAL VASOCONSTRICTION SYNDROME[6 13 14]

- Acute and severe headache (often thunderclap), with or without focal deficits or seizures
- Uniphasic course without new clinical symptoms more than one month after clinical onset
- Segmental constriction of cerebral arteries on indirect (magnetic resonance or computed tomography) angiography or direct catheter angiography
- No evidence of aneurysmal subarachnoid haemorrhage
- Normal or near normal cerebrospinal fluid results (protein <1 g/L, white blood cells $<15\times10^6$/L, normal glucose)
- Complete or marked normalisation of arteries on follow-up indirect or direct angiography performed within 12 weeks of clinical onset

BOX 4 SECONDARY CAUSES OF THUNDERCLAP HEADACHE

Causes usually detected by plain brain computed tomography (CT)

- Subarachnoid haemorrhage (95% during the 24 hours after bleeding)
- Intracerebral haemorrhage
- Intraventricular haemorrhage
- Acute subdural haemorrhage
- Brain infarct (after three hours)
- Tumour (third ventricle colloid cyst, posterior fossa tumour)
- Hydrocephalus (aqueductal stenosis, Chiari type 1 malformation)
- Acute sinusitis (exclusion diagnosis)

Causes detected by lumbar puncture after normal brain CT

- Subarachnoid haemorrhage
- Meningitis (bacterial or viral)

Causes that may present with normal CT and normal or near normal cerebrospinal fluid

- Dissection of cervical arteries (extracranial, intracranial, carotid, or vertebral)
- Symptomatic aneurysm with mass effect (painful third nerve palsy)
- Reversible cerebral vasoconstriction syndrome
- Posterior reversible encephalopathy syndrome
- Cerebral venous thrombosis (opening pressure may be high)
- Pituitary apoplexy
- Intracranial hypotension (opening pressure is low)
- Brain infarct in patients in whom CT was performed within three hours of onset
- Temporal arteritis
- Myocardial ischaemia
- Aortic dissection

BOX 5 CRITERIA FOR CLUSTER HEADACHE[6]

In patients with daily attacks of strictly unilateral severe headaches and normal test results, assess for cluster headache using the following criteria:

- A At least five attacks fulfilling criteria B through to D
- B Severe or very severe unilateral orbital, supraorbital, or temporal pain lasting 15-180 minutes if untreated
- C Headache is accompanied by at least one of the following:
  - Ipsilateral conjunctival injection or lacrimation (or both)
  - Ipsilateral nasal congestion or rhinorrhoea (or both)
  - Forehead and facial sweating
  - Ipsilateral eyelid edema
  - Ipsilateral forehead and facial sweating
  - Ipsilateral miosis or ptosis (or both)
  - A sense of restlessness or agitation
- D Attacks have a frequency from one every other day to eight per day
- E Not attributed to another disorder (investigations are normal)

Bacterial or viral meningitis accounts for 2% of cases of thunderclap headache.[9] Fever and neck stiffness may be lacking. Meningitis can be identified only by analysis of cerebrospinal fluid.[19] Urgent antibiotic or antiviral treatment is needed.

Causes that can be missed by plain CT and lumbar puncture

A systematic review of observational studies and case series showed that some causes of thunderclap headache cannot be ruled out clinically and can present with normal CT and cerebrospinal fluid results (box 4).[4] Because specific treatments can reduce the risk of complications, early diagnosis in patients with isolated headache is crucial.

About 8% of all patients with cervical artery dissection present with pain as the only symptom; the pain has a thunderclap pattern in 20% of these patients.[20] Diagnosis requires imaging of the cervical and intracranial arteries by CTA or an MRI protocol, particularly cervical fat suppressed T1 weighted sequences, to visualise the mural haematoma. Antithrombotic agents are used to prevent ischaemic events.

Thunderclap headache is the presenting and major clinical feature in 2-16% of patients with cerebral venous thrombosis.[21 22 23] Diagnosis is based on visualisation of the clot on brain MRI (hypersignal on T1 and T2 weighted sequences and hyposignal on echo planar T2* or susceptibility weighted imaging) associated with a missing sinus on CT or magnetic resonance venography. Treatment is based on heparin.

Posterior reversible leucoencephalopathy syndrome (PRES)—an acute neurological syndrome—may present with thunderclap headache, usually rapidly followed by confusion, seizures, and visual symptoms. Extreme hypertension is common but not constant. PRES is often associated with RCVS.[12 14 24] MRI shows reversible vasogenic brain oedema (hyperintensity on T2 weighted sequences) and MRA or CTA can detect associated vasospasms.[24] The most common causes of PRES are hypertensive encephalopathy and eclampsia.

Thunderclap headache is the presenting feature in 15% of people with intracranial hypotension.[25] After its sudden onset, the headache becomes a typical positional headache that occurs or worsens while sitting or standing and is relieved by lying down. Most cases occur after dural puncture. Spontaneous intracranial hypotension is more difficult to diagnose. CT is often normal. Opening pressure may be low or unobtainable on lumbar puncture, which is best avoided. Brain MRI with gadolinium is the best diagnostic test but may be normal in the first days. Epidural blood patch is the treatment of choice.

Finally, case reports suggest that thunderclap headache may also be caused by pituitary apoplexy[26] and, rarely, spontaneous retroclival haematoma,[27] myocardial infarction,[28] and aortic dissection.[29] We have also seen a few cases of thunderclap headache in temporal arteritis.

Which investigations are needed?

Plain head CT and, if CT is normal, lumbar puncture are needed.[10 30 31] Despite strong advice from health authorities, lumbar puncture is still often omitted.[32] Because patients with thunderclap headache may have a mass lesion, brain imaging is mandatory before performing lumbar puncture. If the CSF is clear, it is useful to measure the opening pressure because a high pressure may point to cerebral venous thrombosis,[21] and a low pressure to intracranial hypotension.

METHODS BOX

We identified references for this review by searching PubMed up to July 2012 with the terms "thunderclap headache", "acute headache", "sudden headache", "subarachnoid haemorrhage", and "reversible cerebral vasoconstriction". We also searched the reference lists of the identified articles and our own files. Only papers published in English and French, or with an English abstract, were reviewed. The final reference list was generated on the basis of relevance to the broad scope of this review.

QUESTIONS FOR FUTURE RESEARCH

- In cases of isolated thunderclap headache, what is the incidence of the various underlying disorders, especially reversible cerebral vasoconstriction syndrome, cervical artery dissection, and cerebral venous thrombosis?
- In cases of thunderclap headache with normal computed tomography (CT) and cerebrospinal fluid results, what is the diagnostic yield of cervical and cerebral CT angiography, magnetic resonance angiography, and magnetic resonance imaging?
- What are the mechanisms underlying the explosive onset of pain in thunderclap headache according to the various underlying causes?
- What biomarkers could be used as diagnostic screening tools?

Sufficient fluid has to be collected for white and red blood cell counts, Gram staining, protein and glucose concentrations, visual inspection for xanthochromia, and spectrophotometry.

Some authors recommend waiting 12 hours after headache onset to perform lumbar puncture, so that spectrophotometry can be used to differenciate traumatic taps from subarachnoid haemorrhages.[11] Such a delay may be logistically difficult. It exposes patients with meningitis to the risk associated with delayed treatment and those with a ruptured aneurysm to that of early rebleeding, which was seen in just under 14% of cases in the first hours after the initial haemorrhage in a prospective observational study.[33] We therefore do not delay lumbar puncture.

There is still debate about the need for further investigations in patients who have thunderclap headache with normal CT and lumbar puncture results.[30 31] We and others always perform CTA or MRA.[4 13 31] Indeed, in subarachnoid haemorrhage, angiography is needed to detect a ruptured aneurysm. If CT is normal, and CSF is normal, near normal (mild increase in cell counts), or possibly bloodstained due to trauma, cervical and cerebral angiography should be performed to look for alternative diagnoses (box 4). Systematic angiography in such cases can identify incidental unruptured aneurysm, which is present in 2% of the adult population.[11] A multidisciplinary neurovascular team can help decide whether the aneurysm requires treatment. Finally, in thunderclap headache with normal CT, normal CSF, and normal CTA or MRA, brain MRI may show cortical cerebral venous thrombosis, pituitary apoplexy, PRES, or intracranial hypotension (box 4).

Large prospective studies of patients presenting with thunderclap headache are needed to establish the incidence of underlying causes and to evaluate the diagnostic yield of angiography and brain MRI after normal CT and lumbar puncture. However, the wide availability of CTA and MRA means that imaging of the cervical and cerebral vessels is now much easier and more acceptable to patients.

When is four vessel cerebral angiography still necessary?

Conventional angiography is indicated in cases of subarachnoid haemorrhage when non-diagnostic CTA or MRA fails to detect an aneurysm.[3 11] Conventional angiography may be useful in some patients with thunderclap headaches and non-diagnostic MRI, MRA, and CTA, if headache persists or worsens, or if other symptoms appear, to search for occult intracranial arterial dissection, cerebral vasoconstriction syndrome, or vasculitis.

What about primary headache disorders as a cause of thunderclap headache?

Doctors should always look for an underlying cause of thunderclap headache. It can be dangerous to diagnose a primary headache disorder when onset is abrupt or related to cough, exertion, or sexual activity. Rarely, a patient presenting with a first episode of cluster headache might be investigated for recurrent unilateral thunderclap headache, because cluster pain is severe and can peak in one minute. Investigate patients without a history of a similar headache to exclude a secondary cause, especially a carotid dissection. Thereafter, correct diagnosis of cluster headache relies on clinical re-assessment (box 5).[6]

According to the International Classification of Headache Disorders, diagnosis of a primary headache disorder requires the exclusion of a secondary cause.[6] "Primary thunderclap headache" was introduced as a distinct entity in the second version of this classification.[6] However, some doubt whether primary thunderclap headache really exists. We think that all thunderclap headaches are secondary, and that the correct diagnosis can be missed when investigations are performed too early or too late, are incomplete, or lack sensitivity. For example, some cases of RCVS need a repeat CTA or MRA three weeks after headache onset to be detected and others need invasive conventional angiography. Therefore, if the results of all non-invasive investigations are normal and the patient is recurrence-free after a few weeks of follow-up, we use the term "thunderclap headache of undefined origin."[13]

Contributors: AD drafted the manuscript and is guarantor. M-GB and AD revised the manuscript.

Competing interests: All authors have completed the ICMJE uniform disclosure form at www.icmje.org/coi_disclosure.pdf (available on request from the corresponding author) and declare: no support from any organisation for the submitted work; AD has received payment for board membership from Novartis, lecture fees from Almirall, AstraZeneca, GlaxoSmithKline, Merck, and Pfizer, and has received support for travel, accommodation, and meeting expenses from Almirall and Pfizer; M-GB has received support for travel, accommodation, and meeting expenses from Sanofi, Servier, and Moleac; in addition, AD is associate editor of *Cephalalgia*.

Provenance and peer review: Commissioned; externally peer reviewed.

QUESTIONS FOR FUTURE RESEARCH

- In cases of isolated thunderclap headache, what is the incidence of the various underlying disorders, especially reversible cerebral vasoconstriction syndrome, cervical artery dissection, and cerebral venous thrombosis?
- In cases of thunderclap headache with normal computed tomography (CT) and cerebrospinal fluid results, what is the diagnostic yield of cervical and cerebral CT angiography, magnetic resonance angiography, and magnetic resonance imaging?
- What are the mechanisms underlying the explosive onset of pain in thunderclap headache according to the various underlying causes?
- What biomarkers could be used as diagnostic screening tools?

1 Day JW, Raskin NH. Thunderclap headache: symptom of unruptured cerebral aneurysm. *Lancet* 1986;2:1247-8.
2 Landtblom AM, Fridriksson S, Boivie J, Hillman J, Johansson G, Johansson I. Sudden onset headache: a prospective study of features, incidence and causes. *Cephalalgia* 2002;22:354-60.
3 Al-Shahi R, White PM, Davenport RJ, Lindsay KW. Subarachnoid haemorrhage. *BMJ* 2006;333:235-40.
4 Schwedt TJ, Matharu MS, Dodick DW. Thunderclap headache. *Lancet Neurol* 2006;5:621-31.
5 Ducros A, Boukobza M, Porcher R, Sarov M, Valade D, Bousser MG. The clinical and radiological spectrum of reversible cerebral vasoconstriction syndrome. A prospective series of 67 patients. *Brain* 2007;130:3091-101.
6 The international classification of headache disorders. *Cephalalgia* 2004;24:1-160.
7 Dodick DW. Thunderclap headache. *J Neurol Neurosurg Psychiatry* 2002;72:6-11.
8 Linn FH, Rinkel GJ, Algra A, van Gijn J. Headache characteristics in subarachnoid haemorrhage and benign thunderclap headache. *J Neurol Neurosurg Psychiatry* 1998;65:791-3.
9 Linn FH, Wijdicks EF, van der Graaf Y, Weerdesteyn-van Vliet FA, Bartelds AI, van Gijn J. Prospective study of sentinel headache in aneurysmal subarachnoid haemorrhage. *Lancet* 1994;344:590-3.
10 Edlow JA, Caplan LR. Avoiding pitfalls in the diagnosis of subarachnoid hemorrhage. *N Engl J Med* 2000;342:29-36.
11 van Gijn J, Kerr RS, Rinkel GJ. Subarachnoid haemorrhage. *Lancet* 2007;369:306-18.
12 Ducros A, Fiedler U, Porcher R, Boukobza M, Stapf C, Bousser MG. Hemorrhagic manifestations of reversible cerebral vasoconstriction syndrome. Frequency, features, and risk factors. *Stroke* 2010;41:2505-11.
13 Ducros A. Reversible cerebral vasoconstriction syndrome. *Lancet Neurol* 2012;11:906-17.
14 Singhal AB, Hajj-Ali RA, Topcuoglu MA, Fok J, Bena J, Yang D, et al. Reversible cerebral vasoconstriction syndromes: analysis of 139 cases. *Arch Neurol* 2011;68:1005-12.
15 Fugate JE, Ameriso SF, Ortiz G, Schottlaender LV, Wijdicks EF, Flemming KD, et al. Variable presentations of postpartum angiopathy. *Stroke* 2012;43:670-6.
16 Yeh YC, Fuh JL, Chen SP, Wang SJ. Clinical features, imaging findings and outcomes of headache associated with sexual activity. *Cephalalgia* 2010;30:1329-35.
17 Lopes Azevedo L, Breder R, de ASDP, de Freitas GR. Ischemic stroke presenting as thunderclap headache: report of two cases and review of the literature. *Eur Neurol* 2011;66:133-5.
18 McGeeney BE, Barest G, Grillone G. Thunderclap headache from complicated sinusitis. *Headache* 2006;46:517-20.
19 Davenport R. Acute headache in the emergency department. *J Neurol Neurosurg Psychiatry* 2002;72:ii33-ii7.
20 Arnold M, Cumurciuc R, Stapf C, Favrole P, Berthet K, Bousser MG. Pain as the only symptom of cervical artery dissection. *J Neurol Neurosurg Psychiatry* 2006;77:1021-4.
21 De Bruijn SF, Stam J, Kappelle LJ. Thunderclap headache as first symptom of cerebral venous sinus thrombosis. CVST Study Group. *Lancet* 1996;348:1623-5.
22 Cumurciuc R, Crassard I, Sarov M, Valade D, Bousser MG. Headache as the only neurological sign of cerebral venous thrombosis: a series of 17 cases. *J Neurol Neurosurg Psychiatry* 2005;76:1084-7.
23 Timoteo A, Inacio N, Machado S, Pinto AA, Parreira E. Headache as the sole presentation of cerebral venous thrombosis: a prospective study. *J Headache Pain* 2012;13:487-90.
24 Bartynski WS, Boardman JF. Catheter angiography, MR angiography, and MR perfusion in posterior reversible encephalopathy syndrome. *AJNR Am J Neuroradiol* 2008;29:447-55.
25 Schievink WI, Wijdicks EF, Meyer FB, Sonntag VK. Spontaneous intracranial hypotension mimicking aneurysmal subarachnoid hemorrhage. *Neurosurgery* 2001;48:513-6; discussion 6-7.
26 Dodick DW, Wijdicks EF. Pituitary apoplexy presenting as a thunderclap headache. *Neurology* 1998;50:1510-1.
27 Schievink WI, Thompson RC, Loh CT, Maya MM. Spontaneous retroclival hematoma presenting as a thunderclap headache. Case report. *J Neurosurg* 2001;95:522-4.
28 Broner S, Lay C, Newman L, Swerdlow M. Thunderclap headache as the presenting symptom of myocardial infarction. *Headache* 2007;47:724-5.
29 Mistry N, Mathew L, Parry A. Thunderclap headache. *Pract Neurol* 2009;9:294-7.
30 Savitz SI, Edlow J. Thunderclap headache with normal CT and lumbar puncture: further investigations are unnecessary: For. *Stroke* 2008;39:1392-3.
31 Moussouttas M, Mayer SA. Thunderclap headache with normal CT and lumbar puncture: further investigations are unnecessary: Against. *Stroke* 2008;39:1394-5.
32 O'Neill J, McLaggan S, Gibson R. Acute headache and subarachnoid haemorrhage: a retrospective review of CT and lumbar puncture findings. *Scot Med J* 2005;50:151-3.
33 Ohkuma H, Tsurutani H, Suzuki S. Incidence and significance of early aneurysmal rebleeding before neurosurgical or neurological management. *Stroke* 2001;32:1176-80.

Restless legs syndrome

Guy Leschziner, consultant neurologist[1],
Paul Gringras, professor of sleep medicine and neurodisability[2]

[1]Department of Neurology and Sleep Disorders Centre, Guy's and St Thomas' NHS Foundation Trust, London SE1 7EH, UK

[2]Department of Paediatric Neurosciences, Evelina Children's Hospital, London, UK

Correspondence to: G Leschziner guy.leschziner@gstt.nhs.uk

Cite this as: *BMJ* 2012;344:e3056

DOI: 10.1136/bmj.e3056

http://www.bmj.com/content/344/bmj.e3056

Restless legs syndrome is common; it is characterised by an urge to move and usually, but not exclusively, affects the legs. This urge to move is typically accompanied by abnormal sensations, variably described as burning, tingling, aching, or "insects crawling under the skin." These sensations are transiently or partially relieved by movement, and there is a strong circadian influence—symptoms are worse in the evening. It may be idiopathic or secondary to iron deficiency, pregnancy, uraemia, or neurological problems.

Estimates of prevalence of the syndrome range from 1.9% to 15%, depending on case ascertainment,[1] and it affects all age groups, although prevalence increases with age. Prevalence is about twice as high in women as in men.

Restless legs syndrome is a common cause of insomnia related to problems with sleep initiation and sleep maintenance, unrefreshing sleep, and excessive daytime sleepiness, and it may signify an underlying medical condition. Recognition of the condition and appropriate treatment therefore has a large impact on morbidity and quality of life.[2]

What is it?

Restless legs syndrome, which was first described by Ekbom in 1945,[3] is mainly characterised by sensory symptoms or an urge to move. It is now recognised that, in addition to affecting the legs, the syndrome can also affect the arms and even axial segments.[4] [5] The diagnosis is essentially clinical, and there are no specific biological markers. The International Restless Legs Syndrome Study Group refined diagnostic criteria for the condition in 2003.[6] The four essential criteria are: an urge to move the legs, usually accompanied by unpleasant sensations; the urge to move or the sensations worsen during periods of rest or inactivity; the urge to move or the sensations are partially or totally relieved by movement; the urge to move or the sensations are worse in the evening or during the night. Supportive criteria and associated features have also been defined (box).

The diagnosis may be problematic, because patients typically present with disturbed sleep, discomfort, pain, or a non-specific increase in motor activity. They often do not ascribe the sleep disturbance to the symptoms of restless legs syndrome. Furthermore, patients may use a variety of terms to describe the symptoms: a sensation of pulling, jittering, worms or insects moving, tingling, itching, aching, bubbling, fidgeting, electric current sensations, tightness, and throbbing.[7] In some people, pain may be the dominant symptom, and they are often misdiagnosed as having a chronic pain syndrome.

As well as the sensory features, patients may also experience motor features, in addition to the voluntary movements that they make to alleviate discomfort. These involuntary movements may occur in sleep or while awake, and they typically involve brief repetitive movements of the legs, ranging from subtle extension of the hallux to flexion of the hip, knee, and ankle. About 80% of patients with the syndrome experience periodic limb movements of sleep,[8] and these movements can result in arousals, leading to unrefreshing sleep and sleep maintenance insomnia.

Restless legs syndrome is usually a chronic disorder that worsens with time, although it does fluctuate. Periods of remission are common, especially in younger adults.[6] Many patients do not develop daily symptoms until 40-60 years of age.

Who gets it?

The prevalence of restless legs syndrome is controversial. Studies have used a variety of methods to ascertain cases, ranging from a single question such as "Do you have restless legs, or troublesome twitches of the legs?" to more stringent diagnostic criteria and subsequent case review to rule out differential diagnoses. On the basis of a single question, prevalence has been estimated at 9-15%, whereas studies that tried to rule out alternative diagnoses estimated the prevalence as 1.9-4.6%.[1] These prevalence figures are based on a review of 47 peer reviewed published studies of the syndrome in the general population between 1994 and 2010.

The age of onset varies widely, from childhood to over 80 years of age.[9] It occurs in nearly 2% of school age children,[10] and half of these cases have a positive parental history of restless legs syndrome.[11] The disorder is probably underdiagnosed in children, given that 38% of adults have reported the onset of symptoms before age 20 years and 10% before age 10 years.[8] Some children who have been diagnosed as having "growing pains" meet the diagnostic criteria for restless legs syndrome.[12] The sleep disturbance associated with this disorder in childhood can manifest as difficulty falling asleep, bedtime resistance, or night-time awakenings, and symptoms are often associated with attention-deficit/hyperactivity disorder.[13] Diagnostic classifications that require children to describe the sensations in their own words can prove difficult to apply in practice, and other supporting information often needs to be taken into account.[6] Because specialist input is needed in children, this review focuses mainly on adults.

Extensive review of the published literature suggests that prevalence is about two times higher in women than in men and increases with age. It is the most common movement disorder in pregnancy, affecting 13.5-26.6% of pregnant women, and it tends to become more severe and more prevalent over the duration of the pregnancy.[1] Women who experience transient restless legs syndrome in pregnancy

SUMMARY POINTS

- Restless legs syndrome is common in primary and hospital care; it causes great distress and disturbance of sleep
- The syndrome may be idiopathic or secondary to other disease
- Because of its varied presentations, it is often missed or misdiagnosed; diagnostic criteria have now been defined
- Screen all affected patients for iron store status; consider iron supplementation if serum ferritin is below 112 pmol/L (50 µg/L)
- Dopamine agonists are a licensed and proved treatment but are associated with augmentation and impulse control disorders; other unlicensed agents may be efficacious

CRITERIA FOR A DIAGNOSIS OF RESTLESS LEGS SYNDROME

Essential diagnostic criteria

- An urge to move the legs, usually accompanied or caused by uncomfortable or unpleasant sensations in the legs
- Unpleasant sensations or urge to move begin or worsen during periods of rest or inactivity, such as lying or sitting
- Unpleasant sensations or urge to move are partially or totally relieved by movement, at least for as long as the activity continues
- Unpleasant sensations or urge to move are worse during the evening or night than during the day, or they occur only during the evening or night

Supportive criteria

- Positive response to dopaminergic agents
- Periodic limb movements of sleep or during wakefulness
- Positive family history of restless legs syndrome

Associated features

- Onset can be at any age, but patients are usually middle aged or older at presentation
- Leg discomfort or the need to move results in insomnia
- Low serum ferritin (112 pmol/L; <50 μg/L)

have a fourfold increased risk of developing the disorder later in life.[14] Most studies suggest that there is a higher prevalence in Northern Europeans and North Americans than in African, Middle Eastern, Asian, Hispanic, or south eastern Europeans.[15]

Restless legs syndrome may be idiopathic or symptomatic. Idiopathic disease seems to have a strong genetic component, with a family history in 18.5-59.6% of patients.[16 17] Restless legs syndrome has been associated with a wide variety of conditions, most often iron deficiency and uraemia. Other disease associations include cardiovascular disease, obesity, diabetes, rheumatological disorders, peripheral neuropathy, radiculopathy, Parkinson's disease, multiple sclerosis, Charcot-Marie-Tooth disease, and spinal cord lesions. However, many of these described associations were not seen in all studies, and the strengths of these associations are unclear.

What causes restless legs syndrome?

Clinical observation has informed our understanding of the pathophysiology of the syndrome. Dopaminergic drugs alleviate the symptoms and dopamine antagonists can trigger or exacerbate them. However, despite a clear indication of dopamine being implicated in the pathophysiology, its role remains uncertain. Studies in animal models and patients have shown increased tyrosine hydroxylase (the rate limiting enzyme in dopamine synthesis) concentrations in the substantia nigra, decreased numbers of D2 dopamine receptors in the putamen, and increased concentrations of 3-O-methyldopa in the cerebrospinal fluid,[18] which implies that the syndrome is characterised by upregulation of dopaminergic transmission, with postsynaptic desensitisation. Dopaminergic activity shows natural circadian fluctuations, and this is thought to be the underlying mechanism for the characteristic circadian pattern of the symptoms.

Iron deficiency has also been implicated. Although iron deficiency alone is not sufficient to cause restless legs syndrome—and neither is it necessary—precipitation or exacerbation of symptoms with venesection is well described, and serum ferritin correlates inversely with symptom severity. Magnetic resonance imaging and studies of cerebrospinal fluid and autopsy specimens of substantia nigra have shown that brain iron stores are reduced in patients with restless legs syndrome.[19 20] Iron is an essential cofactor for tyrosine hydroxylase and seems to have a crucial role in dopamine metabolism.

The mechanism by which pregnancy worsens or triggers restless legs syndrome has not been elucidated. The symptoms often disappear or dramatically improve after delivery, strongly suggesting a hormonal influence, perhaps through the action of oestradiol or prolactin on dopaminergic transmission.[21] However, iron deficiency in pregnancy may also be important.

Because a family history is common and twin studies have shown hereditability estimates of 54-83%, efforts have been made to identify genetic factors involved in the pathophysiology of restless legs syndrome. Genome-wide association studies have shown associations with variants in four genes, *MEIS1*, *BTBD9*, *MAP2K5/SKOR1*, and *PTPRD*, but the findings have been inconsistent and the roles of these genes remain unclear.[w1-w5] *BTBD9* has also been associated with periodic limb movement of sleep.[w6]

What else could it be?

Several conditions can mimic restless legs syndrome. These include the sensory symptoms associated with peripheral neuropathy, cramps, positional discomfort, akathisia (a feeling of motor restlessness associated with dopamine receptor blocking neuroleptic agents), parkinsonism with sensory symptoms or drug induced dyskinesias, arthritis, hypnic jerks, fibromyalgia, and varicose veins.[7] Careful history taking and a general neurological examination can rule out these differential diagnoses. A diagnosis of restless leg syndrome can then be made if all four essential diagnostic criteria are met (see box).

What impact does restless legs syndrome have on health?

Restless legs syndrome has a large impact on quality of life, similar to that of type 2 diabetes and osteoarthritis.[22 23] Increased symptom severity is associated with serious psychological impairment in multiple psychological domains.[w7] Patients with the disorder have longer adjusted sleep latencies and a higher arousal index than controls,[2] and they report difficulty initiating sleep, difficulty maintaining sleep, and unrefreshing sleep two to three times more often than controls.[1]

Emerging evidence also suggests that restless legs syndrome is associated with metabolic dysregulation, autonomic dysfunction, and risk of cardiovascular disease. A recent extensive systematic review of 629 sources concluded that the syndrome is strongly and positively related to cardiovascular disease, is probably associated with diabetes and impaired glucose tolerance, and may be modestly associated with body mass index and dyslipidaemia.[24] However, the direction of the association is unclear. The syndrome may lead to increased risk for these disorders, perhaps via chronic activation of the sympathetic nervous system and the hypothalalmic-pituitary-adrenal axis; these conditions may increase the risk for the syndrome; or restless legs syndrome may be linked to these conditions through shared risk factors.

How is restless legs syndrome managed?

The treatment of restless legs syndrome in children requires specialist expertise so we will focus on the management of adults. In the past few years, evidence based guidelines have been published by taskforces for the Movement Disorders Society,[25] the European Federation of Neurological Sciences,[26] and the European Restless Legs Syndrome Study Group (EURLSSG),[7] with the last of these focusing on algorithms for treatment in primary care.

Management comprises the recognition and reversal of causes or exacerbators and symptom control. For patients with mild or infrequent symptoms, non-drug based options may be sufficient to provide symptom relief.

Measure serum ferritin in all patients with symptoms of restless legs syndrome. Anaemia is not sufficiently sensitive a marker for iron deficiency. Patients with a serum ferritin of less than 112 pmol/L (50 µg/L) should be started on iron supplements. Take a drug history to screen for exacerbating agents, such as antipsychotics, antidepressants (especially selective serotonin reuptake inhibitors and serotonin noradrenaline reuptake inhibitors), antihistamines, dopamine receptor blocking agents such as metoclopramide and prochlorperazine, and diphenhydramine.[27]

Not all patients need treatment, and only about 20% require drugs.[28] Non-drug based measures include avoidance of alcohol, caffeine, and smoking; good sleep hygiene; moderate regular exercise; avoidance of overexertion, stress, or sleep deprivation; and brief walking or other motor activities, hot baths, or leg massage before bedtime.[w8]

Consider drugs in patients with symptoms that seriously impair quality of life, sleep, or daytime functioning despite reversal of iron deficiency, removal of possible exacerbators, and exclusion of secondary restless legs syndrome. Choice of agent should be guided by the nature of the symptoms,[7] but the dopamine agonists—ropinirole, pramipexole, and rotigotine—are the only agents licensed in the United Kingdom, although in the United States the Food and Drug Administration recently approved a slow release preparation of gabapentin enacarbil, a prodrug of gabapentin.

What problems are associated with dopamine agonists?

A recent Cochrane review showed that dopamine agonists were superior to placebo in randomised controlled trials with up to seven months' follow-up,[29] and a further meta-analysis of 35 trials also showed moderate improvements in symptom severity, self rated sleep quality, and disease specific quality of life.[30] Although these meta-analyses clearly show efficacy, treatment with these drugs has certain problems. These agents can be associated with the phenomenon of augmentation—the onset of symptoms earlier in the day; increased severity of symptoms; or the spread of symptoms to different body parts, such as the arms, trunk, or even face.[31] Augmentation should be distinguished from early morning rebound of symptoms related to declining plasma concentrations of the drug or the slow natural progression of symptoms. Augmentation rates seem to be particularly high with levodopa but are also a problem with licensed dopamine agonists. Recommendations include keeping dosages low because of the association between higher doses and augmentation; monitoring ferritin because low ferritin is associated with clinically significant augmentation[32]; and monitoring lifestyle and drug factors that might have an effect on symptom exacerbation. At present, no direct head to head trials of licensed agents have examined augmentation systematically, and most studies have not been sufficiently long in duration to evaluate augmentation fully.

The other important problem with dopamine agonists is that of impulse control disorders. Several of these disorders have been described after the use of dopamine agonists in Parkinson's disease, including pathological gambling, compulsive shopping, hypersexuality, and compulsive eating. It has recently been shown that these problems are also common in patients with restless legs syndrome treated with these drugs,[33] and that they are associated with higher dose, history of experimental drug use, female sex, and a family history of gambling disorders.[34] Impulse control disorders affect as many as one in five patients with restless legs syndrome who are taking dopamine agonists.

How do I choose between different dopamine agonists?

Currently, insufficient strong evidence is available to allow direct comparison of efficacy, safety and adverse effects such as augmentation and impulse control disorders. Evidence based guidelines do not suggest any particular dopamine agonist, although the EURLSSG taskforce recommends rotigotine, which is administered as a patch and provides therapeutic plasma levels over the entire 24 hour period for

SOURCES AND SELECTION CRITERIA

We searched Medline, the Cochrane Library, and the National Institute for Health and Clinical Excellence website with the search term "restless legs syndrome". We used evidence from published articles and guidelines on the management and treatment of restless legs syndrome by the International Restless Legs Syndrome Study Group, the European Restless Legs Study Group, and the Movement Disorders Society taskforces. Priority was given to evidence obtained from well conducted systematic reviews and meta-analyses.

TIPS FOR NON-SPECIALISTS

- Online algorithms are available for the diagnosis of restless legs syndrome
- Ensure that exacerbators—such as poor sleep hygiene, caffeine, alcohol, smoking, and drugs such as antidepressants, neuroleptics, and other dopamine blocking agents—have been withdrawn or minimised if possible
- Always use the minimum dose of dopamine agonist in an effort to avoid augmentation and impulse control disorders
- Consider avoiding dopamine agonists in patients with a history of impulsive or compulsive behaviour and counsel all patients on the risks of pathological gambling, compulsive shopping, hypersexuality, and compulsive eating

ADDITIONAL EDUCATIONAL RESOURCES

Resources for healthcare professionals

- BMJ Best Practice (http://bestpractice.bmj.com/best-practice/monograph/65.html)—BMJ Best Practice module on restless legs syndrome
- European RLS Study Group (www.eurlssg.org/)—Website with an online algorithm for the diagnosis of restless legs syndrome and sleep diary templates

Resources for patients

- Restless Legs Syndrome Foundation (www.rls.org)—US based charity providing information about the condition and ongoing research
- RLS-UK/Ekbom Syndrome Association (www.rls-uk.org)—UK based organisation providing information and support to patients

patients with severe daytime symptoms.[7] Extended release preparations of other dopamine agonists have not yet been licensed for restless legs syndrome.

Ergot derived dopamine agonists are not recommended because of the risks of cardiac valvular fibrosis and other fibrotic side effects.

What other drugs are available?

No other agents are licensed for restless legs syndrome. However, the Movement Disorders Society taskforce evidence based review of all published studies before 2007 found evidence that gabapentin is efficacious (at least two positive randomised controlled trials with defined outcome measures); that oxycodone, carbamazepine, sodium valproate, and clonidine are probably efficacious (one positive randomised controlled trial without contradictory evidence); but that tramadol, methadone, clonazepam, zolpidem, topiramate, and minerals and vitamins such as folate and magnesium are still under investigation (positive results from controlled clinical trials, observational controlled studies, or case series only).[25] This review also found that intravenous iron is probably efficacious in end stage renal failure but remains investigational in patients with normal renal function.

However, opioid-like drugs such as codeine and tramadol, gabapentin, and pregabalin are recommended as second line treatment by the EURLSSG taskforce,[7] although these are all off-label. Clonazepam, again off-label, is suggested as an option for intermittent symptoms that disturb sleep. These recommendations are based on consensus by European experts in restless legs syndrome and primary care practitioners.

More recently, two very short randomised double blinded placebo controlled trials found pregabalin to be helpful,[35 36] but there are inadequate data to support its long term efficacy.

Whom should I refer to a specialist?

Refer patients to a neurologist or sleep specialist if treatment is unsuccessful. The EURLSSG taskforce defines unsuccessful treatment as[7]:

- An insufficient initial response despite adequate duration and dose of treatment; adequate duration depends on the drug in question and can extend to 10 days for ropinirole
- Response to treatment becomes insufficient despite an increased dose
- The side effects are intolerable
- The maximum recommended dosage is no longer effective
- Augmentation develops.

The taskforce also recommends that children should not be treated in primary care.

Contributors: Both authors helped write the article. GL revised the manuscript and is guarantor.

Competing interests: All authors have completed the ICMJE uniform disclosure form at www.icmje.org/coi_disclosure.pdf (available on request from the corresponding author) and declare: no support from any organisation for the submitted work; GL has received an honorarium from UCB Pharma for an advisory board; no other relationships or activities that could appear to have influenced the submitted work.

Provenance and peer review: Commissioned; externally peer reviewed.

1 Ohayon MM, O'Hara R, Vitiello MV. Epidemiology of restless legs syndrome: A synthesis of the literature. *Sleep Med Rev* 2011; published online 25 July.
2 Winkelman JW, Redline S, Baldwin CM, Resnick HE, Newman AB, Gottlieb DJ. Polysomnographic and health-related quality of life correlates of restless legs syndrome in the Sleep Heart Health Study. *Sleep* 2009;32:772-8.
3 Ekbom KA. Restless legs: a clinical study. *Acta Med Scand* 1945;158(suppl):1-122.
4 Michaud M, Chabli A, Lavigne G, Montplaisir J. Arm restlessness in patients with restless legs syndrome. *Mov Disord* 2000;15:289-93.
5 Pérez-Díaz H, Iranzo A, Rye DB, Santamaría J. Restless abdomen: a phenotypic variant of restless legs syndrome. *Neurology* 2011;77:1283-6.
6 Allen RP, Picchietti D, Hening WA, Trenkwalder C, Walters AS, Montplaisir J. Restless legs syndrome: diagnostic criteria, special considerations, and epidemiology. A report from the restless legs syndrome diagnosis and epidemiology workshop at the National Institutes of Health. *Sleep Med* 2003 Mar;4(2):101-19.
7 Garcia-Borreguero D, Stillman P, Benes H, Buschmann H, Chaudhuri KR, Gonzalez Rodríguez VM, et al. Algorithms for the diagnosis and treatment of restless legs syndrome in primary care. *BMC Neurol* 2011;11:28.
8 Montplaisir J, Boucher S, Poirier G, Lavigne G, Lapierre O, Lespérance P. Clinical, polysomnographic, and genetic characteristics of restless legs syndrome: a study of 133 patients diagnosed with new standard criteria. *Mov Disord* 1997;12:61-5.
9 Winkelmann J, Wetter TC, Collado-Seidel V, Gasser T, Dichgans M, Yassouridis A, et al. Clinical characteristics and frequency of the hereditary restless legs syndrome in a population of 300 patients. *Sleep* 2000;23:597-602.
10 Picchietti D, Allen RP, Walters AS, Davidson JE, Myers A, Ferini-Strambi L. Restless legs syndrome: prevalence and impact in children and adolescents—the Peds REST study. *Pediatrics* 2007;120:253-66.
11 Picchietti DL, Rajendran RR, Wilson MP, Picchietti MA. Pediatric restless legs syndrome and periodic limb movement disorder: parent-child pairs. *Sleep Med* 2009;10:925-31.
12 Walters AS. Is there a subpopulation of children with growing pains who really have restless legs syndrome? A review of the literature. *Sleep Med* 2002;3:93-8.
13 Chervin RD, Archbold KH, Dillon JE, Pituch KJ, Panahi P, Dahl RE, et al. Associations between symptoms of inattention, hyperactivity, restless legs, and periodic leg movements. *Sleep* 2002;25:213-8.
14 Cesnik E, Casetta I, Turri M, Govoni V, Granieri E, Strambi LF, et al. Transient RLS during pregnancy is a risk factor for the chronic idiopathic form. *Neurology* 2010;75:2117-20.
15 Yeh P, Walters AS, Tsuang JW. Restless legs syndrome: a comprehensive overview on its epidemiology, risk factors, and treatment. *Sleep Breath* 2011; published online 26 October.
16 Rangarajan S, Rangarajan S, D'Souza GA. Restless legs syndrome in an Indian urban population. *Sleep Med* 2007;9:88-93.
17 Vogl FD, Pichler I, Adel S, Pinggera GK, Bracco S, De Grandi A, et al. Restless legs syndrome: epidemiological and clinicogenetic study in a South Tyrolean population isolate. *Mov Disord* 2006;21:1189-95.
18 Salas RE, Gamaldo CE, Allen RP. Update in restless legs syndrome. *Curr Opin Neurol* 2010;23:401-6.
19 Earley CJ, Allen RP, Beard JL, Connor JR. Insight into the pathophysiology of restless legs syndrome. *J Neurosci Res* 2000;62:623-8.
20 Connor JR, Boyer PJ, Menzies SL, Dellinger B, Allen RP, Ondo WG, et al. Neuropathological examination suggests impaired brain iron acquisition in restless legs syndrome. *Neurology* 2003;61:304-9.
21 Dzaja A, Wehrle R, Lancel M, Pollmächer T. Elevated estradiol plasma levels in women with restless legs during pregnancy. *Sleep* 2009;32:169-74.
22 Allen RP, Walters AS, Montplaisir J, Hening W, Myers A, Bell TJ, et al. Restless legs syndrome prevalence and impact: REST general population study. *Arch Intern Med* 2005;165:1286-92.
23 Happe S, Reese JP, Stiasny-Kolster K, Peglau I, Mayer G, Klotsche J, et al. Assessing health-related quality of life in patients with restless legs syndrome. *Sleep Med* 2009;10:295-305.
24 Innes KE, Selfe TK, Agarwal P. Restless legs syndrome and conditions associated with metabolic dysregulation, sympathoadrenal dysfunction, and cardiovascular disease risk: a systematic review. *Sleep Med Rev* 2011; published online 4 July.
25 Trenkwalder C, Hening WA, Montagna P, Oertel WH, Allen RP, Walters AS, et al. Treatment of restless legs syndrome: an evidence-based review and implications for clinical practice. *Mov Disord* 2008;23:2267-302.
26 Vignatelli L, Billiard M, Clarenbach P, Garcia-Borreguero D, Kaynak D, Liesiene V, et al; EFNS Task Force. EFNS guidelines on management of restless legs syndrome and periodic limb movement disorder in sleep. *Eur J Neurol* 2006;13:1049-65.
27 Winkelman JW. Considering the causes of RLS. *Eur J Neurol* 2006;13(suppl 3):8-14.
28 Byrne R, Sinha S, Chaudhuri KR. Restless legs syndrome: diagnosis and review of management options. *Neuropsych Dis Treat* 2006;2:155-64.
29 Scholz H, Trenkwalder C, Kohnen R, Riemann D, Kriston L, Hornyak M. Dopamine agonists for restless legs syndrome. *Cochrane Database Syst Rev* 2011;3:CD006009.
30 Hornyak M, Trenkwalder C, Kohnen R, Scholz H. Efficacy and safety of dopamine agonists in restless legs syndrome. *Sleep Med* 2012; published online 24 January.
31 García-Borreguero D, Williams AM. Dopaminergic augmentation of restless legs syndrome. *Sleep Med Rev* 2010;14:339-46.
32 Trenkwalder C, Högl B, Benes H, Kohnen R. Augmentation in restless legs syndrome is associated with low ferritin. *Sleep Med* 2008;9:572-4.

33 Cornelius JR, Tippmann-Peikert M, Slocumb NL, Frerichs CF, Silber MH. Impulse control disorders with the use of dopaminergic agents in restless legs syndrome: a case-control study. *Sleep* 2010;33:81-7.
34 Voon V, Schoerling A, Wenzel S, Ekanayake V, Reiff J, Trenkwalder C, et al. Frequency of impulse control behaviours associated with dopaminergic therapy in restless legs syndrome. *BMC Neurol* 2011;11:117.
35 Garcia-Borreguero D, Larrosa O, Williams AM, Albares J, Pascual M, Palacios JC, et al. Treatment of restless legs syndrome with pregabalin: a double-blind, placebo-controlled study. *Neurology* 2010;74:1897-904.
36 Allen R, Chen C, Soaita A, Wohlberg C, Knapp L, Peterson BT, et al. A randomised, double-blind, 6-week, dose-ranging study of pregabalin in patients with restless legs syndrome. *Sleep Med* 2010;11:512-9.

Neuropathic pain: mechanisms and their clinical implications

Steven P Cohen, professor[1], professor of anesthesiology and physical medicine and rehabilitation[2], Jianren Mao, professor of anesthesia research and vice chair for research[3]

[1]Departments of Anesthesiology and Critical Care Medicine and Physical Medicine and Rehabilitation, Johns Hopkins School of Medicine, Baltimore, MD 21029, USA

[2]Uniformed Services University of the Health Sciences, Bethesda, MD, USA

[3]Massachusetts General Hospital, Harvard Medical School, Boston, MA, USA

Correspondence to: S P Cohen scohen40@jhmi.edu

Cite this as: *BMJ* 2014;348:f7656

DOI: 10.1136/bmj.f7656

http://www.bmj.com/content/348/bmj.f7656

ABSTRACT

Neuropathic pain can develop after nerve injury, when deleterious changes occur in injured neurons and along nociceptive and descending modulatory pathways in the central nervous system. The myriad neurotransmitters and other substances involved in the development and maintenance of neuropathic pain also play a part in other neurobiological disorders. This might partly explain the high comorbidity rates for chronic pain, sleep disorders, and psychological conditions such as depression, and why drugs that are effective for one condition may benefit others. Neuropathic pain can be distinguished from non-neuropathic pain by two factors. Firstly, in neuropathic pain there is no transduction (conversion of a nociceptive stimulus into an electrical impulse). Secondly, the prognosis is worse: injury to major nerves is more likely than injury to non-nervous tissue to result in chronic pain. In addition, neuropathic pain tends to be more refractory than non-neuropathic pain to conventional analgesics, such as non-steroidal anti-inflammatory drugs and opioids. However, because of the considerable overlap between neuropathic and nociceptive pain in terms of mechanisms and treatment modalities, it might be more constructive to view these entities as different points on the same continuum. This review focuses on the mechanisms of neuropathic pain, with special emphasis on clinical implications.

Introduction

Pain is a survival mechanism that serves as a warning sign of ongoing or impending tissue damage. According to an Institute of Medicine report released in 2011, one in three Americans experiences chronic pain—more than the total number affected by heart disease, cancer, and diabetes combined.[1] In Europe, the prevalence of chronic pain is 25-30%.[2] About a fifth of people who report chronic pain are thought to have predominantly neuropathic pain.[3 4]

Rationale for mechanism based treatment

One reason for the high prevalence rate of chronic pain, and neuropathic pain in particular, is the absence of effective treatments. Unlike opioids and non-steroidal anti-inflammatory drugs, which form the cornerstone of drug treatment for nociceptive pain, the adjuvants used to treat neuropathic pain tend to have only a modest effect and in a minority of patients. The main reason for this is the inability to target underlying mechanisms precisely; this is why syndromes (such as fibromyalgia), which lack distinct pathophysiological mechanisms, tend to be associated with lower treatment success rates than diseases.[5]

SUMMARY POINTS

- Neuropathic pain, defined as pain caused by a lesion or disease of the somatosensory nervous system, tends to be more refractory to treatment than other forms of pain
- As more accurate instruments have been developed to identify neuropathic pain, estimates of its prevalence and socioeconomic impact have increased
- The development of neuropathic pain requires a plethora of different mechanisms that extend from the periphery to the central nervous system where they involve the spinal cord, brain, and descending modulation systems
- Although conceptually appealing, the mechanism based treatment of pain is challenging to implement
- Many drugs shown to be effective in preclinical models of neuropathic pain fail in clinical studies, mostly because animal models tend to emphasize evoked, rather than spontaneous, pain and do not account for the emotional aspects of pain
- In view of the large degree of overlap between neuropathic and nociceptive pain in terms of mechanisms and treatment response, many experts view them as different points on a chronic pain continuum, rather than distinct entities

Generally, mechanism based treatments, which target specific pain mechanisms, are superior to disease based or cause based treatments, which target less proximate causes. This may be one reason why so many drugs that are successful in preclinical studies fail in clinical trials.[6] As a general rule, painful conditions such as inflammatory arthritis, in which the mechanisms have been clearly identified, have more effective treatments.[7] But in clinical practice, elucidating the pain mechanisms responsible for neuropathic symptoms can be difficult. One method for identifying mechanisms and predicting treatment outcomes is the use of intravenous infusion tests, such as intravenous ketamine to predict response to dextromethorphan or other NMDA (N-methyl-D-aspartate) receptor antagonists. However, studies that have evaluated these treatments have been methodologically flawed and usually have reported only modest predictive value.[8]

In the past decade, several reviews have been written on the mechanisms of neuropathic pain, most of which are directed at neuroscientists. Yet it is essential that clinicians understand the mechanisms too, because such an understanding can steer future research and guide clinical practice.

Search methods

In September 2013, we searched the databases on Medline via PubMed and Ovid, Embase, and CINAHL Plus using the keywords "neuropathic pain", "sensitization", "neuroplasticity", "mechanisms", "reorganization", "sympathetically maintained", "antinociceptive", and "descending modulation", with no date restrictions. For individual sections, keywords relating to specific topics and mechanisms were identified from the initial search (for example, "ion channel expression", "cytokine", "glial cell") and searched using the same databases. Additional articles and prime references were obtained by cross referencing all search terms with "review article" and searching through reference lists. We considered animal studies, experimental and clinical trials, and review articles published in English.

Physiology and classification

The generation of pain in response to tissue injury involves four basic elements:

- Transduction: a function of nociceptors that converts noxious stimulation to nociceptive signals
- Transmission: a process that sends nociceptive signals along nerve fibers from the site of injury to the central nervous system (CNS)
- Transformation or plasticity: a mechanism that modulates nociceptive signals at synaptic sites and at the level of the CNS through ascending, descending, or regional facilitation and inhibition
- Perception: a key component of the clinical pain experience that integrates cognitive and affective (emotional) responses.

In evolutionary terms the activation of high threshold mechanical nociceptors or other types of specialized nociceptor served a protective role, acting as a warning system for dangerous stimuli. But whereas inflammatory pain is adaptive, evolution has failed to account for our enhanced ability to survive trauma, disease, or iatrogenic trauma intended to prolong or enhance quality of life (such as surgery). In these contexts pain no longer serves a useful function but becomes the disease itself.

Although it is easy to conceptualize pain as a homogeneous entity, this is overly simplistic. In reality there are several different types, each with distinct neurobiological and pathophysiological mechanisms. The most common categorization divides pain into two main types: neuropathic and nociceptive pain (table 1). This distinction is important because it not only reflects the cause of pain but also informs treatment.

Nociceptive pain can be classified as somatic (for example, muscles, joints) or less often visceral (internal organs). Because of the high concentration of nociceptors in somatic tissues, chronic somatic pain is typically well localized and often results from degenerative processes (such as arthritis). By contrast, internal organs are usually unresponsive to classic painful stimuli, such as cutting and burning, but respond to ischemia (for example, angina), inflammation (appendicitis), or occlusion of flow that results in capsular distension (bowel obstruction).

Neuropathic pain is defined as pain caused by a lesion or disease of the somatosensory nervous system.[9] In neuropathic pain, tissue damage directly affects the nervous system, resulting in the generation of ectopic discharges that bypass transduction.[10] One subtype of neuropathic pain is central pain (for example, as a result of spinal cord injury), which manifests as a constellation of signs and symptoms that follows an insult to the CNS as a necessary, but not always sufficient, inciting event. Although many forms of nociceptive pain, and some forms of neuropathic

Table 1 Classification of neuropathic and nociceptive pain

Clinical characteristic	Neuropathic pain	Nociceptive pain
Cause	Injury to the nervous system, often accompanied by maladaptive changes in the nervous system	Damage or potential damage to tissues
Descriptors	Lancinating, shooting, electric-like, stabbing pain	Throbbing, aching, pressure-like pain
Sensory deficits	Common—for example, numbness, tingling, pricking	Uncommon; if present they have a non-dermatomal or non-nerve distribution
Motor deficits	Neurological weakness may be present if a motor nerve is affected; dystonia or spasticity may be associated with central nervous system lesions and sometimes peripheral lesions (such as complex regional pain syndrome)	May have pain induced weakness
Hypersensitivity	Pain often evoked by non-painful (allodynia) or painful (exaggerated response) stimuli	Uncommon except for hypersensitivity in the immediate area of an acute injury
Character	Distal radiation common	Distal radiation less common; proximal radiation more common
Paroxysms	Exacerbations common and unpredictable	Exacerbations less common and often associated with activity
Autonomic signs	Color changes, temperature changes, swelling, or sudomotor (sweating) activity occur in a third to half of patients	Uncommonv

Table 2 Comparison of pain in animal models and clinical pain

Variable	Animal models	Clinical pain
Study methods	Deficiencies in blinding, randomization, and power calculation (low numbers) are common	Greater attention to methodological quality in large scale clinical trials
Time course of development	Minutes to hours to days; largely coincides with the time course of tissue damage	Weeks to months to years; usually outlasts the time course of tissue damage
Hallmark	Increased neuronal excitability, decreased nociceptive threshold, and expanded receptive fields	Altered pain quality with or without neurological deficits (such as numbness, weakness)
Pattern	Correlations between tissue damage and cellular responses; near uniformity in response patterns; sustainability of neuronal responses not confirmed	Considerable individual variations in pain experience; dynamic changes in pain intensity, timing, location, modality, and quality
Presentation	Mainly hyperalgesia and allodynia; rarely contralateral behavioral changes	Usually spontaneous pain; often extends beyond a single nerve or dermatome distribution; contralateral responses may be present; behavioral responses common
Affective component	Absent or unknown	Powerful contributor to the pain experience; has a strong influence on treatment outcome
Intervention	Behavioral changes can be prevented or reversed (or both) by blocking key cellular elements	Similar approaches (blocking key cellular elements) have had mostly negative outcomes in clinical trials; long interval between positive results and implementation of intervention in practice
Outcomes	Considered over the course of days or weeks; treatment response rates are higher than in clinical trials	Considered over the course of weeks or months for clinical trials, and months or years in practice; success rates are lower than in animal models, especially in clinical practice

pain, may confer evolutionary benefits, chronic neuropathic pain is always maladaptive.

Compared with previous studies, estimates of the prevalence of neuropathic pain have significantly increased over the past decade since the development of instruments designed to identify such pain.[11] Around 15-25% of people with chronic pain are currently thought to have neuropathic pain.[3 4] However, the prevalence of neuropathic pain may belie its socioeconomic impact, because studies have found that it is associated with a greater negative impact on quality of life than nociceptive pain.[12]

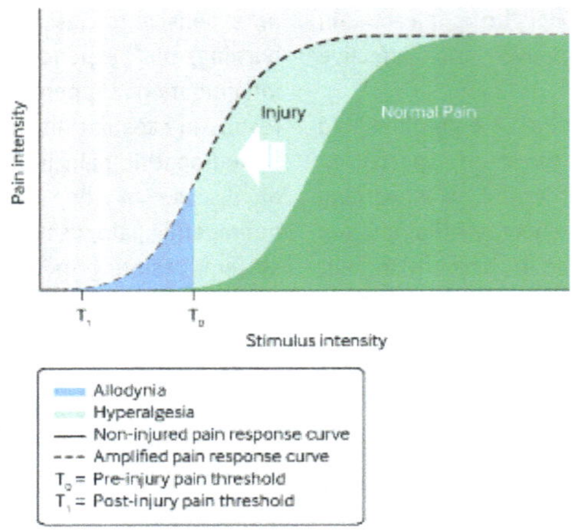

Fig 1 Diagram depicting normally perceived pain, as well as allodynia and hyperalgesia after injury

Emotional versus physiological aspects

A common misconception is that pain is purely a physiological phenomenon. In fact, "pain" represents a final integrative package, the components of which consist of neurophysiological processes as well as contextual, psychological, and sociocultural factors. This is one reason for the discrepancies between preclinical studies (which measure increased tolerance to painful stimuli in animals (anti-nociception)), clinical studies (which assess efficacy), and clinical practice, which measures effectiveness (table 2).

KEY RESEARCH QUESTIONS

- Is it possible to devise a valid animal model that accounts for the "affective-motivational" (emotional) aspect of pain as well as the "sensory-discriminative" (physio-anatomical) aspect?
- Are there any measures that can be taken before (pre-emptive analgesia) or during the early phase after nerve injury that can prevent the transition to chronic neuropathic pain?
- Is neuropathic pain represented differently in the brain than other chronic pain conditions?
- Can we develop better animal models to reflect spontaneous pain, rather than those that emphasize stimulus dependent pain (for example, allodynia), which may be less relevant in clinical practice?
- Although the concept of mechanism based pain treatment is intellectually enticing, can this be routinely incorporated into clinical practice?

DEFINITIONS

- Allodynia: Painful response to a normally innocuous stimulus
- Central pain: A subset of neuropathic pain caused by a lesion or disease of the central somatosensory nervous system
- Central sensitization: Increased responsiveness of nociceptive neurons in the central nervous system to normal or subthreshold sensory input
- Deafferentation pain: Pathological pain condition associated with a partial or complete loss of sensory input from a part of the body after lesions in somatosensory pathways, often as a result of reorganization in the central nervous system. Common examples include phantom limb pain and brachial plexopathy
- Descending modulation: The process by which pathways that descend from the brain to the spinal cord modify incoming somatosensory information so that the perception of and reactions to somatosensory stimuli are altered, resulting in increased or decreased pain
- Ectopic discharge: Trains of ongoing electrical nerve impulses that occur spontaneously without stimulation or originate at sites other than the normal location (or both). This phenomenon typically occurs after nerve injury
- Ephaptic transmission: The phenomenon by which two independent nerves communicate with each other through an artificial synapse, which often develops after injury to the insulating myelin sheath that normally prevents crosstalk between parallel nerves
- Hyperalgesia: Increased pain response to a normally painful stimulus
- Neuropathic pain: Pain caused by a lesion or disease of the somatosensory nervous system
- Neuroplasticity: Changes in neural pathways and synapses that result from bodily injury or changes in behavior, the environment, or neural processes. This is consistent with the concept that the brain is a dynamic organ that constantly changes in response to internal and outside events throughout life
- Nociception: The neural responses of encoding and processing noxious stimuli
- Nociceptive pain: Pain that arises from the activation of peripheral nerve endings (nociceptors) that respond to noxious stimulation. Nociceptive pain arises from actual or potential damage to non-neural tissue and can be categorized as visceral or somatic
- Noxious stimulus: A stimulus that damages or threatens to damage normal tissues
- Peripheral sensitization: A lowering of the stimulus (pain) threshold for nociceptor activation and an increased frequency of nerve impulse firing in response to stimulation (hyperexcitability). Peripheral sensitization is often found at the site of tissue damage or inflammation
- Sympathetically maintained pain: Pain that is enhanced or maintained by a functional abnormality of the sympathetic nervous system, such as functional sympathetic afferent coupling or increased expression of adrenergic receptors at the peripheral terminals of nociceptive afferent fibers
- Windup: Progressive increase in the frequency and magnitude of firing of dorsal horn neurons produced by repetitive activation of C fibers above a critical threshold, leading to a perceived increase in pain intensity

Partly because of these factors and the neurophysiological differences between individuals, the degree of pathology tends to correlate poorly with the intensity of pain for conditions such as back pain.[13] To illustrate, conditions such as fibromyalgia have high reported pain scores despite the absence of overt disease.

Secondary order neurons arising in the spinal cord transmit nociceptive input to the thalamus through ascending pathways such as the spinothalamic tract, which functions as a relay station to higher cortical centers. These centers include:

- The anterior cingulate cortex, which is involved in anxiety, anticipation of pain, attention to pain, and motor responses
- The insular cortex, which may play a role in the sensory discriminative and affective aspects of pain that contribute to the negative emotional responses and behaviors associated with painful stimuli[14]

Table 3 Evidence for pharmacotherapy based on mechanisms of neuropathic pain

Mechanism	Symptoms	Target	Treatment	Evidence
Phosphorylation of TRPV-1 by protein kinase C	Hyperalgesia, burning, and other spontaneous pain	TRPV-1	Capsaicin	Strong evidence for peripheral neuropathic pain
Release of proinflammatory cytokines from immune cells	Spontaneous pain, hyperalgesia, inflammation	Cytokines, such as TNF-α, IL-1β, IL-6, and other interleukins	Cytokine inhibitors (such as etanercept, infliximab)	Strong evidence for inflammatory arthritis; conflicting results in human studies for neuropathic pain
Release of nerve growth factor and other neurotrophins from mast cells	Hyperalgesia, burning and other spontaneous pain, inflammation	Nerve growth factor and its receptors (trkA/p75)	Nerve growth factor inhibitors (such as tanezumab)	Moderate clinical evidence for inflammatory pain (such as arthritis), evidence for neuropathic pain in preclinical studies
Release of substance P in the dorsal horn	Hyperalgesia	NK1 receptor	NK1 receptor antagonists (such as aprepitant)	Evidence in preclinical but not clinical studies
Proliferation of and redistribution of sodium channels	Spontaneous pain, Tinel's sign	Tetrodotoxin sensitive and resistant sodium channels	Membrane stabilizers (such as carbamazepine, lamotrigine) and anti-arrhythmics (such as systemic lidocaine, mexiletine)	Moderate to strong evidence for peripheral neuropathic pain
Increased expression of cannabinoid receptors in the peripheral and central nervous systems, and in glial cells	Hyperalgesia	CB1 and CB2	Natural and synthetic cannabinoids (such as cannabis, dronabinol)	Strong preclinical and clinical evidence for a modest effect for central and peripheral neuropathic pain, and inflammatory pain
Activation of spinal NMDA receptors	Hyperalgesia, opioid tolerance	NMDA receptor	NMDA receptor antagonists (such as ketamine, dextromethorphan, memantine)	Strong evidence in preclinical and clinical trials for peripheral and central neuropathic pain; conflicting results for reduction of opioid tolerance
Increased expression of voltage gated calcium channels at dorsal root ganglia and presynaptic terminals	Spontaneous pain, hyperalgesia	N-type, L-type, and T-type calcium channels	Calcium channel antagonists (such as gabapentin, pregabalin, ziconotide)	Strong evidence for peripheral and central neuropathic pain
Increased release of CGRP from primary afferents	Hyperalgesia, spontaneous pain, inflammation	CGRP inhibitors	CGRP receptor antagonists (such as olcegepant and telcagepant)	Evidence in preclinical studies; in clinical studies, strong evidence only for migraine
Increased expression and sensitivity of α adrenoceptors, sympathetic sprouting	Spontaneous pain, pain exacerbated by cold and stress	Sympathetic ganglia, sympathetic nervous system	Phentolamine, clonidine, sympathetic blocks	Weak evidence for short term effect for peripheral neuropathic pain
Reduced descending inhibition/facilitated transmission	Hyperalgesia, spontaneous pain, anxiety	Opioid receptors, CB2 receptor, serotonin and norepinephrine reuptake, adenosine	μ opioid agonists, GABA agonists, antidepressants and serotonin/norepinephrine reuptake inhibitors, adenosine reuptake inhibitors	Strong evidence for opioids and antidepressants. Weak, negative or conflicting evidence for other drug classes in neuropathic pain
Diminished spinal inhibition	Hyperalgesia, spontaneous pain, anxiety	GABA and glycine receptors	GABA A and GABA B antagonists (such as benzodiazepines, baclofen)	Negative or weak positive (baclofen) evidence in clinical studies
Glial cell activation	Hyperalgesia, opioid tolerance	Phosphodiesterase enzyme	Phosphodiesterase inhibitors (such as pentoxifylline, propentofylline, ibudilast)	Evidence in preclinical, but not clinical studies for neuropathic pain
Activation of p38 mitogen activated protein kinase/ microglial activation	Hyperalgesia, opioid tolerance	P38 mitogen activated protein kinase	Microglial inhibitors, such as dilmapimod, losmapimod	Evidence in preclinical studies, but mostly negative evidence in clinical trials

CB=cannabinoid; CGRP=calcitonin gene related peptide; GABA=γ-aminobutyric acid; IL=interleukin; NK=neurokinin; NMDA=N-methyl-D-aspartate; TNF-α=tumor necrosis factor α; trkA=tropomyosin related kinase A; TRPV-1=transient receptor potential cation channel subfamily V member 1 or vanilloid receptor subtype 1.

- The prefrontal cortex, which is important for sensory integration, decision making, memory retrieval, and attention processing in relation to pain[15]
- The primary and secondary somatosensory cortices that localize and interpret noxious stimuli[16]
- The nucleus accumbens, which is involved in placebo analgesia[17]
- The amygdala, hippocampus, and other parts of the limbic system, which are involved in the formation and storage of memories associated with emotional events, affect, arousal, and attention to pain and learning. The limbic system may also be partially responsible for the fear that accompanies pain.[18]

Because pain is multidimensional experience, it is not surprising that psychosocial factors such as depression, somatization, poor coping skills, social stressors, and negative job satisfaction can predict the development of chronic pain after an acute episode.[19] [20] In addition, the context in which a painful stimulus occurs affects how we perceive it. This is why an injury that occurs during a football game may be less painful than a similar injury that occurs while walking to school, and why acute pain, which we anticipate will get better, is better tolerated than chronic pain.

Peripheral mechanisms

Peripheral sensitization

Once injury occurs, inflammation and reparatory processes ensue, leading to a hyperexcitable state known as peripheral sensitization. In most patients, this state resolves as healing occurs and inflammation subsides. However, when nociception persists because of repeated stimulation from ongoing injury or disease (for example, in diabetes), the changes in primary afferent neurons may persist.

Several factors can contribute to peripheral sensitization. Inflammatory mediators such as calcitonin gene related peptide and substance P, which are released from nociceptive terminals, increase vascular permeability, leading to localized edema and the escape of the byproducts of injury, such as prostaglandins, bradykinin, growth factors, and cytokines. These substances can sensitize as well as excite nociceptors, resulting in lowered firing thresholds and ectopic discharges. The fact that multiple substances can sensitize nociceptors may partly explain why no drug is universally effective and there is a ceiling effect for antagonists that work at only one receptor (such as non-steroidal anti-inflammatory drugs (NSAIDs)).

Ectopic discharges can give rise to spontaneous pain and may originate from the dorsal root ganglion, other points along an injured nerve, or even uninjured adjacent fibers.[21] The process by which adjacent uninjured nerve fibers become excited as a result of non-synaptic "cross talk" is known as ephaptic transmission. Allodynia refers to pain produced by a normally non-painful stimulus, and it may result from decreased stimulation thresholds. Allodynia can be classified as mechanical (pain in response to light touch) or thermal, and it can readily be detected on physical examination. An example is a patient with diabetic neuropathy whose feet are sensitive to putting on socks.

Hyperalgesia refers to exaggerated pain perception as a result of damaged peripheral pain fibers, and it can be categorized as primary or secondary. Primary hyperalgesia occurs in injured tissue as a result of sensitization of peripheral nociceptors (for example, tenderness after a cut), whereas secondary hyperalgesia is seen in adjacent undamaged tissue owing to sensitization within the CNS and can be assessed with a sharp object. In part, this may be caused by ephaptic transmission or the expansion of receptive fields of injured nerves (or both). A clinical example of hyperalgesia might be an amputee who is unable to use a prosthesis because of tenderness overlying the stump. Both allodynia and hyperalgesia are forms of evoked, or stimulus dependent, pain. Although spontaneous neuropathic pain is often more common and distressing than evoked pain in clinical practice, preclinical studies usually measure evoked pain (fig 1).[22] It is still not clear whether animals that develop evoked pain incited by models of peripheral nerve injury experience spontaneous pain.

Expression of ion channels

One contributor to spontaneous firing of nerve fibers after injury is the increased expression of sodium channels in dorsal root ganglia and around the terminal injury site (neuroma) of injured axons.[23] Since this discovery, further preclinical studies have shown that a variety of sodium channels are involved in pain. After nerve injury, the expression of some of these channels increases de novo, the expression of others diminishes, and some translocate into different cellular compartments.[24] The proliferation of heterotopic sodium channels, such as Nav1.3, Nav1.7, and Nav1.8, may lower the stimulation threshold and provoke ectopic discharge, resulting in spontaneous pain. In addition, the spread of sodium channels may trigger central sensitization, leading to allodynia. Several adjuvant drugs, such as carbamazepine, act through the blockade of sodium channels. Yet, because none of these drugs is selective for channel subtypes involved in pain, all have low therapeutic indices and many side effects.

Certain types of calcium channels (N-type, T-type, and L-type), and to a lesser extent potassium channels (hyperpolarization activated cyclic nucleotide gated channels), also play a role in neuropathic pain. After nerve injury, the expression of $\alpha 2\delta$ calcium channels increases in and around the dorsal root ganglia, increasing excitability.[25] These voltage gated calcium channels are the primary site of action for gabapentinoids, a first-line treatment for neuropathic pain,[26] which have been shown in preclinical studies to reduce hyperalgesia and spontaneous pain (table 3).[27]

Phenotypic switch

Differentiated neurons have different properties from undifferentiated ones, which enable them to perform specific functions (Aδ and C fibers transmit pain). After nerve injury, hundreds of genes that affect nerve function are upregulated or downregulated, and this can affect excitability, as well as transduction and transmission properties. Because gene expression affects cellular characteristics, this can result in a change in the phenotype of the nerve fiber, such that neuromodulators usually expressed in C fibers (such as calcitonin gene related peptide, substance P) are now expressed in other fibers.[28] This may theoretically result in stimuli that are usually innocuous being perceived as painful.

Sensory denervation and sprouting of collateral nerve fibers

After injury to a sensory nerve, atrophic changes (wallerian degeneration) cause a decrease in the size of the cell body and the axon diameter, and eventually neuronal death. This leads to a decreased density of intraepidermal nociceptors. Depending on the type of nerve injury, this may cause loss of sensation or, paradoxically, hyperalgesia and increased pain (deafferentation pain).[29] Severing the link between a nerve and its end organ also deprives the nerve of nerve growth factor and other neurotrophins, which are essential for growth and maintenance and serve as signaling molecules. One example of deafferentation pain is phantom limb pain after amputation. Although electrodiagnostic studies may be normal in people with a loss of small pain transmitting nerve fibers, a decreased density of C fibers can be seen on skin biopsy. In response to local release of nerve growth factor, collateral sprouting may follow neuronal loss.

Sympathetically maintained pain

Sympathetically maintained pain is pain that is enhanced or maintained by an abnormality in the sympathetic nervous system. Functional coupling between the sympathetic nervous system and somatosensory nerves after nerve injury has been noted since the American civil war. Although the concept of sympathetically maintained pain is most commonly linked to complex regional pain syndrome, the same principles apply to other pain conditions, such as postherpetic neuralgia.[8] The interaction between the anatomically distinct autonomic and somatosensory systems is complex but probably includes the expression of α adrenoceptors on primary afferent sensory fibers, sympathetic sprouting into dorsal root ganglia, and impaired

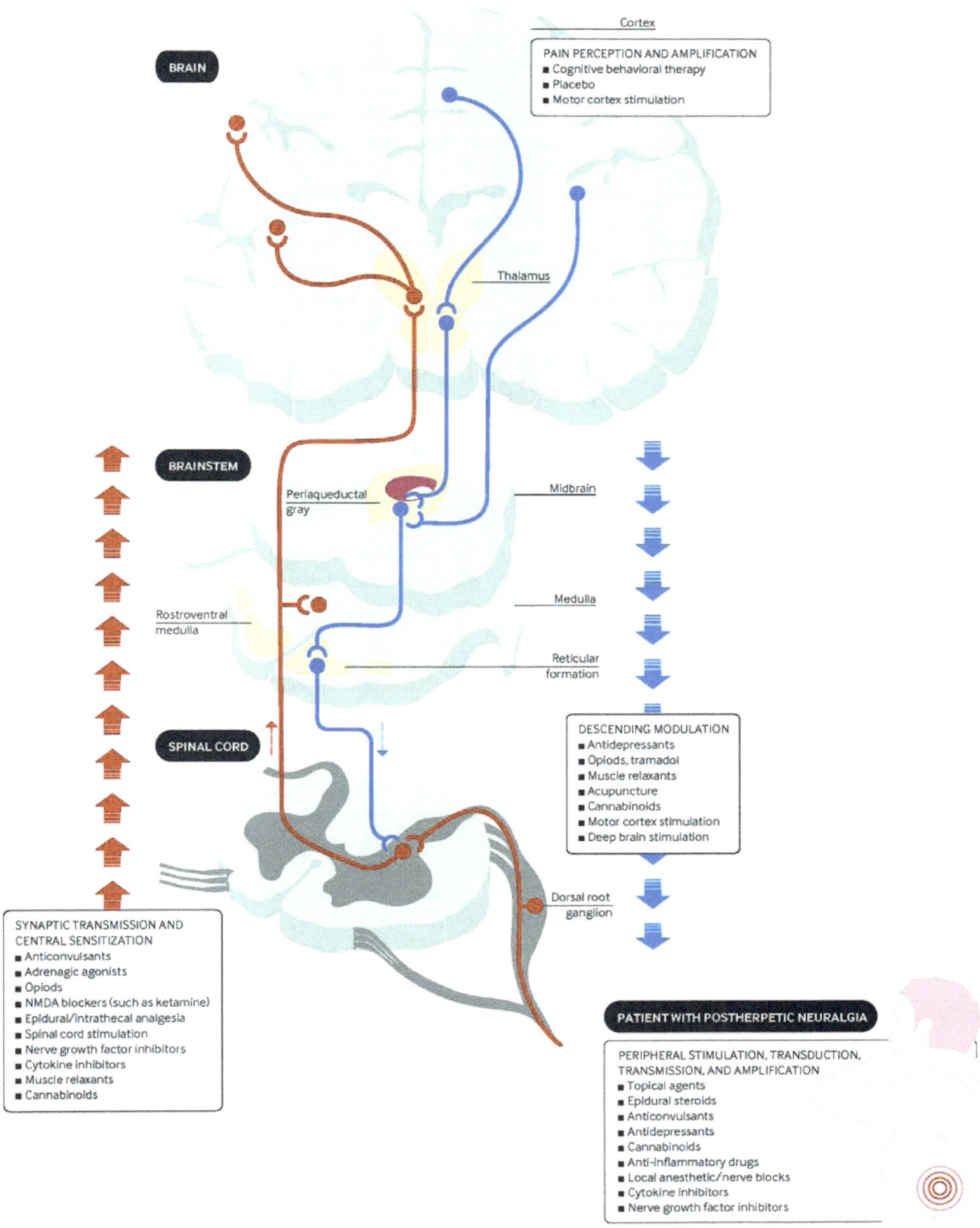

Fig 2 Diagram showing the site(s) of action of various classes of analgesics. NMDA=N-methyl-D-aspartate

oxygenation and nutrition in response to sympathetically mediated vasoconstriction.[30] Clinically, sympathetically maintained pain may manifest as temperature or color changes (or both) in an affected extremity, swelling or atrophy, and pain worsened by cold weather or stress, which enhances sympathetic outflow. Among the various diagnostic tests used to detect sympathetically maintained pain, clinical studies have found that sympathetic blocks are more sensitive but less specific than intravenous infusion of phentolamine.[31]

Spinal mechanisms

An important spinal component of neuropathic pain mechanisms is synaptic plasticity in the form of temporal and spatial summation (increased neuronal responses to repeated noxious stimulation in a time and region dependent manner).[32] Other components include expanded receptive fields of nociceptors and second order neurons,[33] and increased neuronal excitability of ascending nociceptive pathways that send pain signals to supraspinal regions.[34] These neuroplastic changes take place along nociceptive pathways in the spinal cord and in multiple brain regions.[35]

In the neural circuit, nociceptive signals generated by nerve damage are modulated by supraspinal descending inhibition or facilitation that converges onto dorsal horn neurons (or both).[36] At the cellular level, transmission of nociceptive signals within the central nervous system is regulated by cellular and intracellular elements that include[37 38]:

- Ion (Na^+, Ca^{++}, K^+) channels
- Ionotropic and metabotropic receptors such as glutamatergic, GABA (γ-aminobutyric acid)ergic, serotoninergic, adrenergic, neurokinin, and vanilloid receptors
- Inflammatory cytokines released from activated glial cells
- Nerve growth factors
- Intracellular regulators such as protein kinases (for example, protein kinase C) and transcriptional factors (such as nuclear factor-κB).

Spinal glutamatergic regulation

Peripheral nerve injury increases neuronal excitability in the spinal cord by activating excitatory glutamate receptors.[39] Nerve injury also induces downregulation of spinal glutamate transporters responsible for maintaining synaptic glutamate homeostasis. Increased regional glutamate availability secondary to loss of glutamate transporters can result in persistent and enhanced activation of both ionotropic (for example, NMDA and AMPA (α-amino-3-hydroxy-5-methyl-4-isoxazolepropionic acid)) and metabotropic glutamate receptors (such as metabotropic glutamate receptor 2), leading to lower activation thresholds and increased neuronal excitability and neurotoxicity.[40 41]

The term "windup" refers to the progressive increase in the frequency and magnitude of firing of dorsal horn neurons produced by repetitive activation of C fibers, a phenomenon that requires glutamatergic NMDA receptor activity. Spinal glutamatergic activity can in turn initiate intracellular signaling cascades, including activation of protein kinase C, that result in long-lasting neuroplastic changes in the spinal cord.[42] Similar to the role of central glutamatergic mechanisms in the pathogenesis of other neurological disorders such as epilepsy and Alzheimer's disease, glutamate receptors are integral to the development of central sensitization, and blockade of both NMDA and non-NMDA receptors has been shown to attenuate neuropathic pain in animal models.[43] Because of its primary role in neuroplasticity and excitotoxicity, the NMDA receptor has been implicated in such diverse areas as memory, opioid tolerance, and opioid induced hyperalgesia—the phenomenon whereby opioid use paradoxically increases pain sensitivity.[44] In clinical practice, the use of NMDA receptor antagonists to prevent opioid tolerance and hyperalgesia has been disappointing.[45] The long-term use of these drugs to treat chronic neuropathic pain has also had mixed results, and their use may be limited by side effects, particularly psychomimetic ones, which seem to increase in proportion to potency. The use of ketamine infusions as a treatment for refractory neuropathic pain has generated intense interest, although studies are limited by methodological flaws and lack of long term follow-up (table 3).[46] The rationale behind these infusions is that high doses may "reset" the nervous system back to its pre-injury state, in essence reversing central sensitization.

Glial activation and proinflammatory cytokines

The role of glial activation and cytokines in neuropathic pain has been extensively studied. Proinflammatory cytokines including interleukin 1β (IL-1β), IL-6, and tumor necrosis factor α (TNF-α) are produced peripherally and centrally in response to nerve injury.[47] These proinflammatory cytokines play a crucial role in inflammatory responses after nerve injury through intracellular mediators such as protein kinase C and 3',5'-cAMP.[48] Proinflammatory cytokines also play an important role in sensitization of the CNS and may contribute to allodynia, hyperalgesia, and neuroma formation.[49 50 51] In animal models, administration of cytokine inhibitors before nerve injury reduces neuropathology and pain-related behaviors.[52 53] However, in controlled clinical trials, most of which were performed in patients with radiculopathy, the use of systemic and neuraxial cytokine inhibitors has been largely disappointing.[54 55]

Glial cells comprise about 70% of the central nervous system and play an important role in maintenance and homeostasis. Microglia are activated within 24 hours of nerve injury, and astrocytes follow shortly thereafter, with activation persisting for up to 12 weeks. Glial cells undergo structural and functional transformation after injury, with astrocytes releasing a host of different pronociceptive factors, such as prostaglandins, excitatory amino acids, and cytokines.[56]

Microglial cells comprise less than 20% of spinal glial cells under normal conditions but proliferate rapidly at the dorsal root ganglia and spinal cord after nerve injury.[56 57] On activation, microglial cells stimulate the complement component of the immune system and release cytokines, chemokines, and cytotoxic substances such as nitric oxide and free radicals.[56 58 59] This proinflammatory milieu begins at synaptic sites in the brain stem and the site of nerve injury but spreads to more distant sites. The ensuing release of cytokines from astrocytes and microglia induces an array of cellular responses such as upregulation of glucocorticoid and glutamate receptors, leading to spinal excitation and neuroplastic changes.[60] IL-1β also enhances conditioned "fear memory" (conditioned fear related memories associated with behavioral responses) through glucocorticoids,[61] suggesting that proinflammatory cytokines may participate in the affective experience of pain. Drugs that modulate microglia, such as minocycline, pentoxifylline, and propentofylline, have shown some efficacy in preclinical models of neuropathic pain but have not proved effective in a clinical context (table 3; fig 2).[62]

Supraspinal mechanisms

Nociceptive signals can also be altered at supraspinal levels. The brains of patients with chronic pain are different from those without pain, with variations in metabolism and regional concentrations of neurotransmitters occurring in areas such as the thalamus and cingulate cortex. These differences vary according to the type of pain experienced (for example, acute pain or allodynia).[63] In patients with neuropathic pain, cortical reorganization occurs after injury, and the extent of the changes seems to correlate with the degree of pain. For example, in upper extremity amputees with phantom limb pain, because of the close proximity of their somatotopic representations, the area of the brain responsible for moving the lips transgresses into the hand movement area of the motor cortex; this phenomenon does not occur in amputees without phantom limb pain.[64] The observation that these changes occur after injury suggests that disinhibition may not only be a consequence of nerve injury, but may render patients susceptible to chronic pain.[65]

Preclinical studies demonstrating changes in gene expression after nerve injury have provided insight into how changes in signal transduction and neuroprotection/apoptosis contribute to neuropathic pain.[66 67] Changes that occur in supraspinal regions may explain the strong association between neuropathic pain and mood disorders.

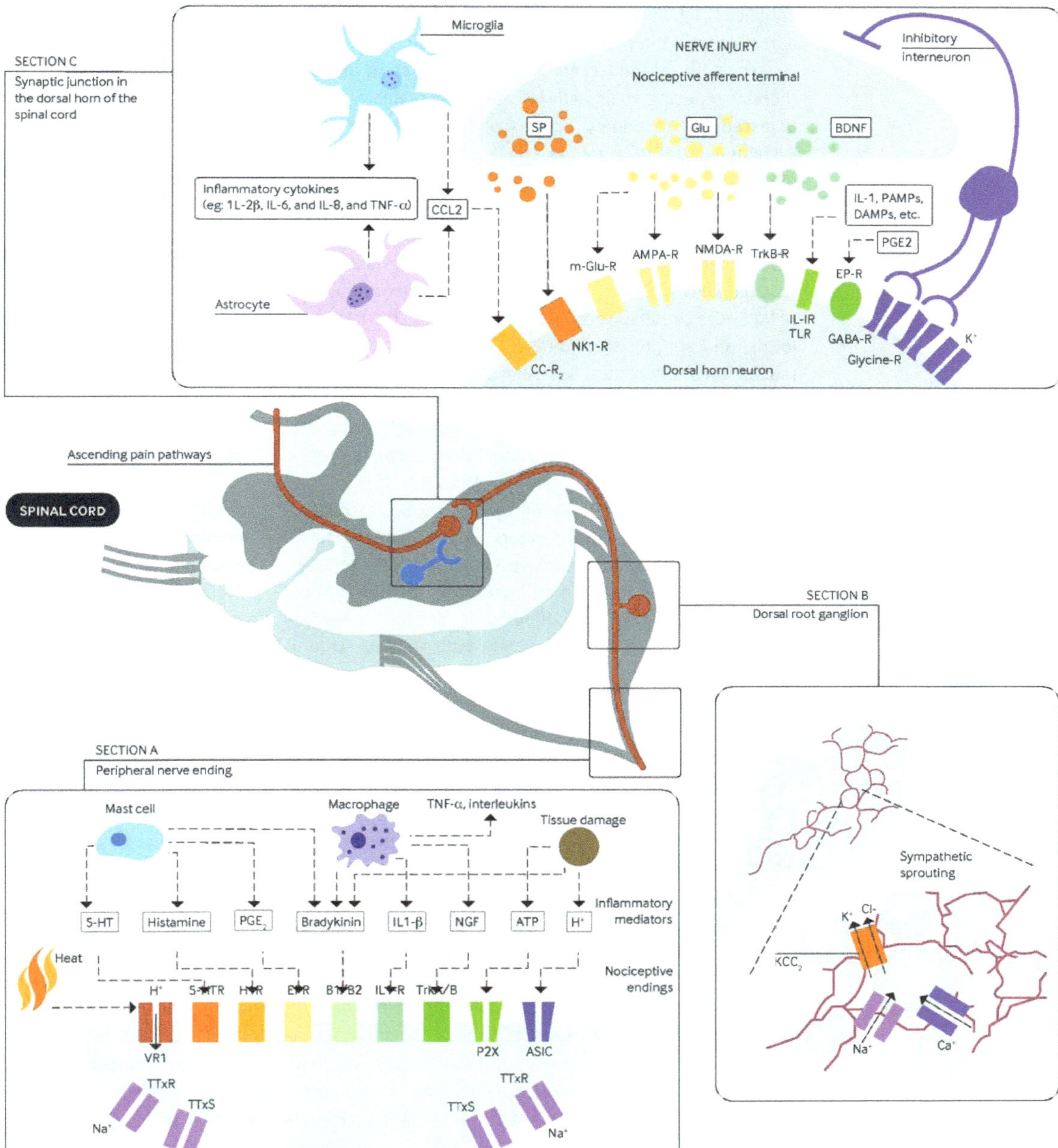

BMJ 2014;348:f7656

Fig 3 Diagram showing the various mechanisms involved in neuropathic pain at different sites in the nociceptive pathway. AMPA=α-amino-3-hydroxy-5-methyl-4-isoxazolepropionic acid; ASIC=acid sensing ion channel; B1/B2=bradykinin receptor 1/2; BDNF=brain derived neurotrophic factor; CCL=chemokine (C-C motif) ligand; CC-R2=CC-chemokine receptor; DAMPs=danger associated molecular patterns; EPR=prostaglandin E2 sensitive receptor; GABA: γ-aminobutyric acid; Glu=glutamate; H1R=histamine receptor; 5-HT=5-hydroxytryptamine; IL=interleukin; KCC=potassium-chloride cotransporter; m-Glu=metabatropic glutamate; NGF=nerve growth factor; NK=neurokinin; NMDA=N-methyl-D-aspartate; PAMPs: pathogen associated molecular patterns; PG=prostaglandin; P2X=purinergic receptor channel; -R=receptor; SP=substance P; TLR=toll-like receptor; TNF=tumor necrosis factor; Trk=tyrosine kinase; TTxR=tetrodotoxin resistant sodium channel; TTxS=tetrodotoxin sensitive sodium channel; VR=vanilloid receptor (transient receptor potential cation channel subfamily V member 1 TRPV-1)

Investigators recently found that altered corticotropin releasing factor signaling in the limbic system, an area involved in emotions, may play a role in the development of neuropathic pain.[68] Patients with chronic pain have also been shown to have reduced gray matter compared with control patients, and this can be partially reversed by treatment.[69]

Disinhibition

Spinal cord level

Once a nociceptive stimulus is transmitted to higher cortical centers, a series of events occurs that results in the activation of inhibitory neurons that attenuate pain. At the spinal cord level, there is increased release of GABA and glycine from primary afferent terminals, and enhanced activity in inhibitory GABAergic and glycinergic dorsal horn interneurons. These spinal interneurons synapse with central terminals of primary afferent neurons, thereby reducing their activity, and also regulate activity in ascending secondary order neurons. Spinal inhibitory systems may exert a greater effect on the development of mechanical hyperalgesia than on thermal hyperalgesia.[70 71]

After nerve injury, a loss of inhibitory currents occurs as a result of dysfunctional GABA production and release mechanisms; impaired intracellular homeostasis from reduced activity of K^+Cl^- cotransporter or increased activity of $Na^+K^-Cl^-$ cotransporter (or both), leading to increased Cl^- levels; and apoptosis of spinal inhibitory interneurons.[72 73] Loss of inhibitory control has been shown to provoke tactile allodynia and hyperalgesia,[74] and to facilitate structural changes that increase transmission from Aβ fibers that normally transmit non-painful stimuli to nociceptive specific secondary order neurons in the dorsal horn.[75]

After nerve injury, dorsal root ganglia exhibit decreased expression of μ opioid receptors and secondary spinal neurons become less responsive to opioids.[76] By contrast, inflammation may result in an increase in the number and affinity of opioid receptors, thereby enhancing the efficacy of opioids.[77] This may explain why patients with chronic neuropathic pain require higher doses of opioids than those with acute and chronic nociceptive pain.[78] In preclinical studies, the administration of NMDA receptor antagonists, protein kinase Cγ inhibitors, and GABA-A agonists has been shown to reverse allodynia and hyperalgesia.[75 79] Clinical trials provide evidence for a small effect size for ketamine in neuropathic pain, although the high doses given make it difficult to identify the precise mechanism responsible for analgesia.[8 46] There is some evidence to support the use of the GABA-B agonist baclofen for trigeminal neuralgia, but most of the evidence in favor of benzodiazepines as analgesics is anecdotal (table 3).[79 80]

Descending inhibition plays an important role in determining how people experience pain. Recently, it has been shown that descending modulation can be both inhibitory and facilitatory, with conflicting signals often arising from the same regions.[81] The balance between inhibition and amplification is dynamic and influenced by context, behavior, emotions, expectations, timing, and pathology. After injury, there is an initial spike mediated by changes in the activation and gene expression of NMDA and AMPA excitatory glutaminergic receptors, and a subsequent decrease in the excitability of neurons in the rostral ventromedial medulla, which lead to facilitation and inhibition, respectively.[82] The evolutionary advantage of these changes is that the initial stimulus is reinforced to ensure that it is given priority, but once this occurs the brain seeks to mitigate the consequences.

Expectations and context also play a role in descending modulation. In one randomized study,[83] 20 healthy subjects were subjected to painful electrical stimulation of the sural nerve after immersion of an arm in cold water. Half the subjects were told that the immersion would decrease the pain, whereas the other half were told that it would exacerbate the pain. Normally, exposure to a spatially distinct noxious stimulus should decrease the response to pain, a concept known as "descending (or diffuse) noxious inhibitory control." The study found that the analgesia expectancy group experienced a 77% decrease in pain intensity during immersion compared with no significant reduction in pain in the group that anticipated hyperalgesia. Moreover, corresponding changes in activity levels were noted in cortical areas involved in descending inhibition and placebo analgesia.[84] These findings agree with other studies that have found that a host of psychosocial factors such as emotions, expectations, and attention affect our intrinsic ability to inhibit pain.[84 85] This may explain why positive expectations tend to result in better treatment outcomes and a higher placebo response rate, and why we are less likely to perceive pain when an injury occurs while we are preoccupied (for example, during a sports game rather than at bedtime).[86]

Supraspinal level

Descending pathways that modulate transmission of nociceptive signals originate in the periaqueductal gray, locus coeruleus, anterior cingulate gyrus, amygdala, and hypothalamus, and are relayed through brainstem nuclei in the periaqueductal gray and medulla to the spinal cord. The inhibitory transmitters involved in these pathways include norepinephrine (noradrenaline), 5-hydroxytryptamine, dopamine, and endogenous opioids. After nerve injury, several processes take place that mitigate the normal pain attenuating pathways. These include a diminution in tonic noradrenergic inhibition and a shift from a predominantly inhibitory role to a facilitative function for descending serotonergic modulation.[87] The manifold roles of these neurotransmitters to affect pain, mood, and sleep may partially explain the high comorbidity rates between pain, depression, anxiety, and sleep disturbances.[88] Monoamine reuptake inhibitors such as tricyclic antidepressants are not only effective for neuropathic pain and depression but also alleviate anxiety and improve sleep (fig 3).[89]

Neuropathic versus nociceptive pain: different entities or part of the same continuum?

It is generally acknowledged that neuropathic and non-neuropathic pain are distinct entities, but some experts dispute this assertion, considering it part of our natural tendency to categorize things. There are two main factors that distinguish neuropathic pain from nociceptive pain:

- Nociceptive pain requires transduction to convert a non-electrical signal (for example, mechanical) to an electrochemical one, whereas neuropathic pain involves direct nerve stimulation
- Different prognosis: most people with nociceptive pain (for example, after surgery) recover, but injury to a major nerve (for example, plexopathy or limb amputation) often results in persistent pain.[90]

Even the requirement for "nerve injury" in neuropathic pain is contentious. After a nociceptive stimulus, we feel pain because microscopic nerve fibers are embedded in the injured tissue. The difference between neuropathic and non-neuropathic pain might therefore be considered one of scope (large *v* small nerve injury), although many forms of neuropathic pain, such as small fiber neuropathy, also do not involve discrete nerve injury.

Neuroscientists use distinct models for non-neuropathic (for example, Carrageenan) and neuropathic pain, and even different models (>40) of neuropathic pain to reflect myriad causes (for example, chronic constriction injury, spared nerve injury models).[91] Yet, the same neurotransmitters, neuropeptides, cytokines, and enzymes are implicated in both types of pain, with a large degree of overlap. NMDA receptor antagonists are often considered to be effective for neuropathic pain only, being intricately involved in the process of central sensitization, but preclinical and clinical studies have shown that they alleviate nociceptive pain too.[46 92 93] Similarly, the voltage gated calcium channel subunit α-2δ-1 is upregulated in injured dorsal root ganglion neurons but not in inflammatory pain.[25] However, drugs that block these channels, such as gabapentin, are effective in both preclinical models of nociceptive pain[94] and in preventing chronic postsurgical pain when given pre-emptively.[95] Conversely, drugs widely acknowledged to be effective only for nociceptive pain may also alleviate neuropathic pain. NSAIDs are so widely viewed as being ineffective for neuropathic pain that no major guidelines even mention them in their algorithm.[26] But preclinical and clinical studies have demonstrated efficacy for NSAIDs in neuropathic pain states,[96 97] and they are commonly prescribed for neuropathic pain (tables 2 and 3).[98]

It is important to note that ascending spinal pathways, supraspinal regions that process these signals, and descending modulation pathways are essentially the same for neuropathic and non-neuropathic pain. This creates a difference between the taxonomic classification of pain and the functional and practical classification. Considering the large overlap between neuropathic and nociceptive pain, similar to the classification of other neurological disorders (such as tension-type and migraine headaches) that share pathophysiological mechanisms and overlap in their response to treatment,[99] the different types of chronic pain might best be viewed as points on the same continuum.

Emerging treatments

It is anticipated that translational pain research will play an important role in understanding pain mechanisms, formulating treatment and research paradigms, and developing new analgesics in the next decade. To facilitate this, several emerging developments must unfold.

Firstly, new animal models should account for the influence of clinical comorbidities such as depression on nociceptive behaviors.[100] This will be challenging, because animal models for emotional outcomes tend to be less studied than those for physiological parameters.

Secondly, behavioral assessment tools should be capable of measuring the various dimensions of pain experiences, such as the use of conditional place preference or aversion (forms of pavlovian conditioning used to measure the motivational effects of positive and negative experiences) and behavioral coding in preclinical studies.[101 102] For example, because the relief of pain is a reward in itself, analgesic agents that are not rewarding in the absence of pain should become rewarding only in the presence of pain.

Thirdly, the association between brain reorganization seen on advanced imaging and the chronicity of pain should be further explored, with emphasis on how changes on imaging relate to pain behaviors and response to treatment.[103]

Lastly, the identification of biomarkers and the genotyping or phenotyping of pain characteristics may provide tools that enable us to understand better the heterogeneity of clinical pain and formulate individualized treatment regimens.[104 105]

These research advances, together with the development of newer drugs tailored to individual patients and specific pain mechanisms, will probably improve the treatment of neuropathic pain in the coming years.

Conclusions

Injury to the peripheral or central nervous system results in maladaptive changes in neurons along the nociceptive pathway that can cause neuropathic pain. Unlike acute pain, chronic neuropathic pain confers no individual or evolutionary advantage and is often considered to be a disease in itself. The myriad mechanisms involved in neuropathic pain overlap considerably with non-neuropathic pain and other neurological conditions. Although treatment based on the mechanism(s) of pain is widely accepted to be theoretically better than treatment based on the cause of pain, or empirical treatment, this paradigm can be difficult to implement in clinical practice. The multitude of different mechanisms, and the affective-motivational component of chronic pain that distinguishes "human pain" from nociception tested in preclinical pain models, make neuropathic pain notoriously refractory to treatment. This in turn has resulted in chronic pain being considered not only a medical problem but also a socioeconomic concern that requires urgent attention.

Thanks to Srinivasa Raja and Tony Yaksh for their help.

Contributors: SPC conceived, designed, partly wrote, and reviewed the article and tables, and helped with the figures. JM wrote part of the article and tables and critically reviewed the article.

Funding: Funded in part by the Centers for Rehabilitation Sciences Research, Uniformed Services University of the Health Sciences, Bethesda, MD, USA.

Competing interests: We have read and understood the BMJ Group policy on declaration of interests and declare the following interests: None.

The opinions or assertions contained herein are the private views of the authors and must not be construed as official or as reflecting the views of the US Department of the Army or the Department of Defense.

Provenance and peer review: Commissioned; externally peer reviewed.

1 Institute of Medicine Report from the Committee on Advancing Pain Research, Care, and Education. Relieving pain in America. A blueprint for transforming prevention, care, education and research. National Academies Press, 2011. http://books.nap.edu/openbook.php?record_id=13172&page=1.
2 Leadley RM, Armstrong N, Lee YC, Allen A, Kleijnen J. Chronic diseases in the European Union: the prevalence and health cost implications of chronic pain. *J Pain Palliat Care Pharmacother* 2012;26:310-25.
3 Torrance N, Smith BH, Bennett MI, Lee AJ. The epidemiology of chronic pain of predominantly neuropathic origin. Results from a general population survey. *J Pain* 2006;7:281-9.
4 Bouhassira D, Lantéri-Minet M, Attal N, Laurent B, Touboul C. Prevalence of chronic pain with neuropathic characteristics in the general population. *Pain* 2008;136:380-7.
5 Henningsen P, Zipfel S, Herzog W. Management of functional somatic syndromes. *Lancet* 2007;369:946-55.
6 Woolf CJ, Max MB. Mechanism-based pain diagnosis: issues for analgesic drug development. *Anesthesiology* 2001;95:241-9.
7 Walsh DA, McWilliams DF. Pain in rheumatoid arthritis. *Curr Pain Headache Rep* 2012;16:509-17.
8 Cohen SP, Kapoor SG, Rathmell JP. Intravenous infusion tests have limited utility for selecting long-term drug therapy in patients with chronic pain: a systematic review. *Anesthesiology* 2009;111:416-31.

9 Treede RD, Jensen TS, Campbell JN, Cruccu G, Dostrovsky JO, Griffin JW, et al. Neuropathic pain: Redefinition and a grading system for clinical and research purposes. *Neurology* 2008;70:1630-5.
10 Devor M. Neuropathic pain and injured nerve: peripheral mechanisms, *Br Med Bull* 1991;47:619-30.
11 Freynhagen R, Baron R, Gockel U, Tolle TR. painDETECT: a new screening questionnaire to identify neuropathic components in patients with back pain. *Curr Med Res Opin* 2006;22:1911-20.
12 Smith BH, Torrance N, Bennett MI, Lee AJ. Health and quality of life associated with chronic pain of predominantly neuropathic origin in the community. *Clin J Pain* 2007;23:143-9.
13 Jarvik JG, Deyo RA. Diagnostic evaluation of low back pain with emphasis on imaging. *Ann Intern Med* 2002;137:586-97.
14 Giesecke T, Gracely RH, Grant MA, Nachemson A, Petzke F, Williams DA, et al. Evidence of augmented central pain processing in idiopathic chronic low back pain. *Arthritis Rheum* 2004;50:613-23.
15 Bornhovd K, Quante M, Glauche V, Bromm B, Weiller C, Buchel C. Painful stimuli evoked different stimulus-reponse functions in the amygdala, prefrontal, insula and somatosensory cortex: a single-trial fMRI study. *Brain* 2002;125:1326-36.
16 Chen JI, Ha B, Bushnell MC, Pike B, Duncan GH. Differentiating noxious- and innocuous-related activation of human somatosensory cortices using temporal analysis of fMRI. *J Neurophysiol* 2002;88:464-74.
17 Zubieta JK, Stohler CS. Neurobiological mechanisms of placebo response. *Ann NY Acad Sci* 2009;1156:198-210.
18 Jaggi AS, Singh N. Role of different brain areas in peripheral nerve injury-induced neuropathic pain. *Brain Res* 2011;1381:187-201.
19 Pincus T, Burton A, Vogel S, Field AP. A systematic review of psychosocial factors as predictors of chronicity/disability in prospective cohorts of low back pain. *Spine* 2002;27:E109-120.
20 Shipton EA. The transition from acute to chronic post surgical pain. *Anaesth Intensive Care* 2011;39:824-36.
21 Wall PD, Devor M. Sensory afferent impulses originate from dorsal root ganglia as well as from the periphery in normal and nerve injured rats. *Pain* 1983;17:321-39.
22 Rasmussen PV, Sindrup SH, Jensen TS, Bach FW. Symptoms and signs in patients with suspected neuropathic pain. *Pain* 2004;1‑0:461-9.
23 Devor M, Keller CH, Deerinck TJ, Levinson SR, Ellisman MH. Na^+ channel accumulation on axolemma of afferent endings in nerve end neuromas in Apteronotus. *Neurosci Lett* 1989;102:149-54.
24 Levinson SR, Luo S, Henry MA. The role of sodium channels in chronic pain. *Muscle Nerve* 2012;46:155-65.
25 Luo ZD, Chaplan SR, Higuera ES, Sorkin LS, Stauderman KA, Williams ME, et al. Upregulation of dorsal root ganglion (alpha)2(delta) calcium channel subunit and its correlation with allodynia in spinal nerve-injured rats. *J Neurosci* 2001;21:1868-75.
26 Attal N, Cruccu G, Baron R, Haanpää M, Hansson P, Jensen TS, et al. EFNS guidelines on the pharmacological treatment of neuropathic pain: 2010 revision. *Eur J Neurol* 2010;17:1113-e88.
27 Field MJ, McCleary S, Hughes J, Singh L. Gabapentin and pregabalin, but not morphine and amitriptyline, block both static and dynamic components of mechanical allodynia induced by streptozocin in the rat. *Pain* 1999;80:391-8.
28 Ueda H. Molecular mechanisms of neuropathic pain-phenotypic switch and initiation mechanisms. *Pharmacol Ther* 2006;109:57-77.
29 Schüning J, Scherens A, Haussleiter IS, Schwenkreis P, Krumova EK, Richter H, et al. Sensory changes and loss of intraepidermal nerve fibers in painful unilateral nerve injury. *Clin J Pain* 2009;25:683-90.
30 Nickel FT, Seifert F, Lanz S, Maihofner C. Mechanisms of neuropathic pain. *Eur J Neuropsychopharmacol* 2012;22:81-91.
31 Wehnert Y, Muller B, Larsen B, Kohn D: Sympathetically maintained pain (SMP): phentolamine test vs sympathetic nerve blockade. Comparison of two diagnostic methods [in German]. *Orthopade* 2002;31:1076-83.
32 Price DD. Psychological and neural mechanisms of the affective dimension of pain. *Science* 2000;288:1769-72.
33 Willis WD Jr. Role of neurotransmitters in sensitization of pain responses. *Ann NY Acad Sci* 2001:933:142-56.
34 Dougherty PM, Willis WD. Enhanced responses of spinothalamic tract neurons to excitatory amino acids accompany capsaicin-induced sensitization in the monkey. *J Neurosci* 1992;12:883-94.
35 Zhuo M. Glutamate receptors and persistent pain: targeting forebrain NR2B subunits. *Drug Discov Today* 2002;7:259-67.
36 Gebhart GF. Descending modulation of pain. *Neurosci Biobehav Rev* 2004;27:729-37.
37 Porreca F, Lai J, Bian D, Wegert S, Ossipov MH, Eglen RM, et al. A comparison of the potential role of the tetrodotoxin-insensitive sodium channels, PN3/SNS and NaN/SNS2, in rat models of chronic pain. *Proc Natl Acad Sci U S A* 1999;96:7640-4.
38 Watkins LR, Maier SF. Glia: a novel drug discovery target for clinical pain. *Nat Rev Drug Discov* 2003;2:973-85.
39 Guo W, Zou S, Guan Y, Ikeda T, Tal M, Dubner R, et al. Tyrosine phosphorylation of the NR2B subunit of the NMDA receptor in the spinal cord during the development and maintenance of inflammatory hyperalgesia. *J Neurosci* 2002;22:6208-17.
40 Miller KE, Hoffman EM, Sutharshan M, Schechter R. Glutamate pharmacology and metabolism in peripheral primary afferents: physiological and pathophysiological mechanisms. *Pharmacol Ther* 2011;130:283-309.
41 Sung B, Lim G, Mao J. Altered expression and uptake activity of spinal glutamate transporters after nerve injury contribute to the pathogenesis of neuropathic pain in rats. *J Neurosci* 2003;23:2899-910.
42 Malmberg AB, Chen C, Tonegawa S, Basbaum AI. Preserved acute pain and reduced neuropathic pain in mice lacking PKC gamma. *Science* 1997;278:279-83.
43 Mao J, Mayer DJ, Hayes RL, Lu J, Price DD. Differential roles of NMDA and non-NMDA receptor activation in induction and maintenance of thermal hyperalgesia in rats with painful peripheral mononeuropathy. *Brain Res* 1992;598:271-8.
44 Mao J, Sung B, Ji RR, Lim G. Chronic morphine induces downregulation of spinal glutamate transporters: implications in morphine tolerance and abnormal pain sensitivity. *J Neurosci* 2002;22:8312-23.
45 Liu Y, Zheng Y, Gu X, Ma Z. The efficacy of NMDA receptor antagonists for preventing remifentanil-induced increase in postoperative pain and analgesic requirement: a meta-analysis. *Minerva Anesthesiol* 2012;78:653-67.
46 Cohen SP, Liao W, Gupta A, Plunkett A. Ketamine in pain management. *Adv Psychosom Med* 2011;30:139-61.
47 Vallejo R, Tilley DM, Vogel L, Benyamin R. The role of glia and the immune system in the development and maintenance of neuropathic pain. *Pain Pract* 2010;10:167-84.
48 Barkhudaryan N, Dunn AJ. Molecular mechanisms of actions of interleukin-6 on the brain, with special reference to serotonin and the hypothalamo-pituitary-adrenocortical axis. *Neurochem Res* 1999;24:1169-80.
49 Sorkin LS, Doom CM. Epineurial application of TNF elicits an acute mechanical hyperalgesia in the awake rat. *J Peripher Nerv Syst* 2000;5:96-100.
50 Leung L, Cahill CM. TNF-alpha and neuropathic pain—a review. *J Neuroinflammation* 2010;7:27.
51 Lu G, Beuerman RW, Zhao S, Sun G, Nguyen DH, Ma S, et al. Tumor necrosis factor-alpha and interleukin-1 induce activation of MAP kinase in human neuroma fibroblasts. *Neurochem Int* 1997;30:401-10.
52 Olmarker K, Rydevik B. Selective inhibition of tumor necrosis factor-alpha prevents nucleus pulposus-induced thrombus formation, intraneural edema, and reduction of nerve conduction velocity. Possible implications for future pharmacologic treatment strategies of sciatica. *Spine* 2001;26:863-9.
53 Quintao NL, Balz D, Santos AR, Campos MM, Calixto JB. Long-lasting neuropathic pain induced by brachial plexus injury in mice: role triggered by the pro-inflammatory cytokine, tumour necrosis factor alpha. *Neuropharmacology* 2006;50:614-20.
54 Korhonen T, Karppinen J, Paimela L, Malmivaara A, Lindgren KA, Bowman C, et al. The treatment of disc-herniation-induced sciatica with infliximab: one-year follow-up results of FIRST II, a randomized controlled trial. *Spine (Phila Pa 1976)* 2006;31:2759-66.
55 Cohen SP, White RL, Kurihara C, Larkin TM, Chang A, Griffith SR, et al. Epidural steroids, etanercept, or saline in subacute sciatica: a multicenter randomized trial. *Ann Intern Med* 2012;156:551-9.
56 Mika J, Zychowska M, Popiolek-Barczyk K, Rojewska E, Przewlocka B. Importance of glial activation in neuropathic pain. *Eur J Pharmacol* 2013; published online 13 Mar.
57 Mika J, Rojewska E, Makuch W, Przewlocka B. Minocycline reduces the injury-induced expression of prodynorphin and pronociceptin in DRG in a rat model of neuropathic pain. *Neuroscience* 2010;165:1420-8.
58 Johnston IN, Milligan ED, Wieseler-Frank J, Frank MG, Zapata V, Campisi J, et al. A role for proinflammatory cytokines and fractalkine in analgesia, tolerance, and subsequent pain facilitation induced by chronic intrathecal morphine. *J Neurosci* 2004;24:7353-65.
59 Opree A, Kress M. Involvement of the proinflammatory cytokines tumor necrosis factor-alpha, IL-1beta, and IL-6 but not IL-8 in the development of heat hyperalgesia: effects on heat-evoked calcitonin gene-related peptide release from rat skin. *J Neurosci* 2000;20:6289-93.
60 Wang S, Lim G, Zeng Q, Yang L, Sung B, Mao J. Central glucocorticoid receptors modulate the expression and function of spinal NMDA receptors after peripheral nerve injury. *J Neurosci* 2005;25:488-95.
61 Song C, Phillips AG, Leonard B. Interleukin 1 beta enhances conditioned fear memory in rats: possible involvement of glucocorticoids. *Eur J Neurosci* 2003;18:1739-43.
62 Landry RP, Jacobs VL, Romero-Sandoval EA, DeLeo JA. Propentofylline, a CNS glial modulator does not decrease pain in post-herpetic neuralgia patients: in vitro evidence for differential responses in human and rodent microglia and macrophages. *Exp Neurol* 2012;234:340-50.
63 Apkarian AV, Baliki MN, Geha PY. Towards a theory of chronic pain. *Prog Neurobiol* 2009;87:81-97.
64 Lotze M, Grodd W, Birbaumer N, Erb M, Huse E, Flor H. Does use of a myoelectric prosthesis prevent cortical reorganization and phantom limb pain? *Nat Neurosci* 1999;2:501-2.
65 Moseley GL, Flor H. Targeting cortical representations in the treatment of chronic pain: a review. *Neurorehabil Neural Repair* 2012;26:646-52.
66 Tang Y, Chu GY, He HX, Yu CP, An JX, Guo XY. Screening of differentially expressed genes in the hypothalamus of a rat neuropathic pain model following sciatic nerve injury. *Chin Med J (Engl)* 2009;122:2893-7.
67 Kõks S, Fernandes C, Kurrikoff K, Vasar E, Schalkwyk LC. Gene expression profiling reveals upregulation of Tlr4 receptors in Cckb receptor deficient mice. *Behav Brain Res* 2008;188:62-70.

68 Rouwette T, Vanelderen P, Roubos EW, Kozicz T, Vissers K. The amygdala, a relay station for switching on and off pain. *Eur J Pain* 2012;16:782-92.

69 Seminowicz DA, Wideman TH, Naso L, Hatami-Khoroushahi Z, Fallatah S, Ware MA, et al. Effective treatment of chronic low back pain in humans reverses abnormal brain anatomy and function. *J Neurosci* 2011;31:7540-50.

70 Yaksh TL. Behavioral and autonomic correlates of the tactile evoked allodynia produced by spinal glycine inhibition: effects of modulatory receptor systems and excitatory amino acid antagonists. *Pain* 1989;37:111-23.

71 Polgár E, Hughes DI, Riddell JS, Maxwell DJ, Puskár Z, Todd AJ. Selective loss of spinal GABAergic or glycinergic neurons is not necessary for development of thermal hyperalgesia in the chronic constriction injury model of neuropathic pain. *Pain* 2003;104:229-39.

72 Janssen SP, Truin M, Van Kleef M, Joosten EA. Differential GABAergic disinhibition during the development of painful peripheral neuropathy. *Neuroscience* 2011;184:183-94.

73 Moore KA, Kohno T, Karchewski LA, Scholz J, Baba H, Woolf CJ. Partial peripheral nerve injury promotes a selective loss of GABAergic inhibition in the superficial dorsal horn of the spinal cord. *J Neurosci* 2002;22:6724-31.

74 Drew GM, Siddall PJ, Duggan AW. Mechanical allodynia following contusion injury of the rat spinal cord is associated with loss of GABAergic inhibition in the dorsal horn. *Pain* 2004;109:379-88.

75 Miraucourt LS, Dallel R, Voisin DL. Glycine inhibitory dysfunction turns touch into pain through PKC gamma interneurons. *PLoS One* 2007;2:e1116.

76 Kohno T, Ji RR, Ito N, Allchorne AJ, Befort K, Karchewski LA, et al. Peripheral axonal injury results in reduced mu opioid receptor pre- and post-synaptic action in the spinal cord. *Pain* 2005;117:77-87.

77 Przewłocki R, Przewłocka B. Opioids in chronic pain. *Eur J Pharmacol* 2001;429:79-91.

78 Benedetti F, Vighetti S, Amanzio M, Casadio C, Oliaro A, Bergamasco B, et al. Dose-response relationship of opioids in nociceptive and neuropathic postoperative pain. *Pain* 1998;74:205-11.

79 Zeilhofer HU, Benke D, Yevenes GE. Chronic pain states: pharmacological strategies to restore diminished inhibitory spinal pain control. *Annu Rev Pharmacol Toxicol* 2012;52:111-33.

80 Zakrzewska JM, McMillan R. Trigeminal neuralgia: the diagnosis and management of this excruciating and poorly understood facial pain. *Postgrad Med J* 2011;87:410-6.

81 Zhuo M, Gebhart GF. Biphasic modulation of spinal nociceptive transmission from the medullary raphe nuclei in the rat. *J Neurophysiol* 1997;78:746-58.

82 Dubner R. The neurobiology of persistent pain and its clinical implications. *Suppl Clin Neurophysiol* 2004;57:3-7.

83 Goffaux P, Redmond WJ, Rainville P, Marchand S. Descending analgesia–when the spine echoes what the brain expects. *Pain* 2007;130:137-43.

84 Wager TD, Rilling JK, Smith EE, Sokolik A, Casey KL, Davidson RJ, et al. Placebo-induced changes in fMRI in the anticipation and experience of pain. *Science* 2004;303:1162-7.

85 Valet M, Sprenger T, Boecker H, Willoch F, Rummeny E, Conrad B, et al. Distraction modulates connectivity of the cingulo-frontal cortex and the midbrain during pain–an fMRI analysis. *Pain* 2004;109:399-408.

86 Enck P, Benedetti F, Schedlowski M. New insights into the placebo and nocebo responses. *Neuron* 2008;59:195-206.

87 Wei F, Dubner R, Zou S, Ren K, Bai G, Wei D, et al. Molecular depletion of descending serotonin unmasks its novel facilitatory role in the development of persistent pain. *J Neurosci* 2010;30:8624-36.

88 Bannister K, Bee LA, Dickenson AH. Preclinical and early clinical investigations related to monoaminergic pain modulation. *Neurotherapeutics* 2009;6:703-12.

89 McCleane G. Antidepressants as analgesics. *CNS Drugs* 2008;22:139-56.

90 Ciaramitaro P, Mondelli M, Logullo F, Grimaldi S, Battiston B, Sard A, et al; Italian Network for Traumatic Neuropathies. Traumatic peripheral nerve injuries: epidemiological findings, neuropathic pain and quality of life in 158 patients. *J Peripher Nerv Syst* 2010;15:120-7.

91 Barrot M. Tests and models of nociception and pain in rodents. *Neuroscience* 2012;211:39-50.

92 Quintero GC, Herrera J, Bethancourt J. Cortical NR2B NMDA subunit antagonism reduces inflammatory pain in male and female rats. *J Pain Res* 2011;4:301-8.

93 Siu A, Drachtman R. Dextromethorphan: a review of N-methyl-d-aspartate receptor antagonist in the management of pain. *CNS Drug Rev* 2007;13:96-106.

94 Yoon MH, Yaksh TL. The effect of intrathecal gabapentin on pain behavior and hemodynamics on the formalin test in the rat. *Anesth Analg* 1999;89:434-9.

95 Clarke H, Bonin RP, Orser BA, Englesakis M, Wijeysundera DN, Katz J. The prevention of chronic postsurgical pain using gabapentin and pregabalin: a combined systematic review and meta-analysis. *Anesth Analg* 2012;115:428-42.

96 Vo T, Rice AS, Dworkin RH. Non-steroidal anti-inflammatory drugs for neuropathic pain: how do we explain continued widespread use? *Pain* 2009;143:169-71.

97 Cohen KL, Harris S. Efficacy and safety of nonsteroidal anti-inflammatory drugs in the therapy of diabetic neuropathy. *Arch Int Med* 1987;147:1442-4.

98 Dieleman JP, Kerklaan J, Huygen FJ, Bouma PA, Sturkenboom CJ. Incidence rates and treatment of neuropathic pain conditions in the general population. *Pain* 2008;137:681-8.

99 Schulman EA. Overview of tension-type headache. *Curr Pain Headache Rep* 2001;5:454-62.

100 Seminowicz DA, Laferriere AL, Millecamps M, Yu JS, Coderre TJ, Bushnell MC. MRI structural brain changes associated with sensory and emotional function in a rat model of long-term neuropathic pain. *Neuroimage* 2009;47:1007-14.

101 King T, Vera-Portocarrero L, Gutierrez T, Vanderah TW, Dussor G, Lai J, et al. Unmasking the tonic-aversive state in neuropathic pain. *Nat Neurosci* 2009;12:1364-6.

102 Langford DJ, Bailey AL, Chanda ML, Clarke SE, Drummond TE, Echols S, et al. Coding of facial expressions of pain in the laboratory mouse. *Nat Methods* 2010;7:447-9.

103 Baliki MN, Petre B, Torbey S, Herrmann KM, Huang L, Schnitzer TJ, et al. Corticostriatal functional connectivity predicts transition to chronic back pain. *Nat Neurosci* 2012;15:1117-9.

104 Goodsaid F. Challenges of biomarkers in drug discovery and development. *Expert Opin Drug Discov* 2012;7:457-61.

105 Lariviere WR, Mogil JS. The genetics of pain and analgesia in laboratory animals. *Methods Mol Biol* 2010;617:261-78.

BPP UNIVERSITY SCHOOL OF HEALTH BMJ

Management of lumbar spinal stenosis

Jon Lurie, associate professor[1], Christy Tomkins-Lane, associate professor[2]

[1]Department of Medicine, Dartmouth Medical School, Dartmouth Hitchock Medical Center, NH, USA

[2]Department of Health and Physical Education, Mount Royal University, Calgary, Canada

Correspondence to: J Lurie jon.d.lurie@hitchcock.org

Cite this as: *BMJ* 2016;352:h6234

DOI: 10.1136/bmj.h6234

http://www.bmj.com/content/352/bmj.h6234

ABSTRACT

Lumbar spinal stenosis (LSS) affects more than 200 000 adults in the United States, resulting in substantial pain and disability. It is the most common reason for spinal surgery in patients over 65 years. Lumbar spinal stenosis is a clinical syndrome of pain in the buttocks or lower extremities, with or without back pain. It is associated with reduced space available for the neural and vascular elements of the lumbar spine. The condition is often exacerbated by standing, walking, or lumbar extension and relieved by forward flexion, sitting, or recumbency. Clinical care and research into lumbar spinal stenosis is complicated by the heterogeneity of the condition, the lack of standard criteria for diagnosis and inclusion in studies, and high rates of anatomic stenosis on imaging studies in older people who are completely asymptomatic. The options for non-surgical management include drugs, physiotherapy, spinal injections, lifestyle modification, and multidisciplinary rehabilitation. However, few high quality randomized trials have looked at conservative management. A systematic review concluded that there is insufficient evidence to recommend any specific type of non-surgical treatment. Several different surgical procedures are used to treat patients who do not improve with non-operative therapies. Given that rapid deterioration is rare and that symptoms often wax and wane or gradually improve, surgery is almost always elective and considered only if sufficiently bothersome symptoms persist despite trials of less invasive interventions. Outcomes (leg pain and disability) seem to be better for surgery than for non-operative treatment, but the evidence is heterogeneous and often of limited quality.

Introduction

Lumbar spinal stenosis (LSS) is a degenerative condition in which changes in the discs, ligamentum flavum, and facet joints with aging cause narrowing of the spaces around the neurovascular structures of the spine. These changes lead to pain in the legs and back, as well as impaired ambulation and other disabilities.[1]

LSS is the most common indication for spinal surgery in people older than 65 years.[2] However, there is no single objective standard for identifying LSS and diagnosis relies on complex judgments that integrate symptoms, signs, imaging findings, and comorbid conditions. Clinical care and research in LSS are complicated by the heterogeneity of the condition and the lack of standard criteria for diagnosis and for inclusion in studies.[3]

Central stenosis with associated neurogenic claudication, lateral stenosis with radiculopathy, and combined syndromes are sometimes included under the label of LSS or evaluated separately, which can make interpretation of the literature challenging. Similarly, subgroups of LSS can be lumped together to create heterogeneous cohorts. Such subgroups include—but are not limited to—LSS related to degenerative changes but with normal spinal alignment, LSS associated with isolated degenerative spondylolisthesis, and LSS with some associated degenerative scoliosis. Recent studies have begun to focus on more clearly defined cohorts but much more work is needed to obtain the most clinically relevant data to guide care. The aims of this review are to organize and summarize the vast and diverse literature on the diagnosis and management of LSS. The impact of this condition is expected to grow as the aging population rises, while overall the available evidence remains of low to moderate quality at best.

Incidence and prevalence

LSS affects more than 200 000 people in the United States, resulting in substantial pain and disability, and it is the most common reason for spinal surgery in patients over 65 years.[4] In 2007 more than 37 000 laminectomies for spinal stenosis were performed in Medicare alone with an aggregated hospital bill for these procedures of nearly $1.65bn (£1.1bn; €1.55bn).[5] Data from the national ambulatory medical care survey and the National Spine Network indicate that 13-14% of patients with low back problems who see a specialist and 3-4% who see a general physician may have spinal stenosis.[6] In the Framingham population study, 19-47% of Americans over age 60 had evidence of anatomic spinal stenosis on cross sectional imaging, depending on the criteria used.[7] The prevalence of diagnosed LSS is expected to continue to increase with the aging of the population and increased use of advanced imaging.[8]

Sources and selection criteria

We searched the Cochrane Library and PubMed database using the search term "lumbar spinal stenosis", with a filter for systematic reviews in PubMed. We identified systematic reviews published from January 2000 to May 2015 and screened the reference lists from these reviews for additional relevant articles. Clinical articles with lumbar spinal stenosis in the title were considered for inclusion. The breadth of the topic precluded a formal systematic review.

Definition

LSS may have been described as early as the 1880s,[9] but the modern description dates back to 1949, when Verbiest reported "a particular form of narrowing of the lumbar vertebral canal not associated with any other anomaly of the spine . . . On walking and standing these patients presented signs of disturbance of the cauda equina: bilateral radicular pains, disturbances of sensation and impairment of motor power in the legs. When the patient was recumbent the symptoms immediately disappeared and neurological examination during rest revealed nothing abnormal . . . Myelography showed a block with the appearance of extradural compression."[10] LSS is currently recognized as "a clinical syndrome of buttock or lower extremity pain, which may occur with or without back pain, associated with diminished space available for the neural and vascular elements in the lumbar spine" associated with certain characteristic provocative and palliative features.[11]

Causes

In LSS a narrowing of the central spinal canal, lateral recesses, or intervertebral foramen (or a combination thereof) causes compression of associated neurovascular structures. LSS can be classified as congenital (developmental) or acquired (or both).

Congenital stenosis is an uncommon condition (2.6-4.7% in the Framingham study),[7] which involves spinal canal narrowing caused by abnormalities or disorders in postnatal development.[12] Most cases of LSS are degenerative, resulting from changes in the spine with aging.[13] Changes of the spine that may lead to LSS include facet joint hypertrophy, loss of intervertebral disc height, disc bulging, osteophyte formation, and hypertrophy of the ligamentum flavum (fig 1).

It has been suggested that the degenerative process underlying stenosis often begins with changes in the intervertebral discs (loss of disc height and bulging) and then moves to the facet joints.[14] Acquired degenerative stenosis can also be caused by excess scar tissue or proliferation of bone after surgery, or as a result of infection or trauma.[12] Although anatomic narrowing of the spinal canal or foramen is a necessary component of LSS, it is not sufficient for the clinical syndrome to be expressed—the degree of narrowing must be such that the compression of the neurovascular structures compromises nerve or vascular function.[13]

LSS also has an important dynamic component.[15] The association between standing or walking and leg symptoms and relief of symptoms when sitting down or bending forward correlate with dynamic changes in the spine with positioning. This is because extension of the lumbar spine reduces the size of the lumbar spinal canal, as does axial loading.[16] These changes occur in normal spines and the effects are magnified in degenerated spines with baseline narrowing.[17]

Symptoms and signs

Pain is often the main symptom and main reason for seeking care.[18 19 20] The most common sites of reported pain are the lower back, buttocks, thighs, and legs. The discomfort associated with LSS is often described as a cramping or burning feeling.[13] Symptom patterns vary from a gradual onset of dull aching pain in the sacroiliac area and posterolateral thighs to sharp radicular pain in the thighs, legs, and feet.[21] In people with central canal LSS the pain may be bilateral but usually not entirely symmetrical. By contrast, patients with exclusively foraminal or lateral recess stenosis often report symptoms resembling unilateral radiculopathy.[22]

Patient also commonly report problems with balance,[23] sensory loss (numbness or tingling), and weakness of the muscles of the lower extremities.[19 24] Patients with LSS nearly always have low back pain, but low back pain alone, with no leg symptoms, is usually not thought to be caused by LSS even in the presence of severe anatomic stenosis, although in some cases this is controversial. Nearly all the studies considered here required patients to have leg symptoms, either neurogenic claudication or radicular pain, and confirmation of stenosis by imaging.

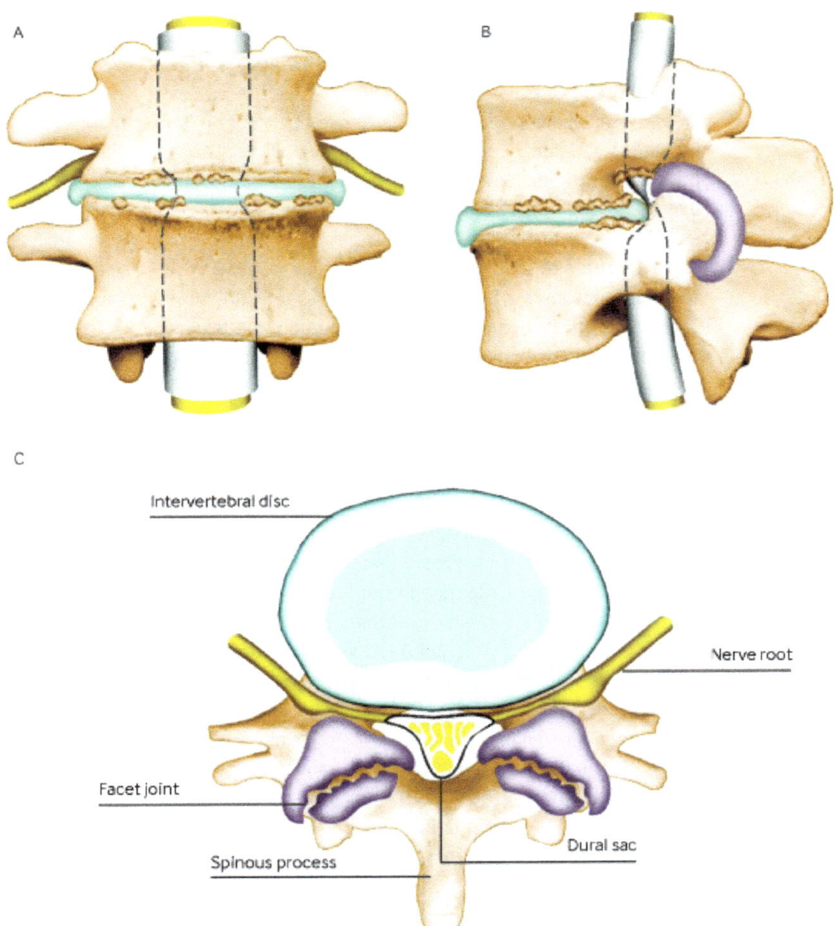

Fig 1 Degenerative spinal stenosis: frontal (A), sagittal (B), and axial views (C). Thickening of the tissue surrounding the dural sac is shown in purple. The axial figure depicts only a relatively minor degree of stenosis to allow visualization of the different structures. Reproduced with permission from the department of orthopedic surgery at Dartmouth-Hitchcock Medical Center

The cardinal manifestation and most specific symptom of central LSS is neurogenic claudication.[25] Neurogenic claudication consists of the progressive onset of pain, numbness, weakness, and tingling in the low back, buttocks, and legs, which is initiated by standing, walking, or lumbar extension.[26] Symptoms are posture dependent, appearing with standing and lumbar extension, exacerbated by walking, and relieved by sitting or forward flexion.[21] The "shopping cart sign," with the patient walking in a flexed or stooped position to relieve or reduce symptoms, is a common indicator of neurogenic claudication. This stooped posture or the inability to stand fully upright may be the presenting problem.

A key diagnostic challenge is differentiating neurogenic claudication caused by LSS from vascular claudication related to peripheral vascular disease, both of which present with leg pain during walking. In general, the distinction centers around the difference between exacerbation of symptoms with posture versus exertion. Patients with vascular claudication often improve with rest while standing, whereas those with neurogenic claudication need to sit down or lean over. A recent study found that the combination of triggering of symptoms with standing, relief with sitting, symptoms located above the knees, and a positive shopping cart sign provided strong evidence for neurogenic claudication (likelihood ratio of 13). Conversely, the alleviation of symptoms with standing (stopping walking but remaining upright) and symptoms located below the knees provided strong evidence for vascular claudication (likelihood ratio of 20).[27]

The symptoms of LSS can have a substantial impact on mobility, functional autonomy, and performance (physical activity in daily life). Most people with symptomatic LSS have limited walking capacity; they may require walking aids and may even avoid walking altogether.[28 29 30 31] This limitation can have repercussions for overall health and physical performance, with most patients exhibiting varying degrees of sedentary behavior.[32]

Natural course of LSS

The natural course of untreated LSS is largely unknown, given that most people with the condition, particularly those with severe symptoms, seek some sort of treatment.[33] However, the frequent misconception that LSS is a "degenerative" condition that inexorably worsens over time is not supported by evidence.

The North American Spine Society (NASS) clinical guidelines concluded that the natural course is favorable in a third to a half of patients with clinically mild to moderate LSS.[11] Other reviews suggest that the condition may deteriorate in some patients and improve in about a third, with most patients remaining unchanged for up to eight years of follow-up.[33 34 35] Rapid or catastrophic neurological decline seems to be rare in mild to moderate stenosis.[11] A recent study that followed 34 patients with LSS diagnosed by magnetic resonance imaging for 10 years concluded that 60% of patients did not progress dramatically, despite progressive anatomic changes.[36] Others suggest that clinical spinal stenosis is a fluctuating and potentially improving continuum,[37] where the current function of patients predicts their future function.

Pathophysiology

The physiological mechanism behind neurogenic claudication is unclear. The two main theories are the ischemic theory and the venous stasis theory,[13] which are both based to some degree on the mechanical compression of nervous and vascular structures during lumbar extension.

The ischemic theory suggests that compression of the microvasculature causes nerve root ischemia, which leads to symptoms including paresthesias, pain, and weakness.[38 39] By contrast, the venous stasis theory suggests that the underlying mechanism is inadequate oxygenation and accumulation of metabolites in the cauda equina due to venous pooling in multilevel stenosis.[26 40 41] In addition to neurogenic claudication, LSS may present with postural aggravation of radiculopathy as a direct result of compression of the neural elements.[42] Of note, there is no strong evidence for acute inflammation as a cause for the symptoms of spinal stenosis.[43]

As discussed in more detail below, anatomic narrowing and neurovascular compression are fundamental to the pathogenesis of LSS; however, these imaging findings are often seen in asymptomatic people and the association between anatomic narrowing and clinical symptoms is unclear.[44] Similarly, symptoms typically wax and wane over time, whereas the degree of anatomic narrowing, with the exception of the dynamic components related to posture, remains relatively stable or gradually worsens over time.

A possible link between venous congestion from cardiovascular disease and symptoms of stenosis has been suggested.[45] Overall, the lack of a detailed understanding of the underlying pathophysiology linking anatomic stenosis to patients' symptoms remains a key barrier to advancing research and clinical care in LSS.

Diagnosis

There is no objective standard for the clinical diagnosis of LSS.[46] In the absence of valid objective criteria it has been suggested that expert opinion be considered the "gold standard" in diagnosis.[29] The clinical syndrome of LSS is generally diagnosed using a combination of clinical signs from the history, physical examination, and imaging.[47]

The most useful findings from the history are age, radiating leg pain that is exacerbated by standing up or walking, the absence of pain when seated, the improvement of symptoms when bending forward, and a wide based gait.[48] Balance impairment, neuromuscular deficits in the lower extremities including decreased strength (weakness), sensory deficits (numbness), and absent or decreased reflexes (Achilles tendon and patellar) are also highly associated with LSS.[29] Although neurogenic claudication is the cardinal symptom of LSS, it is usually seen when a patient is walking. In the past, observational tests of walking have not been used in clinical diagnosis, but this type of assessment is becoming more popular when assessing functional capacity. Tests used for this purpose include treadmill protocols,[31 49 50 51 52 53 54 55] the gait loading test,[56] and the self paced walking test.[55] Tests of lumbar extension loading have also been proposed for use in the diagnosis of LSS.[57]

Researchers have also recently begun to assess the impact of LSS on daily physical activities and on gait characteristics using accelerometry. Preliminary reports suggest that changes in gait parameters, including postural sway, associated with claudication during continuous walking, can be detected using accelerometers.[58] Although the gait and performance parameters specific to LSS have yet to be fully defined, these techniques may be useful for diagnosis in the future.[59]

Electrodiagnostics

Electrodiagnostic methods including electromyography may also be used in the differential diagnosis of LSS,[60] and in assessing the physiological consequences of stenosis. Electromyography is not used routinely but is most useful when the clinical picture and imaging results do not correlate and in differentiating the condition from diseases with a similar presentation, including peripheral vascular disease (vascular claudication), hip osteoarthritis, and spinal cord lesions.[61]

One quantitative electromyographic protocol called paraspinal mapping has been shown to be useful in the diagnosis of LSS, showing statistically significant differences between people with clinical stenosis and those with mechanical back pain and asymptomatic volunteers.[62] In one study, this technique was found to be 93% sensitive in the diagnosis of radiologically confirmed symptomatic LSS.[63] A recent study focusing on lateral stenosis found that paraspinal electromyographic findings correlate significantly with lateral stenosis seen on magnetic resonance imaging (MRI) and with patient symptoms, including pain and disability.[64] This study concluded that electromyography may be useful in detecting lateral LSS.

However, several other conditions can increase paraspinal mapping scores, including inflammatory radiculopathy, polyneuropathy, myopathy, motor neuron diseases, and previous surgery, thereby decreasing the specificity in clinical practice.[63] To date, the diagnostic accuracy of other techniques, including dermatomal somatosensory evoked potentials and magnetic stimulation remain unclear.[48]

Imaging

Current LSS guidelines state that imaging provides the most definitive diagnostic information for patients with symptoms thought to be related to LSS.[48] Yet imaging is generally reserved for diagnostic confirmation and procedure planning for patients considering invasive interventions for LSS rather than as a routine part of the initial evaluation.

MRI, which allows examination of the size, shape, and anatomic associations between spinal and neural elements,[21] is currently the recommended method for confirming the diagnosis of LSS.[48] Computed tomography is recommended when MRI is contraindicated or unavailable. MRI is used because of its outstanding soft tissue contrast, but a systematic review found no evidence that it was more accurate than computed tomography in the diagnosis of LSS.[65] Myelography has been used extensively in the past, but it is not recommended because it is invasive and is no more accurate than MRI.[48]

Although a Delphi study conducted in 2012 found that there are no standard quantitative criteria for defining anatomic LSS on imaging,[66] a systematic review found 10 parameters that are currently used to quantify LSS.[67] The parameters reported most often for central stenosis were anteroposterior diameter (<10 mm) and cross sectional area (<70 mm^2) of the spinal canal, whereas height and depth of the lateral recess were measured for lateral stenosis and neuroforaminal diameter for foraminal stenosis.[67] The two qualitative imaging criteria rated most important as diagnostic indicators in the Delphi study were disc protrusion and perineural intraforaminal fat.[66] A study conducted to determine clinically relevant MRI measurements at the spinal level defined developmental LSS as anteroposterior diameter of <20 mm at L1, <19 mm at both L2 and L3, <17 mm at L4, and <16 mm at L5 and S1.[68]

A review found that MRI had a sensitivity of 87-96% and specificity of 68-75% for the diagnosis of LSS.[69] One study found that MRI showed substantial reliability for assessment of the central canal, but poor to substantial reliability for assessment of the subarticular and foraminal zones, respectively.[70] Newer semi-quantitative grading schemes based on dural sac morphology and the relation of cerebrospinal fluid to nerve roots in the central canal have shown initial promise for assessing the severity of LSS.[71 72]

Recent research has found that the "sedimentation sign"—the absence of posterior nerve root settling on supine MRI—has excellent reliability and may be useful in the diagnosis of severe LSS, although more research is needed to fully understand its role in the evaluation of LSS.[73 74 75] A systematic review identified 14 different qualitative and semi-quantitative criteria that have been used with remarkable variability in individual definitions.[76] Standardization and vigorous evaluation of the clinical and prognostic significance of imaging parameters with respect to treatment outcomes should be a high research priority.[77]

Although the presence of anatomic narrowing and neurovascular compression on imaging is needed for the diagnosis of LSS, it is not sufficient. Spinal stenosis is a clinical syndrome, not an anatomic or radiological finding. An estimated 21% of people with anatomic stenosis on MRI are asymptomatic.[78] In fact, although a large proportion of older people show some degree of spinal stenosis on imaging, most are symptom free.[78] Imaging must therefore be combined with history and clinical presentation before a diagnosis can be made.[13 46]

To date, research on the relation between clinical symptoms and findings on imaging has produced inconsistent results, with some studies finding an association,[49] and others not.[52 79 80 81 82] The lack of association might partly be explained by most imaging studies being conducted with the patient supine, whereas symptoms of LSS generally present during standing or walking.[46] Nonetheless, the exact mechanism by which a constrained canal or nerve foramina manifests itself in symptoms has yet to be elucidated.

Clinical prediction rules

Three clinical prediction rules have been developed for LSS.[83 84 85 86] A systematic review found that older age, pain with standing and walking, and relief with sitting or bending were common independent predictors of LSS across all prediction rules.[87] Only one of these prediction rules has been validated.[84 85] Using this tool, a score of 7 or more provides a positive likelihood ratio of just 1.6 (95% confidence interval 1.3 to 2.0), suggesting that this rule would have little effect in clinical practice.[87]

A consensus on criteria to define and classify lumbar spinal stenosis is needed.[48] Preliminary findings from a Delphi study involving an international group of 68 experts suggest that the six most important factors in the diagnosis of LSS are "leg pain while walking," "flex forward while walking to relieve symptoms," "sit down or bend forward to relieve pain," "normal foot pulses," "relief with rest, and "lower extremity weakness."[88]

Management

Non-surgical options

The many options for non-surgical management of LSS include drugs, physiotherapy, spinal injections, lifestyle modification, and multidisciplinary rehabilitation. Few high quality randomized trials have investigated these non-operative management strategies for LSS. A systematic review published in 2013 on non-operative treatments for patients with neurogenic claudication and imaging confirmed LSS concluded that there was insufficient evidence to recommend any specific type of non-surgical treatment for LSS.[89] It also concluded that a lack of clear descriptions of non-surgical treatment protocols hinders proper analysis of treatment outcomes. There is a clear need for large well designed trials examining different non-surgical management strategies for LSS, with clearly articulated treatment protocols. Several ongoing trials may provide greater insight to guide appropriate recommendations. One trial is comparing usual medical care with individualized manual therapy and rehabilitative exercise versus community based group exercise.[90] The other is examining the effects of a pedometer and nutrition lifestyle intervention compared with usual care.[51 92]

Despite the lack of consensus around treatment recommendations, most patients who seek care for neurogenic claudication are treated conservatively, and a course of conservative treatment is typically recommended before surgical intervention.[89] The main categories of non-surgical treatment are drugs, physiotherapy, and injections.

Drugs

Although various over-the-counter and prescription drugs are used to treat LSS, the evidence to guide choices is limited. Single small trials suggest that some drugs, including prostaglandins, gabapentin, and vitamin B1 improve pain and walking distance, although evidence is of low or very low quality.[90] Evidence from several small trials and a recent meta-analysis suggests that calcitonin is no better than placebo or acetaminophen (paracetamol) in the treatment of LSS.[93 94 95 96]

Given their analgesic and anti-inflammatory properties, non-steroidal anti-inflammatory drugs (NSAIDs) ought to be effective in LSS, but the evidence suggests they are no more effective than acetaminophen.[25 97] Opioids and muscle relaxants are also prescribed for pain control in LSS, although they have not been shown to be more effective than acetaminophen or NSAIDs in well controlled studies.[25 97]

The role of long term opioid use in LSS is currently unclear.[25] It has also been suggested that prostaglandin E1 may improve symptoms by improving blood flow to the cauda equina and nerve roots through vasodilation and antiplatelet aggregation effects. A recent review concluded that overall prostaglandin E1 improved clinical outcome measures including pain, Japanese Orthopedic Association score, and walking distance, although most of the studies had only short term follow-up.[98]

Finally, although both corticosteroids and antidepressants are often prescribed for patients with LSS, their efficacy remains unclear because of the lack of well controlled studies.

Physiotherapy

Physiotherapy is an accepted treatment for LSS. Physiotherapy related treatments include, but are not limited to:

- Exercise (aerobic, strength, flexibility)
- Specific exercises in lumbar flexion (cycling)
- Body weight supported treadmill walking
- Muscle coordination training
- Balance training
- Lumbar semi-rigid orthosis
- Braces and corsets
- Pain relieving treatments (heat, ice, electrical stimulation, massage, ultrasound)
- Spinal manipulation
- Postural instruction.

One study found that treatments most commonly used by patients are massage (27%), strengthening exercises (23%), flexibility exercises (18%), and heat or ice (14%), whereas physiotherapists most often advocate flexibility exercises (87%), stabilization exercises (86%), strengthening exercises (83%), heat or ice (76%), acupuncture (63%), and joint mobilization (62%).[99]

Unfortunately, there has been very little rigorous research into the efficacy of physiotherapy for LSS. A recent systematic review of non-operative treatments for patients with neurogenic claudication and imaging confirmed LSS found low quality evidence from a single trial that exercise provides short term benefit for leg pain and function compared with no treatment.[93] The review also found that walking and stationary cycling provide similar, limited results. No trials have shown a strong effect of physiotherapy on walking capacity or performance. To date, evidence that physiotherapy is better than no treatment, oral diclofenac (non-steroidal anti-inflammatory) plus home exercises, or combined manual therapy plus exercise at improving walking ability is of very low to low quality.[93]

A systematic review published in 2013 found that no conclusions could be drawn about which physiotherapy treatments are best for LSS.[100] The review found low quality evidence that physiotherapy interventions have no additional effect over exercise alone.[100] When physiotherapy was compared with surgical interventions, surgery led to better long term (two year) outcomes for pain and disability but not walking distance.

Finally, a secondary analysis of the non-randomized Spine Patient Outcomes Research Trial (SPORT) found that use of physiotherapy was associated with no improvement in pain but some improvement in self reported physical function and a reduced likelihood of patients receiving surgery within one year.[101]

A subsequent randomized trial published in 2015 compared surgical decompression with a standardized physiotherapy regimen of lumbar flexion, conditioning exercises, and patient education.[102] It found no difference in results at one or two years; however, 57% of the patients assigned to physiotherapy crossed over to surgery, which made it difficult to interpret the effects of physiotherapy.

Given the dynamic aspects of posture relative to spinal canal diameter, flexion exercise may improve the underlying pathophysiology of LSS; alternatively, the main role of physiotherapy may be to improve patients' function with LSS rather than improve the LSS itself. Although the therapeutic effects may not be manifested at the level of the spinal pathology directly, the effects of these interventions may be sufficient to meet the goals and expectations of some patients with LSS. To this end, preliminary results from an ongoing randomized controlled trial (RCT) investigating a lifestyle intervention for LSS suggest that increased physical activity and weight loss may improve function and reduce symptoms in people with LSS. Although the mechanisms of these effects are unclear, this type of treatment warrants further investigation.

Injections

The results of trials on the effects of epidural injections for LSS vary. A systematic review published in 2013 found very low quality evidence from a single trial that epidural steroid injections improve pain, function, and quality of life for two weeks after injection when compared with home exercise or inpatient physiotherapy.[103] However, two trials showed no effect compared with placebo.[103] A more recent meta-analysis published in 2015 found that epidural steroid injections provide limited short term and long term improvement in pain and walking distance in patients with LSS.[104] Minimal evidence shows that epidural steroid injections are better than local anesthetic injections alone, regardless of the mode of epidural injection.[104] Another review of injections for central LSS concluded that epidural injections with local anesthetic alone, or local anesthetic with steroids, offer some relief of low back pain and lower extremity pain for central LSS. It also suggested that the interlaminar approach is superior to the caudal approach although the caudal approach is superior to the transforaminal one.[105]

A randomized trial published in 2014 that investigated epidural injections for LSS received much attention in the media and in the scientific community.[106] This large double blinded controlled trial found no evidence of a treatment effect at six weeks with injection of glucocorticoids plus lidocaine, compared with lidocaine alone. These results suggest that the addition of glucocorticoids does not improve short term outcome, although it can increase the risks, as highlighted by an outbreak of fungal meningitis caused by contamination of a steroid preparation used for epidural injections.[107] The most recent systematic review found immediate improvements in pain and function with epidural corticosteroid injections for radiculopathy but limited evidence of a lack of effectiveness in spinal stenosis (fig 2).[108]

Other non-surgical options

Many older people with low back pain seek out complementary and alternative medicine, and although studies have not always clearly defined the diagnoses some of these people probably have spinal stenosis. However, little rigorous data are available on the efficacy of these alternative treatments in LSS. In the past, LSS with severe degenerative changes was considered to be a contraindication to spinal manipulation.[15] However, several studies have recently looked at the effects of flexion distraction manipulation in LSS. A review of chiropractic treatment in LSS from 2009 found limited evidence of potential benefit but the evidence was of extremely low quality.[109] More rigorous comparative studies are looking at this question,[110 111] but currently there is no high quality evidence of the efficacy of spinal manipulation in LSS. Similarly, a systematic review published in 2013 of acupuncture in LSS found "that current evidence for the use of acupuncture in patients with LSS is limited, due to the scarcity of existing clinical trials and high risk of bias" and was therefore unable to draw any conclusions regarding its effectiveness.[112]

Surgical options

Several different surgical procedures are used to treat patients with LSS who do not improve with non-operative treatments. Given the rarity of rapid deterioration and that the disease often waxes and wanes then gradually improves, surgery is almost always an elective procedure that is considered only if sufficiently bothersome symptoms persist despite trials of less invasive interventions,[113] and clinical practice varies widely.

Between 1979 and 1992, the rate of surgery for LSS increased almost eightfold and then plateaued.[5 114] In recent years, although overall rates of surgery have been fairly stable, at one to two per 1000, the rates of operations that include lumbar fusion have increased dramatically.[115 116] Rates vary widely across geographic regions—an eightfold variation in rates of decompression surgery and 14-20-fold variation in the use of fusion surgery.[115 116] This variability occurs within the context of a lack of consensus among surgeons regarding indications for surgery and evidence that decision making in practice is often driven by surgeons' preferences and enthusiasm rather than patient characteristics.[8] In addition, there is no evidence of benefit for fusion in LSS without spondylolisthesis or scoliosis.[117 118]

Decompression

The primary goal of surgical intervention in LSS is to decompress the neural structures that are being encroached upon, theoretically relieving symptoms and improving function.

The specific details of the surgical approach vary according to the location of the stenosis, number of segments affected, associated deformity or spinal instability, history

Outcome	Estimate (95% CI)	Trials (N)
	WEIGHTED MEAN DIFFERENCE (0-100)	
Pain		
Immediate follow-up	−22.0 (−36.0 to −8.00)	1
Short term follow-up	0.62 (−2.87 to 4.11)	5
Intermediate term follow-up	3.73 (−0.81 to 8.26)	3
Long term follow-up	4.00 (−2.87 to 10.9)	1
Function		
Intermediate term follow-up	2.81 (−0.44 to 6.06)	3
Long term follow-up	2.78 (−1.24 to 6.79)	2
	STANDARDIZED MEAN DIFFERENCE	
Function		
Immediate follow-up	−0.32 (−0.85 to 0.22)	2
Short term follow-up	−0.03 (−0.31 to 0.26)	5
SUCCESS/COMPOSITE OUTCOMES	RELATIVE RISK	
Pain		
Short term follow-up	0.98 (0.84 to 1.15)	3
Intermediate term follow-up	0.98 (0.78 to 1.24)	2
Long term follow-up	0.97 (0.74 to 1.28)	3
Function		
Short term follow-up	0.91 (0.70 to 1.18)	3
Intermediate term follow-up	0.96 (0.74 to 1.25)	2
Long term follow-up	0.95 (0.71 to 1.26)	2
Surgery		
Long term follow-up	0.76 (0.38 to 1.54)	1

Fig 2 Pooled results of epidural steroid injections versus placebo interventions for spinal stenosis[108]

of previous surgery, and the surgeon's preferences.[113] The various approaches to achieving decompression include traditional laminectomy, bilateral laminotomies, bilateral decompression through unilateral laminotomy, and different forms of laminoplasty.[113]

Current evidence does not allow strong conclusions to be drawn about the comparative effectiveness of these approaches.[119] A systematic review of three newer techniques for surgical decompression in LSS found no significant difference in self care abilities and leg pain compared with conventional laminectomy. However, the quality of evidence was low or very low because of the limited number of studies available for review and the poor study designs.[120] The studies considered here typically involved different sites of stenosis; in addition, the exact method and extent of decompression was determined by the operating surgeon. This reflects the heterogeneity that complicates the interpretation of the literature in LSS.

Decompression of the neural structures generally focuses on relieving the leg symptoms (claudication or radiculopathy) associated with LSS and less on improving any accompanying back pain. Therefore, although back pain does improve, the improvement in leg pain is usually greater.[121] Patients with LSS and predominant leg pain have better surgical outcomes and a greater relative improvement in surgical rather than non-operative outcomes than do patients with predominant back pain or equally bothersome pain in the legs and the back.[122]

Several randomized trials and systematic reviews have compared the efficacy of surgery versus non-operative treatment for LSS. A small RCT of patients with moderate sciatic symptoms and stenosis confirmed by imaging found a small persistent advantage for the surgery group at 10 years but provided no formal statistical analysis.[18] The long term outcomes of a high quality RCT of moderate LSS found a significant early advantage for surgery; this advantage narrowed by six years but was still significant when viewed over the entire six years.[123] SPORT was the largest study to compare surgery and non-operative treatment in LSS. It found no differences in the intent to treat analyses in the randomized component of the study, but high rates of treatment crossover greatly limited the conclusions that could be drawn.[121 124] As-treated analyses of both the randomized and concurrent observational cohorts from SPORT showed a significant early benefit to surgery, although in the randomized cohort this advantage decreased over time and was no longer significant at six to eight years of follow-up.[125]

A recent review of reviews evaluating surgery compared with non-operative treatment for LSS concluded that "surgery appears to result in better outcomes (leg pain and disability) with regard to conservative interventions, but the evidence is heterogeneous and the underlying methodology is of low quality."[105] Similarly, an updated systematic review found very low quality evidence from a meta-analysis of two trials that compared direct decompression (with or without fusion) with multimodal non-operative care for the outcome of pain related disability, as measured by the Oswestry disability index.[121 126] There was no significant difference at six months (mean difference −3.66, −10.12 to 2.80) or one year (−6.18, −15.03 to 2.66), but at 24 months a significant difference was found favoring decompression (−4.43, −7.91 to −0.96). Longer term follow-up data were available but a combined analysis could not be performed for those end points.[127]

A recent trial, published since these reviews, compared surgical decompression with a standardized physiotherapy regimen of lumbar flexion, conditioning exercises, and patient education.[102] This trial reported no difference in results between the surgery and physiotherapy groups at one or two years; however, 57% of the patients assigned to physiotherapy crossed over to surgery, which is even higher than the 43% seen in SPORT.[102 128] These crossover rates complicate the comparison of outcomes between the two treatment groups. However, all patients in both studies were considered candidates for surgery before randomization, which suggests that expert non-operative therapy in patients with LSS who are considered to be suitable for surgery could reduce the rate of surgery with good patient outcomes.

A systematic review of predictors of postoperative outcomes in LSS found that depression, cardiovascular comorbidity, disorders that affected walking ability, and scoliosis predicted poorer subjective outcomes. By contrast, better walking ability, better self rated health, higher income, less overall comorbidity, and pronounced central stenosis predicted better subjective outcomes.[129] However, it is unclear whether these same factors would also predict non-operative outcomes. In a study of predictors of the treatment effect of surgery, smoking emerged as a major predictor of worse surgical outcomes and a smaller surgical treatment effect. Other predictors of a poor response included baseline disability, neuroforaminal stenosis, predominant leg pain, not lifting at work, and presence of a baseline neurological deficit.[130]

Role of postoperative rehabilitation

Although the general consensus is that surgery probably has better outcomes than non-operative treatment for LSS, only 60-70% of patients are satisfied with their symptoms after surgery.[124] A systematic review of postoperative rehabilitation in LSS found moderate quality evidence that postoperative active rehabilitation after decompression surgery for lumbar spinal stenosis is more effective than usual care in improving both short term and long term (back related) functional status. Similar findings were noted for secondary outcomes, including short term improvement in low back pain and long term improvement in both low back pain and leg pain.[131]

Role of fusion

One of the major controversies about surgery for spinal stenosis is the role of spinal fusion. Spinal arthrodesis with the goal of achieving spinal fusion has generally been recommended for spinal stenosis associated with degenerative spondylolisthesis, recurrent stenosis after previous decompression, instability, or scoliosis.[113] A recent clinical practice guideline recommended that "in the absence of deformity or instability, lumbar fusion has not been shown to improve outcomes in patients with isolated stenosis, and therefore it is not recommended (grade C recommendation).[132] Similarly, guidelines from the North American Spine Society recommend that in the absence of associated scoliosis or spondylolisthesis, "decompression alone is suggested for patients with leg predominant symptoms without instability (grade B)."[133]

Despite this lack of evidence of an advantage for fusion in the absence of deformity or instability, and recommendations against it, epidemiological data suggest marked increases in the use of fusion in patients receiving surgery for isolated spinal stenosis, and a 14-fold variation in rates across the US.[115] Increases and variability in rates are even more marked for complex fusions involving multiple levels or combinations of anterior and posterior fusion.[5] Fusions, particularly complex fusions, however, are also independently associated with increased perioperative mortality, major complications, readmission to hospital, and cost.[5 134]

Interspinous spacers

Interspinous spacer devices are an alternative intervention in spinal stenosis designed to separate the spinous processes at the stenotic levels, thereby preventing the narrowing associated with loading and lumbar extension. They are inserted between the spinous processes using a minimally invasive technique and are designed to limit extension and decompress the nerves.

Biomechanical studies in cadaveric spines have shown a significant reduction in the motion from flexion into extension at levels implanted with a spacer with no significant effect on the kinematics of the adjacent levels.[135] Additional studies in cadaveric spines showed that the device increased the spinal canal area during extension of the spine by 18%, the foraminal area by 25%, and the foraminal width by 41%.[136] A neurophysiologic study showed similar improvement in transcranial motor evoked potential with interspinous distraction in severe single level spinal stenosis to that seen with decompressive laminectomy.[137] A claims based analysis in the US showed that a spacer was inserted in about 6% of US Medicare beneficiaries receiving surgery for LSS.

One large randomized clinical trial compared an interspinous spacer device with continued non-operative therapy consisting of at least one epidural injection and drugs or physiotherapy (or both) in 191 patients.[138] At two years, 48% of the spacer group and only 5% of the non-operative group met a composite success measure of improved symptom severity, improved physical function scores, and satisfaction with the treatment. Side effects were reported by 11% of those who underwent interspinous spacer implantation and 1.1% of the control group; these included spinous process fracture, coronary ischemia, respiratory distress, hematoma, and death from pulmonary edema.[139]

Recently, three RCTs from the Netherlands, Sweden, and Norway compared interspinous spacer implantation with decompressive surgery for LSS.[140 141 142] They all found lower rates of complications but higher rates of re-operation in the spacer group (25-29% *v* 5-8% in the laminectomy group), although outcomes were similar between groups at two years. In the US claims analysis, patients receiving a spacer alone had fewer major medical complications than those undergoing decompression or fusion surgery (1.2% *v* 1.8% and 3.3%, respectively), but had significantly higher rates of further inpatient lumbar surgery (16.7% *v* 8.5% for decompression and 9.8% for fusion at two years).[143] Two recent systematic reviews and meta-analyses both found that although interspinous spacers may provide some benefit, they are associated with a higher incidence of reoperation and higher cost compared with decompressive laminectomy, and that the indications, risks, and benefits of using these devices should be carefully considered before surgery.[144 145]

The MILD procedure

The minimally invasive lumbar decompression (MILD) procedure is an image guided minimally invasive procedure for treatment of degenerative central canal LSS with ligamentum flavum hypertrophy through percutaneous decompression of the hypertrophic ligamentum flavum.[146] A randomized study of 38 patients showed no significant difference at six weeks in the Oswestry disability index for patients treated with MILD versus those treated with epidural steroid injections (mean difference 5.70, 0.57 to 10.83), although improvements in pain were greater in the MILD decompression group (2.40, 1.92 to 2.88). At 12 weeks there were many crossovers, which prevented further analysis, and no safety differences were observed.[147] A systematic review found that current evidence on MILD is of low quality with risk of bias, although the procedure seems to be relatively safe in the treatment of symptomatic LSS.[148] However, evidence for the relative safety and comparative effectiveness of MILD compared with standard decompression is lacking.

Associated conditions affecting treatment

Degenerative spondylolisthesis

Degenerative spondylolisthesis is a type of degenerative spinal deformity in which one vertebral body slips forward relative to the one below (fig 3) although the neural arch remains intact.[149] This malalignment can cause narrowing of the central canal, lateral recesses, and neuroforamina, resulting in symptomatic spinal stenosis. Degenerative spondylolisthesis is more likely than LSS with normal vertebral alignment to occur in women and to present with stenosis at a single level.[150] Evidence on the efficacy or comparative effectiveness of different non-operative treatments for this condition is limited and there are no rigorous guidelines. Generally recommended non-operative treatments for LSS with associated degenerative spondylolisthesis include patient education, analgesics, flexion strengthening and stabilizing exercises, and physical and cognitive treatments focused on function and activities of daily living.[149]

Many studies of LSS include patients with degenerative spondylolisthesis but only SPORT evaluated the outcomes of surgery versus non-operative treatment in patients with LSS and degenerative spondylolisthesis and those with normal alignment separately.[121 151] As with LSS, the study found no difference in intention to treat analyses between randomized groups, but the high rates of crossover complicated the interpretation of the results. Observational analyses (as treated) in the randomized and observational cohorts showed a significant advantage for surgery at two and four years.[151 152] A combined analysis directly comparing results between the degenerative spondylolisthesis and isolated LSS cohorts found similar baseline levels of symptom severity and disability between the groups, greater improvement with surgery in the degenerative spondylolisthesis cohort, and similar non-operative outcomes between the two cohorts. It concluded that surgical treatment had a greater effect in patients with degenerative spondylolisthesis.[150]

As mentioned above, in contrast to isolated LSS, current recommendations on the surgical treatment of degenerative spondylolisthesis include decompression and fusion.[133] This recommendation is mainly based on a prospective study from 1991 that showed better outcomes in people treated with laminectomy and arthrodesis rather than laminectomy alone.[153] However, with the development of less extensive decompression techniques, interest in the use of decompression alone has been renewed.[154] In SPORT, 6% of patients with degenerative spondylolisthesis had decompression alone.[155]

Another controversy in the surgical treatment of degenerative spondylolisthesis is the appropriate role of instrumentation when an arthrodesis is performed. A randomized trial comparing instrumented and non-instrumented fusion in degenerative spondylolisthesis found a significant increase in fusion rate with instrumentation but no difference in clinical outcomes.[156] Long term follow-up of patients having non-instrumented posterolateral fusion found that those with a pseudo-arthrosis had a worse outcome than those who achieved solid fusion. However, because this case series had no comparison group with instrumented fusion, it provides no direct evidence on the question of instrumentation.[157] In SPORT, 21% of patients with degenerative spondylolisthesis had non-instrumented fusion, 56% had fusion with the use of posterior instrumentation, and 17% had a circumferential fusion; clinical outcomes were similar between the three groups.[155] Current clinical practice guideline recommendations (grade B) on the use of instrumentation in the treatment of degenerative spondylolisthesis state that the addition of instrumentation is thought to improve fusion rates but not clinical outcomes in patients with symptomatic LSS and degenerative spondylolisthesis.[133]

In a study of predictors of surgical treatment effect in degenerative spondylolisthesis, age less than 67 years, female sex, absence of stomach problems, neurogenic claudication, baseline reflex deficit, opioid use, not taking antidepressants, dissatisfaction with symptoms, and patient anticipation of a high likelihood of being pain free after surgery predicted a greater relative benefit from surgery.[158] These predictors, however, have not been replicated or validated in other studies. An international panel attempted to define criteria for surgery in degenerative spondylolisthesis using the Rand appropriateness criteria. The main criteria associated with a clinical scenario being rated as appropriate for surgery were the presence of severe disability, severe neurological abnormalities, and the absence of severe psychosocial comorbidities. Few scenarios with back pain only—that is, without accompanying neurogenic claudication or radiculopathy—were considered appropriate for surgery.[159] However, these criteria need to be validated in clinical practice.

Degenerative scoliosis

Adult scoliosis, which includes patients with curvature of the spine of varying degrees that is caused or affected by degenerative disc and joint disease, is a common disorder in the aging population. It has an important effect on quality of life and may be contribute to symptomatic spinal stenosis in some cases. Both the prevalence and severity of lumbar scoliosis increase steadily with age. Evidence based guidelines for the treatment of adult degenerative scoliosis are lacking and treatment decisions largely depend on the healthcare provider's clinical expertise and practice patterns as well as the patient's preferences. An ongoing clinical trial sponsored by the National Institutes of Health comparing surgical and non-operative treatments for adult symptomatic lumbar scoliosis (Clinicaltrials.gov; NCT00854828) may help provide some insight into the management of this complex disorder in the future. Complication rates approaching 60% have been reported for long fusion procedures used to treat degenerative scoliosis.[160] The pros and cons of extensive reconstructive surgery with high complication rates versus more limited intervention with the risk of progressive deformity and the need for further surgery are controversial. However, discussion of the management of LSS patients with severe concurrent scoliosis is beyond the scope of this review.

Conclusion

LSS is a common and often debilitating condition in older people. It is characterized by degenerative changes that cause encroachment of the soft tissues into spaces around the neural structures and lead to symptoms of neurogenic claudication or radiculopathy, or both. The high rate of anatomic spinal stenosis on imaging in asymptomatic older people, the often vague and variable symptoms of spinal stenosis, and the heterogeneity across the spectrum of LSS make this condition complex to diagnose and treat. Over-reliance on imaging findings probably results in overdiagnosis of LSS so should be avoided.

Many of the treatments lack a strong evidence base and even those with the strongest evidence base, such as decompressive surgery, may be only modestly successful and carry potential risks. Given the marked heterogeneity in LSS and the trade-offs involved in different treatment approaches, a shared decision making approach is needed. This should focus on providing patients with standardized information on the treatment options, eliciting and clarifying patients' personal values and goals, and tailoring treatment

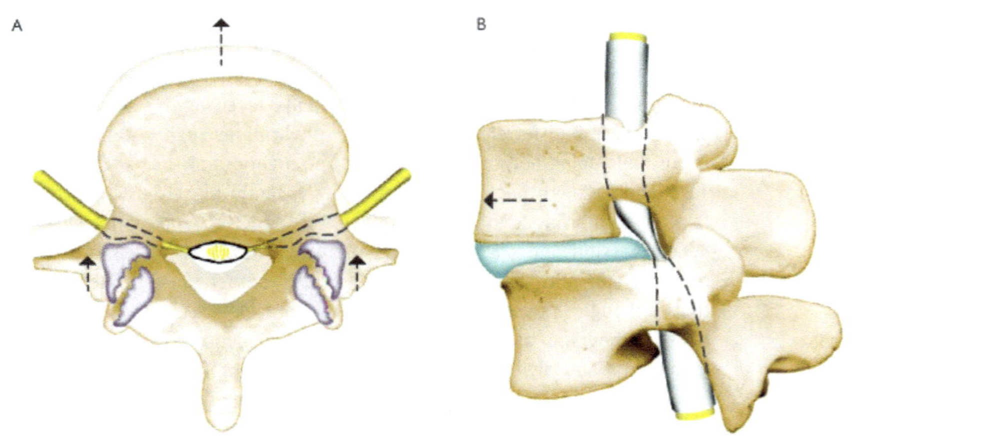

Fig 3 Degenerative spondylolisthesis: frontal (A) and sagittal (B) views. Forward slippage of one vertebra over the other may cause narrowing of the central canal, lateral recesses, and neuroforamina, thereby contributing to lumbar spinal stenosis. Reproduced with permission from the department of orthopedic surgery at Dartmouth-Hitchcock Medical Center

to achieve patients' symptomatic and functional goals. Key information for patients includes the typical waxing and waning but generally favorable natural course of the disease, in contrast to the rapid and progressive deterioration that many of them fear, along with the expected outcomes and risks of the various treatment options. Formal decision aids for spinal stenosis, both video[161] and paper based,[115] are available to help inform and engage patients in decision making. More evidence on well defined homogeneous phenotypes within the broad spectrum of LSS could provide more tailored evidence on the likely outcomes for individual patients.

Contributors: Both authors participated fully in the planning, conduct, and reporting of the work described in the article, and are responsible for the overall content as guarantors.

Competing interests: We have read and understood BMJ policy on declaration of interests and declare the following interests: CTL: none; JDL: consulting for FzioMed and the Informed Medical Decisions Foundation and stock options from NewVert; FzioMed and NewVert produce products related to surgery for intervertebral disc herniation but not for spinal stenosis. This work was supported in part by the Multidisciplinary Clinical Research Center in Musculoskeletal Diseases at Dartmouth, funded by NIAMS (P60-AR048094 and P60-AR062799).

Provenance and peer review: Commissioned; externally peer reviewed.

1 Katz JN, Harris MB. Clinical practice. Lumbar spinal stenosis. N Engl J Med2008;358:818-25.
2 Deyo RA. Treatment of lumbar spinal stenosis: a balancing act. Spine J 2010;10:625-7.
3 Genevay S, Atlas SJ, Katz JN. Variation in eligibility criteria from studies of radiculopathy due to a herniated disc and of neurogenic claudication due to lumbar spinal stenosis: a structured literature review. Spine2010;35:803-11.
4 Deyo RA, Gray DT, Kreuter W, et al. United States trends in lumbar fusion surgery for degenerative conditions. Spine 2005;30:1441-5; discussion 1446-7.
5 Deyo RA, Mirza SK, Martin BI, et al. Trends, major medical complications, and charges associated with surgery for lumbar spinal stenosis in older adults. JAMA2010;303:1259-65.
6 ECRI Health Technology Assessment Group. Treatment of degenerative lumbar spinal stenosis: summary. 2001. www.ncbi.nlm.nih.gov/books/NBK11855/.
7 Kalichman L, Cole R, Kim DH, et al. Spinal stenosis prevalence and association with symptoms: the Framingham Study. Spine J2009;9:545-50.
8 Deyo RA. Treatment of lumbar spinal stenosis: a balancing act. Spine J 2010;10:625-7.
9 Szpalski M, Gunzburg R. Lumbar spinal stenosis in the elderly: an overview. Eur Spine J2003;12:S170-5.
10 Verbiest H. A radicular syndrome from developmental narrowing of the lumbar vertebral canal. J Bone Joint Surg Br1954;36-B:230-7.
11 Watters WC, Baisden J, Gilbert TJ, et al. Degenerative lumbar spinal stenosis: an evidence-based clinical guideline for the diagnosis and treatment of degenerative lumbar spinal stenosis. Spine J 2008;8:305-10.
12 Ciricillo SF, Weinstein PR. Lumbar spinal stenosis. West J Med1993;158:171-7.
13 Chad DA. Lumbar spinal stenosis. Neurol Clin2007;25:407-18.
14 Arbit E, Pannullo S. Lumbar stenosis: a clinical review. Clin Orthop2001;384:137-43.
15 Fritz JM, Delitto A, Welch WC, et al. Lumbar spinal stenosis: a review of current concepts in evaluation, management, and outcome measurements. Arch Phys Med Rehabil1998;79:700-8.
16 Schönström N, Lindahl S, Willén J, et al. Dynamic changes in the dimensions of the lumbar spinal canal: an experimental study in vitro. J Orthop Res 1989;7:115-21.
17 Penning L. Functional pathology of lumbar spinal stenosis. Clin Biomech (Bristol Avon)1992;7:3-17.
18 Amundsen T, Weber H, Nordal HJ, et al. Lumbar spinal stenosis: conservative or surgical management?: a prospective 10-year study. Spine2000;25:1424-35; discussion 1435-6.
19 Iversen MD, Katz JN. Examination findings and self-reported walking capacity in patients with lumbar spinal stenosis. Phys Ther2001;81:1296-306.
20 Lin S-I, Lin R-M. Disability and walking capacity in patients with lumbar spinal stenosis: association with sensorimotor function, balance, and functional performance. J Orthop Sports Phys Ther2005;35:220-6.
21 Binder DK, Schmidt MH, Weinstein PR. Lumbar spinal stenosis. Semin Neurol2002;22:157-66.
22 Lee CK, Rauschning W, Glenn W. Lateral lumbar spinal canal stenosis: classification, pathologic anatomy and surgical decompression. Spine1988;13:313-20.
23 Tomkins-Lane CC, Battié MC. Predictors of objectively measured walking capacity in people with degenerative lumbar spinal stenosis. J Back Musculoskelet Rehabil2013;26:345-52.
24 Johnsson KE, Rosén I, Udén A. Neurophysiologic investigation of patients with spinal stenosis. Spine1987;12:483-7.
25 Atlas SJ, Delitto A. Spinal stenosis: surgical versus nonsurgical treatment. Clin Orthop2006;443:198-207.
26 Porter RW. Spinal stenosis and neurogenic claudication. Spine1996;21:2046-52.
27 Nadeau M, Rosas-Arellano M, Gurr K, et al. The reliability of differentiating neurogenic claudication from vascular claudication based on symptomatic presentation. Can J Surg2103;56:372-7.
28 Conway J, Tomkins CC, Haig AJ. Walking assessment in people with lumbar spinal stenosis: capacity, performance, and self-report measures. Spine J 2011;11:816-23.
29 Katz JN, Dalgas M, Stucki G, et al. Degenerative lumbar spinal stenosis. Diagnostic value of the history and physical examination. Arthritis Rheum1995;38:1236-41.
30 Tomkins-Lane CC, Conway J, Hepler C, et al. Changes in objectively measured physical activity (performance) after epidural steroid injection for lumbar spinal stenosis. Arch Phys Med Rehabil2012;93:2008-14.
31 Whitehurst M, Brown LE, Eidelson SG, et al. Functional mobility performance in an elderly population with lumbar spinal stenosis. Arch Phys Med Rehabil2001;82:464-7.
32 Tomkins-Lane CC, Holz SC, Yamakawa KS, et al. Predictors of walking performance and walking capacity in people with lumbar spinal stenosis, low back pain, and asymptomatic controls. Arch Phys Med Rehabil2012;93:647-53.
33 Benoist M. The natural history of lumbar degenerative spinal stenosis. J Bone Spine Rev Rhum2002;69:450-7.
34 Hurri H, Slätis P, Soini J, et al. Lumbar spinal stenosis: assessment of long-term outcome 12 years after operative and conservative treatment. J Spinal Disord1998;11:110-5.
35 Johnsson KE, Rosén I, Udén A. The natural course of lumbar spinal stenosis. Clin Orthop1992;279:82-6.
36 Minamide A, Yoshida M, Maio K. The natural clinical course of lumbar spinal stenosis: a longitudinal cohort study over a minimum of 10 years. J Orthop Sci 2013;18:693-8.
37 Haig AJ, Tong HC, Yamakawa KSJ, et al. Predictors of pain and function in persons with spinal stenosis, low back pain, and no back pain. Spine2006;31:2950-7.
38 Evans JG. Neurogenic intermittent claudication. BMJ1964;2:985-7.
39 Watanabe R, Parke WW. Vascular and neural pathology of lumbosacral spinal stenosis. J Neurosurg1986;64:64-70.
40 Ooi Y, Mita F, Satoh Y. Myeloscopic study on lumbar spinal canal stenosis with special reference to intermittent claudication. Spine1990;15:544-9.
41 Porter RW, Ward D. Cauda equina dysfunction. The significance of two-level pathology. Spine1992;17:9-15.
42 Binder DK, Schmidt MH, Weinstein PR. Lumbar spinal stenosis. Semin Neurol2002;22:157-66.
43 Genevay S, Atlas SJ. Lumbar spinal stenosis. Best Pract Res Clin Rheumatol2010;24:253-65.
44 Andreisek G, Hodler J, Steurer J. Uncertainties in the diagnosis of lumbar spinal stenosis. Radiology2011;261:681-4.
45 Frymoyer JW. Degenerative spondylolisthesis: diagnosis and treatment. J Am Acad Orthop Surg1994;2:9-15.
46 Haig AJ, Tomkins CC. Diagnosis and management of lumbar spinal stenosis. JAMA2010;303:71-2.
47 Suri P, Rainville J, Kalichman L, et al. Does this older adult with lower extremity pain have the clinical syndrome of lumbar spinal stenosis? JAMA2010;304:2628-36.
48 De Schepper EIT, Overdevest GM, Suri P, et al. Diagnosis of lumbar spinal stenosis: an updated systematic review of the accuracy of diagnostic tests. Spine2013;38:E469-81.
49 Barz T, Melloh M, Staub L, et al. The diagnostic value of a treadmill test in predicting lumbar spinal stenosis. Eur Spine J 2008;17:686-90.
50 Deen HG, Zimmerman RS, Lyons MK, et al. Measurement of exercise tolerance on the treadmill in patients with symptomatic lumbar spinal stenosis: a useful indicator of functional status and surgical outcome. J Neurosurg1995;83:27-30.
51 Deen HG, Zimmerman RS, Lyons MK, et al. Use of the exercise treadmill to measure baseline functional status and surgical outcome in patients with severe lumbar spinal stenosis. Spine1998;23:244-8.
52 Herno A, Saari T, Suomalainen O, et al. The degree of decompressive relief and its relation to clinical outcome in patients undergoing surgery for lumbar spinal stenosis. Spine1999;24:1010-4.
53 Jensen OH, Schmidt-Olsen S. A new functional test in the diagnostic evaluation of neurogenic intermittent claudication. Clin Rheumatol1989;8:363-7.
54 Tenhula J, Lenke LG, Bridwell KH, et al. Prospective functional evaluation of the surgical treatment of neurogenic claudication in patients with lumbar spinal stenosis. J Spinal Disord2000;13:276-82.
55 Tomkins CC, Battié MC, Rogers T, et al. A criterion measure of walking capacity in lumbar spinal stenosis and its comparison with a treadmill protocol. Spine2009;34:2444-9.
56 Kim Y-S, Park S-J, Oh I-S, et al. The clinical effect of gait load test in two level lumbar spinal stenosis. Asian Spine J2009;3:96-100.
57 Takahashi N, Kikuchi S, Yabuki S, et al. Diagnostic value of the lumbar extension-loading test in patients with lumbar spinal stenosis: a cross-sectional study. BMC Musculoskelet Disord2014;15:259.

58 Nagai K, Aoyama T, Yamada M, et al. Quantification of changes in gait characteristics associated with intermittent claudication in patients with lumbar spinal stenosis. J Spinal Disord Tech2014;27:E136-42.
59 Tomkins-Lane CC, Haig AJ. A review of activity monitors as a new technology for objectifying function in lumbar spinal stenosis. J Back Musculoskelet Rehabil2012;25:177-85.
60 Kalff R, Ewald C, Waschke A, et al. Degenerative lumbar spinal stenosis in older people. Dtsch Ärztebl Int2013;110:613-24.
61 Haig AJ, Tong HC, Yamakawa KSJ, et al. The sensitivity and specificity of electrodiagnostic testing for the clinical syndrome of lumbar spinal stenosis. Spine2005;30:2667-76.
62 Haig AJ, Tong HC, Yamakawa KS, et al. Spinal stenosis, back pain, or no symptoms at all? A masked study comparing radiologic and electrodiagnostic diagnoses to the clinical impression. Arch Phys Med Rehabil2006;87:897-903.
63 Yagci I, Gunduz OH, Ekinci G, et al. The utility of lumbar paraspinal mapping in the diagnosis of lumbar spinal stenosis. Am J Phys Med Rehabil 2009;88:843-51.
64 Kuittinen P, Sipola P, Aalto TJ, et al. Correlation of lateral stenosis in MRI with symptoms, walking capacity and EMG findings in patients with surgically confirmed lateral lumbar spinal canal stenosis. BMC Musculoskelet Disord2014;15:247.
65 De Graaf I, Prak A, Bierma-Zeinstra S, et al. Diagnosis of lumbar spinal stenosis: a systematic review of the accuracy of diagnostic tests. Spine2006;31:1168-76.
66 Mamisch N, Brumann M, Hodler J, et al. Radiologic criteria for the diagnosis of spinal stenosis: results of a Delphi survey. Radiology2012;264:174-9.
67 Steurer J, Roner S, Gnannt R, et al. Quantitative radiologic criteria for the diagnosis of lumbar spinal stenosis: a systematic literature review. BMC Musculoskelet Disord2011;12:175.
68 Cheung JP-Y, Samartzis D, Shigematsu H, et al. Defining clinically relevant values for developmental spinal stenosis: a large-scale magnetic resonance imaging study. Spine2014;39:1067-76.
69 Wassenaar M, van Rijn RM, van Tulder MW, et al. Magnetic resonance imaging for diagnosing lumbar spinal pathology in adult patients with low back pain or sciatica: a diagnostic systematic review. Eur Spine J 2012;21:220-7.
70 Lurie JD, Tosteson AN, Tosteson TD, et al. Reliability of readings of magnetic resonance imaging features of lumbar spinal stenosis. Spine2008;33:1605-10.
71 Lee S, Lee JW, Yeom JS, et al. A practical MRI grading system for lumbar foraminal stenosis. AJR Am J Roentgenol2010;194:1095-8.
72 Schizas C, Theumann N, Burn A, et al. Qualitative grading of severity of lumbar spinal stenosis based on the morphology of the dural sac on magnetic resonance images. Spine2010;35:1919-24.
73 Barz T, Melloh M, Staub LP, et al. Nerve root sedimentation sign: evaluation of a new radiological sign in lumbar spinal stenosis. Spine2010;35:892-7.
74 Moses RA, Zhao W, Staub LP, et al. Is the sedimentation sign associated with spinal stenosis surgical treatment effect in SPORT? Spine2015;40:129-36.
75 Tomkins-Lane CC, Quint DJ, Gabriel S, et al. Nerve root sedimentation sign for the diagnosis of lumbar spinal stenosis: reliability, sensitivity, and specificity. Spine2013;38:E1554-60.
76 Andreisek G, Imhof M, Wertli M, et al. A systematic review of semiquantitative and qualitative radiologic criteria for the diagnosis of lumbar spinal stenosis. Am J Roentgenol2013;201:W735-46.
77 Andreisek G, Deyo RA, Jarvik JG, et al. Consensus conference on core radiological parameters to describe lumbar stenosis—an initiative for structured reporting. Eur Radiol2014;24:3224-32.
78 Boden SD, Davis DO, Dina TS, et al. Abnormal magnetic-resonance scans of the lumbar spine in asymptomatic subjects. A prospective investigation. J Bone Joint Surg Am1990;72:403-8.
79 Amundsen T, Weber H, Lilleås F, et al. Lumbar spinal stenosis. Clinical and radiologic features. Spine1995;20:1178-86.
80 Geisser ME, Haig AJ, Tong HC, et al. Spinal canal size and clinical symptoms among persons diagnosed with lumbar spinal stenosis. Clin J Pain2007;23:780-5.
81 Herno A, Airaksinen O, Saari T. Computed tomography after laminectomy for lumbar spinal stenosis. Patients' pain patterns, walking capacity, and subjective disability had no correlation with computed tomography findings. Spine1994;19:1975-8.
82 Lohman CM, Tallroth K, Kettunen JA, et al. Comparison of radiologic signs and clinical symptoms of spinal stenosis. Spine2006;31:1834-40.
83 Cook C, Brown C, Michael K, et al. The clinical value of a cluster of patient history and observational findings as a diagnostic support tool for lumbar spine stenosis. Physiother Res Int J Res Clin Phys Ther2011;16:170-8.
84 Kato Y, Kawakami T, Kifune M, et al. Validation study of a clinical diagnosis support tool for lumbar spinal stenosis. J Orthop Sci 2009;14:7118.
85 Konno S, Hayashino Y, Fukuhara S, et al. Development of a clinical diagnosis support tool to identify patients with lumbar spinal stenosis. Eur Spine J 2007;16:1951-7.
86 Sugioka T, Hayashino Y, Konno S, et al. Predictive value of self-reported patient information for the identification of lumbar spinal stenosis. Fam Pract2008;25:237-44.
87 Haskins R, Osmotherly PG, Rivett DA. Diagnostic clinical prediction rules for specific subtypes of low back pain: a systematic review. J Orthop Sports Phys Ther2015;45:61-76.
88 Sandella DE, Haig AJ, Tomkins-Lane C, et al. Defining the clinical syndrome of lumbar spinal stenosis: a recursive specialist survey process. PM R2013;5:491-5; quiz 495.
89 Ammendolia C, Stuber KJ, Rok E, et al. Nonoperative treatment for lumbar spinal stenosis with neurogenic claudication. Cochrane Database Syst Rev2013;8;CD010712.
90 Schneider M, Ammendolia C, Murphy D, et al. Comparison of non-surgical treatment methods for patients with lumbar spinal stenosis: protocol for a randomized controlled trial. Chiropr Man Ther2014;22:19.
91 Tomkins-Lane CC, Lafave LMZ, Parnell JA, et al. The spinal stenosis pedometer and nutrition lifestyle intervention (SSPANLI) randomized controlled trial protocol. BMC Musculoskelet Disord2013;14:322.
92 Tomkins-Lane CC, Lafave LMZ, Parnell JA, et al. The spinal stenosis pedometer and nutrition lifestyle intervention (SSPANLI): development and pilot. Spine J 2014; published online 22 Oct.
93 Ammendolia C, Stuber K, de Bruin LK, et al. Nonoperative treatment of lumbar spinal stenosis with neurogenic claudication: a systematic review. Spine2012;37:E609-16.
94 Coronado-Zarco R, Cruz-Medina E, Arellano-Hernández A, et al. Effectiveness of calcitonin in intermittent claudication treatment of patients with lumbar spinal stenosis: a systematic review. Spine2009;34:E818-22.
95 Podichetty VK, Segal AM, Lieber M, et al. Effectiveness of salmon calcitonin nasal spray in the treatment of lumbar canal stenosis: a double-blind, randomized, placebo-controlled, parallel group trial. Spine2004;29:2343-9.
96 Peng K, Chen L, Peng J, et al. Effects of calcitonin on lumbar spinal stenosis: a systematic review and meta-analysis. Int J Clin Exp Med2015;8:2536-44.
97 Van Tulder MW, Scholten RJ, Koes BW, et al. Non-steroidal anti-inflammatory drugs for low back pain. Cochrane Database Syst Rev2000;2:CD000396.
98 Yoshihara H. Prostaglandin E1 treatment for lumbar spinal canal stenosis: review of the literature. Pain Pract 2015; published online 7 Jan.
99 Tomkins CC, Dimoff KH, Forman HS, et al. Physical therapy treatment options for lumbar spinal stenosis. J Back Musculoskelet Rehabil2010;23:31-7.
100 Macedo LG, Hum A, Kuleba L, et al. Physical therapy interventions for degenerative lumbar spinal stenosis: a systematic review. Phys Ther2013;93:1646-60.
101 Fritz JM, Lurie JD, Zhao W, et al. Associations between physical therapy and long-term outcomes for individuals with lumbar spinal stenosis in the SPORT study. Spine J 2014;14:1611-21.
102 Delitto A, Piva SR, Moore CG, et al. Surgery versus nonsurgical treatment of lumbar spinal stenosis: a randomized trial. Ann Intern Med2015;162:465-73.
103 Ammendolia C, Stuber KJ, Rok E, et al. Nonoperative treatment for lumbar spinal stenosis with neurogenic claudication. Cochrane Database Syst Rev2013;8:CD010712.
104 Liu K, Liu P, Liu R, et al. Steroid for epidural injection in spinal stenosis: a systematic review and meta-analysis. Drug Des Dev Ther2015;9:707-16.
105 Manchikanti L, Singh V, Pampati V, et al. Comparison of the efficacy of caudal, interlaminar, and transforaminal epidural injections in managing lumbar disc herniation: is one method superior to the other? Korean J Pain2015;28:11-21.
106 Friedly JL, Comstock BA, Turner JA, et al. A randomized trial of epidural glucocorticoid injections for spinal stenosis. N Engl J Med2014;371:11-21.
107 Centers for Disease Control and Prevention (CDC). Multistate outbreak of fungal infection associated with injection of methylprednisolone acetate solution from a single compounding pharmacy—United States, 2012. MMWR Morb Mortal Wkly Rep2012;61:839-42.
108 Chou R, Hashimoto R, Friedly J, et al. Epidural corticosteroid injections for radiculopathy and spinal stenosis: a systematic review and meta-analysis. Ann Intern Med2015;163:373-81.
109 Stuber K, Sajko S, Kristmanson K. Chiropractic treatment of lumbar spinal stenosis: a review of the literature. J Chiropr Med2009;8:77-85.
110 Cambron JA, Schneider M, Dexheimer JM, et al. A pilot randomized controlled trial of flexion-distraction dosage for chiropractic treatment of lumbar spinal stenosis. J Manipulative Physiol Ther2014;37:396-406.
111 Schneider M, Ammendolia C, Murphy D, et al. Comparison of non-surgical treatment methods for patients with lumbar spinal stenosis: protocol for a randomized controlled trial. Chiropr Man Ther2014;22:19.
112 Kim KH, Kim T-H, Lee BR, et al. Acupuncture for lumbar spinal stenosis: A systematic review and meta-analysis. Complement Ther Med2013;21:535-56.
113 Sengupta DK, Herkowitz HN. Lumbar spinal stenosis. Treatment strategies and indications for surgery. Orthop Clin North Am2003;34:281-95.
114 Ciol MA, Deyo RA, Howell E, et al. An assessment of surgery for spinal stenosis: time trends, geographic variations, complications, and reoperations. J Am Geriatr Soc1996;44:285-90.
115 Dartmouth Institute. Variation in the care of surgical conditions: spinal stenosis. 2014. www.dartmouthatlas.org/downloads/reports/Spinal_stenosis_report_10_29_14.pdf.
116 Weinstein JN, Lurie JD, Olson PR, et al. United States' trends and regional variations in lumbar spine surgery: 1992-2003. Spine2006;31:2707-14.

117 Kreiner DS, Shaffer WO, Baisden JL, et al. An evidence-based clinical guideline for the diagnosis and treatment of degenerative lumbar spinal stenosis (update). Spine J2013;13:734-43.
118 Resnick DK, Watters WC III, Mummaneni PV, et al. Guideline update for the performance of fusion procedures for degenerative disease of the lumbar spine. Part 10: Lumbar fusion for stenosis without spondylolisthesis. J Neurosurg Spine2014;21:62-6.
119 Jacobs WCH, Rubinstein SM, Koes B, et al. Evidence for surgery in degenerative lumbar spine disorders. Best Pract Res Clin Rheumatol2013;27:673-84.
120 Overdevest GM, Jacobs W, Vleggeert-Lankamp C, et al. Effectiveness of posterior decompression techniques compared with conventional laminectomy for lumbar stenosis. Cochrane Database Syst Rev2015;3:CD010036.
121 Weinstein JN, Tosteson TD, Lurie JD, et al. Surgical versus nonsurgical therapy for lumbar spinal stenosis. N Engl J Med2008;358:794-810.
122 Pearson A, Blood E, Lurie J, et al. predominant leg pain is associated with better surgical outcomes in degenerative spondylolisthesis and spinal stenosis: results from the Spine Patient Outcomes Research Trial (SPORT). Spine2011;36:219-29.
123 Slätis P, Malmivaara A, Heliövaara M, et al. Long-term results of surgery for lumbar spinal stenosis: a randomised controlled trial. Eur Spine J2011;20:1174-81.
124 Weinstein JN, Tosteson TD, Lurie JD, et al. Surgical versus nonoperative treatment for lumbar spinal stenosis four-year results of the Spine Patient Outcomes Research Trial. Spine2010;35:1329-38.
125 Lurie JD, Tosteson TD, Tosteson A, et al. Long-term outcomes of lumbar spinal stenosis: eight-year results of the Spine Patient Outcomes Research Trial (SPORT). Spine2015;40:63-76.
126 Malmivaara A, Slätis P, Heliövaara M, et al. Surgical or nonoperative treatment for lumbar spinal stenosis? A randomized controlled trial. Spine2007;32:1-8.
127 Zaina F, Tomkins-Lane C, Carragee E, et al. Surgical versus non-surgical treatment for lumbar spinal stenosis. Cochrane Database Syst Rev [forthcoming].
128 Weinstein JN, Tosteson TD, Lurie JD, et al. Surgical versus nonsurgical therapy for lumbar spinal stenosis. N Engl J Med2008;358:794-810.
129 Aalto TJ, Malmivaara A, Kovacs F, et al. Preoperative predictors for postoperative clinical outcome in lumbar spinal stenosis: systematic review. Spine2006;31:E648-63.
130 Pearson A, Lurie J, Tosteson T, et al. Who should have surgery for spinal stenosis? Treatment effect predictors in SPORT. Sp ine2012;37:1791-802.
131 McGregor AH, Probyn K, Cro S, et al. Rehabilitation following surgery for lumbar spinal stenosis. A Cochrane review. Spine2014;39:1044-54.
132 Resnick DK, Watters WC III, Mummaneni PV, et al. Guideline update for the performance of fusion procedures for degenerative disease of the lumbar spine. Part 10: lumbar fusion for stenosis without spondylolisthesis. J Neurosurg Spine2014;21:62-6.
133 Kreiner DS, Shaffer WO, Baisden JL, et al. An evidence-based clinical guideline for the diagnosis and treatment of degenerative lumbar spinal stenosis (update). Spine J2013;13:734-43.
134 Carragee EJ. The increasing morbidity of elective spinal stenosis surgery: is it necessary? JAMA2010;303:1309.
135 Lindsey DP, Swanson KE, Fuchs P, et al. The effects of an interspinous implant on the kinematics of the instrumented and adjacent levels in the lumbar spine. Spine2003;28:2192-7.
136 Richards JC, Majumdar S, Lindsey DP, et al. The treatment mechanism of an interspinous process implant for lumbar neurogenic intermittent claudication. Spine2005;30:744-9.
137 Schizas C, Pralong E, Tzioupis C, et al. Interspinous distraction in lumbar spinal stenosis: a neurophysiological perspective. Spine2013;38:2113-7.
138 Zucherman JF, Hsu KY, Hartjen CA, et al. A prospective randomized multi-center study for the treatment of lumbar spinal stenosis with the X STOP interspinous implant: 1-year results. Eur Spine J 2004;13:22-31.
139 Zucherman JF, Hsu KY, Hartjen CA, et al. A multicenter, prospective, randomized trial evaluating the X STOP interspinous process decompression system for the treatment of neurogenic intermittent claudication: two-year follow-up results. Spine2005;30:1351-8.
140 Lønne G, Johnsen LG, Aas E, et al. Comparing cost-effectiveness of X-stop to minimally invasive decompression in lumbar spinal stenosis: a randomized controlled trial. Spine2015; published online 20 Jan.
141 Strömqvist BH, Berg S, Gerdhem P, et al. X-stop versus decompressive surgery for lumbar neurogenic intermittent claudication: randomized controlled trial with 2-year follow-up. Spine2013;38:1436-42.
142 Moojen WA, Arts MP, Jacobs WCH, et al. Interspinous process device versus standard conventional surgical decompression for lumbar spinal stenosis: randomized controlled trial. BMJ2013;347:f6415.
143 Deyo RA, Martin BI, Ching A, et al. Interspinous spacers compared with decompression or fusion for lumbar stenosis: complications and repeat operations in the Medicare population. Spine2013;38:865-72.
144 Hong P, Liu Y, Li H. Comparison of the efficacy and safety between interspinous process distraction device and open decompression surgery in treating lumbar spinal stenosis: a meta analysis. J Investig Surg 2015;28:40-9.
145 Wu A-M, Zhou Y, Li Q-L, et al. Interspinous spacer versus traditional decompressive surgery for lumbar spinal stenosis: a systematic review and meta-analysis. PloS One2014;9:e97142.
146 Deer TR, Kapural L. New image-guided ultra-minimally invasive lumbar decompression method: the mild procedure. Pain Physician2010;13:35-41.
147 Brown LL. A double-blind, randomized, prospective study of epidural steroid injection vs the mild procedure in patients with symptomatic lumbar spinal stenosis. Pain Pract 2012;12:333-41.
148 Kreiner DS, MacVicar J, Duszynski B, et al. The mild procedure: a systematic review of the current literature. Pain Med Malden Mass2014;15:196-205.
149 Kalichman L, Hunter DJ. Diagnosis and conservative management of degenerative lumbar spondylolisthesis. Eur Spine J2008;17:327-35.
150 Pearson A, Blood E, Lurie J, et al. Degenerative spondylolisthesis versus spinal stenosis: does a slip matter? Comparison of baseline characteristics and outcomes (SPORT). Spine2010;35:298-305.
151 Weinstein JN, Lurie JD, Tosteson TD, et al. Surgical versus nonsurgical treatment for lumbar degenerative spondylolisthesis. N Engl J Med2007;356:2257-70.
152 Weinstein JN, Lurie JD, Tosteson TD, et al. Surgical compared with nonoperative treatment for lumbar degenerative spondylolisthesis. four-year results in the Spine Patient Outcomes Research Trial (SPORT) randomized and observational cohorts. J Bone Joint Surg Am2009;91:1295-304.
153 Herkowitz HN, Kurz LT. Degenerative lumbar spondylolisthesis with spinal stenosis. A prospective study comparing decompression with decompression and intertransverse process arthrodesis. J Bone Joint Surg Am1991;73:802-8.
154 Eismont FJ, Norton RP, Hirsch BP. Surgical management of lumbar degenerative spondylolisthesis. J Am Acad Orthop Surg2014;22:203-13.
155 Abdu WA, Lurie JD, Spratt KF, et al. Degenerative spondylolisthesis: does fusion method influence outcome? Four-year results of the spine patient outcomes research trial. Spine2009;34:2351-60.
156 Fischgrund JS, Mackay M, Herkowitz HN, et al. Degenerative lumbar spondylolisthesis with spinal stenosis: a prospective, randomized study comparing decompressive laminectomy and arthrodesis with and without spinal instrumentation. Spine1997;22:2807-12.
157 Kornblum MB, Fischgrund JS, Herkowitz HN, et al. Degenerative lumbar spondylolisthesis with spinal stenosis: a prospective long-term study comparing fusion and pseudarthrosis. Spine2004;29:726-33; discussion 733-4.
158 Pearson AM, Lurie JD, Tosteson TD, et al. Who should undergo surgery for degenerative spondylolisthesis? Treatment effect predictors in SPORT. Spine2013;38:1799-811.
159 Mannion AF, Pittet V, Steiger F, et al. Development of appropriateness criteria for the surgical treatment of symptomatic lumbar degenerative spondylolisthesis (LDS). Eur Spine J 2014;23:1903-17.
160 Wang G, Hu J, Liu X, et al. Surgical treatments for degenerative lumbar scoliosis: a meta analysis. Eur Spine J2015;24:1792-9.
161 Phelan EA, Deyo RA, Cherkin DC, et al. Helping patients decide about back surgery: a randomized trial of an interactive video program. Spine2001;26:206-11; discussion 212.

BPP UNIVERSITY SCHOOL OF HEALTH BMJ

Opioids for low back pain

Richard A Deyo, professor[1,2], Michael Von Korff, senior investigator[3], David Duhrkoop, volunteer regional director[4]

[1]Departments of Family Medicine, Internal Medicine, and Public Health and Preventive Medicine and Oregon Institute for Occupational Health Sciences, Oregon Health and Science University, Portland, OR 97239, USA

[2]Center for Health Research, Kaiser Permanente Northwest, Portland, OR, USA

[3]Group Health Research Institute, Seattle, WA, USA

[4]American Chronic Pain Association, Rocklin, CA, USA

Correspondence to: R A Deyo Department of Family Medicine, Mail Code FM, Oregon Health and Science University, Portland, OR 97239, USA deyor@ohsu.edu

Cite this as: *BMJ* 2015;350:g6380

DOI: 10.1136/bmj.g6380

http://www.bmj.com/content/350/bmj.g6380

ABSTRACT

Back pain affects most adults, causes disability for some, and is a common reason for seeking healthcare. In the United States, opioid prescription for low back pain has increased, and opioids are now the most commonly prescribed drug class. More than half of regular opioid users report back pain. Rates of opioid prescribing in the US and Canada are two to three times higher than in most European countries. The analgesic efficacy of opioids for acute back pain is inferred from evidence in other acute pain conditions. Opioids do not seem to expedite return to work in injured workers or improve functional outcomes of acute back pain in primary care. For chronic back pain, systematic reviews find scant evidence of efficacy. Randomized controlled trials have high dropout rates, brief duration (four months or less), and highly selected patients. Opioids seem to have short term analgesic efficacy for chronic back pain, but benefits for function are less clear. The magnitude of pain relief across chronic non-cancer pain conditions is about 30%. Given the brevity of randomized controlled trials, the long term effectiveness and safety of opioids are unknown. Loss of long term efficacy could result from drug tolerance and emergence of hyperalgesia. Complications of opioid use include addiction and overdose related mortality, which have risen in parallel with prescription rates. Common short term side effects are constipation, nausea, sedation, and increased risk of falls and fractures. Longer term side effects may include depression and sexual dysfunction. Screening for high risk patients, treatment agreements, and urine testing have not reduced overall rates of opioid prescribing, misuse, or overdose. Newer strategies for reducing risks include more selective prescription of opioids and lower doses; use of prescription monitoring programs; avoidance of co-prescription with sedative hypnotics; and reformulations that make drugs more difficult to snort, smoke, or inject.

Introduction

Back pain affects most adults, is a leading cause of activity limitation and work disability worldwide, and is among the most common reasons for seeking healthcare.[1 2 3 4 5] It has an enormous impact on individuals, healthcare systems, and national economies, and treatment approaches have important consequences for patients, clinicians, and society.

In the United States, the prescription of opioids for low back pain has increased.[5] Insurance claims data suggest that the opioids are the most commonly prescribed class of drug for back pain,[6] and more than half of regular opioid users report back pain.[7] Unfortunately, increased drug misuse, complications, and fatal overdoses have accompanied this rise in opioid use.[8] Clinicians must therefore weigh the possible analgesic benefits of opioid therapy against the risks. Figure 1 details useful precautions that should be taken when prescribing opioids for low back pain.

The aims of this review are to examine trends and variations in the use of opioids for back pain; assess the evidence for opioid efficacy in acute and chronic back pain; summarize new data on the adverse effects of long term opioids; and make recommendations for judicious prescribing. The review is interspersed with commentary from a patient with back pain and extensive experience with opioid therapy.

Despite some evidence from randomized controlled trials (RCTs) on the efficacy of opioids in the short term treatment of low back pain, little evidence is available on long term efficacy and safety.[9] Because clinical trials in this area may not generalize well to routine care and provide no evidence on long term use, we also considered selected observational data.

Sources and selection criteria

We identified reviews of opioid efficacy for back pain published between 2000 and April 2014 in the PubMed database using the search terms low back pain and opioids, with a filter for systematic reviews. Because efficacy may differ for back pain relative to other pain conditions (such as neuropathic pain, headache, and fibromyalgia), we focused on reviews that separated back pain from other causes.

Patients with mood disorders or a history of substance misuse are often excluded from RCTs of opioids, but they are more likely to receive opioids in routine care.[10 11 12] No RCTs of opioids for back pain have lasted for more than four months,[9] although many patients receive treatment for longer. Thus, we also examined relevant cohort studies from primary care or employed populations.

Relevant RCTs have been too small, brief, and selective to adequately assess less common complications, those occurring with long term use, and those related to comorbid conditions or drug interactions. We therefore conducted a separate PubMed search for studies on the prevalence of opioid misuse in patients receiving long term prescriptions using the terms opioids, abuse, and prevalence, with a filter for systematic reviews. We considered systematic reviews published in 2007 and 2008, as well as articles published since 2007 that were based in primary care, observed patients for at least a year, and used standardized measures of opioid misuse or dependence.

We examined observational studies for other adverse events during long term treatment with opioids, using reference lists of other retrieved articles and our personal knowledge. We considered studies published since 2000 with comparators (opioids *v* no opioids, or high dose *v* low dose opioids).

Incidence and prevalence of low back pain

Prevalence of symptoms

The US national health interview survey reported that 28% of adults had experienced low back pain that lasted a whole day or more during the past three months.[13] About half of all adults experience some back pain over a one year period, with 20% reporting "frequent" back pain. The prognosis is good for acute back pain in primary care: within a month,

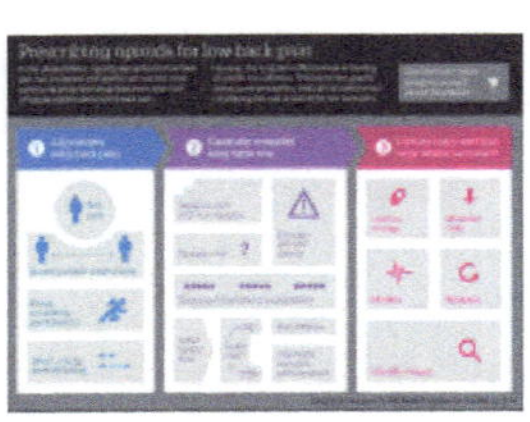

Fig 1 Use our interactive graphic as a guide to prescribing opioids for low back pain. See www.bmj.com/content/350/bmj.g6380/infographic

pain and disability scores improve by an average of 58%,[14] but recurrence is common.[15] Only 10% of patients develop chronic pain (longer than three months), but these patients have higher healthcare and disability compensation costs.[2]

Prevalence of pathophysiologic changes

The differential diagnosis of back pain is broad, including degenerative conditions in the intervertebral discs and vertebrae and musculoligamentous conditions. However, degenerative radiologic findings are common in pain-free individuals, so the cause of pain is often unclear.[16] Degenerative conditions often coexist, increasing uncertainty. Chronic pain itself can induce structural and functional changes in the central nervous system, perpetuating the perception of pain.[17,18,19] Mood disorders and workplace factors often influence the evolution of, and the adaptation to, chronic back pain.[10,11,12] Thus, a biopsychosocial model of back pain is widely accepted, and a meaningful anatomical diagnosis remains uncertain for many patients.

Serious systemic diseases such as metastatic cancer, spinal infections, and inflammatory spondylopathies each account for less than 1% of patients with back pain in primary care.[20] Therefore, we focused on opioid treatment of back pain without underlying serious systemic disease.

Trends in opioid prescribing

Opioid prescribing has increased worldwide, with US opioid sales quadrupling between 1999 and 2010.[21] This was in part a response to undertreatment of patients receiving cancer care, palliative care, or treatment for acute pain. However, opioid therapy for chronic musculoskeletal pain, including back pain, also grew substantially and disproportionately.[7,22] As US opioid sales quadrupled, admissions to substance misuse treatment programs and opioid related overdose deaths also increased fourfold.[8,21] Similarly, deaths in England and Wales involving methadone or codeine doubled between 2005 and 2009.[23]

US national survey data showed a 660% increase in expenditure on opioids for spine problems from 1997 to 2006 owing to increasing prices and increasing use.[24] From 1999 to 2010, the proportion of visits to ambulatory physician practices for back and neck pain that resulted in prescription of an opioid increased from 19% to 29%.[25] In a per person analysis of privately insured employed people, 42% of patients received a prescription within a year of index diagnosis.[6]

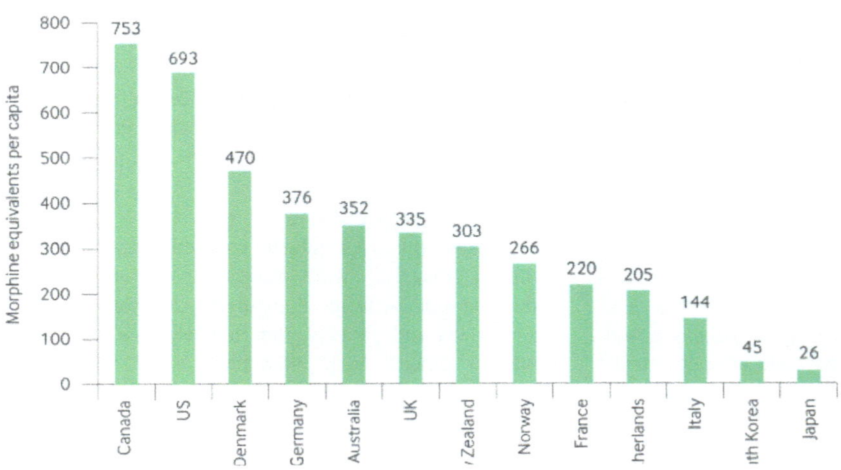

Fig 2 International use of six powerful opioids—fentanyl, hydromorphone, methadone, morphine, oxycodone, and pethidine (meperidine)—during 2010 (www.painpolicy.wisc.edu)

Opioids are mostly prescribed for chronic pain. In one US health plan, 87% of all morphine equivalents for pain were dispensed to patients receiving long term opioids.[26] Patients with back pain seem to be more likely than patients with other common pain diagnoses to receive high doses.[27]

Substantial geographic variations in opioid prescribing may reflect limited professional consensus on appropriate use. Per capita use of potent opioids is higher in North America than in other developed countries: twice the rate seen in the United Kingdom; three times that in the Netherlands; and 26 times that in Japan (fig 2). Even within the US, per capita opioid prescription varied 23-fold among state run low income insurance programs.[28]

Several factors account for North America's increased use of opioids. In the 1980s, on the basis of a small case series and an inpatient sample, pain experts argued that opioids were underused and that the risks of misuse were minimal.[29,30] Starting in the mid-1990s, drug industry marketing assumed an important role, with extensive sponsorship of pain specialty societies, continuing medical education programs, and guidelines.[23,31,32,33] The prescription of potent opioids quickly increased (fig 3),[34] However, some marketing was misleading: The manufacturer of OxyContin (oxycodone hydrochloride) and its three top executives pleeded guilty to criminal charges for misbranding the drug with claims of lower risk of misuse than for other opioids.[23,31]

The growth in opioid prescribing for back pain belies a paucity of evidence for efficacy, safety, and optimal prescribing. For example, US pain society guidelines for chronic non-cancer pain summarized data from short term opioid RCTs, but of 25 recommendations, 21 were based on "low quality evidence."[35]

PATIENT COMMENTARY

"Why do people seek opioids? By the time pain becomes chronic, most patients have tried less potent drugs and they seek relief from a stronger prescribed source. We're a society of bad backs, and people don't want their backs to hurt. So they're looking to their doctors for a silver bullet."

Efficacy and effectiveness of opioids for low back pain

Acute low back pain

The analgesic efficacy of opioids for acute pain is well established, but there is a paucity of data on back pain in particular. A systematic review by the American Pain Society and the American College of Physicians found no

PATIENT INVOLVEMENT BOX

David Duhrkoop is a patient with chronic back pain who chairs a patient advisory committee for one of Dr Von Korff's research grants. He was recommended for this role by the director of the American Chronic Pain Association, a patient organization he has been involved with for many years. On a volunteer basis, Mr Duhrkoop has extensive experience in facilitating groups that help patients develop their abilities to effectively manage chronic pain. He reviewed and added to our initial outline of the manuscript and suggested topics on which he might comment. He offered novel ideas about our approach to developing the manuscript. He reviewed drafts of the manuscript as it evolved and offered his agreement with the content. He then prepared reactions and responses to the various components of the manuscript, offering personal experiences and those of other patients with whom he has worked. He reviewed and approved the final version of the paper for intellectual content.

RCTs comparing opioids with placebo for acute low back pain. Instead, they reported "fair" evidence based on trials for other acute pain conditions.[36] However, it is uncertain how opioids compare with non-steroidal anti-inflammatory drugs (NSAIDs), muscle relaxants, or other alternatives. It is also unclear whether opioid prescribing for acute back pain hastens recovery or return to work and how often it leads to long term use.

In a state-wide observational study of patients with acute work related back injuries (n=1843), a third of patients received an opioid prescription within six weeks, most at the first medical visit. After adjusting for pain, injury, and functional severity, patients who received more than seven days of opioids were twice as likely to remain work disabled at one year.[37] A national study found that opioid prescribing within 15 days of injury was associated with longer work disability, even after adjusting for the severity of injury, demographic characteristics, and job tenure. Longer work disability was also associated with higher doses of opioid.[38] It may be that opioids worsen outcomes—for example, by promoting physical deactivation and apathetic mood. Alternatively, patients prescribed opioids may simply be at higher risk of poor outcomes independent of medication. Regardless, these studies do not suggest that opioids expedite the return to work.

In a UK study of 715 primary care patients with low back pain, two thirds had acute pain and one third received opioids. Those receiving opioids had worse pain, functioning, self efficacy, catastrophizing, fear of movement, and depression. Even after adjusting for these and other baseline variables, patients who received opioids had worse functioning after six months than those who did not—an association not found among patients who received NSAIDs.[39] As with the return to work studies, the causal pathways are uncertain, but opioid prescribing at baseline was not linked to improved functional outcomes.

Prescription of opioids for acute pain may inadvertently lead to long term use if prescribers provide a large supply or simply continue to refill the prescription. This can lead to drug dependence and long term use.[40]

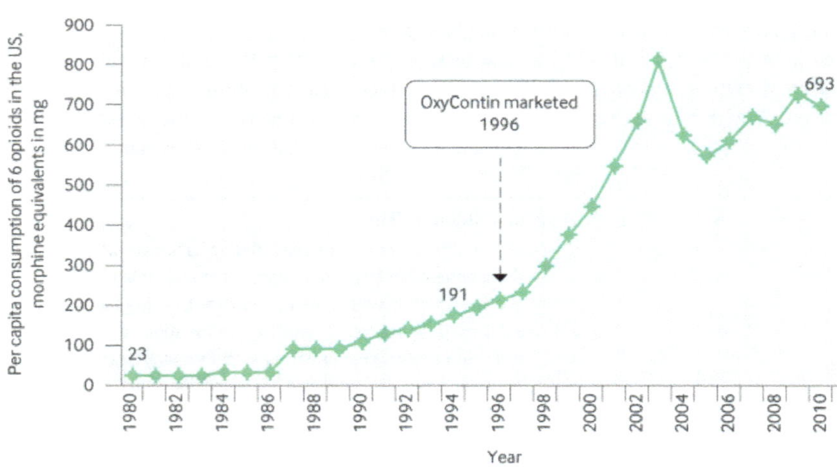

Fig 3 Per capita consumption of fentanyl, hydromorphone, methadone, morphine, oxycodone, pethidine (meperidine) in the United States. This figure does not include all opioids, and hydrocodone, in particular, is not included. Data from the US Centers for Disease Control indicate that total opioid sales in the US continued to rise consistently at least through 2010[21]

Chronic low back pain

Opioids versus placebo

Most RCTs of opioids for back pain have assessed chronic pain. Even here the evidence is meager and inconclusive. No trials lasted beyond four months,[9 41] and all had high dropout rates (>20%), mostly because of adverse effects or inefficacy.[9]

To reduce dropouts some opioid RCTs used an "enriched enrollment randomized withdrawal design," excluding patients who did not respond to treatment or had unacceptable adverse effects. Potential participants received the study drug before randomization and were included only if they benefited and tolerated side effects. Participants were then randomized to opioid withdrawal or continued treatment. This design underestimates adverse effects and risks overestimating efficacy.[42]

Many RCTs excluded patients with a history of substance misuse or mental disorders. Clinical guidelines typically caution against long term opioid prescribing for such patients. However, in routine care these patients are most likely to receive and sustain opioid use, a phenomenon called "adverse selection."[10 11 12 43] They are also more likely to receive higher doses and concurrent treatment with a sedative hypnotic drug.[10] Thus, safety data from clinical trials may generalize poorly to routine care.

Systematic reviews largely agree that opioids have greater short term analgesic efficacy than placebo, but that benefits for function are less clear.[9 36 41 44 45 46 47] They also agree that the evidence is sparse and of low quality. The mean magnitude of pain relief across a variety of chronic non-cancer pain conditions is about 30%.[47] Given the short duration of available studies, the reviews conclude that the effectiveness and safety of long term opioid use is unknown.

Of 15 RCTs in the most recent systematic review,[9] five examined the weak opioid agonist tramadol.[48 49 50 51 52] The reviewers found "low quality evidence" that tramadol was better than placebo at reducing pain, and "moderate quality evidence" that it was better at improving functional outcomes.

Two studies in this review assessed transdermal buprenorphine.[53 54] The reviewers found "very low quality evidence" that this drug was better than placebo for pain or functional outcomes.[9]

Seven RCTs compared long acting strong opioids (tapentadol, morphine, oxymorphone, hydromorphone, and oxycodone) with placebo (fig 4).[55 56 57 58 59 60 61] Five were industry sponsored, and three tested withdrawal of the drugs using the "enriched enrollment" design. The review found "moderate quality" evidence that these drugs are better than placebo in reducing pain and improving function, again in the short term.[9]

Opioids versus other drugs

For regulatory purposes, industry sponsored trials generally compare analgesics with placebo.[9 41] However, trials comparing opioids with alternatives are more relevant for clinicians and patients. Unfortunately, few RCTs have compared opioids with alternatives such as NSAIDs, antidepressants, or muscle relaxants.

One small RCT (n=55) for lumbar radiculopathy compared morphine, the tricyclic antidepressant nortriptyline, or a combination of both of these drugs with placebo (fig 4).[57] By the end of this crossover trial with four study groups almost 50% of participants had dropped out. Morphine and nortriptyline had similar analgesic effects and only the combination of the two drugs worked significantly better than placebo.

Two identical RCTs (total n=1598) compared a fixed dose of celecoxib with a fixed dose of tramadol.[62] At six weeks, significantly more patients achieved 30% pain relief with celecoxib than with tramadol (63% *v* 50% in study 1; 64% *v* 55% in study 2).

One small RCT compared the strong opioid oxycodone (or a combination of oxycodone plus morphine) with naproxen.[63] Both opioid groups had greater analgesia than the naproxen group, but no differences were seen in patient activity levels.

Together, these trials provide only weak evidence but suggest that NSAIDs may have analgesic efficacy intermediate between tramadol and stronger opioids, with similar effects on functioning.

Observational studies for chronic back pain

Given the short duration of available RCTs, observational studies provide the only evidence on the long term efficacy of opioids for back pain. In a study of work related back injuries, 38% of patients received an opioid at an early medical visit (n=694), but only 16% of them (n=111) received opioids for four calendar quarters. Among these long term users, a quarter experienced a 30% improvement in pain, but only 16% had improvement in function.[64] Average opioid doses increased each calendar quarter, except among the few patients with functional improvement.

A Danish population survey found that people taking long term opioids for non-cancer pain reported worse pain and quality of life than those with chronic pain who were not taking opioids.[65] People taking opioids may have had worse initial pain, but the drug did not achieve pain relief or quality of life comparable even to others with chronic pain. Thus, despite modest short term efficacy for chronic pain, it is unclear whether long term opioid therapy has meaningful therapeutic benefits.

Reasons for potential loss of efficacy

It has been proposed that loss of efficacy with long term use of opioids may be the result of tolerance and hyperalgesia (increased pain sensitivity).[66] Opioid tolerance—a need for increasing doses to achieve a desired effect—is seen in experimental pain (artificially induced pain, often with heat or cold) and after one month of oral morphine in patients with back pain.[56 67] Tolerance is seen in animal studies and in routine care when higher than usual doses are needed for acute pain in patients receiving long term opioids.[66] Tolerance may account for the common need to increase the dose with longer term use of opioids.[64 68]

Hyperalgesia is a common feature of opioid withdrawal that also occurs with experimental pain when opioids are stopped.[69] However, hyperalgesia may occur during opioid therapy, with both animal models and experimental pain models suggesting this effect.[66 70] Thus, repeated opioid use may spur both the development of tolerance (desensitization to opioids) and a pro-nociceptive process (sensitization to pain).

Responses to opioid tapering

The phenomena of tolerance and hyperalgesia raise the possibility that many patients receiving long term opioids would fare as well or better without them. This possibility has been tested in multidisciplinary pain treatment programs that include opioid cessation, which have reported success among participants who taper the dose over three weeks.[71 72 73] On average, these patients reported less pain after completing the program. The degree of improvement

Trial	Patient sample	Treatment groups	"Enriched enrollment"	Industry sponsor	Duration, FU rate	Results by group; P value
Chu (2012)[56]	**N=139** LBP ≥6 months; low dose opioids okay *Exclusions*: History of substance misuse, psychiatric disease, pain outside low back	Group 1: Long acting morphine Group 2: Placebo	● (no)	● (no)	1 month 74% FU	Average pain improvement: Group 1: 44% Group 2: 23% P<0.001
Hale (2010)[61]	**N=268** LBP≥6 months; already receiving ≥60 MEQ daily opioid; titrated on hydromorphone before randomization *Exclusions*: Depression, other pain conditions	Group 1: Hydromorphone ER Group 2: Placebo (hydromorphone discontinued)	● (yes)	● (yes)	12 weeks Overall: 41.4% FU Group 1: 49.6% FU Group 2: 33.1% FU	Worsening on 11 point scale: Group 1: 0.2 units Group 2: 1.6 units P<0.001
Buynak (2010)[55]	**N=981** Chronic LBP ≥3 months; must be taking analgesics for ≥3 months *Exclusions*: Psychiatric diseases	Group 1: Tapentadol ER Group 2: Oxycodone controlled release Group 3: Placebo	● (no)	● (yes)	Titration phase +12 weeks Group 1: 47.6% FU Group 2: 52.2% FU Group 3: 40.5% FU	≥30% improvement in pain: Group 1: 39.7% Group 2: 30.4% Group 3: 27.0% Group 1 *v*3: P=0.016
Khoromi (2007)[57]	**N=55** Lumbar radiculopathy ≥3 months *Exclusions*: Substance misuse, depression, unwilling to taper off opioids for 2 weeks	Group 1: Long acting morphine + inert placebo Group 2: Nortriptyline + inert placebo Group 3: Both active drugs Group 4: Active placebo*	● (no)	● (no)†	1 month on each regimen (crossover) 51% FU	≥30% improvement in pain: Group 1: 42% Group 2: 40% Group 3: 67% 4) 37% Only group 3 significantly better than placebo
Hale (2007)[58]	**N=143** LBP ≥3 months; already receiving ≥60 MEQ daily opioid *Exclusions*: Radiculopathy	Group 1: Oxymorphone ER Group 2: Placebo (oxymorphone discontinued)	● (yes)	● (yes)	12 weeks Group 1: 70% FU Group 2: 25% FU	Worsening on VAS pain score: Group 1: 8.7 mm Group 2: 31.6 mm P<0.0001
Katz (2007)[59]	**N=205** LBP ≥3 months; titrated on oxymorphone before randomization *Exclusions*: Radiculopathy	Group 1: Oxymorphone ER Group 2: Placebo (oxymorphone discontinued)	● (yes)	● (yes)	12 weeks Group 1: 68% FU Group 2: 47% FU	Worsening on VAS pain score: Group 1: 10.0 mm Group 2: 26.9 mm P<0.0001
Webster (2006)[60]	**N=719** LBP ≥6 months; any opioids discontinued *Exclusions*: History of substance misuse, litigation	Group 1: Placebo Group 2: Oxycodone four times daily Group 3: Oxycodone + naltrexone 1 μg four times daily Group 4: Combination twice daily	● (no)	● (yes)	Titration phase + 12 weeks 46% FU (2/3 of dropouts during titration phase)	% improvement in pain score: Group 1: 32% Group 2: 46% Group 3: 41% Group 4: 42% Groups 2-4 better than placebo, P<0.05

● = yes, ● = no

*The "active placebo" group received benztropine, which has no known effect on neuropathic pain but causes side effects that mimic those of morphine and nortriptyline, with the intent of producing more effective blinding than inert placebo. † No industry sponsorship, but MS Contin placebo tablets were a gift from Purdue Pharma.

Fig 4 Randomized trials of strong opioids versus placebo for chronic low back pain or sciatica included in a systematic review.[20] ER=extended release; FU=follow-up; LBP=lower back pain; MEQ=morphine equivalents; VAS=visual analogue scale

was similar whether or not participants were receiving opioids when they started. Mean depression scores and physical functioning improved substantially over the three week treatment period—for patients with back pain, in particular, and among those with or without previous spine surgery.[73 74] It is uncertain how these results generalize to patients who declined participation or did not complete the program. Nonetheless, these results suggest that many patients with persistent back pain can achieve favorable pain and function outcomes after stopping opioids in a multidisciplinary intervention.

PATIENT COMMENTARY

"Once patients start using opioids long term they are likely to continue, even if the doctor suspects it's not doing them much good—because patients expect it and feel it's important to their quality of life. Too often doctor and patient do not discuss whether opioids are improving the patient's overall quality of life, and patients often report that they do not understand the risks of continued opioid use."

Adverse effects of opioid treatment for low back pain

Opioid dependency, misuse, and addiction

Dependency

Most patients prescribed opioids continue to take them for days or weeks only. Acute pain may subside, many patients experience side effects, and others find the drugs unhelpful. However, insurance data show that more than half of patients who continue to take opioids for at least three months are still taking them years later.[75]

With prolonged use of these drugs many patients develop opioid dependence, meaning that cessation causes an unpleasant withdrawal syndrome (such as agitation, insomnia, diarrhea, rhinorrhea, piloerection, and hyperalgesia). Physical dependence results from compensatory adaptations in parts of the brain that control somatic functions, especially in the locus coeruleus. Psychological dependence refers to unpleasant emotional effects on withdrawal, including anhedonia, dysphoria, and the motivational effect of craving opioids.[66] Experimentally, withdrawal symptoms can be reliably induced with even a single parenteral dose of morphine or hydromorphone, followed by the opioid antagonist naloxone.[76]

Clinically important opioid dependence—as opposed to experimentally induced dependence—may emerge at different times in different patients. Evidence from a clinical trial for back pain suggests that dependence can emerge with just one to three months of daily use.[60] In this trial, patients underwent an opioid washout period before randomization. One study arm then received oxycodone, titrated to achieve pain relief. Patients who took the drug for at least four weeks before stopping completed the short opiate withdrawal scale, which measures the severity of 10 withdrawal symptoms (mostly physical symptoms), producing a score of 0-30. The day after stopping, 24% of patients in the oxycodone group scored over 5 and 12% scored over 10, whereas only 3.5% of the placebo group had scores over 5 and no scores over 10.

Although physical dependence is distinct from addiction, it can still be problematic for patients wishing to end long term treatment with opioids. For patients who continue to take opioids, dependence can cause withdrawal symptoms if they are unable to obtain a refill.

Problem use of prescription opioids

Problem use of prescription opioids ranges from overuse (occasionally using more than prescribed), to misuse (use that is potentially harmful or dangerous), to opioid use disorder (or addiction). Addiction is characterized by repeated compulsive drug seeking (psychological dependence) and continued use despite adverse social, psychological, or physical consequences. Physical dependence can occur in patients receiving long term opioids with or without an opioid use disorder.

Although conceptually distinct, these terms may be part of a continuum of "opioid use disorder." This is how they are used in the American Psychiatric Association's new

Table 1 Prevalence of opioid "dependency," "abuse," or "misuse" among patients receiving prescription opioids

Patients	Type of dependency, misuse, or abuse; criteria	Prevalence
Opioid dependence or abuse		
n=801; primary care practices of 235 physicians[81]	Current (30 day) dependence or abuse, DSM-4 and ICD-10 criteria*	3.7%
n=705; 9 primary care and 3 specialty clinics[80]	Current dependence, DSM-4 criteria	26%
Heterogeneous studies that excluded previous substance abuse[83]	Variable criteria	0.19%
Studies that did not exclude previous substance abuse[83]	Variable criteria	5.0%
Opioid misuse		
Primary care[81]	Purposeful oversedation	24%
	Requested early refills	45%
	Increased dose on own	37%
	Medication lost or stolen	30%
	Obtained extra opioids from other doctors	8%
	Used opioids for purposes other than pain	16%
	Drank alcohol to relieve pain	20%
n=100; primary care[82]	Abusive behaviors: lost or stolen medications, documented use of other sources of medications, requests for 2 or more early refills	24-31%
Heterogeneous studies that did not exclude previous substance abuse[83]	"Adverse drug related behaviors"	11.2%
Urine drug screens		
Heterogeneous studies[83]	Non-prescribed opioid in urine or no opioid in urine	20.4%
Primary care[81]	Any illicit drug (mostly marijuana)	24.0%

**DSM-4=Statistical Manual of Mental Disorders, fourth edition; ICD-10=International Statistical Classification of Diseases and Related Health Problems, tenth revision. Both sets of criteria for "dependence" incorporate features commonly associated with addiction.*

Diagnostic and Statistical Manual of Mental Disorders, fifth edition (DSM-5).[77] However, in DSM-5, tolerance and dependence are removed as criteria for opioid use disorder when considering prescribed opioids, because they are expected iatrogenic consequences of regular opioid use. In the earlier DSM-4, criteria for dependence and opioid misuse were distinct, although the criteria for "dependence" included many features typically associated with addiction.[78]

These terms are used variably, often with implicit criteria, and often without uniform application to a study population. Furthermore, DSM-4, DSM-5, and ICD-10 (international classification of diseases, 10th revision) do not use the term "addiction."[79] However, many clinicians and researchers use the term for what these manuals label "substance use disorder" or "dependence." Confusion regarding these concepts has made it difficult to reliably determine the prevalence of opioid use disorder from existing research.

Prevalence of problem use

The reported prevalence of opioid addiction among long term opioid users in routine care varies widely. Few studies have used formal diagnostic criteria. One study in primary care used a diagnostic interview to assess DSM-4 criteria for opioid "dependence" (similar to addiction). Among those who received four or more opioid prescriptions in a year (n=705), 26% met criteria for "dependence" (table 1).[80] However, another primary care study using similar methods reported only a 3.7% prevalence of opioid "dependence" or "abuse" among patients receiving daily opioids for at least three months (with 96% using for more than a year) (table 1).[81] Serious opioid misuse was substantially more common (table 1), and 9.7% met criteria for dependence or abuse of any substance. Similarly, another study reported misuse (lost or stolen medications, use of multiple sources of medication, multiple early refill requests) in 24-31% of patients receiving long term opioids for non-cancer pain.[82]

Studies of urine drug screens have reported aberrant findings, including no opioid in the urine (possibly indicating diversion of prescribed opioids for non-medical use, such as sale on the street), a non-prescribed opioid, or an illicit drug (table 1). Rates of unexpected findings are typically greater than 20%, which is substantially higher than patient self reports.[81 83] However, accurate interpretation requires more clinical information.

Despite guideline cautions, patients with a history of substance misuse or mood disorders are among those most likely to receive long term opioids in routine care.[10 11 12] These disorders are risk factors for opioid misuse, prompting the term "adverse selection."[43] By contrast, patients with a history of substance misuse or mood disorders are usually excluded from opioid RCTs for ethical, efficacy, and safety reasons. As a result, evidence from RCTs probably underestimates the rate of misuse in community practice.

A systematic review of heterogeneous studies with variable diagnostic criteria supported this concern. The lowest rates of substance misuse came from studies in which patients with previous alcohol or illicit drug use were excluded, resulting in typical misuse rates of 0.19%. Among studies without such exclusions, rates averaged more than an order of magnitude higher (5.0%).[83] Informal evidence of misuse, in turn, appears several-fold greater (table 1).

The increase in admissions to addiction treatment programs highlights the risk of addiction with prescribed opioids. As opioid prescribing quadrupled in the US, so did addiction therapy, with prescription opioids as a reason for admission second only to marijuana.[8]

PATIENT COMMENTARY

"What I've learned from working with patients with chronic pain is that many don't decide to become long term opioid users, they slide into it instead. There's a significant habitual side to it.

Still, most patients have no idea they're becoming dependent on opioids—until for some reason they run out or can't get more. Then the withdrawal symptoms begin, and that's very painful.

I went through some times when I was taking too much and running out early. You can't go to your doctor and say you've been taking four pills a day instead of two. So you end up lying to your doctor. I found myself in that position many times, and I've heard similar stories from dozens of patients over the years.

It took a shock to realize that what I was doing was affecting my family. I didn't notice because I was high. I used to take my family for a drive after taking my meds. Then one day I was holding my granddaughter on the beach, and I realized I might not ever hold her again. I knew I was taking too much medicine and feared that sooner or later I'd fall asleep and not wake up. My wife and two daughters confronted me that weekend. They said that I'd become a completely different person and that they missed the old me. My wife told me she wanted her husband back. I realized I had to change or I wasn't going to be around to enjoy the many things I had. That was my turning point. I decided to go to rehab to get myself back."

Overdose and mortality risks

By 2010, deaths related to prescription opioid overdose had reached 16651 a year in the US, far exceeding deaths from cocaine or heroin.[84 85] Deaths from prescription opioids have also increased in the UK.[23] Respiratory depression is the usual cause.

It was traditionally thought that there is no upper limit to opioid dosing for patients in pain, as long as increases are gradual. However, recent large studies suggest that opioid overdose and mortality risks increase in a dose related manner.[86 87 88] Compared with patients receiving 20 mg or less of morphine equivalents per day, the risk of serious or fatal overdose increased 1.9-3.7-fold in those receiving 50-100 mg per day. In those receiving more than 100-200 mg per day the risk increased 2.9-8.9-fold.

Opioid overdoses often involve multiple drugs, and certain combinations pose particular risks. For example, one study reported a threefold increase in serious overdoses in

Table 2 Common short term side effects of opioids compared with placebo in short term trials[47]

Side effect	Trials (n)	Occurring with opioid (%)*	Occurring with placebo (%)*	Relative risk (95% CI)	NNH†
Constipation	8	41	11	3.6 (2.7 to 4.7)	3.4
Nausea	8	32	12	2.7 (2.1 to 3.6)	5.0
Sedation	7	29	10	3.3 (2.4 to 4.5)	5.3
Vomiting	7	15	3	6.1 (3.3 to 11)	8.1
Dizziness	8	20	7	2.8 (2.0 to 4.0)	8.2
Itching	6	15	7	2.2 (1.4 to 3.3)	13
Dry mouth	7	13	9	1.5 (1.0 to 2.1)	Not calculated
Discontinued treatment because of a side effect	8	24	15	1.4 (1.1 to 1.9)	12
Any adverse event	4	80	56	1.4 (1.3 to 1.6)	4.2

Total number of patients experiencing the symptom divided by total number receiving treatment summed across studies.

†NNH=number needed to harm

patients receiving concurrent opioids and benzodiazepines.[87] Surprisingly, these coprescriptions occur more often with increasing dose and duration of opioid therapy.[68 89 90]

Many patients continue long term opioid treatment even after spinal surgery.[91 92] In a cohort study of patients who had lumbar fusion operations, opioid related overdose was the most common cause of death in the three years after surgery.[93]

Although patients receiving daily opioids have the highest risk of overdose, they accounted for only a quarter of overdoses in an insured population. More patients receive less than daily opioids and they accounted for a larger proportion of overdoses.[68] Similarly, in a workers' compensation system, most opioid overdoses occurred in patients who were not receiving high dose or long term opioids.[94] Thus, efforts to reduce overdose risks may need to extend to all patients receiving prescription opioids.

Some guidelines have recommended opioids as a safer choice than NSAIDs for pain in older people (mainly those aged 75 years or more), given the gastrointestinal, renal, and cardiovascular risks associated with NSAIDs.[95] However, a cohort study found higher all cause mortality among older people using opioids for arthritis than among those using NSAIDs.[96] Rates of heart disease, fractures, and bowel obstruction were particularly high among opioid users. Thus, comparative safety remains uncertain.

Other adverse effects

The common short term side effects often make opioids unappealing to patients (table 2).[47] Most cause no permanent harm and some improve with time. Constipation is an exception and often requires long term management. In short term trials, the number needed to harm, considering all the side effects in table 2, was 4.2.[47]

Sedation and dizziness

Sedation and dizziness seem to contribute to dose related increases in falls and fractures, especially in older people.[97 98 99 100 101] Sedation may also contribute to a possible increased risk of motor vehicle crashes in drivers using prescription opioids, with a relative increase of 20-50%.[102 103] Studies conflict, however, and pain, other drugs, or comorbid conditions may also contribute.[104 105] Nonetheless, patients receiving long term opioids (median dose, 60 mg morphine equivalents) for pain showed reduced reaction time, attention, and psychomotor speed in laboratory testing.[106]

Depression

Depression may be another important central nervous system side effect of opioids. Causality is difficult to assess, however, because patients with depression are more likely to use opioids than those without depression. Cross sectional studies report more depression with increasing dose and duration of opioid therapy.[89] Furthermore, a cohort study of patients without a diagnosis of depression who started treatment with opioids suggested an increased likelihood of depression during treatment and greater risk with a longer duration of treatment.[107]

Endocrine effects

Long term opioid treatment is linked to important endocrine side effects, with hypogonadism being recognized in the 1970s among men on methadone maintenance.[108 109] More recent studies detected hypogonadism in patients receiving oral opioids for chronic pain.[110 111 112] The mechanism is suppression of gonadotropin releasing hormone secretion by the hypothalamus.[113 114] This suppresses pituitary gonadotropins, which fall acutely with opioid ingestion. This in turn reduces sex steroid synthesis in the testes and ovaries.

Decreased testosterone levels have been reported in men receiving long acting opioid analgesics or opioids for at least a year.[110 112] Amenorrhea or oligomenorrhea can occur in premenopausal women receiving such treatment; both testosterone and estradiol are reduced.[111 112] Estimates of the prevalence of hypogonadism with opioid treatment range from 0% (small, short term randomized trials) to almost 90% (self selected patients on long acting opioids).[111 112]

Although erectile dysfunction in men with back pain may have multiple causes, the use of drugs for the condition is associated with both the dose and duration of opioid treatment.[115] Among men with back pain taking long term opioids at a daily dose of at least 120 morphine equivalents, 19% used drugs for erectile dysfunction or testosterone replacement. Among those with back pain but no opioid use, 7% used such drugs, with an adjusted odds ratio of 1.45 for long term opioid use. Symptoms of sexual dysfunction may have a gradual onset, and neither patient nor clinician may consider medication as a cause. Furthermore, patients are often reluctant to report sexual problems, so they may go unrecognized and untreated.

Interference with other treatments

Interference with other treatments is a growing concern. Success rates of lumbar facet denervation for back pain were lower in patients receiving opioids.[116] After multidisciplinary rehabilitation for back pain, opioid dependent patients were less likely to return to work and more likely to seek new sources of care.[117] It is unclear whether these problems result from the pharmacologic effects of opioids, characteristics of patients most likely to receive them, or some combination.

PATIENT COMMENTARY

"I have had low back pain for over 22 years. I have had eight low back operations and two cervical fusions. I have taken opioids in several forms for over 20 years. My experience led me to become a patient advocate and to join the American Chronic Pain Association, where I've led dozens of patient groups and helped people in seeking hospital or emergency room care. It's alarming how many patients don't ask anything about the meds or the side effects. They don't take the time to find out about the risks—like overdose and addiction. A common perspective among patients with chronic pain is that they just want to rely on their doctors for decisions and information. But most doctors don't have a lot of time to inform patients of the up and down sides of these meds."

Reducing risks of opioid therapy

Screening

Efforts to maximize the safety of opioids have centered on screening patients for a high risk of misuse; use of "pain contracts" to specify expectations and limits on prescribing; and use of routine urine drug screening. However, a systematic review found only weak evidence to support the effectiveness of opioid treatment agreements and urine

PRACTICAL PRINCIPLES IN PRESCRIBING OPIOIDS FOR LOW BACK PAIN[145]

For all patients with back pain

- Emphasize that self care is the foundation of effective back care and that it is usually more important to remain physically active and continue rewarding activities rather than rely on medical prescriptions
- An empathetic supportive doctor-patient relationship can encourage effective self care
- Rather than monitoring progress by changes in reported pain alone, it may be more effective to guide care towards participation in activities
- Differentiate goals of short term pain relief from those of long term effectiveness. For long term use, opioids have unproven benefits and substantial risks

For patients in whom long term opioid use is considered

- Use stepped care with non-opioid drugs before considering a trial of opioids for long term use. This may include non-steroidal anti-inflammatory drugs, tricyclic antidepressants, and topical analgesics
- Put safety first, placing patient and clinician on common ground. Adverse effects, including addiction, overdose, dependence, depression, cognitive impairment, sexual dysfunction, chronic constipation, motor vehicle accidents, and fractures due to falls, should all be discussed
- Systematically evaluate risk but do not overestimate your ability to identify high risk patients. Minimize "adverse selection" by using extra caution in patients with a history of substance misuse (opioids or others) or mood disorders such as depression or anxiety. If a prescription drug monitoring program is available, it should be checked before prescribing
- Consider intermittent opioid prescription, with clear expectations for short duration of use. Prescription of a few days to a week of short acting opioids may reduce risks of tolerance, dependence, and dose related adverse effects
- Avoid long term opioid use without decisive benefits. Place a one month time limit on an initial opioid trial. Involve the patient in choosing functional goals for the trial. If goals are not met, discontinue opioids and try alternative approaches. If opioids are continued, obtain informed consent regarding known risks and uncertain benefits. A pain contract can help establish expectations: a single prescriber, one designated pharmacy, regular monitoring, and precautions to prevent diversion

For patients in whom long term use is initiated

- Keep the opioid dose as low as possible. When the dose reaches 50-100 mg morphine equivalents per day, re-evaluate treatment and consider specialist consultation. Higher doses have unproven benefits and increased risks, and make discontinuation more difficult
- Because of the risk of overdose, avoid concurrent opioids, sedative-hypnotic drugs, and alcohol
- Closely monitor use, inquiring about misuse and adverse behavioral or medical effects. Check urine drug screens and prescription drug monitoring program data regularly
- Regularly reassess whether the opioid dose can be reduced or discontinued. High risk misuse or drug diversion requires discontinuation; non-fatal overdose requires reduction or tapering off
- Identify and treat opioid misuse: misuse or addiction should be treated rather than result in discharge from care. Addiction referral options should be identified

testing for reducing opioid misuse in patients with chronic pain.[118]

Other systematic reviews used structured interviews, observation, and self report questionnaires to identify high risk patients. They concluded that the psychometric properties of risk screening tools are weak and that study samples were small and unrepresentative.[119 120] Personal history of alcohol or drug misuse was the strongest predictor of risk; pain severity was not a predictor. No single method can reliably identify patients who are unsuitable for opioid treatment or who require closer monitoring.[120] The screening of patients may stigmatize them or leave them feeling abandoned if opioids are withheld.[121]

Opioid prescription, misuse, and overdose have all increased despite guidelines that recommend screening tools, treatment agreements, and urine testing. It is unclear whether this is because the recommendations are difficult to implement and inconsistently used or because they are ineffective.[118 122] The acknowledgment that these measures

PATIENT COMMENTARY

"Once I decided to start cutting back and talked with my doctor about it, I came to the conclusion that opioids had little to do with pain and more to do with habit. Opioids took control over my life because the habit of taking them was the most important thing. Now I take only what is prescribed—not more or less. I've learned to follow the rules. I know now that even when the physical cause of pain is clear, the feeling of pain is subjective. It is related to anxiety, stress, work, family, relationships—all these can cause a person to have more pain, and it becomes an Achilles heel.

I've observed that many people who take opioids don't see this reality or take responsibility for their meds. They don't like taking these drugs, but they're afraid not to. Some realize it's bad for them, but they underestimate the power they have to beat this problem. When patients realize that they're responsible for how they use these meds—that's when I've seen them change their lives."

seem insufficient may shift attention from trying to identify "risky patients" to broader awareness of inherent drug risks.[121]

Newer safety strategies

Many argue that alternative treatments for back pain should be more readily available and affordable,[123] with easier access and better insurance coverage. Systematic reviews suggest that services such as exercise therapy and cognitive behavioral therapy benefit patients with back pain. Exercise seems to reduce pain, risk of recurrence, and work disability.[124 125 126] Cognitive behavioral therapy seems to improve pain scores and enhance the effects of exercise.[127 128 129] Both approaches support long term self care strategies. Systematic reviews also suggest that spinal manipulation, acupuncture, and massage may be at least as effective as conventional primary care, with advantages in safety.[130 131 132 133]

Prescription drug monitoring programs

Such programs are emerging in North America. Most are web based databases to which all pharmacies in a state report prescriptions filled for controlled substances. Clinicians can access these data to identify patients with overlapping opioid prescriptions, prescriptions from multiple clinicians or pharmacies, or risky coprescriptions. The information may influence prescribing decisions or referrals for addiction treatment and occasionally results in law enforcement actions for illegal prescribing or drug diversion. Limited data from these programs suggest that they may reduce the risk of overdose.[134 135]

Evidence on dose related overdose risk has prompted recommendations for maximum opioid dosing. For example, in 2007 Washington state public insurance agencies (Medicaid, workers' compensation, public employees, prison health) developed prescribing guidelines that warned against doses exceeding 120 mg per day of morphine equivalents and advised consultation with a pain specialist before prescribing higher doses. The guideline included a web based calculator to determine daily morphine equivalents for any opioid drug (http://agencymeddirectors.wa.gov/mobile.html). The number of opioid prescriptions and the mean daily dose in the workers' compensation system plateaued, then fell in 2009 and 2010. Opioid related deaths rose through 2009, then fell sharply in 2010.[136]

Reformulation
Another strategy for reducing misuse and diversion is to reformulate long acting opioids to prevent them being crushed or dissolved, making them more difficult to snort, smoke, or inject. After extended release oxycodone was reformulated in 2010, surveillance suggested a reduction in misuse and diversion.[137 138]

Emerging treatments
There is a growing sense that the management of back pain should focus on return to normal activities more than pain relief because a reduction in pain often follows improved function. For example, the Subgroups for Targeted Treatment (STarT Back) trial offered the highest risk patients a program of psychologically informed physical therapy, which resulted in improved outcomes and reduced cost.[139] High risk for prolonged pain was identified and treated by non-drug based management—a distinctly different approach from adverse selection of high risk patients into long term opioid therapy. The generalizability of this approach is being tested in diverse settings and countries.

Guidelines
Although guidelines from the UK National Institute for Health and Care Excellence (NICE) and joint guidelines from the American College of Physicians and the American Pain Society (ACP/APS) recommend paracetamol (acetaminophen) as the first line drug,[140 141] a recent study did not support its efficacy for back pain.[142] The NICE guideline then recommends either NSAIDs or weak opioids such as codeine. Strong opioids are recommended only as short term treatment for severe pain. Specialist assessment is recommended when considering long term use of strong opioids.

The ACP-APS guideline is similar, recommending opioids or tramadol as an option after a trial of NSAIDs and advocating careful consideration of benefits and potential harms. If a patient does not respond to a time limited course of opioids, alternative treatments or specialist referral should be considered. Both guidelines recommend tricyclic antidepressants, exercise, cognitive behavioral therapy, spinal manipulation, acupuncture, and massage as treatment options.

Several guidelines have assessed opioid therapy for chronic pain in general, and a systematic review of 13 guidelines is available.[143] Only two were judged to be of high quality: one from the American Pain Society and the American Academy of Pain Medicine,[35] and another from a Canadian national opioid use guideline group.[144] Most guidelines recommend avoiding doses greater than 90-200 mg of morphine equivalents per day. Despite weak evidence, most recommend the use of opioid risk assessment tools, written treatment agreements, and urine drug testing. Ten of the guidelines note that opioids and benzodiazepines are a high risk combination. Ten also name a history of substance misuse or mental health disorders as the leading risk factors for overdose or misuse.

Conclusion
Clinicians must treat back pain as effectively as possible while minimizing the associated risks, and the box outlines the practical principles in prescribing opioids for low back pain.[145] As clinicians' perceptions of the effectiveness and safety of opioids shifted over the past two decades, prescribing increased dramatically. However, the effectiveness of long term opioid therapy for back pain remains unclear, and surveillance data have shown markedly increased rates of opioid overdose and addiction. Patients at the highest risk of these major adverse outcomes are the most likely to receive long term opioids. Other long term complications of opioid treatment include falls, fractures, motor vehicle crashes, and other injuries; cognitive and mood effects; and hypogonadism and sexual dysfunction.

There is no evidence that opioids improve return to work or reduce the use of other treatments. They may even limit the effectiveness of other treatments. Clinicians may want to monitor treatment success on the basis of functional ability, in addition to self reported pain severity.

Short term opioid use has analgesic benefits, but it may be necessary to avoid the adverse selection of patients with past substance misuse or mood disorders and to set limits on the duration of prescription to avoid inadvertently initiating long term use. An effective strategy for reducing misuse, diversion, and overdose would be to limit patients' exposure to opioids. Canadian and American researchers have argued that "many physicans and patients have had unreasonable expectations of opioids and have seriously underestimated their risks. It is time to collectively lower expectations and prescribe these drugs less readily, to fewer patients, at lower doses, and for shorter periods."[146]

In current practice, patients at highest risk of adverse effects are most likely to receive opioids. Thus, support for alternative treatments should be strengthened. One promising approach is to improve access to psychologically informed interventions that support return to meaningful life activities, with more intensive intervention for patients at the highest prognostic risk.

FUTURE RESEARCH QUESTIONS
- Relative to alternatives, how safe and effective are opioids for long term management of back pain?
- Can a subset of patients with chronic back pain in whom long term opioid use is safe and effective be accurately identified?
- How common are serious adverse effects of long term opioid use, including addiction, drug induced mood disorders, behavioral deactivation, hyperalgesia, sexual dysfunction, fractures, and motor vehicle injuries?
- Are there mitigation strategies that appreciably reduce the risks of adverse events in patients using long term opioids, such as frequent monitoring visits; rotation of opioid preparations; or use of low or intermittent dosing regimens?

PATIENT COMMENTARY
"I have good days and bad days, like everyone else. What's different now is that I'm not seeking an answer out of a medicine bottle. I start by analyzing my situation, what's causing my stress, what's making me want to take more meds today. What I have to do is understand that this is a normal process, and that I must take responsibility for it. Then I find a way to manage the stress rather than take something to mask it. Now I have 12 years of experience working with patients in chronic pain groups. I've learned that, with the support of others, there's a better way to live—even with chronic pain. Taking more meds than prescribed isn't a solution, it's just the beginning of a disastrous cycle. I've learned to accept my pain because I know it's my reality and that I can still be productive and enjoy life."

Thanks to Jessica Ridpath for invaluable editorial advice.

Contributors: RAD and MVK both conducted the literature searches and summarized the scientific content. DD helped to plan the manuscript, reviewed and approved multiple drafts, and contributed the patient commentary. RAD and MVK are both guarantors.

Competing interests: We have read and understood BMJ policy on declaration of interests and declare the following interests: RAD receives honorariums from UpToDate for authoring topics on low back pain. He benefits from an endowment to his university from Kaiser Permanente. He has been a member of the board of directors for the Informed Medical Decisions Foundation, a non-profit organization. MVK has several research grants from Pfizer awarded to the Group Health Research Institute. He is also a co-investigator on Food and Drug Administration mandated post-marketing surveillance studies of opioid safety funded by a consortium of drug companies.

Provenance and peer review: Commissioned; externally peer reviewed.

1 Hoy D, March L, Brooks P, Blyth F, Woolf A, Bain C, et al. The global burden of low back pain: estimates from the Global Burden of Disease 2010 study. *Ann Rheum Dis* 2014;73: 968-74.
2 Andersson GBJ. Epidemiological features of chronic low-back pain. *Lancet* 1999;354;581-5.
3 Lawrence RC, Felson DT, Helmick CG, Arnold LM, Choi H, Deyo RA, et al. Estimates of the prevalence of arthritis and other rheumatic conditions in the United States, part II. *Arth Rheum* 2008;58:26-35.
4 National Ambulatory Medical Care Survey: 2010 summary tables. www.cdc.gov/nchs/data/ahcd/namcs_summary/2010_namcs_web_tables.pdf.
5 Martin BI, Deyo RA, Mirza SK, Turner JA, Comstock BA, Hollingworth W, et al. Expenditures and health status among adults with back and neck problems. *JAMA* 2008;299:656-64.
6 Ivanova JI, Birnbaum GH, Schiller M, Kantor E, Johnstone BM, Swindle RW. Real-world practice patterns, health-care utilization, and costs in patients with low back pain: the long road to guideline-concordant care. *Spine J* 2011;11:622-32.
7 Hudson TJ, Edlund MJ, Steffick DE, Tripathi SP, Sullivan MD. Epidemiology of regular prescribed opioid use: results from a national, population-based survey. *J Pain Sympt Mgmt* 2008;36:280-8.
8 Okie S. A flood of opioids, a rising tide of deaths. *N Engl J Med* 2010;363:1981-5.
9 Chaparro LE, Furlan AD, Deshpande A, Mailis-Gagnon A, Atlas S, Turk DC. Opioids compared with placebo or other treatments for chronic low back pain: an update of the Cochrane review. *Spine* 2014;39:556-63.
10 Weisner CM, Campbell CI, Ray GT, Saunders K, Merrill JO, Banta-Green C, et al. Trends in prescribed opioid therapy for non-cancer pain for individuals with prior substance use disorders. *Pain* 2009;145:287-93.
11 Braden JB, Sullivan MD, Ray GT, Saunders K, Merrill J, Silverberg MJ, et al. Trends in long-term opioid therapy for noncancer pain among persons with a history of depression. *Gen Hosp Psychiatr* 2009;31:564-70.
12 Edlund MJ, Martin BC, Devries A, Fan Ming-Yu, Braden JB, Sullivan MD. Trends in use of opioids for chronic noncancer pain among individuals with mental health and substance use disorders: the TROUP study. *Clin J Pain* 2010;26:1-8.
13 US Department of Health and Human Services. Summary health statistics for US adults: national health interview survey, 2012. *Vital and Health Statistics* Series 10. No 260. 2014. www.cdc.gov/nchs/data/series/sr_10/sr10_260.pdf.
14 Pengel LH, Herbert RD, Maher CG, Refshauge KM. Acute low back pain: systematic review of its prognosis. *BMJ* 2003;327:323.
15 Von Korff M, Saunders K. The course of back pain in primary care. *Spine* 1996;21:2833-7.
16 Jensen MC, Brant-Zawadzki MN, Obuchowski N, Modic MT, Malkasian D, Ross JS. Magnetic resonance imaging of the lumbar spine in people without low back pain. *N Engl J Med* 1994;331:69-73.
17 Baliki MN, Petre B, Torbey S, Herrmann KM, Huang L, Schnitzer TJ, et al. Corticostriatal functional connectivity predicts transition to chronic back pain. *Nat Neurosci* 2012;15:1117-9.
18 Rodriguez-Raecke R, Niemeier A, Ihle K, Ruether W, May A. Structural brain changes in chronic pain reflect probably neither damage nor atrophy. *PLoS One* 2013;8:e54475.
19 Seminowicz DA, Wideman TH, Naso L, Hatami-Khoroushahi Z, Fallatah S, Ware MA, et al. Effective treatment of chronic low back pain in humans reverses abnormal brain anatomy and function. *J Neurosci* 2011;31:7540-50.
20 Henschke N, Maher CG, Refshauge KM, Herbert RD, Cumming RG, Bleasel J, et al. Prevalence of and screening for serious spinal pathology in patients presenting to primary care settings with acute low back pain. *Arthritis Rheum* 2009;60:3072-80.
21 Paulozzi LJ, Jones CM, Mack KA, Rudd RA. Vital signs: overdoses of prescription opioid pain relievers, United States, 1999-2008. *MMWR Morb Mortal Wkly Rep* 2011;60:1487-92.
22 Boudreau D, Von Korff M, Rutter CM, Saunders K, Ray GT, Sullivan MD, et al. Trends in long-term opioid therapy for chronic non-cancer pain. *Pharmacoepidemiol Drug Safety* 2009;18:1166-75.
23 Dhalla IA, Persaud N, Juurlink DN. Facing up to the prescription opioid crisis. *BMJ* 2011;343:d5142.
24 Martin BI, Turner JA, Mirza SK, Lee MJ, Comstock BA, Deyo RA. Trends in health care expenditures, utilization, and health status among US adults with spine problems, 1997-2006. *Spine* 2009;34:2077-84.
25 Mafi JN, McCarthy EP, Davis RB, Landon BE. Worsening trends in the management and treatment of back pain. *JAMA Intern Med* 2013;173:1573-81.
26 Von Korff M, Kolodny A, Deyo RA, Chou R. Long-term opioid therapy reconsidered. *Ann Intern Med* 2011;155:325-8.
27 Morasco BJ, Duckart JP, Carr TP, Deyo RA, Dobscha SK. Clinical characteristics of veterans prescribed high doses of opioid medications for chronic non-cancer pain. *Pain* 2010;151:625-32.
28 Zerzan JT, Morden NE, Soumerai S, Ross-Degnan D, Roughead E, Zhang F, et al. Trends and geographic variation of opiate medication use in state Medicaid fee-for-service programs, 1996 to 2002. *Med Care* 2006;44:1005-10.
29 Portenoy RK, Foley KM. Chronic use of opioid analgesics in non-malignant pain: report of 38 cases. *Pain* 1986;25:171-86.
30 Porter J, Jick H. Addiction rare in patients treated with narcotics. *N Engl J Med* 1980;302:123.
31 Van Zee A. The promotion and marketing of OxyContin: commercial triumph, public health tragedy. *Am J Pubic Health* 2009;99:221-7.
32 Ballantyne JC. Pain medicine: repairing a fractured dream. *Anesthesiology* 2011;114:243-6.
33 General Accounting Office. Prescription drugs: OxyContin abuse and diversion and efforts to address the problem. 2003. www.gao.gov/new.items/d04110.pdf.
34 International Narcotics Control Board. Opioid consumption data. Annual reports. www.painpolicy.wisc.edu/opioid-consumption-data.
35 Chou R, Fanciullo GJ, Fine PG, Adler JA, Ballantyne JC, Davies P, et al. Clinical guidelines for the use of chronic opioid therapy in chronic noncancer pain. *J Pain* 2009;10:113-30.
36 Chou R, Huffman LH. Medications for acute and chronic low back pain: a review of the evidence for an American Pain Society/American College of Physicians clinical practice guideline. *Ann Intern Med* 2007;147:505-14.
37 Franklin GM, Stover BD, Turner JA, Fulton-Kehoe D, Wickizer TM. Early opioid prescription and subsequent disability among workers with back injuries: the Disability Risk Identification Study Cohort. *Spine* 2008;33:199-204.
38 Webster BS, Verma SK, Gatchel RJ. Relationship between early opioid prescribing for acute occupational low back pain and disability duration, medical costs, subsequent surgery, and late opioid use. *Spine* 2007;32:2127-32.
39 Ashworth J, Green DJ, Dunn KM, Jordan KP. Opioid use among low back pain patients in primary care: is opioid prescription associated with disability at 6-month follow-up? *Pain* 2013;154:1038-44.
40 Von Korff M, Saunders K, Ray GT, Boudreau D, Campbell C, Merrill J, et al. De facto long-term opioid therapy for noncancer pain. *Clin J Pain* 2008;24:521-7.
41 Martell BA, O'Connor PG, Kerns RD, Becker WC, Morales KH, Kosten TR, et al. Systematic review: opioid treatment for chronic back pain: prevalence, efficacy, and association with addiction. *Ann Intern Med* 2007;146:116-27.
42 Furlan AD, Chaparro LE, Irvin E, Mailis-Gagnon A. A comparison between enriched and nonenriched enrollment randomized withdrawal trials of opioids for chronic noncancer pain. *Pain Res Manage* 2011;16:337-51.
43 Sullivan MD, Howe CQ. Opioid therapy for chronic pain in the United States: promises and perils. *Pain* 2013;154:S94-100.
44 Kuipers T, van Middelkoop M, Rubinstein SM, Ostelo R, Verhagen A, Koes BW, et al. A systematic review on the effectiveness of pharmacological interventions for chronic non-specific low-back pain. *Eur Spine J* 2011;20:40-50.
45 Chung JWY, Zeng Y, Wong TKS. Drug therapy for the treatment of chronic nonspecific low back pain: systematic review and meta-analysis. *Pain Physician* 2013;16:E685-704.
46 Kroenke K, Krebs EE, Bair MJ. Pharmacotherapy of chronic pain: a synthesis of recommendations from systematic reviews. *Gen Hosp Psychiatry* 2009;31:206-19.
47 Kalso E, Edwards JE, Moore RA, McQuay HJ. Opioids in chronic non-cancer pain: systematic review of efficacy and safety. *Pain* 2004;112:372-80.
48 Schnitzer TJ, Gray WL, Paster RZ, Kamin M. Efficacy of tramadol in treatment of chronic low back pain. *J Rheumatol* 2000;27:772-8.
49 Uberall MA, Mueller-Schwefe GH, Terhaag B. Efficacy and safety of flupirtine modified release for the management of moderate to severe chronic low back pain: results of SUPREME, a prospective randomized, double-blind, placebo- and active-controlled parallel-group phase IV study. *Curr Med Res Opin* 2012;28:1617-34.
50 Vorsanger GJ, Xiang J, Gana TJ, Pascual ML, Fleming RR. Extended-release tramadol (tramadol ER) in the treatment of chronic low back pain. *J Opioid Manage* 2008;4:87-97.
51 Peloso PM, Fortin L, Beaulieu A, Kamin M, Rosenthan N; Protocol TRP-CAN-1 Study Group. Analgesic efficacy and safety of tramadol/acetaminophen combination tablets (Ultracet) in treatment of chronic low back pain: a multicenter, outpatient, randomized, double blind, placebo controlled trial. *J Rheumatol* 2004;31:2454-63.
52 Ruoff GE, Rosenthal N, Jordan D, Karim R, Kamin M; Protocol CAPSS-112 Study Group. Tramadol/acetaminophen combination tablets for the treatment of chronic lower back pain: a multicenter, randomized, double-blind, placebo-controlled outpatient study. *Clin Ther* 2003;25:1123-41.
53 Gordon A, Callaghan D, Spink D, Cloutier C, Dzongowski P, O'Mahony W, et al. Buprenorphine transdermal system in adults with chronic low back pain: a randomized, double-blind, placebo-controlled crossover study, followed by an open-label extension phase. *Clin Ther* 2010;32:844-60.

54 Steiner DJ, Sitar S, Wen W, Sawyerr G, Munera C, Ripa SR, et al. Efficacy and safety of the seven-day buprenorphine transdermal system in opioid-naive patients with moderate to severe chronic low back pain: an enriched, randomized, double-blind, placebo-controlled study. *J Pain Symptom Manage* 2011;42:903-17.
55 Buynak R, Shapiro DY, Okamoto A, Van Hove I, Rauschkolb C, Steup A, et al. Efficacy and safety of tapentadol extended release for the management of chronic low back pain: results of a prospective, randomized, double-blind, placebo- and active-controlled Phase III study. *Expert Opin Pharmacother* 2010;11:1787-804.
56 Chu LF, D'Arcy N, Brady C, Zamora AK, Young CA, Kim JE, et al. Analgesic tolerance without demonstrable opioid-induced hyperalgesia: a double-blinded, randomized, placebo-controlled trial of sustained-release morphine for treatment of chronic nonradicular low back pain. *Pain* 2012;153:1583-92.
57 Khoromi S, Cui L, Nackers L, Max MB. Morphine, nortriptyline and their combination vs placebo in patients with chronic lumbar root pain. *Pain* 2007;130:66-75.
58 Hale ME, Ahdieh H, Ma T, Rauck R; Oxymorphone ER Study Group 1. Efficacy and safety of OPANA ER (oxymorphone extended release) for relief of moderate to severe chronic low back pain in opioid-experienced patients: a 12-week, randomized, double-blind, placebo-controlled study. *J Pain* 2007;8:175-84.
59 Katz N, Rauck R, Ahdieh H, Ma T, van der Hoop RG, Kerwin R, et al. A 12-week, randomized, placebo-controlled trial assessing the safety and efficacy of oxymorphone extended release for opioid-naive patients with chronic low back pain. *Curr Med Res Opin* 2007;23:117-28.
60 Webster LR, Butera PG, Moran LV, Wu N, Burns LH, Friedmann N. Oxytrex minimizes physical dependence while providing effective analgesia: a randomized controlled trial in low back pain. *J Pain* 2006;7:937-46.
61 Hale M, Khan A, Kutch M, Li S. Once-daily OROS hydromorphone ER compared with placebo in opioid-tolerant patients with chronic low back pain. *Curr Med Res Opin* 2010;26:1505-18.
62 O'Donnell JB, Ekman EF, Spalding WM, Bhadra P, McCabe D, Berger MF. The effectiveness of a weak opioid medication versus a cyclo-oxygenase-2 (COX-2) selective nonsteroidal anti-inflammatory drug in treating flare-up of chronic low back pain: results from two randomized, double-blind, 6-week studies. *J Int Med Res* 2009;37:1789-802.
63 Jamison RN, Raymond SA, Slawsby EA, Nedeljkovic SS, Katz NP. Opioid therapy for chronic noncancer back pain. A randomized prospective study. *Spine (Phila Pa 1976)* 1998;23:2591-600.
64 Franklin GM, Rahman EA, Turner JA, Daniell WE, Fulton-Kehoe D. Opioid use for chronic low back pain: a prospective, population-based study among injured workers in Washington state, 2002-2005. *Clin J Pain* 2009;25:743-51.
65 Eriksen J, Sjogren P, Bruera E, Ekholm O, Rasmussen NK. Critical issues on opioids in chronic non-cancer pain: an epidemiological study. *Pain* 2006;125:172-9.
66 Ballantyne JC, Shin NS. Efficacy of opioids for chronic pain: a review of the evidence. *Clin J Pain* 2008;24:469-78.
67 McQuay H. Opioids in pain management. *Lancet* 1999;353:2229-32.
68 Paulozzi LJ, Zhang K, Jones CM, Mack KA. Risk of adverse health outcomes with increasing duration and regularity of opioid therapy. *J Am Board Fam Med* 2014;27:329-38.
69 Compton P, Athanasos P, Elashoff D. Withdrawal hyperalgesia after acute opioid physical dependence in nonaddicted humans: a preliminary study. *J Pain* 2003;4:511-9.
70 Brush DE. Complications of long-term opioid therapy for management of chronic pain: the paradox of opioid-induced hyperalgesia. *J Med Toxicol* 2012;8:387-92.
71 Murphy JL, Clark ME, Banou E. Opioid cessation and multidimensional outcomes after interdisciplinary chronic pain treatment. *Clin J Pain* 2013;29:109-17.
72 Townsend CO, Kerkvliet JL, Bruce BK, Rome JD, Hooten WM, Luedtke CA, et al. A longitudinal study of the efficacy of a comprehensive pain rehabilitation program with opioid withdrawal: comparison of treatment outcomes based on opioid use status at admission. *Pain* 2008;140:177-89.
73 Baron MJ, McDonald PW. Significant pain reduction in chronic pain patients after detoxification from high-dose opioids. *J Opioid Manage* 2006;2:277-82.
74 Crisostomo RA, Schmidt JE, Hooten WM, Kerkvliet JL, Townsend CO, Bruce BK. Withdrawal of analgesic medication for chronic low-back pain patients: improvement in outcomes of multidisciplinary rehabilitation regardless of surgical history. *Am J Phys Med Rehabil* 2008;87:527-36.
75 Martin BC, Fan MY, Edlund MJ, Devries A, Braden JB, Sullivan MD. Long-term chronic opioid therapy discontinuation rates from the TROUP study. *J Gen Intern Med* 2011;26:1450-7.
76 Compton P, Miotto K, Elashoff D. Precipitated opioid withdrawal across acute physical dependence induction methods. *Pharmacol Biochem and Behav* 2004;77:263-8.
77 American Psychiatric Association. Diagnostic and statistical manual of mental disorders. Fifth ed. 2013. www.dsm.psychiatryonline.org.
78 American Psychiatric Association. Diagnostic and statistical manual of mental disorders. 4th ed. Text revision (DSM-IV-TR). APA, 2000.
79 WHO. ICD-10 classification of mental and behavioural disorders: clinical descriptions and diagnostic guidelines. www.who.int/substance_abuse/terminology/ICD10ClinicalDiagnosis.pdf.
80 Boscarino JA, Rukstalis M, Hoffman SN, Han JJ, Erlich PM, Gerhard GS, et al. Risk factors for drug dependence among out-patients on opioid therapy in a large US health-care system. *Addiction* 2010;105:1776-82.
81 Fleming MF, Balousek SL, Klessig CL, Mundt MP, Brown DD. Substance use disorders in a primary care sample receiving daily opioid therapy. *J Pain* 2007;8:573-82.
82 Reid MC, Engles-Horton LL, Weber MB, Kerns RD, Rogers EL, O'Connor PG. Use of opioid medications for chronic noncancer pain syndromes in primary care. *J Gen Intern Med* 2002;17:173-9.
83 Fishbain DA, Cole B, Lewis J, Rosomoff HL, Rosomoff RS. What percentage of chronic nonmalignant pain patients exposed to chronic opioid analgesic therapy develop abuse/addiction and/or aberrant drug related behaviors? A structured evidence-based review. *Pain Med* 2008;9:444-59.
84 Paulozzi LJ, Jones CM, Mack KA, Rudd RA. Vital signs: overdoses of prescription opioid pain relievers, United States, 1999-2008. *MMWR Morb Mortal Wkly Rep* 2011;60:1487-92.
85 Jones CM, Mack KA, Paulozzi LJ. Pharmaceutical overdose deaths, United States, 2010. *JAMA* 2013;309:657-9.
86 Bohnert AS, Valenstein M, Bair MJ, Ganoczy D, McCarthy JF, Ilgen MA, et al. Association between opioid prescribing patterns and opioid overdose-related deaths. *JAMA* 2011;305:1315-21.
87 Dunn KM, Saunders KW, Rutter CM, Banta-Green CJ, Merrill JO, Sullivan MD, et al. Opioid prescriptions for chronic pain and overdose: a cohort study. *Ann Intern Med* 2010;152:85-92.
88 Gomes T, Mamdani MM, Dhalla IA, Paterson JM, Juurlink DN. Opioid dose and drug-related mortality in patients with nonmalignant pain. *Arch Intern Med* 2011;171:686-91.
89 Deyo RA, Smith DH, Johnson ES, Donovan M, Tillotson CJ, Yang X, et al. Opioids for back pain patients: primary care prescribing patterns and use of services. *J Am Board Fam Med* 2011;24:717-27.
90 Kobus AM, Smith DH, Morasco BJ, Johnson ES, Yang X, Petrik AF, et al. Correlates of higher-dose opioid medication use for low back pain in primary care. *J Pain* 2012;13:1131-8.
91 Blumenthal S, McAfee PC, Guyer RD, Hochschuler SH, Geisler FH, Holt RT, et al. A prospective, randomized, multicenter Food and Drug Administration investigational device exemptions study of lumbar total disc replacement with the CHARITE artificial disc versus lumbar fusion. Part I: evaluation of clinical outcomes. *Spine* 2005;30:1565-75.
92 Zigler J, Delamarter R, Spivak JM, Linovitz RJ, Danielson GO 3rd, Haider TT, et al. Results of the prospective, randomized, multicenter Food and Drug Administration investigational device exemption study of the ProDisc-L disc replacement versus circumferential fusion for the treatment of 1-level degenerative disc disease. *Spine* 2007;32:1155-62.
93 Juratli SM, Mirza SK, Fulton-Kehoe D, Wickizer TM, Franklin GM. Mortality after lumbar fusion surgery. *Spine* 2009;34:740-7.
94 Fulton-Kehoe D, Garg RK, Turner JA, Bauer AM, Sullivan MD, Wickizer TM, et al. Opioid poisonings and opioid adverse effects in workers in Washington state. *Am J Ind Med* 2013;56:1452-62.
95 American Geriatrics Society Panel. Pharmacological management of persistent pain in older persons. *J Am Geriatr Soc* 2009;57:1331-46.
96 Solomon DH, Rassen JA, Glynn RJ, Lee J, Levin R, Schneeweiss S. The comparative safety of analgesics in older adults with arthritis. *Arch Intern Med* 2010;170:1968-78.
97 Li L, Setoguchi S, Cabral H, Jick S. Opioid use for noncancer pain and risk of fracture in adults: a nested case-control study using the general practice research database. *Am J Epidemiol* 2013;178:559-69.
98 Vestergaard P, Rejnmark L, Mosekilde L. Fracture risk associated with the use of morphine and opiates. *J Intern Med* 2006;260:76-87.
99 Miller M, Sturmer T, Azrael D, Levin R, Solomon DH. Opioid analgesics and the risk of fractures in older adults with arthritis. *J Am Geriatr Soc* 2011;59:430-8.
100 Takkouche B, Montes-Martinez A, Gill SS, Etminan M. Psychotropic medications and the risk of fracture: a meta-analysis. *Drug Saf* 2007;30:171-84.
101 Saunders KW, Dunn KW, Merrill JO, Sullivan M, Weisner C, Braden JB, et al. Relationship of opioid use and dosage levels to fractures in older chronic pain patients. *J Gen Intern Med* 2010;25:310-5.
102 Gomes T, Redelmeier DA, Juurlink DN, Dhalla IA, Camacho X, Mamdani MM. Opioid dose and risk of road trauma in Canada: a population-based study. *JAMA Intern Med* 2013;173:196-201.
103 Meuleners LB, Duke J, Lee AH, Palamara P, Hildebrand J, Ng JQ. Psychoactive medications and crash involvement requiring hospitalization for older drivers: a population-based study. *J Am Geriatr Soc* 2011;59:1575-80.
104 Monarrez-Espino J, Moller J, Berg HY, Kalani M, Laflamme L. Analgesics and road traffic crashes in senior drivers: an epidemiological review and explorative meta-analysis on opioids. *Accid Anal Prev* 2013;57:157-64.
105 Strand MC, Fjeld B, Arnestad M, Morland J. Can patients receiving opioid maintenance therapy safely drive? A systematic review of epidemiological and experimental studies on driving ability with a focus on concomitant methadone or buprenorphine administration. *Traffic Inj Prev* 2013;14:26-38.
106 Sjogren P, Thomsen AB, Olsen AK. Impaired neuropsychological performance in chronic nonmalignant pain patients receiving long-term oral opioid therapy. *J Pain Symptom Manage* 2000;19:100-8.

107 Scherrer JF, Svrakic DM, Freedland KE, Chrusciel T, Balasubramanian S, Bucholz KK, et al. Prescription opioid analgesics increase the risk of depression. *J Gen Intern Med* 2014;29:491-9.
108 Cicero TJ, Bell RD, Wiest WG, Allison JH, Polakoski K, Robins E. Function of the male sex organs in heroin and methadone users. *N Engl J Med* 1975;292:882-7.
109 Mendelson JH, Mendelson JE, Patch VD. Plasma testosterone levels in heroin addiction and during methadone maintenance. *J Pharmacol Exp Ther* 1975;192:211-7.
110 Daniell HW. Hypogonadism in men consuming sustained-action oral opioids. *J Pain* 2002;3:377-84.
111 Daniell HW. Opioid endocrinopathy in women consuming prescribed sustained-action opioids for control of nonmalignant pain. *J Pain* 2008;9:28-36.
112 Fraser LA, Morrison D, Morley-Forster P, Paul TL, Tokmakejian S, Nicholson RL, et al. Oral opioids for chronic non-cancer pain: higher prevalence of hypogonadism in men than in women. *Exp Clin Endocrinol Diabetes* 2009;117:38-43.
113 Cicero TJ, Schainker BA, Meyer ER. Endogenous opioids participate in the regulation of the hypothalamus-pituitary-luteinizing hormone axis and testosterone's negative feedback control of luteinizing hormone. *Endocrinology* 1979;104:1286-91.
114 Giri M, Kaufman JM. Opioidergic modulation of in vitro pulsatile gonadotropin-releasing hormone release from the isolated medial basal hypothalamus of the male guinea pig. *Endocrinology* 1994;135:2137-43.
115 Deyo RA, Smith DH, Johnson ES, Tillotson CJ, Donovan M, Yang X, et al. Prescription opioids for back pain and use of medications for erectile dysfunction. *Spine* 2013;38:909-15.
116 Cohen SP, Williams KA, Kurihara C, Nguyen C, Shields C, Kim P, et al. Multicenter, randomized comparative cost-effectiveness study comparing 0, 1, and 2 diagnostic medial branch (facet joint (facet joint nerve) block treatment paradigms before lumbar facet radiofrequency denervation. *Anesthesiology* 2010;113:395-405.
117 Mayer TG, Gatchel RJ, Brede E, Theodore BR. Lumbar surgery in work-related chronic low back pain: can a continuum of care enhance outcomes? *Spine J* 2014;14:263-73.
118 Starrels JL, Becker WC, Alford DP, Kapoor A, Williams AR, Turner BJ. Systematic review: treatment agreements and urine drug testing to reduce opioid misuse in patients with chronic pain. *Ann Intern Med* 2010;152:712-20.
119 Turk DC, Swanson KS, Gatchel RJ. Predicting opioid misuse by chronic pain patients: a systematic review and literature synthesis. *Clin J Pain* 2008;24:497-508.
120 Sehgal N, Manchikanti L, Smith HS. Prescription opioid abuse in chronic pain: a review of opioid abuse predictors and strategies to curb opioid abuse. *Pain Physician* 2012;15 (3 suppl):ES67-92.
121 Dowell D, Kunins HV, Farley TA. Opioid analgesics—risky drugs, not risky patients. *JAMA* 2013;309:2219-20.
122 Krebs EE, Ramsey DC, Miloshoff JM, Bair MJ. Primary care monitoring of long-term opioid therapy among veterans with chronic pain. *Pain Med* 2011;12:740-6.
123 Coffin P, Banta-Green C. The dueling obligations of opioid stewardship. *Ann Intern Med* 2014;160:207-8.
124 Van Middelkoop M, Rubinstein SM, Verhagen AP, Ostelo RW, Koes BW, van Tulder MW. Exercise therapy for chronic nonspecific low-back pain. *Best Pract Res Clin Rheumatol* 2010;24:193-204.
125 Oesch P, Kool J, Hagen KB, Bachmann S. Effectiveness of exercise on work disability in patients with non-acute non-specific low back pain: systematic review and meta-analysis of randomized controlled trials. *J Rehabil Med* 2010;42:193-205.
126 Choi BKL, Verbeek JH, Tam WW-S, Jiang JY. Exercises for prevention of recurrences of low-back pain. *Cochrane Database Syst Rev* 2010;1:CD006555.
127 Monticone M, Ferrante S, Rocca B, Baiardi P, Dal Farra F, Foti C. Effect of a long-lasting multidisciplinary program on disability and fear-avoidance behaviors in patients with chronic low back pain: results of a randomized controlled trial. *Clin J Pain* 2013;29:929-38.
128 Henschke N, Ostelo RWJG, van Tulder MW, Vlaeyen JW, Morley S, Assendelft WJ, et al. Behavioural treatment for chronic low-back pain. *Cochrane Database Syst Rev* 2010;7:CD002014.
129 Lamb SE, Hansen Z, Lall R, Castelnuovo E, Withers EJ, Nichols V, et al. Group cognitive behavioural treatment for low-back pain in primary care: a randomised controlled trial and cost-effectiveness analysis. *Lancet* 2010;375:916-23.
130 Vickers AJ, Cronin AM, Maschino AC, Lewith G, MacPherson H, Foster NE, et al. Acupuncture for chronic pain. Individual patient data analysis. *Arch Intern Med* 2012;172:1444-53.
131 Rubinstein SM, Terwee CB, Assendelft WJ, de Boer MR, van Tulder MW. Spinal manipulative therapy for acute low back pain: an update of the Cochrane review. *Spine* 2013;38:E158-77.
132 Rubinstein SM, van Middelkoop M, Assendelft WJ, de Boer MR, van Tulder MW. Spinal manipulative therapy for chronic low-back pain: an update of a Cochrane review. *Spine* 2011;36:E825-46.
133 Kumar S, Beaton K, Hughes T. The effectiveness of massage therapy for the treatment of nonspecific low back pain: a systematic review of systematic reviews. *Int J Gen Med* 2013;6:733-41.
134 Dormuth CR, Miller TA, Huang A, Mamdani MM, Juurlink DN. Effect of a centralized prescription network on inappropriate prescriptions for opioid analgesics and benzodiazepines. *CMAJ* 2012;184:E852-6.
135 Deyo RA, Irvine JM, Millet LM, Beran T, O'Kane N, Wright DA, et al. Measures such as interstate cooperation would improve the efficacy of programs to track controlled drug prescriptions. *Health Affairs* 2013;32:603-13.
136 Franklin GM, Mai J, Turner J, Sullivan M, Wickizer T, Fulton-Kehoe D. Bending the prescription opioid dosing and mortality curves: impact of the Washington State opioid dosing guideline. *Am J Indust Med* 2012;55:325-31.
137 Severtson SG, Bartelson BB, Davis JM, Munoz A, Schneider MF, Chilcoat H, et al. Reduced abuse, therapeutic errors, and diversion following reformulation of extended-release oxycodone in 2010. *J Pain* 2013;14:1122-30.
138 Butler SF, Cassidy TA, Chilcoat H, Black RA, Landau C, Budman SH, et al. Abuse rates and routes of administration of reformulated extended-release oxycodone: initial findings from a sentinel surveillance sample of individuals assessed for substance abuse treatment. *J Pain* 2013;14:351-8.
139 Hill JC, Whitehurst DG, Lewis M, Bryan S, Dunn KM, Foster NE, et al. Comparison of stratified primary care management for low back pain with current best practice (STarT Back): a randomised controlled trial. *Lancet* 2011;378:1560-71.
140 National Institute for Health and Care Excellence. Low back pain: early management of persistent non-specific low back pain. Clinical guideline 88. 2009. www.nice.org.uk/guidance/cg88.
141 Chou R, Qaseem A, Snow V, Casey D, Cross JT, Shekelle P, et al. Diagnosis and treatment of low back pain: a joint clinical ractice guideline from the American College of Physicians and the American Pain Society. *Ann Intern Med* 2007;147:478-91.
142 Williams CM, Maher CG, Latimer J, McLachlan AJ, Hancock MJ, Day RO, et al. Efficacy of paracetamol for acute low-back pain: a double-blind, randomized controlled trial. *Lancet* 2014; published online 23 Jul.
143 Nuckols TK, Anderson L, Popescu I, Diamant AL, Doyle B, Di Capua P, et al. Opioid prescribing: a systematic review and critical appraisal of guidelines for chronic pain. *Ann Intern Med* 2014;160:38-47.
144 Furlan AD, Reardon R, Weppler C; National Opioid Use Guideline Group. Opioids for chronic noncancer pain; a new Canadian practice guideline. *CMAJ* 2010;182:923-30.
145 Von Korff MR. Long-term use of opioids for complex chronic pain. *Best Pract Res Clin Rheumatol* 2013;27:663-72.
146 Juurlink DN, Dhalla IA, Nelson LS. Improving opioid prescribing: the New York City recommendations. *JAMA* 2013;309:879-80.

Trigeminal neuralgia

Joanna M Zakrzewska, professor of pain medicine in relation to oral medicine[1], Mark E Linskey, professor of neurological surgery[2]

[1]Facial Pain Unit, Eastman Dental Hospital, UCLH NHS Foundation Trust, London WC1X 8LD, UK

[2]Department of Surgery, University of California, Irvine, Orange, CA, USA

Correspondence to: J M Zakrzewska j.zakrzewska@ucl.ac.uk

Cite this as: *BMJ* 2014;348:g474

DOI: 10.1136/bmj.g474

http://www.bmj.com/content/348/bmj.g474

Trigeminal neuralgia is a rare, episodic facial pain that is unilateral, electric shock-like, and provoked by light touch. At first, it is often mistaken as a tooth problem owing to its presentation in the two lower branches of the trigeminal nerve. Patients may undergo unnecessary—and sometimes irreversible—dental treatment before the condition is recognised. Initially, a small dose of an antiepileptic drug (such as carbamazepine) rather than any analgesic drug can provide excellent pain relief. However, up to 10% of patients will not respond to antiepileptic drugs,[1] and in rare instances trigeminal neuralgia can be secondary to a brain tumour, multiple sclerosis, or vascular anomalies, which will be identified only on neuroimaging.[2] If quality of life becomes impaired and symptoms are uncontrolled with drug treatment, patients should be referred to a neurosurgeon for consideration of surgical management. Studies in Europe have shown that trigeminal neuralgia results in considerable interference with activities of daily living that is comparable to other neuropathic pain conditions,[3] and could lead to suicide.[4] This review aims to highlight the key features of trigeminal neuralgia and familiarise readers with both the medical and surgical management of this condition, which remains based on limited evidence and expert opinion.

How common is trigeminal neuralgia?

Trigeminal neuralgia is rare, and hence it is difficult to obtain high quality epidemiological data. Data from the United States and validated in the 1990s provided a crude annual incidence of 5.7 per 100 000 women and 2.5 per 100 000 men.[5] Peak incidence lies between age 50 and 60 years, with prevalence increasing with age. A general practice based survey in London of neurological diseases showed an incidence of 8 (95% confidence interval 4 to 13) per 10 000 people per year and a lifetime prevalence of 0.7 (0.4 to 1) per 100 000 people per year.[6] Subsequent studies examining general practice databases reported an incidence of 27 per 100 000 person years in the United Kingdom,[7] and this figure was also noted in Holland. However, when trained specialists checked the data in Holland, the number fell to 12.6 per 100 000 person years.[8] A community based study in Germany using face to face interviews with trained neurologists reported a lifetime prevalence of 0.3%.[9]

SUMMARY POINTS

- Trigeminal neuralgia is a severe, unilateral, episodic pain of the face that is provoked by light touch; it should be differentiated from dental causes of pain
- Magnetic resonance imaging (MRI) can distinguish between patients having secondary trigeminal neuralgia related to tumours and that related to multiple sclerosis
- The first line drug for treatment is either carbamazepine or oxcarbazepine, and doses should be slowly escalated. Neurosurgical options should be discussed at an early stage, but surgery may not be required until quality of life is compromised
- Microvascular decompression is a major neurosurgical procedure that provides the longest period of pain relief and aims to preserve function of the nerve
- Percutaneous, palliative destructive procedures and stereotactic radiosurgery can provide temporary relief, but at the risk of facial numbness, which increases with repetition of the procedure

Who are most at risk of having trigeminal neuralgia?

Data from the US have found that women were more at risk than men of trigeminal neuralgia, but the association was not as strong if correction was made for women living longer than men.[5] The strongest association of having trigeminal neuralgia is with multiple sclerosis, which has been seen in both epidemiological data and in data for multiple sclerosis.[10] There could also be an association with hypertension[5] and stroke,[11] but this could be due to chance because the epidemiology is similar between hypertension and other degenerative diseases.

What is the underlying pathophysiology of trigeminal neuralgia?

Large surgical series from many different centres have confirmed that microvascular decompression of the trigeminal nerve root is the most effective and durable treatment for trigeminal neuralgia. Strong empirical evidence indicates that vascular compression of the trigeminal nerve root is associated with trigeminal neuralgia in about 95% of patients.[12] However, the exact pathophysiology of how vascular compression leads to trigeminal neuralgia remains speculative. Popular hypotheses include a combination of central demyelination of the nerve root entry zone and reinforcing electrical excitability (the ignition hypothesis).[13 14 15 16 17] Recent studies suggest that this demyelination then leads to an impairment of the nociceptive system. Those patients with more background pain seem to have a loss of central inhibition of the nociceptive system[18]; even after successful surgery, some form of abnormality of somatosensory function remains.[19] Other factors including predisposing biology on a genetic basis are likely to be important because although rare, familial clusters do exist.[20]

The remaining small subset of trigeminal neuralgia cases are associated with multiple sclerosis plaques or lacunar infarctions within the brain stem trigeminal system or cerebellopontine mass lesions.[21 22] Demyelinating multiple sclerosis plaques have been reported involving brain stem trigeminal nuclei. However, in a study of consecutive patients with multiple sclerosis, MRI showed that the only lesion localisation common to all patients was the intrapontine course of fibres in the fascicular trigeminal nerve root,[23] lending further support to the role of demyelination at the central nerve root in trigeminal neuralgia.

How is trigeminal neuralgia diagnosed?

The box shows the key clinical features and red flags of trigeminal neuralgia. The diagnosis of trigeminal neuralgia and other episodic, unilateral neuralgiform pain is based nearly entirely on the history. However, the diagnostic criteria have not been validated by case-control studies and remain based on expert consensus, mainly from headache neurologists and epidemiological studies from the 1990s.[24] Trigeminal neuralgia often starts suddenly with a memorable onset. The periods of remission tend to get shorter with time and the attacks of pain often get longer; 65% of patients newly diagnosed with trigeminal neuralgia will have a second episode within five years, and 77% within 10 years.[5] Fifty per cent of patients will have remissions of at least six months' duration. Patients can have as few as three or four attacks a day, but they could have as many as 70 per day. At times the attacks of pain come so quickly that it is impossible to determine whether there is a gap between each attack. There is often a refractory period when the pain cannot be triggered. Pain can occur at night in a third of patients. It is unusual to have trigeminal neuralgia in the first ophthalmic division of the trigeminal nerve only.

Some patients continue to have a background pain of lower intensity for 50% of the time. This condition has variously been called atypical trigeminal neuralgia, type 2[25] or—in the new International Classification for Headache Disorders—trigeminal neuralgia with concomitant persistent facial pain.[26] Some patients might also have autonomic features such as conjunctival injection, lacrimation, nasal congestion or rhinorrhoea, eye lid oedema, ptosis, or facial sweating.[26] In the presence of autonomic symptoms, it can be difficult to determine whether this is still trigeminal neuralgia or a variant known as short unilateral neuralgiform pain with autonomic symptoms (SUNA) or short unilateral neuralgiform pain with conjunctival injection and lacrimation (SUNCT). A retrospective study of patients who had undergone a microvascular decompression indicated that up to 67% reported one autonomic symptom and 14% had four or more, and that those with autonomic features were more likely to have a poorer response to surgery.[27]

It is important to carefully examine the face and oral cavity, including an examination of the cranial nerves, because any abnormalities could indicate alternative causes that would necessitate referral to a specialist.

What investigations should be done?

Trigeminal neuralgia itself is a purely clinical diagnosis. However, investigations could be required especially if red flags are noted (box) and the indications for them are based on case reports. These investigations are targeted towards identifying other craniofacial pain syndromes within a differential diagnosis of trigeminal neuralgia, identifying non-vascular compressive causes of trigeminal neuralgia, and obtaining baseline laboratory test values to assist with toxicity monitoring before starting pharmacological treatment.

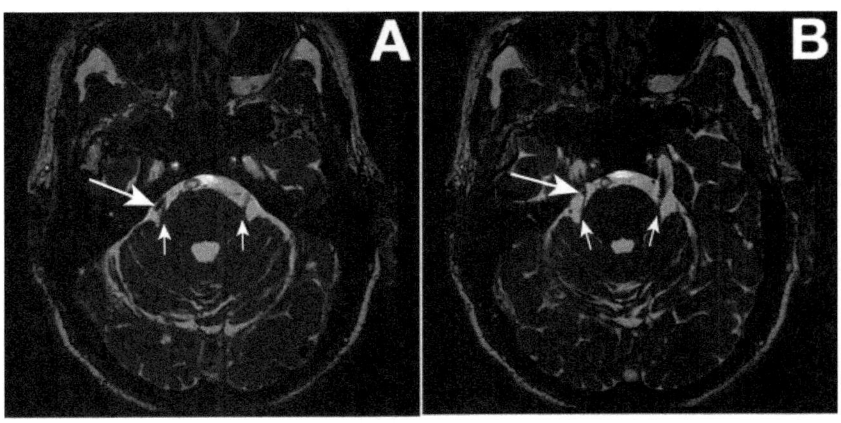

Fig 1 MRI of the posterior fossa of the brain showing neurovascular compression. Sequential, 0.8 mm, fine cut axial images from a volumetric T2 MRI acquisition on a patient with right sided trigeminal neuralgia. Caudal (A) and rostral (B) axial images shown. Origin of the trigeminal nerve from the brainstem on both sides is indicated by small arrows positioned along the course of the nerve. Inferior and lateral compression of the right trigeminal nerve route by a flow void representing the superior cerebellar artery is indicated by large arrows positioned perpendicular to the nerve course. The trigeminal nerve root is not only contacted but also displaced medially in its cisternal course by the superior cerebellar artery (B)

Patients' self assessment tools could develop in time to the point when they allow for a sensitive and specific diagnosis of trigeminal neuralgia, but evidence so far is sparse. In small studies of patients with trigeminal neuralgia or atypical facial pain, the McGill Pain questionnaire (a general tool for use in all pain conditions) was able to predict the correct diagnosis in 90% of the patients.[28 29] In another study, an extended version of the Brief Pain Inventory identified the difference in effect on daily living between 114 patients with classic trigeminal neuralgia and 42 patients with atypical trigeminal neuralgia.[30] Both of these tools have yet to be externally validated in a larger series of patients with trigeminal neuralgia.

Imaging

The most useful investigation is an MRI scan of the brain with and without contrast, which is used to rule out other potential causes of pain if the diagnosis is not clear cut or if red flags are present.[31 32] MRI is very sensitive in identifying the following features:

- Sinusitis
- Extracranial masses along the course of the trigeminal nerve
- Pathological enhancement of the trigeminal nerve that could indicate perineural spread of malignancy
- Cavernous sinus masses
- Demyelination plaques that might indicate multiple sclerosis
- Intrinsic brain lesions in the thalamus or trigeminal brain stem pathways such as lacunar infarctions
- Cerebellopontine angle mass lesions such as tumour, epidermoid, dermoid, or arachnoid cyst, aneurysm, or arteriovenous malformation.

MRI is the most sensitive screening and diagnostic test available for detecting multiple sclerosis and has the highest positive predictive value.[33 34] Although rare, brain tumours can be associated with trigeminal neuralgia.[2 35] Posterior fossa tumours are the tumours most likely to be associated with typical trigeminal neuralgia pain characteristics, and are most commonly vestibular schwannomas, meningiomas, or epidermoid cysts.[35] It is tempting to order an MRI scan to assess the trigeminal nerve for vascular compression, and in our experience, it is sometimes requested by patients once

TIPS FOR NON-SPECIALISTS

- Rule out dental causes for the pain, but also remember that trigeminal neuralgia can present as toothache and result in unnecessary dental treatment
- Careful history taking should detect signs of symptomatic trigeminal neuralgia; if there are red flags, imaging should be used. Carbamazepine or oxcarbazepine are highly effective but need to be titrated up slowly because they cause significant side effects to the central nervous system
- Patients will have periods of remission, but it is important that they continue to have access to their drugs and learn to titrate the drugs themselves with the use of pain diaries
- Untreated or poorly treated trigeminal neuralgia could result in weight loss and depression, and can lead to suicide; thus prompt referral to multidisciplinary teams with an interest in this condition (neurosurgeons, neurologists, pain specialist) is important
- Refer patients with uncontrolled symptoms for consideration of surgical procedures
- Opioids do not control this pain, and lidocaine injected into trigger points is much more effective in patients who develop severe unremitting pain

they have been diagnosed with trigeminal neuralgia and have done some research on the subject. MRI can detect vascular contact with the trigeminal nerve; however, this contact is best seen with specialised T2 and T1 volumetric acquisition techniques with fine slicing in all three planes (fig 1).

These techniques are expensive and not usually included as standard MRI head protocol, and will be available only in specialist settings. In addition, because the vessels in question are normal blood vessels and vascular contact with cranial nerves is a normal variant found in many patients without trigeminal neuralgia, an image showing vascular contact could be read as "normal" by the radiologist reading the study. A multidisciplinary evidence based review of the published literature by the American Academy of Neurology and the European Federation of Neurological Societies concluded that MRI is currently too insensitive for detecting vascular compression of the trigeminal nerve to recommend routine use.[31 32] Some small studies with more sophisticated technology have suggested improved correlations but these technologies are not available routinely at present.[36] However, more sophisticated techniques have been used recently, as reported in small series, which have shown actual changes in the trigeminal nerve.[37 38]

Biochemical investigations

Depending on the drugs chosen to treat trigeminal neuralgia, particularly among antiepileptic drugs, issues related to reductions in white blood cell count, elevation in liver transaminases, and hyponatraemia are well documented. Thus, depending on the treatment planned, a complete blood count at baseline with differential, serum electrolytes, and liver function tests are needed to monitor for potential drug toxicity over time. Regular blood test monitoring is not recommended unless there is a clinical indication. For patients taking enzyme inducing drugs, the National Institute for Health and Care Excellence (NICE) recommends a full blood count, measurements of electrolytes, liver enzymes, and vitamin D levels, and other tests of bone metabolism (for example, serum calcium and alkaline phosphatase) every two to five years.[39]

What are the medical options for treatment?

All drugs currently used to treat trigeminal neuralgia were initially developed for other indications, principally for epilepsy. Only a handful of small randomised controlled trials have investigated drug treatments for trigeminal neuralgia, many of which are old and have methodological flaws. International guidelines,[31 32] Cochrane systematic

QUESTIONS FOR FUTURE RESEARCH

- What is the natural history of trigeminal neuralgia and are there associated risk factors?
- Is there a genetic basis?
- Are there objective biomarkers to confirm the clinical diagnosis, and can they be used to predict prognosis?
- What are the best care pathways to optimise quality of life and when should treatment change from medical to surgical management?
- What novel trial designs should be used to evaluate new drugs and different surgical procedures?
- How do we improve decision making for patients and ensure they give informed consent?

DIAGNOSTIC CRITERIA FOR TRIGEMINAL NEURALGIA AND RED FLAGS

Site
- Pain is unilateral in the distribution of the trigeminal nerve, bilateral in only 3% of patients, and rarely is the pain active on both sides at the same time

Periodicity
- Episodic and sudden onset of pain, lasting a few seconds to minutes and stopping suddenly, with many attacks a day. There is a refractory period between each attack. Pain might then go into remission for weeks or months; pain-free intervals gradually shorten between episodes

Character
- Electric shock-like, sharp, shooting

Severity
- Very severe attacks, but attacks can get milder when patients are given drug treatment

Factors affecting pain
- Can be provoked by light touch to the face, eating, cold winds, or vibrations

Associated factors
- Rarely associated with history of other chronic pain or migraine. Some forms have more continued aching background pain after main attack. Rarely associated with autonomic features

Red flags
- Sensory changes, deafness or other ear problems, difficulty achieving pain control, poor response to carbamazepine, history of any skin lesions or oral lesions that could lead to perineural spread, ophthalmic division only or bilateral as suggestive of benign or malignant lesions or multiple sclerosis, age of onset under 40 years, optic neuritis, family history of multiple sclerosis

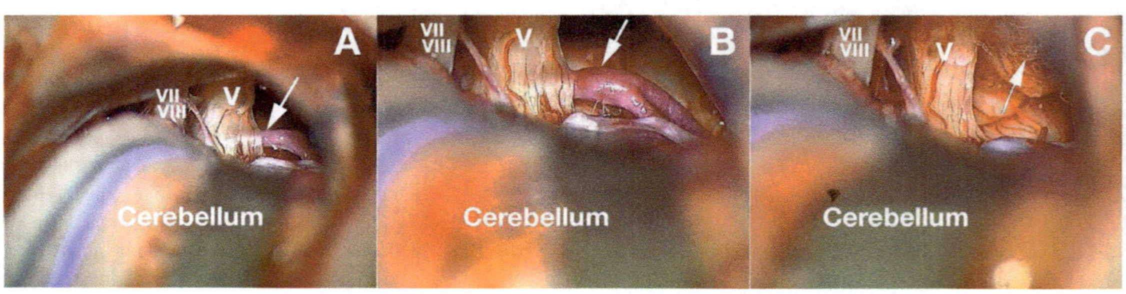

Fig 2 Compression of the trigeminal nerve in the posterior fossa and microvascular decompression. Intraoperative photographs taken during a microvascular decompression for left sided trigeminal neuralgia via a supralateral, cerebellar retrosigmoid approach. (A) Low power view showing severe proximal ventral trigeminal nerve compression of the trigeminal nerve (V) by the superior cerebellar artery (white arrow). (B) Higher power view showing the vascular interaction with the trigeminal nerve. (C) High power view of trigeminal nerve (V) after microvascular decompression, with superior cerebellar artery displaced rostrally (out of view) and held in position by shredded Teflon felt (white arrow). VII and VIII=cranial nerve VII and VIII complex

reviews,[40 41 42] and *Clinical Evidence*[43] have highlighted the key treatments (table).

In the UK, the only drug licensed specifically for trigeminal neuralgia is carbamazepine, but drugs licensed for use in neuropathic pain are often used (trigeminal neuralgia is considered a neuropathic condition). However, updated NICE guidelines[44] for management of neuropathic pain state that in primary care only carbamazepine should be used and if it fails patients should be referred for specialist care. The guidelines specifically exclude use of other neuropathic drugs for trigeminal neuralgia in primary care. All the drugs should be started at low doses and gradually escalated every three to seven days to determine the best pain control with lowest side effects. Careful monitoring is needed initially and if drug doses become high.

The preferred drug remains to be carbamazepine (based on four small randomised controlled trials of poor quality), which provides initially 100% pain relief in 70% of patients.[40] However, many patients will have side effects, mainly affecting the central nervous system—such as tiredness and poor concentration—and there is a high risk of drug interactions. The second drug of choice is oxcarbazepine, a keto derivative of carbamazepine that has shown similar efficacy to carbamazepine but increased tolerability and fewer drug interactions. The evidence is based on three randomised controlled trials including a total of 130 participants, but only one has been published in full (with the rest in abstract form only).[31 32]

If a patient develops allergies to these drugs, international recommendations suggest the use of baclofen and lamotrigine.[31 32] In a randomised controlled trial of 10 participants that lasted only seven days, Fromm and colleagues[45] showed a benefit of baclofen. However, owing to its limitations, the trial was excluded by a Cochrane systematic review.[42] A crossover randomised controlled trial of 14 participants showed that lamotrigine in combination with carbamazepine or phenytoin was slightly more effective than placebo.[46 41] These two drugs also have a high incidence of side effects, and lamotrigine must be escalated slowly to avoid rashes. A small randomised controlled trial combining gabapentin with regular ropivicane injections into trigger sites showed improved pain control and quality of life, but these results have not been replicated.[47] A prospective, open label study of 53 patients followed up for one year reports the effectiveness of pregablin.[48] No trials of combination therapies such as those used in epilepsy have been conducted so far.

What are the surgical options?

Surgical options for trigeminal neuralgia fall into two categories: palliative destructive procedures (one of four procedures) and microvascular decompression. Microvascular decompression aims to decompress the trigeminal nerve, and deals with the cause of trigeminal neuralgia in the 95% of cases not caused by other lesional causes (fig 2).[12]

Palliative destructive procedures involve partly controlled damage to the trigeminal nerve root with the aim to relieve pain, although there could be a risk of trigeminal numbness resulting from the planned nerve damage. They can be performed for all causes of trigeminal neuralgia, including non-vascular decompression. Common procedures damage the nerve through heating (radiofrequency lesioning),[49] chemically (with a viscous glycerol called glycerol rhizolysis),[50] and mechanically (by crushing the nerve against surrounding bone and dural reflections called balloon compression).[51] All procedures involve a trans foramen ovale approach to the retrogasserian portion of the trigeminal nerve using a percutaneous needle. The latest technique is stereotactic radiosurgery, most commonly performed with the Gamma Knife, which damages the nerve root with a high and concentrated dose of radiation (fig 3).[52] There is very limited evidence for the use of peripheral treatments such as cryotherapy, neurectomy, or alcohol blocks.[53]

Only three randomised controlled trials of reasonable quality have investigated surgical procedures although they do not include microvascular decompression.[53] Furthermore, there is considerable variation in the quality of many

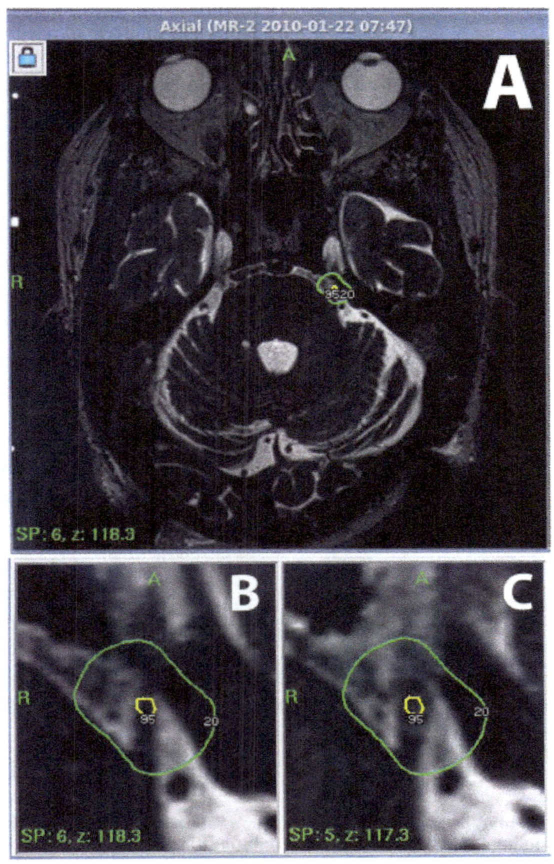

Fig 3 Targeting the trigeminal nerve with stereotactic radiosurgery using the Gamma Knife. Fine cut, 1 mm, axial T2 targeting images of a rhizotomy to the left trigeminal nerve root in a patient with trigeminal neuralgia. (A) Overview of the pons and the posterior fossa anatomy. (B-C) Sequential high magnification views of the trigeminal nerve root in relation to the dose plan. Inner circle=95% isodose line (76 Gy for an 80 Gy maximum treatment dose); outer circle=20% isodose line (16 Gy for an 80 Gy maximum treatment dose). In this case, two sector blocks were used to custom sculpt the radiation fall-off so that the surface of the brain stem received a dose no greater than 16 Gy

Most common drugs used for the medical management of trigeminal neuralgia*

Drug	Comments
Carbamazepine	Beware drug interactions; only drug licensed for trigeminal neuralgia in the UK
Oxcarbazepine	Results in hyponatraemia at higher doses; equipotencies of carbamazepine and oxcarbazepine is about 1:1.5
Baclofen	Useful in multiple sclerosis and when combined with carbamazepine
Lamotrigine	Start treatment very slowly from 25 mg daily; can be used with carbamazepine or oxcarbazepine
Gabapentin	Only one small randomised controlled trial shows effectiveness
Pregablin	Long term cohort study shows effectiveness

**Only carbamazepine should be initiated in primary care.*

cohort data studies.[54] According to large surgical series from multiple sites, microvascular decompression provides patients with about 80% chance of being pain-free without need for further treatment for trigeminal neuralgia, with a recurrence rate of about 10% over 10-20 years.[12 31 32 55 56 57] According to a systematic review for trigeminal neuralgia, the best surgical results in the short term (≤4 years) are achieved with microvascular decompression; the next best results come from the palliative destructive procedures, which have roughly equivalent results.[58 59] A meta-analysis suggested that radiofrequency lesioning had a slight outcome advantage for patients with a higher incidence of treatment induced numbness.[55] Although all surgical procedures for trigeminal neuralgia have roughly equal chances of achieving pain relief without the need for drug treatment, microvascular decompression has a recurrence rate of about 4% per year which plateaus to about 1-2% per year by year six;[56] the palliative destructive procedures have a recurrence rate of about 50% after three to five years, increasing linearly thereafter.[55]

Even in experienced hands, microvascular decompression does carry the risk of a patient having to undergo general anaesthesia, a risk (<3%) of hearing loss, as well as the risks (<1%) common to elective open cranial microsurgery.[31 32 60] Percutaneous procedures (radiofrequency lesioning, glycerol rhizolysis, and balloon compression) all require brief periods of heavy sedation and are associated with autonomic responses of trigeminal-vagal nerve reflex, which may be important considerations for patients with significant cardiac disease. Large case series report that radiofrequency lesioning has the highest risk of facial numbness (often an intended consequence), and that balloon compression has a risk of temporary motor weakness in the trigeminal nerve.[59] Stereotactic radiosurgery has the lowest risk of numbness, but does not take effect immediately, taking an average of four to six weeks for the onset of pain relief.

No randomised clinical trials have compared the outcomes of surgical procedures for trigeminal neuralgia. But in two prospective cohort trials, microvascular decompression provided better results for pain relief as well as a lower recurrence rate than the Gamma Knife.[61 62]

What to do in a crisis?

Patients who develop severe unremitting pain often attend emergency departments and are usually given opioids, although there have been no reported trials investigating this. However, opioids anecdotally have no effect on this pain, and they have not been recommended by NICE guidelines.[44] Clinical experience shows that local anaesthesia injected into a trigger area can help pain relief. This technique was used in a randomised controlled trial combining ropivacaine and gabapentin, and even those patients who only had ropivacaine showed short term reduction in pain.[47] In a randomised controlled trial of 25 patients with second division pain, those given an 8% spray of lidocaine as opposed to saline had a statistically significant decrease in pain for a mean of four hours.[63]

There is one report of three patients responding to intravenous infusion of fosphenytoin,[64] although this should be performed only under specialist supervision because hospital admission and cardiac monitoring are required. This procedure can help to break the cycle and should

ADDITIONAL EDUCATIONAL RESOURCES

Resources for healthcare professionals

- NICE clinical knowledge summaries (http://cks.nice.org.uk/trigeminal-neuralgia)—provides evidence based material on the diagnosis and management of trigeminal neuralgia in primary care guideline 173, November 2013. Free, no registration
- American Academy for Neurology guidelines (https://www.aan.com/Guidelines/)—search for trigeminal neuralgia provides materials in various formats, with patient summaries. Free, no registration needed
- E-learning 20 minute session on trigeminal neuralgia hosted by the Cardiff University Community Centre (www.paincommunitycentre.org/article/diagnosis-and-treatment-trigeminal-neuralgia)—prepared under the e-learning for healthcare scheme, it is targeted at primary care doctors and dentists, has short video clips on diagnosis, and a section on management and multiple choice questions. Free, no registration
- PIER trigeminal neuralgia module from the American College of Physicians (http://smartmedicine.acponline.org/content.aspx?gbosId=299)—comprehensive evidence based review of trigeminal neuralgia. Must be a member to access
- Professional sections on website for trigeminal neuralgia support groups (see below)

Resources for patients

- Trigeminal Neuralgia Association UK (www.tna.org.uk)—also includes information for professionals, listing higher quality published articles and many links to other organisations for patients and professionals. Some information is freely available but members have access to a forum and more details
- Facial Pain Association (formerly the Trigeminal Neuralgia Association) (www.fpa-support.org/ and www.endthepain.org)—the association caters for people with trigeminal neuropathic pain. Registration needed for free access
- Trigeminal Neuralgia Association Australia (www.tnaaustralia.org.au)—provides basic information on trigeminal neuralgia for free, but there is also a members' area and regular e-newsletter that provides research updates and details on each support group
- Trigeminal Neuralgia Association of Canada (www.tnac.org/)—provides basic information for free but also has a members' area. This site provides clear pictures of surgical procedures (www.umanitoba.ca/cranial_nerves/trigeminal_neuralgia/manuscript/medications.html)
- Weigel G, Casey KE. Striking back: the trigeminal neuralgia and face pain handbook. Trigeminal Neuralgia Association, 2003—written by a patient with input from a neurosurgeon, it provides comprehensive material on trigeminal neuralgia that is jargon free
- Zakrzewska, JM. Insights facts and stories behind trigeminal neuralgia. Trigeminal Neuralgia Association , 2006—written by a doctor for patients, it has contributions from over 100 patients and provides a comprehensive review from both patients' and professionals' perspectives
- Brain and Spine Foundation (www.brainandspine.org.uk/)—covers a wide range of neurological and neurosurgical conditions, and includes free download of booklet on head and face pain that provides details of trigeminal neuralgia and other related facial pain conditions

SOURCES AND SELECTION CRITERIA

We used Medline and Embase and the search terms "trigeminal neuralgia" and "tic dolloureux." One author (JZ) has done Cochrane reviews on both medical and surgical outcomes for trigeminal neuralgia, and the search strategy is shown in those publications. We searched the Cochrane Neuromuscular Disease Group specialised register, Cochrane Library, Medline, and Embase using the search terms "trigeminal neuralgia/facial neuralgia/tic douloureux," "tic dolloureux," "tic doloreux," or "tic douloreux" with no language exclusion. Clinical knowledge summaries and international guidelines for trigeminal neuralgia were published in 2008, and the search strategy can be found on www.aan.com. We also used our own extensive archives of references.

be followed up by an increase of oral drug treatments. Patients sometimes need to be admitted for rehydration and possible management of hyponatraemia if they have used high doses of antiepileptic drugs. Good oral hygiene needs to be maintained to prevent any additional dental pain, and a hygienist may be needed to provide more detailed instructions. Patients in a crisis should be kept calm because they can feel overwhelmed by the pain and its continuation, which can induce more attacks.[65]

What other support is available for patients with trigeminal neuralgia?

In view of the rarity of trigeminal neuralgia, few general practitioners have experience of dealing with these patients, who can feel isolated and live in fear of developing a severe pain attack. Patient support groups have been shown to be helpful.[66] Meeting other healthcare professionals and fellow patients can help decision making about treatment choices, which is difficult because of the paucity of high quality evidence.[66 67]

Contributors: JMZ and ML conceived and designed the article, drafted the manuscript, and approved the final version of the manuscript to be published. JMZ is guarantor of the article.

Competing interests: We have read and understood the BMJ Group policy on declaration of interests and declare the following interests: JMZ is partly funded by University College London and University College London Hospital Trust, which received a proportion of funding from the Department of Health (via the Biomedical Research Centre funding scheme from the National Institute for Health Research), and receives consultancy fees from Convergence pharmaceuticals; ML has no competing interests.

Provenance and peer review: Commissioned; externally peer reviewed.

1 Sato J, Saitoh T, Notani K, Fukuda H, Kaneyama K, Segami N. Diagnostic significance of carbamazepine and trigger zones in trigeminal neuralgia. *Oral Surg Oral Med Oral Pathol Oral Radiol Endod* 2004;97:18-22.
2 Cheng TM, Cascino TL, Onofrio BM. Comprehensive study of diagnosis and treatment of trigeminal neuralgia secondary to tumors. *Neurology* 1993;43:2298-302.
3 Tolle T, Dukes E, Sadosky A. Patient burden of trigeminal neuralgia: results from a cross-sectional survey of health state impairment and treatment patterns in six European countries. *Pain Practice* 2006;6:153-160.
4 Zakrzewska JM. Insights: facts and stories behind trigeminal neuralgia. Trigeminal Neuralgia Association, 2006.
5 Katusic S, Beard CM, Bergstralh E, Kurland LT. Incidence and clinical features of trigeminal neuralgia, Rochester, Minnesota, 1945-1984. *Ann Neurol* 1990;27:89-95.
6 MacDonald BK, Cockerell OC, Sander JW, Shorvon SD. The incidence and lifetime prevalence of neurological disorders in a prospective community-based study in the UK. *Brain* 2000;123:665-76.
7 Hall GC, Carroll D, Parry D, McQuay HJ. Epidemiology and treatment of neuropathic pain: the UK primary care perspective. *Pain* 2006;122:156-62.
8 Koopman JS, Dieleman JP, Huygen FJ, de Mos M, Martin CG, Sturkenboom MC. Incidence of facial pain in the general population. *Pain* 2009;147:122-7.
9 Mueller D, Obermann M, Yoon MS, Poitz F, Hansen N, Slomke MA, et al. Prevalence of trigeminal neuralgia and persistent idiopathic facial pain: a population-based study. *Cephalalgia* 2011;31:1542-8.
10 Cruccu G, Biasiotta A, Di Rezze S, Fiorelli M, Galeotti F, Innocenti P, et al. Trigeminal neuralgia and pain related to multiple sclerosis. *Pain* 2009;143:186-91.
11 Pan SL, Chen LS, Yen MF, Chiu YH, Chen HH. Increased risk of stroke after trigeminal neuralgia--a population-based follow-up study. *Cephalalgia* 2011;31:937-42.
12 Zakrzewska JM, Coakham HB. Microvascular decompression for trigeminal neuralgia: update. *Curr Opin Neurol* 2012;25:296-301.
13 Devor M, Amir R, Rappaport ZH. Pathophysiology of trigeminal neuralgia: the ignition hypothesis. *Clin J Pain* 2002;18:4-13.
14 Calvin WH, Devor M, Howe JF. Can neuralgias arise from minor demyelination? Spontaneous firing, mechanosensitivity, and afterdischarge from conducting axons. *Exp Neurol* 1982;75:755-63.
15 Gardner WJ. Concerning the mechanism of trigeminal neuralgia and hemifacial spasm. *J Neurosurg* 1962;19:947-58.
16 Hamlyn PJ, King TT. Neurovascular compression in trigeminal neuralgia: a clinical and anatomical study. *J Neurosurg* 1992;76:948-54.
17 Sindou M, Howeidy T, Acevedo G. Anatomical observations during microvascular decompression for idiopathic trigeminal neuralgia (with correlations between topography of pain and site of the neurovascular conflict). prospective study in a series of 579 patients. *Acta Neurochir (Wien)* 2002;144:1-13.
18 Obermann M, Yoon MS, Ese D, Maschke M, Kaube H, Diener HC, et al. Impaired trigeminal nociceptive processing in patients with trigeminal neuralgia. *Neurology* 2007;69:835-841.
19 Blatow M, Nennig E, Sarpaczki E, Reinhardt J, Schlieter M, Herweh C, et al. Altered somatosensory processing in trigeminal neuralgia. *Hum Brain Mapp* 2009;30:3495-508.
20 El OH, Moutaouakil F, Fadel H, Slassi I. [Familial trigeminal neuralgia]. *Rev Neurol (Paris)* 2008;164:384-7.
21 Brisman R. Trigeminal neuralgia and multiple sclerosis. *Arch Neurol* 1987;44:379-81.
22 Jensen TS, Rasmussen P, Reske-Nielsen E. Association of trigeminal neuralgia with multiple sclerosis: clinical and pathological features. *Acta Neurol Scand* 1982;65:182-9.
23 Gass A, Kitchen N, MacManus DG, Moseley IF, Hennerici MG, Miller DH. Trigeminal neuralgia in patients with multiple sclerosis : lesion localisation with magnetic resonance imaging. *Neurology* 1997;49:1142-4.
24 Zakrzewska JM. Diagnosis and differential diagnosis of trigeminal neuralgia. *Clin J Pain* 2002;18:14-21.
25 Limonadi FM, McCartney S, Burchiel KJ. Design of an artificial neural network for diagnosis of facial pain syndromes. *Stereotact Funct Neurosurg* 2006;84:212-20.
26 Anon. The international classification of headache disorders, 3rd ed (beta version). *Cephalalgia* 2013;33:629-808.
27 Simms HN, Honey CR. The importance of autonomic symptoms in trigeminal neuralgia. Clinical article. *J Neurosurg* 2011;115:210-6.
28 Melzack R, Terrence C, Fromm G, Amsel R. Trigeminal neuralgia and atypical facial pain: use of the McGill pain questionnaire for discrimination and diagnosis. *Pain* 1986;27:297-302.
29 Zakrzewska JM. Trigeminal neuralgia. 1st ed. WB Saunders, 1995:76-9.
30 Lee JY, Chen HI, Urban C, Hojat A, Church E, Xie SX, et al. Development of and psychometric testing for the brief pain inventory-facial in patients with facial pain syndromes. *J Neurosurg* 2010;113:516-23.
31 Cruccu G, Gronseth G, Alksne J, Argoff C, Brainin M, Burchiel K, et al. AAN-EFNS guidelines on trigeminal neuralgia management. *Eur J Neurol* 2008;15:1013-28.
32 Gronseth G, Cruccu G, Alksne J, Argoff C, Brainin M, Burchiel K, et al. Practice parameter: the diagnostic evaluation and treatment of trigeminal neuralgia (an evidence-based review): report of the quality standards subcommittee of the American Academy of Neurology and the European Federation of Neurological Societies. *Neurology* 2008;71:1183-90.
33 Lee KH, Hashimoto SA, Hooge JP, Kastrukoff LF, Oger JJ, Li DK, et al. Magnetic resonance imaging of the head in the diagnosis of multiple sclerosis: a prospective 2-year follow-up with comparison of clinical evaluation, evoked potentials, oligoclonal banding, and CT. *Neurology* 1991;41:657-60.
34 Paty DW, Oger JJ, Kastrukoff LF, Hashimoto SA, Hooge JP, Eisen AA, et al. MRI in the diagnosis of MS: a prospective study with comparison of clinical evaluation, evoked potentials, oligoclonal banding, and CT. *Neurology* 1988;38:180-5.
35 Bullitt E, Tew JM, Boyd J. Intracranial tumors in patients with facial pain. *J Neurosurg* 1986;64:865-71.
36 Zeng Q, Zhou Q, Liu Z, Li C, Ni S, Xue F. Preoperative detection of the neurovascular relationship in trigeminal neuralgia using three-dimensional fast imaging employing steady-state acquisition (FIESTA) and magnetic resonance angiography (MRA). *J Clin Neurosci* 2013;20:107-11.
37 Hodaie M, Chen DQ, Quan J, Laperriere N. Tractography delineates microstructural changes in the trigeminal nerve after focal radiosurgery for trigeminal neuralgia. *PLoS One* 2012;7:e32745.
38 Liu Y, Li J, Butzkueven H, Duan Y, Zhang M, Shu N, et al. Microstructural abnormalities in the trigeminal nerves of patients with trigeminal neuralgia revealed by multiple diffusion metrics. *Eur J Radiol* 2013;82:783-6.
39 National Institute for Health and Care Excellence. The epilepsies: the diagnosis and management of the epilepsies in adults and children in primary and secondary care. NICE, 2013:1-636.

40 Wiffen PJ, Derry S, Moore RA, McQuay HJ. Carbamazepine for acute and chronic pain in adults. *Cochrane Database Syst Rev* 2011;1:CD005451.

41 Wiffen PJ, Derry S, Moore RA. Lamotrigine for acute and chronic pain. *Cochrane Database Syst Rev* 2011;2:CD006044.

42 Zhang J, Yang M, Zhou M, He L, Chen N, Zakrzewska JM. Non-antiepileptic drugs for trigeminal neuralgia. *Cochrane Database Syst Rev* 2013;12:CD004029.

43 Zakrzewska JM, Linskey ME. Trigeminal neuralgia. *Clin Evid (Online)* 2009;2009:1207.

44 NICE. Neuropathic pain—pharmacological management. The pharmacological management of neuropathic pain in adults in non specialist settings. NICE clinical guideline 173. 2013:1-41.

45 Fromm GH, Terrence CF, Chattha AS. Baclofen in the treatment of trigeminal neuralgia: double-blind study and long-term follow-up. *Ann Neurol* 1984;15:240-4.

46 Zakrzewska JM, Chaudhry Z, Nurmikko TJ, Patton DW, Mullens EL. Lamotrigine (lamictal) in refractory trigeminal neuralgia: results from a double-blind placebo controlled crossover trial. *Pain* 1997;73:223-30.

47 Lemos L, Flores S, Oliveira P, Almeida A. Gabapentin supplemented with ropivacain block of trigger points improves pain control and quality of life in trigeminal neuralgia patients when compared with gabapentin alone. *Clin J Pain* 2008;24:64-75.

48 Obermann M, Yoon MS, Sensen K, Maschke M, Diener HC, Katsarava Z. Efficacy of pregabalin in the treatment of trigeminal neuralgia. *Cephalalgia* 2008;28:174-81.

49 Sweet WH, Wepsic JG. Controlled thermocoagulation of trigeminal ganglion and rootlets for differential destruction of pain fibres, part 1. Trigeminal neuralgia. *J Neur Surg* 1974;40:143-58.

50 Hakanson S. Trigeminal neuralgia treated by the injection of glycerol into the trigeminal cistern. *Neurosurgery* 1981;9:638-46.

51 Mullan S, Lichtor T. Percutaneous microcompression of the trigeminal ganglion for trigeminal neuralgia. *J Neurosurg* 1983;59:1007-12.

52 Young RF, Vermulen S, Posewitz A. Gamma knife radiosurgery for the treatment of trigeminal neuralgia. *Stereotact Funct Neurosurg* 1998;70(suppl 1):192-9.

53 Zakrzewska JM, Akram H. Neurosurgical interventions for the treatment of classical trigeminal neuralgia. *Cochrane Database Syst Rev* 2011;9:CD007312.

54 Akram H, Mirza B, Kitchen N, Zakrzewska JM. Proposal for evaluating the quality of reports of surgical interventions in the treatment of trigeminal neuralgia: the surgical trigeminal neuralgia score. *Neurosurg Focus* 2013;35:E3.

55 Tatli M, Satici O, Kanpolat Y, Sindou M. Various surgical modalities for trigeminal neuralgia: literature study of respective long-term outcomes. *Acta Neurochir (Wien)* 2008;150:243-55.

56 Barker FG2, Jannetta PJ, Bissonette DJ, Larkins MV, Jho HD. The long-term outcome of microvascular decompression for trigeminal neuralgia. *N Engl J Med* 1996;334:1077-83.

57 Burchiel KJ, Clarke H, Haglund M, Loeser JD. Long-term efficacy of microvascular decompression in trigeminal neuralgia. *J Neurosurg* 1988;69:35-8.

58 Lopez BC, Hamlyn PJ, Zakrzewska JM. Stereotactic radiosurgery for primary trigeminal neuralgia: state of the evidence and recommendations for future reports. *J Neurol Neurosurg Psychiatry* 2004;75:1019-24.

59 Lopez BC, Hamlyn PJ, Zakrzewska JM. Systematic review of ablative neurosurgical techniques for the treatment of trigeminal neuralgia. *Neurosurgery* 2004;54:973-82.

60 Kalkanis SN, Eskandar EN, Carter BS, Barker FG. Microvascular decompression surgery in the United States, 1996 to 2000: mortality rates, morbidity rates, and the effects of hospital and surgeon volumes. *Neurosurgery* 2003;52:1251-61.

61 Linskey ME, Ratanatharathorn V, Penagaricano J. A prospective cohort study of microvascular decompression and Gamma Knife surgery in patients with trigeminal neuralgia. *J Neurosurg* 2008;109(suppl):160-72.

62 Pollock BE, Schoeberl KA. Prospective comparison of posterior fossa exploration and stereotactic radiosurgery dorsal root entry zone target as primary surgery for patients with idiopathic trigeminal neuralgia. *Neurosurgery* 2010;67:633-8.

63 Kanai A, Suzuki A, Kobayashi M, Hoka S. Intranasal lidocaine 8% spray for second-division trigeminal neuralgia. *Br J Anaesth* 2006;97:559-63.

64 Cheshire WP. Fosphenytoin: an intravenous option for the management of acute trigeminal neuralgia crisis. *J Pain Symptom Manage* 2001;21:506-10.

65 Moisset X, Villain N, Ducreux D, Serrie A, Cunin G, Valade D, et al. Functional brain imaging of trigeminal neuralgia. *Eur J Pain* 2011;15:124-31.

66 Zakrzewska JM, Jorns TP, Spatz A. Patient led conferences—who attends, are their expectations met and do they vary in three different countries? *Eur J Pain* 2009;13:486-91.

67 Spatz AL, Zakrzewska JM, Kay EJ. Decision analysis of medical and surgical treatments for trigeminal neuralgia: how patient evaluations of benefits and risks affect the utility of treatment decisions. *Pain* 2007;131:302-10.

Painful diabetic neuropathy

Amanda Peltier, assistant professor of neurology[1], Stephen A Goutman, assistant professor of neurology[2], Brian C Callaghan, assistant professor of neurology[2]

[1]Department of Neurology, Vanderbilt University, Nashville, TN, USA

[2]Department of Neurology, University of Michigan, Ann Arbor, MI 48109, USA

Correspondence to: B Callaghan bcallagh@med.umich.edu

Cite this as: *BMJ* 2014;348:g1799

DOI: 10.1136/bmj.g1799

http://www.bmj.com/content/348/bmj.g1799

ABSTRACT

Diabetes is a worldwide epidemic, and associated neuropathy is its most costly and disabling complication. Given the rising prevalence of painful diabetic neuropathy, it is increasingly important that we understand the best ways to diagnose and treat this condition. Diagnostic tests in this field are evolving rapidly. These include the use of skin biopsies to measure small unmyelinated fibers, as well as even newer techniques that can measure both small unmyelinated fibers and large myelinated fibers in the same biopsy. The main treatments for painful diabetic neuropathy remain management of the underlying diabetes and drugs for the relief of pain. However, emerging evidence points to major differences between type 1 and type 2 diabetes, including the ability of glycemic control to prevent neuropathy. Enhanced glucose control is much more effective at preventing neuropathy in patients with type 1 diabetes than in those with type 2 disease. This dichotomy emphasizes the need to study the pathophysiologic differences between the two types of diabetes, because different treatments may be needed for each condition. The impact of the metabolic syndrome on neuropathy in patients with type 2 diabetes may account for the difference between the two types of diabetes and requires further study. Finally, neuropathic pain is under-recognized and undertreated despite an ever evolving list of effective drugs. Evidence exists to support several drugs, but the optimal sequence and combination of these drugs are still to be determined.

Introduction

Painful diabetic neuropathy is a common condition that will only increase as the diabetes epidemic grows.[2] All physicians need to be aware of this under-recognized condition and be able to diagnose and treat neuropathy using the tests and drugs that have the best levels of evidence. Diagnostic testing continues to evolve, and some of these newer techniques can visualize nerve pathology without the need for a sural nerve biopsy. Randomized controlled trials for neuropathic pain continue to add to the levels of evidence for and against older and newer drugs. Finally, understanding the difference between type 1 and type 2 diabetes, including the role of the metabolic syndrome, has the potential to lead to new therapies for painful diabetic neuropathy that treat the underlying cause of the nerve injury rather than the resulting pain.

Epidemiology

Both type 1 diabetes, caused by insulin deficiency, and type 2 diabetes, caused by insulin resistance, are metabolic diseases that result in hyperglycemia.[3] Diabetes affects 8.5% of people in Europe and 8.3% in the United States, with annual treatment costs of $106bn (£63.4bn; €77bn) in Europe and $174bn in the US.[4 5] The most common complication is diabetic sensorimotor polyneuropathy, which occurs in 10-54% of patients with type 1 diabetes,[6 7] while retinopathy occurs in 26.5% of patients and nephropathy in 32%.[8] Similar rates exist in type 2 disease.[9 10] Symptoms of diabetic sensorimotor polyneuropathy typically manifest earlier in the course of type 2 diabetes than in type 1 disease—8% of patients have neuropathy at the time of diagnosis of type 2 diabetes.[11] A third of patients with diabetic sensorimotor polyneuropathy develop painful diabetic neuropathy, and this condition is more prevalent in type 2 diabetes than in type 1 disease.[1] Painful diabetic neuropathy has a negative impact on physical and mental quality of life (QOL) compared with painless diabetic neuropathy.[12] In painful diabetic neuropathy, most commonly associated with the diabetic sensorimotor polyneuropathy subtype, patients may describe burning, electric, or stabbing pain. Allodynia (painful sensations to innocuous stimuli) and hyperalgesia (increased sensitivity to painful sensations) are other common manifestations of diabetic sensorimotor polyneuropathy. Pain can also occur in other diabetic neuropathies, which are described in more detail below.

Classification

Diabetic sensorimotor polyneuropathy is characterized by symmetric numbness, paresthesias, or pain in the distal lower limbs (or a combination thereof).[13] Examination may disclose stocking and glove sensory loss, impaired vibration and proprioception in the toes, reduced or absent Achilles tendon reflexes, and weakness or atrophy of the intrinsic muscles of the foot, which can result in foot abnormalities such as pes cavus and hammertoes.[13 14 15] Signs and symptoms progress in a centripetal fashion and are not confined to a single nerve or dermatomal distribution.

In 2004, an American Academy of Neurology consensus panel reviewed the literature to develop a case definition of distal symmetric polyneuropathy, with many of the reviewed studies evaluating diabetic sensorimotor polyneuropathy. They proposed that diagnostic accuracy is greatest when multiple neuropathic symptoms (pain, paresthesias, or numbness) and multiple neuropathic examination findings (sensory abnormalities or diminished reflexes) are present and electrodiagnostic studies confirm neuropathy, although sensitivity and specificity were not provided.[15] They also stated that multiple symptoms and multiple signs alone provide modest diagnostic accuracy. The main drawback to these guidelines was a lack of acknowledgment of a small fiber predominant neuropathy, typically in patients with type 2 diabetes. Skin biopsy with epidermal nerve fiber density has since been acknowledged by the European Federation of Neurological Societies as a sensitive measure of both diabetic and non-diabetic small fiber neuropathy (sensitivity was not provided).[2 16]

In 2009, the Toronto consensus panel was convened to update the definition of diabetic sensorimotor polyneuropathy. The panel proposed the following definition: "a symmetrical, length-dependent sensorimotor polyneuropathy attributable to metabolic and microvessel alterations as a result of chronic hyperglycemia exposure and cardiovascular risk covariates."[2] It further defined painful diabetic polyneuropathy as "pain arising as a direct consequence of abnormalities in the peripheral somatosensory system in people with diabetes . . . the symptoms are distal, symmetrical, often associated with nocturnal exacerbations, and commonly described as prickling, deep aching, sharp, like an electric shock, and burning."[2] It proposed that patients with possible neuropathy should be defined as those with neuropathic symptoms, neuropathic sensory examination findings, or abnormal reflexes and patients with probable neuropathy as those with two of these three features. Confirmed clinical neuropathy was considered for those with either neuropathic symptoms or examination findings, including abnormal reflexes with documented abnormalities on nerve conduction studies or skin biopsy.

Small fiber neuropathy is another phenotype of painful diabetic neuropathy. Small diameter myelinated and unmyelinated fibers are affected, resulting in pain such as that seen in "burning feet" syndrome.[17] The Toronto consensus panel defined "possible" small fiber neuropathy as symptoms or signs of small fiber involvement.[2] "Probable" small fiber neuropathy requires the addition of a normal sural nerve sensory response on nerve conduction studies. "Definite" small fiber neuropathy requires the same criteria for probable small fiber neuropathy as well as a confirmatory test such as skin biopsy or quantitative sensory testing. Of note, most patients with diabetes and small fiber neuropathy have concomitant large fiber involvement or develop abnormalities in large fibers, transitioning to typical diabetic sensorimotor polyneuropathy.

Other subtypes of painful diabetic neuropathy include diabetic lumbosacral radiculoplexus neuropathy, mononeuropathy, treatment induced neuropathy, and mononeuritis multiplex (fig 1). Diabetic lumbosacral radiculoplexus neuropathy presents with asymmetric pain and weakness in the proximal lower limb.[18] Weight loss and improved glucose control, such as after starting insulin, can be associated features. Cervical and thoracic subtypes are also described.[19 20] No treatment has been proved to be effective in diabetic lumbosacral radiculoplexus neuropathy or its cervical and thoracic subtypes. Carpal tunnel syndrome is the most common mononeuropathy seen in patients with diabetes.[21] Other mononeuropathies that cause pain and are common in patients with diabetes include ulnar mononeuropathies at the elbow and lateral femoral cutaneous neuropathies (meralgia paresthetica). Treatment induced neuropathy is characterized by the acute onset of pain and autonomic dysfunction in the setting of improved glucose control.[22] This condition can occur after insulin or oral hypoglycemic drugs are started and patients often improve with time, particularly those with type 1 diabetes. Diabetic mononeuritis multiplex results in a stepwise progressive dysfunction of specific nerves and leads to pain, sensory loss, and weakness.[23] Peroneal and ulnar nerves are particularly susceptible. Perivascular infiltrates can be seen on biopsy, supporting an immune mediated vasculopathy.[23]

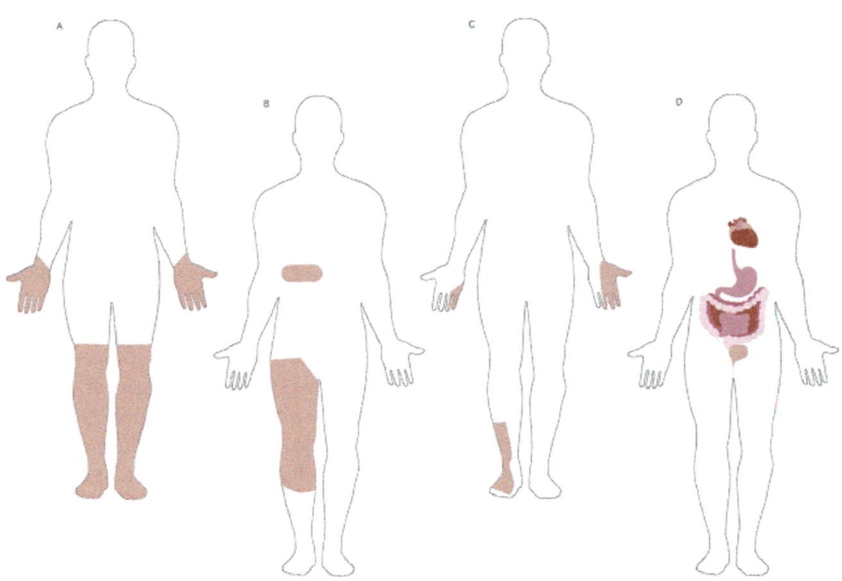

Fig 1 Many patterns of nerve injury are seen in patients with diabetes. The following patterns are shown in the figure: (A) diabetic sensorimotor polyneuropathy, small fiber neuropathy, or treatment induced neuropathy; (B) radiculoplexopathy or radiculopathy; (C) mononeuropathy or mononeuritis multiplex; (D) autonomic neuropathy (the most commonly affected organs are shown) including treatment induced neuropathy. Small fiber neuropathy has the same pattern as diabetic sensorimotor polyneuropathy but neurologic examination and electrodiagnostic studies are different, which can make the diagnosis difficult

Diagnostic studies

Diabetic sensorimotor polyneuropathy is considered in patients with diabetes who have numbness, paresthesias, or pain and in those who present with ulcerations, loss of balance, falls, or injury owing to loss of sensation. The condition may also be recognized in patients with diabetes through screening algorithms that use monofilament testing or other quantitative sensory testing.[24]

For greater specificity, both in clinical practice and in research, the diagnosis of diabetic sensorimotor polyneuropathy often requires abnormalities in at least one diagnostic test. The most commonly performed diagnostic tests are nerve conduction studies, which are reliable when performed by an experienced technician.[25] Such studies survey only large myelinated fibers, and the earliest changes noted are slowing of the conduction velocity of the sural sensory or peroneal motor responses and prolonged F wave latencies.[26] These are followed by a decrease in amplitude of the sural and peroneal responses, as well as prolonged distal latency of the peroneal motor response.

These changes occur after years of hyperglycemia in type 1 diabetes, yet in type 2 diabetes they are often detected before diagnosis, when the patient is in a pre-diabetic state.[27] A recent study found that changes in nerve conduction velocity and amplitude do not occur as fast in patients treated with modern glycemic goals as in those observed in the Diabetes Complications and Control Trial and Rochester diabetes cohort studies.[28] This suggests a change in the natural course of diabetic sensorimotor polyneuropathy secondary to stricter glycemic control goals. Also, owing to the typically short observation period of therapeutic trials in diabetic sensorimotor polyneuropathy, new tests that can detect smaller changes in nerve conduction are needed.

Another common clinical and research diagnostic test is to measure the perception of pressure and light touch with monofilaments of varying weights and stiffness. Protocols for monofilament testing may require the monofilament to be applied to one area (often the dorsum of the great toe), although results are more reliable and sensitive when multiple areas are tested. Both monofilament testing and vibration perception thresholds can reliably identify patients at high risk of having foot ulcers, infections, or amputations.[29 30]

In the past, histologic evaluation of nerves was limited to whole nerve biopsy, typically of the sural nerve. This method is not commonly used as a diagnostic test because of the side effects of the procedure, including a pain syndrome in the lateral part of the foot. In addition, nerve biopsy is rarely used in research studies because it cannot be repeated in the same location, which limits its usefulness as an endpoint in longitudinal studies. Sural nerve biopsy is usually abnormal—showing decreased myelinated nerve fiber density, swelling of axons, and segmental demyelination—even when signs of diabetic sensorimotor polyneuropathy are minimal or absent.[31 32]

Biopsy of hairy skin in the lower extremities, followed by immunostaining and quantification of unmyelinated C fibers in the epidermis (intraepidermal nerve fiber density) is also a sensitive and reliable way to identify patients with diabetic sensorimotor polyneuropathy.[33 34] This method has the advantage of quantifying unmyelinated C fibers and places greater emphasis on the involvement of small unmyelinated fibers in the condition. The measurement of intraepidermal nerve fiber density is particularly important in patients with small fiber neuropathy, whose large fiber nerves are not affected and who therefore have normal nerve conduction studies. Longitudinal studies suggest that in patients with type 2 diabetes or pre-diabetes, loss of C fibers occurs before abnormalities in large myelinated fibers.[35 36]

The major drawback to biopsy of hairy skin is the relative paucity of myelinated fibers in this type of skin. Biopsy of glabrous skin, found on the palms of the hands and soles of the feet, overcomes this obstacle, allowing a more accurate measurement of distal myelinated fiber density.[37 38] This method also shows a significantly greater involvement of myelinated fibers in patients with type 1 diabetes than in those with type 2 disease with similar severity of neuropathy, suggesting a difference in mechanism and natural course of diabetic sensorimotor polyneuropathy between the two type of diabetes.[39]

The diagnosis of diabetic sensorimotor polyneuropathy for research purposes typically uses one of the published neuropathy scores, including the Michigan diabetes neuropathy score,[40] total neuropathy score,[41] and the lower limb neuropathy impairment score.[42] Most neuropathy scores include reflexes, perception of vibrations, monofilament sensation, strength of toe flexion or extension, and pinprick sensation. Scores are heavily biased towards functions associated with large myelinated fibers. An exception is the Utah early neuropathy score, which gives greater point value to loss or reduction of pinprick sensation and considers allodynia, both of which are mediated by small myelinated and unmyelinated fibers.[43]

Screening surveys for neuropathic symptoms, which use questionnaires of symptoms without utilizing examination findings, can also be used. One such example is the Michigan neuropathy screening instrument, which has a sensitivity of 40% and a specificity of 92%.[44] These surveys typically include questions on pain, loss of sensation, common manifestations of allodynia, and distal autonomic impairment.

Quantitative sensory testing is also used for diagnosis in clinical research studies. The most common sensory modalities tested are vibration or thermal perception.[45] These tests are not as useful as clinical tests because they are subjective, dependent on patient cooperation, and may show abnormalities in patients without neuropathy.[46] However, quantitative sensory testing is more sensitive than nerve conduction studies and is highly reliable in research study populations. Unlike nerve conduction studies, these methods test the functionality of unmyelinated C fibers and can also be used for thermal perception.

Other diagnostic methods used to quantify C fiber function in research studies include quantitative sudomotor axon reflex testing, quantitative direct and indirect axon reflex, and sudoscan, which quantify the sudomotor C fibers that innervate sweat glands.[47 48 49] Laser Doppler flare imaging is used to study vasomotor C fibers that innervate superficial small arteries, which are responsible for vasodilation.[50] This imaging modality is abnormal in patients with diabetes and pre-diabetic neuropathy.[51]

SOURCES AND SELECTION CRITERIA

We searched PubMed and Medline for articles on diabetic neuropathy, published from September 2008 to September 2013.

When searching for articles on diabetic neuropathy we used the keywords "diabetes mellitus" and "peripheral nervous system diseases" or "neuropathy." This retrieved 2440 articles. Search criteria for patient oriented outcomes were "quality of life" and "neuropathy" (1213 articles). Search criteria for diagnostic criteria were "guidelines" or "diagnosis" and "neuropathy" (2695 articles). Search criteria for compression mononeuropathies were "mononeuropathy" and "diabetes mellitus" or "carpal tunnel" or "ulnar" or "cubital tunnel" and "diabetes mellitus" (171 articles).

References to trials published earlier than September 2008 were included as needed. Duplicates were excluded.

DRUGS USED FOR NEUROPATHIC PAIN

Antiepileptics

- Pregabalin*
- Gabapentin†
- Carbamazepine
- Oxcarbamazepine
- Sodium valproate or valproic acid†
- Lamotrigine
- Lacosamide

Antidepressants

- Duloxetine*
- Venlafaxine†
- Amitriptyline†
- Nortriptyline
- Imipramine
- Milnacipran

Opioids and others

- Tapentadol*
- Oxycodone†
- Morphine sulfate†
- Tramadol†
- α lipoic acid†
- Capsaicin cream
- Lidocaine cream or patch

**Approved by the Food and Drug Administration for neuropathic pain.*
†Shown to be efficacious in a placebo controlled trial.

Important patient outcomes

The important patient oriented outcomes in painful diabetic neuropathy are pain reduction, side effects of drugs, and QOL. The first two outcomes have been covered in previous sections. The HRQOL, a health related QOL tool developed for peripheral neuropathy, showed that severity of symptoms was more closely associated with QOL than electrophysiologic measures or examination findings.[52] Clinical trials, with limited time for secondary QOL endpoints, typically favor QOL measures that are shorter, with forced choice (Likert)-type answers rather than more individualized QOL scores. Generic QOL tools, such as the Nottingham Health Profile (NHP) and the Sickness Impact Profile (SIP), have also been used to assess the effectiveness of treatments.[52 53] Moreover, several different QOL tools have been developed for clinical trials of painful diabetic neuropathy. These include the Norfolk QOL Questionnaire-Diabetic Neuropathy,[54] Nottingham Health Profile,[55] PN-QOL,[52] and Neuro-QOL.[56] These tools contain 28-97 items that evaluate pain, disruption of daily activities, autonomic symptoms, and sexual functioning, as well as neuropathy specific sensory and motor items.

Patients with painful diabetic neuropathy have significantly decreased QOL scores owing to several factors, including pain, impaired balance and mobility, and frequent falling. Pain in itself has a large effect on QOL, including quality of sleep, mood, energy, and mobility.[57] Among the complications of diabetes, painful diabetic neuropathy was second only to amputation in decreasing QOL.[58] Further studies are needed on whether treatment of painful diabetic neuropathy improves QOL scores in patients with diabetes.

Treatment

Prevention

The treatment of diabetic sensorimotor polyneuropathy is mostly preventive and symptom oriented. Management of the underlying diabetes continues to be the main approach to preventing the onset and delaying the progression of neuropathy. Multiple large clinical trials of patients with type 2 diabetes have shown that intensive glycemic therapy delays the onset of diabetic sensorimotor polyneuropathy to a small degree, although this effect was not significant in a meta-analysis.[59 60] This is in contrast to several studies conclusively showing a large, significant benefit of preventing neuropathy with aggressive glycemic control in type 1 diabetes.[60] The Diabetes Complications and Control Trial also demonstrated the concept of metabolic memory in type 1 diabetes.[58] Patients randomized to intensive treatment continued to have a lower incidence of diabetic sensorimotor polyneuropathy and other microvascular complications than patients on conventional treatment even years after this last group of patients was switched to intensive therapy at trial completion.[56] In fact, patients in the intensive treatment group had a 64% relative risk reduction (45% to 76%) in the incidence of neuropathy compared with the conventional group.[57]

Because compressive mononeuropathies are common in patients with diabetes, multiple surgical releases have been advocated for the treatment of diabetic sensorimotor polyneuropathy.[58] However, data supporting such surgical interventions are limited to uncontrolled case report series. No placebo controlled studies of surgical treatment have been performed, so these interventions are not currently recommended.[61] However, several non-randomized studies suggest that carpal tunnel syndrome and ulnar entrapment at the elbow improve significantly with surgical release.[62 63]

Symptoms

Pain relieving drugs for painful diabetic neuropathy fall into three major categories: antiepileptics, antidepressants that affect norepinephrine (noradrenaline) reuptake, and non-specific analgesics, including opioids (box).

Pregabalin, duloxetine, and tapentadol are the only drugs approved by the US Food and Drug Administration for neuropathic pain in painful diabetic neuropathy. Duloxetine is also licensed in the European Union. Tapentadol is unique in that it has two mechanisms of action: activation of μ-opioid receptors and inhibition of norepinephrine reuptake.[64]

Antiepileptic drugs

In addition to pregabalin, the only other antiepileptic drug with demonstrated efficacy in treatment of diabetic neuropathic pain is gabapentin, which has a similar mechanism of action to pregabalin (binds to calcium channels in the dorsal horn containing the $\alpha 2\delta$ subunit and decreases neurotransmitter release).[65] Gabapentin and pregabalin have similar efficacy, with a number needed to treat (NNT) of 3.9-4.2.[66] Gabapentin is licensed for neuropathic pain in the UK but not in the US.

Most antiepileptic drugs have shown limited benefit in painful diabetic neuropathy. Topiramate was not shown to be efficacious in phase III studies of diabetic neuropathic pain, although phase II studies were promising.[67 68] Placebo controlled studies of oxcarbazepine, lamotrigine, and lacosamide show conflicting results and no placebo controlled studies of carbamazepine exist. This raises questions of the efficacy of these drugs in diabetic neuropathic pain, despite their use in other neuropathic pain conditions.[69 70 71] Sodium valproate demonstrated efficacy in two trials with methodologic concerns, and its side effects and safety profile make it unlikely to be used by most clinicians.[72]

Antidepressants with effects on norepinephrine reuptake

These have consistently shown benefit in the treatment of painful diabetic neuropathy, with a NNT between 2.1 and 5.5 to achieve 50% reduction in pain.[66] Amitriptyline, nortriptyline, and other tricyclic antidepressants have the advantage of once daily dosing, and they are economical owing to generic availability. However, they can have serious side effects, including orthostasis, constipation, somnolence, and erectile dysfunction. The newer serotonin-norepinephrine reuptake inhibitors (SNRIs) venlafaxine and duloxetine are also efficacious in painful diabetic neuropathy.[73 74]

Opioid based drugs

These drugs have known efficacy in the treatment of painful diabetic neuropathy. Placebo controlled studies show that oxycodone, morphine sulfate, tramadol, and tapentadol significantly improve pain in painful diabetic neuropathy (box).[7 75] Important drawbacks to opioid treatment include tolerance, withdrawal symptoms on discontinuation, and risk of misuse. In addition, the need to monitor opioid drugs using electronic prescription databases and urine drug screens makes opioid prescriptions labor intensive for many clinicians.

α lipoic acid

A systematic review of α lipoic acid in the treatment of diabetic neuropathic pain found that this drug may help relieve pain and improve neuropathy,[76] possibly through its potent antioxidant properties and ability to reduce glutathione concentrations.[77] The largest trials included in the review are the SYDNEY, ALADIN, and SYDNEY2 trials. All of these trials showed that this drug provided benefit in patients with painful diabetic neuropathy.[78 79] The NATHAN 1 trial suggested that use of α lipoic acid (600 mg daily) improved neuropathy scores, and possibly delayed progression.[80] However, pain was not a predefined endpoint in these studies and the effect on pain control was only moderate.

Topical treatments

Topical treatments have had limited success in the treatment of painful diabetic neuropathy, largely because of a lack of placebo controlled trials and side effects. Capsaicin cream is approved for topical relief of neuropathic pain but many patients cannot tolerate it because of the initial pain on application.[81] Lidocaine cream or patches can be used for focal areas of pain but are less effective for more diffuse pain. Many pharmacies can produce creams with gabapentin or amitriptyline, which often include ketamine for pain control. These creams are not typically covered by health insurance, have no placebo controlled studies of efficacy, and may be cost prohibitive for some patients. However, for patients with multiple medical problems, these topical treatments may be of some benefit because of reduced drug interactions.[82]

Non-pharmacologic treatments

Two non-randomized studies with a before and after design found that exercise improved pain in pre-diabetic neuropathy and diabetic sensorimotor polyneuropathy as well as improving nerve fiber density on skin biopsy.[83 84] However, because these studies were not all blinded the optimum exercise routine is yet to be determined. Other non-pharmacologic treatments used in painful diabetic neuropathy include transcutaneous electrical nerve stimulation, electromagnetic stimulation, spinal cord stimulation, deep brain stimulation, low level laser treatment, and massage, all of which have failed to demonstrate efficacy.[7 85 86 87] No placebo controlled studies exist for acupuncture.

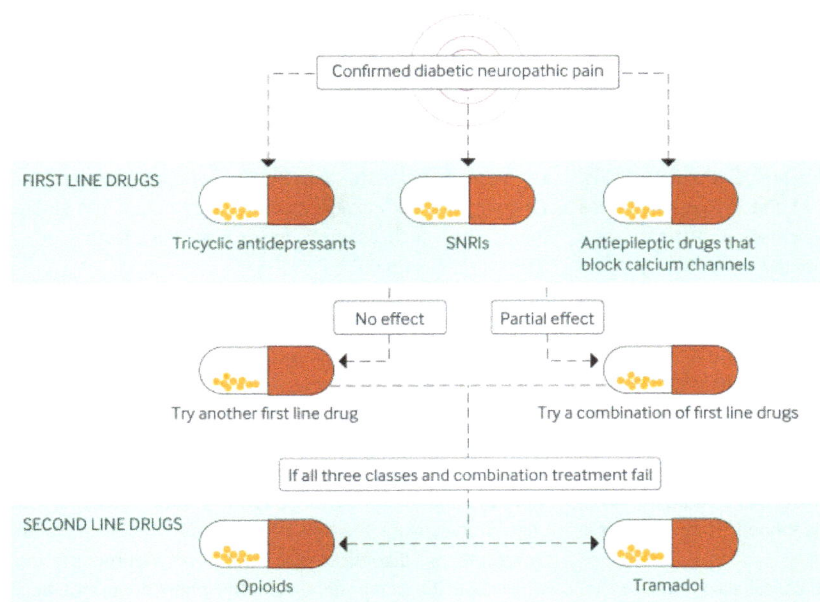

Fig 2 Algorithm for the treatment of painful diabetic neuropathy including first and second line treatments. SNRI=serotonin norepinephrine reuptake inhibitor

Summary of evidence on treatment

Evidence supports the use of antiepileptic drugs that block calcium channels, serotonin norepinephrine reuptake inhibitors, and tricyclic antidepressants as first line drugs for relief of neuropathic pain (fig 2).[5 88 89 90] Opioids can be considered when multiple first line agents alone or in combination do not control pain.[7] However, little evidence exists to compare these strategies and to determine the precise algorithm for their use.

Current evidence on painful diabetic neuropathy is limited by the lack of standardized assessments of pain, side effects, and QOL. Furthermore, longer trials of pain management are needed because most current trials study patients for months only. Trials to evaluate how and when to stop neuropathic drugs are also needed. Finally, the cost effectiveness of these drugs in painful diabetic neuropathy is rarely studied but will become increasingly important as healthcare resources become more limited.

Guidelines and recommendations

American Diabetes Association guidelines recommend screening for diabetic sensorimotor polyneuropathy at diagnosis of type 2 diabetes and five years after the diagnosis of type 1 disease, and then annually. Specifically, they recommend screening with clinical bedside tests of pinprick sensation, vibration perception using a 128 Hz tuning fork, or monofilament pressure sensation with a 10 g monofilament at the distal plantar aspect of both great toes and metatarsal joints, and assessment of ankle reflexes.[91]

The International Diabetes Federation (IDF) also recommends screening with a 128 Hz tuning fork, biothesiometer, non-traumatic pinprick, or monofilament. It also recommends looking for other causes of neuropathy, including alcoholism, vitamin B12 deficiency, renal disease, inherited neuropathies, vasculitis, and chronic inflammatory demyelinating polyneuropathy.[92]

The American Diabetes Association recommends that physicians perform a foot examination, including inspection of the feet for deformities, cuts, ulcerations, and wounds in addition to sensation. Assessment for distal pulses is also recommended, and the ankle brachial index should be measured if peripheral arterial disease needs to be evaluated. Furthermore, patients with diabetes are encouraged to examine their feet daily and wear supportive footwear.[91]

Treatment guidelines for painful diabetic neuropathy focus mainly on drugs for pain relief. Most studies are based on reducing pain on the 11 point Likert or visual analog scales. A reduction in pain of at least 30% is the primary outcome measure for most studies.[93]

Treatment guidelines published by the American Academy of Neurology, Toronto Expert Panel meeting, and European Federation of Neurological Societies suggest that pregabalin, gabapentin, venlafaxine, duloxetine, tricyclic antidepressants, and opioids as the drugs with the best evidence to support their use.[6 7 94] The American Diabetes Association also recommends at least 150 minutes of exercise a week (weight bearing and non-weight bearing) for patients with diabetes, including those with painful diabetic neuropathy or diabetic sensorimotor polyneuropathy. Patients with coexistent diabetic autonomic neuropathy are advised to seek cardiac evaluation before starting an exercise program.

What to discuss with patients

Important items to discuss with patients with painful diabetic neuropathy are treatment of the underlying diabetes and management of the accompanying pain. As discussed earlier, the only known effective disease modifying treatment of painful diabetic neuropathy is enhanced glucose control.[60] The importance of diet and exercise must be emphasized despite obstacles for weight loss, such as long term adherence. Drugs including oral hypoglycemics and insulin need to be considered if diet and exercise do not adequately control glucose levels. Potential side effects of these drugs, such as hypoglycemia, should be explained, with a goal to minimize their occurrence.

Before pain can be managed, physicians must identify those patients who are affected. Observational studies indicate that more than 12% of patients with painful diabetic neuropathy have not talked about their pain with their physician and almost 40% of them have not received treatment for their pain.[95] Physicians should therefore ask all patients with diabetes about pain.

Once the diagnosis of painful diabetic neuropathy has been established, it is essential to discuss which drugs have the best levels of evidence to support their use. SNRIs, tricyclic antidepressants, and antiepileptic drugs that block calcium channels should be considered with a focus on potential treatments of comorbidities, minimizing side effects, and cost to the patient. For example, SNRIs and tricyclic antidepressants can treat concomitant anxiety and depression, so may be favored in patients with these common conditions. Potential side effects are also important to consider. For example, drugs that block calcium channels are metabolized by the kidneys, so they must be used carefully in patients with chronic kidney disease.

Finally, the cost to patients must be considered. Because these drugs have similar evidence of efficacy, newer drugs can be cost prohibitive and may result in non-compliance with treatment.

Other important discussion points include the risk of falls, foot ulceration, and amputation of the lower extremities secondary to loss of protective sensation. Patients with diabetic sensorimotor polyneuropathy are two to three times more likely to fall than patients with diabetes without neuropathy.[96] These falls can lead to fractures and other injuries, especially in elderly people. Appropriate evaluation for ankle foot orthoses and other ambulatory assist devices, in additional to gait therapy, can help prevent falls. Similarly, painful diabetic neuropathy is a major risk factor for the development of foot ulcers and the need for amputation of the lower extremities.[97] Foot care and evaluation by a physician will help reduce the likelihood of these severe outcomes.

In addition, risk factors such as tobacco and alcohol are important. Multiple studies suggest that smoking is a significant risk factor for diabetic sensorimotor polyneuropathy.[98 99] Concurrent use of alcohol also may increase the risk of diabetic sensorimotor polyneuropathy.[100] Counseling about smoking and alcohol cessation should also be included as a therapeutic intervention.

Other causes of neuropathy, such as vitamin B12 deficiency, which can be associated with metformin use, should also be assessed.[101] Furthermore, patients with diabetic sensorimotor polyneuropathy are at high risk of depression, with an odds ratio of 1.7 (1.1 to 2.77).[102] Patients with major depression have a high risk of developing foot ulceration, which is independent of glycemic control.[103 104] Physicians should therefore ask patients about depression and treat as necessary.

Challenging assumptions in diabetic neuropathy

For years, it has been assumed that hyperglycemia is the key driver of nerve injury in diabetic sensorimotor polyneuropathy. However, emerging data have shown that patients with type 1 and type 2 diabetes respond differently to enhanced glucose control.[60] More intensive treatment of hyperglycemia in patients with type 1 diabetes leads to a substantially lower incidence of neuropathy.[57 105] In contrast, enhanced glucose control has a minimal effect on the prevention of neuropathy in patients with type 2 diabetes.[106 107 108 109] These results highlight the fact that type 1 and type 2 diabetes are different diseases that probably have different mechanisms of nerve injury.

In type 1 diabetes, the large effect of glucose control suggests that hyperglycemia is the primary driver of nerve injury, whereas in type 2 disease, the lack of effect implies that factors other than hyperglycemia are important. The metabolic syndrome possibly contributes to nerve injury given that the cardiovascular risk factors that comprise the syndrome often cluster together with diabetes. Two independent research teams have shown an association between the metabolic syndrome and neuropathy using cross sectional designs.[110 111 112] Other investigators have shown associations between individual components of the metabolic syndrome—including obesity, hypertension, low concentration of high density lipoprotein, and hypertriglyceridemia—and neuropathy.[12 98]

Unresolved questions and emerging treatments

The underlying mechanisms involved in diabetic sensorimotor polyneuropathy need to be identified so that disease modifying treatments can be developed. This includes, but is not limited to, understanding the roles of oxidative stress, inflammation, and altered gene expression.[113 114] Emerging literature suggests that inflammation and glucose metabolites such as methylglyoxal are key factors in the development of pain.[115 116]

Attention should also focus on improving our understanding of the differences between type 1 and type 2 diabetes,[59] and the role of modifiable risk factors as a means of controlling both diabetic sensorimotor polyneuropathy and painful diabetic neuropathy. These modifiable factors may include components of the metabolic syndrome such as obesity, insulin resistance, hypertension, hypertriglyceridemia, and dyslipidemia.[117] With this in mind, future studies should investigate the size of the impact of the metabolic syndrome on diabetic sensorimotor polyneuropathy, and which specific components are the main drivers of nerve injury. Better understanding of how the metabolic syndrome relates to diabetic sensorimotor polyneuropathy may provide the basis for effective treatments.[117]

RESEARCH QUESTIONS

- Which diagnostic test(s) should be used to confirm neuropathy in the clinic and in research studies?
- What is the optimal treatment algorithm for painful diabetic neuropathy?
- What are the pathophysiologic differences between type 1 and type 2 diabetes?
- What is the role of metabolic syndrome components in nerve injury?
- What is the natural course of neuropathic pain in painful diabetic neuropathy?

The recently published evidence based guideline for the treatment of painful diabetic neuropathy identified areas for future research into drugs for pain.[7] Firstly, it notes a paucity of class I studies to evaluate the effectiveness of the drugs. Moreover, standardized and formalized scales for pain, QOL, and physical function are needed when comparing drugs against placebo, head to head or in combination with other treatments. In addition, because diabetic sensorimotor polyneuropathy is a chronic disease, trials of longer duration are needed. Finally, a better understanding of the side effects and cost effectiveness of these drugs in treating painful diabetic neuropathy is needed, because chronic use is anticipated.

Conclusions

Diabetic sensorimotor polyneuropathy is encountered by all types of physician and often results in pain. As the diabetic epidemic continues to grow, the prevalence of diabetic sensorimotor polyneuropathy and painful diabetic neuropathy will increase. Diagnostic tests to confirm neuropathy continue to evolve, with nerve conduction studies and skin biopsies the current mainstays of diagnosing large and small fiber nerve dysfunction, respectively. The management of diabetes is the only disease modifying treatment for diabetic sensorimotor polyneuropathy. However, several clinical trials in the past two decades have shown that glucose control is not sufficient to prevent neuropathy in patients with diabetes, especially in those with type 2 disease.[60] These consistent results indicate the need for understanding the differences between the two types of diabetes and of developing new treatments beyond glucose control.

Painful diabetic neuropathy is under-recognized and undertreated, which indicates the opportunity for improved patient care.[95] A growing number of drugs have strong evidence to support their use, but many other drugs have not shown benefit in clinical trials. Current evidence supports the use of antiepileptic drugs that block calcium channels, SNRIs, and tricyclic antidepressants as first line drugs in the treatment of neuropathic pain.[6] [7] However, further studies are needed to develop new drugs and to determine the order and combinations that can best limit neuropathic pain. Limitations of past studies need to be tackled by using standardized assessments of pain, side effects, and QOL; studying drugs for longer periods of time; and evaluating the cost effectiveness of different strategies.

Contributors: All authors helped review the literature, write, and edit the manuscript.

Competing interests: We have read and understood the BMJ Group policy on declaration of interests and declare the following interests: AP and SG have none. BCC received research support from Impeto Medical.

Provenance and peer review: Commissioned; externally peer reviewed.

1 Abbott CA, Malik RA, van Ross ER, Kulkarni J, Boulton AJ. Prevalence and characteristics of painful diabetic neuropathy in a large community-based diabetic population in the U.K. *Diabetes Care* 2011;34:2220-4.
2 Tesfaye S, Boulton AJ, Dyck PJ, Freeman R, Horowitz M, Kempler P, et al. Diabetic neuropathies: update on definitions, diagnostic criteria, estimation of severity, and treatments. *Diabetes Care* 2010;33:2285-93.
3 Powers AC. Diabetes mellitus. In: Longo DL, Fauci AS, Kasper DL, Hauser SL, Jameson JL, Loscalzo J, eds. Harrison's principles of internal medicine. 18th ed. McGraw-Hill, 2012.
4 Centers for Disease Control and Prevention. 2011 National Diabetes Fact Sheet. 2012. www.cdc.gov/diabetes/pubs/factsheet11.htm?loc=diabetes-statistics#citation.
5 International Diabetes Federation. IDF diabetes atlas. 2013. www.idf.org/diabetesatlas.
6 Attal N, Cruccu G, Baron R, Haanpaa M, Hansson P, Jensen TS, et al. EFNS guidelines on the pharmacological treatment of neuropathic pain: 2010 revision. *Eur J Neurol* 2010;17:1113-e88.
7 Bril V, England J, Franklin GM, Backonja M, Cohen J, Del Toro D, et al. Evidence-based guideline: treatment of painful diabetic neuropathy: report of the American Academy of Neurology, the American Association of Neuromuscular and Electrodiagnostic Medicine, and the American Academy of Physical Medicine and Rehabilitation. *Neurology* 2011;76:1758-65.
8 Pambianco G, Costacou T, Ellis D, Becker DJ, Klein R, Orchard TJ. The 30-year natural history of type 1 diabetes complications: the Pittsburgh Epidemiology of Diabetes Complications Study experience. *Diabetes* 2006;55:1463-9
9 Adler AI, Stevens RJ, Manley SE, Bilous RW, Cull CA, Holman RR, et al. Development and progression of nephropathy in type 2 diabetes: the United Kingdom Prospective Diabetes Study (UKPDS 64). *Kidney Int* 2003;63:225-32.
10 Fong DS, Aiello L, Gardner TW, King GL, Blankenship G, Cavallerano JD, et al. Retinopathy in diabetes. *Diabetes Care* 2004;27(suppl 1):S84-7.
11 Partanen J, Niskanen L, Lehtinen J, Mervaala E, Siitonen O, Uusitupa M. Natural history of peripheral neuropathy in patients with non-insulin-dependent diabetes mellitus. *N Engl J Med* 1995;333:89-94.
12 Van Acker K, Bouhassira D, De Bacquer D, Weiss S, Matthys K, Raemen H, et al. Prevalence and impact on quality of life of peripheral neuropathy with or without neuropathic pain in type 1 and type 2 diabetic patients attending hospital outpatients clinics. *Diabetes Metab* 2009;35:206-13.
13 Martin MM. Diabetic neuropathy; a clinical study of 150 cases. *Brain* 1953;76:594-624.
14 Dyck PJ, Karnes JL, O'Brien PC, Litchy WJ, Low PA, Melton LJ 3rd. The Rochester Diabetic Neuropathy Study: reassessment of tests and criteria for diagnosis and staged severity. *Neurology* 1992;42:1164-70.
15 England JD, Gronseth GS, Franklin G, Miller RG, Asbury AK, Carter GT, et al. Distal symmetrical polyneuropathy: a definition for clinical research. A report of the American Academy of Neurology, the American Association of Electrodiagnostic Medicine, and the American Academy of Physical Medicine and Rehabilitation. *Arch Phys Med Rehabil* 2005;86:167-74.
16 Lauria G, Hsieh ST, Johansson O, Kennedy WR, Leger JM, Mellgren SI, et al. European Federation of Neurological Societies/Peripheral Nerve Society guideline on the use of skin biopsy in the diagnosis of small fiber neuropathy. Report of a joint task force of the European Federation of Neurological Societies and the Peripheral Nerve Society. *Eur J Neurol* 2010;17:903-12.
17 Holland NR, Crawford TO, Hauer P, Cornblath DR, Griffin JW, McArthur JC. Small-fiber sensory neuropathies: clinical course and neuropathology of idiopathic cases. *Ann Neurol* 1998;44:47-59.
18 Dyck PJ, Norell JE, Dyck PJ. Microvasculitis and ischemia in diabetic lumbosacral radiculoplexus neuropathy. *Neurology* 1999;53:2113-21.
19 Katz JS, Saperstein DS, Wolfe G, Nations SP, Alkhersam H, Amato AA, et al. Cervicobrachial involvement in diabetic radiculoplexopathy. *Muscle Nerve* 2001;24:794-8.
20 Kikta DG, Breuer AC, Wilbourn AJ. Thoracic root pain in diabetes: the spectrum of clinical and electromyographic findings. *Ann Neurol* 1982;11:80-5.
21 Dyck PJ, Kratz KM, Karnes JL, Litchy WJ, Klein R, Pach JM, et al. The prevalence by staged severity of various types of diabetic neuropathy, retinopathy, and nephropathy in a population-based cohort: the Rochester Diabetic Neuropathy Study. *Neurology* 1993;43:817-24.
22 Gibbons CH, Freeman R. Treatment-induced diabetic neuropathy: a reversible painful autonomic neuropathy. *Ann Neurol* 2010;67:534-41.
23 Kelkar P, Parry GJ. Mononeuritis multiplex in diabetes mellitus: evidence for underlying immune pathogenesis. *J Neurol Neurosurg Psychiatry* 2003;74:803-6.
24 Perkins BA, Orszag A, Ngo M, Ng E, New P, Bril V. Prediction of incident diabetic neuropathy using the monofilament examination: a 4-year prospective study. *Diabetes Care* 2010;33:1549-54.
25 Arezzo JC, Zotova E. Electrophysiologic measures of diabetic neuropathy: mechanism and meaning. *Int Rev Neurobiol* 2002;50:229-55.
26 Dunnigan SK, Ebadi H, Breiner A, Katzberg HD, Lovblom LE, Perkins BA, et al. Conduction slowing in diabetic sensorimotor polyneuropathy. *Diabetes Care* 2013;36:3684-90.
27 Singleton JR, Smith AG, Bromberg MB. Painful sensory polyneuropathy associated with impaired glucose tolerance. *Muscle Nerve* 2001;24:1225-8.

28 Gibbons CH, Freeman R, Tecilazich F, Dinh T, Lyons TE, Gnardellis C, et al. The evolving natural history of neurophysiologic function in patients with well-controlled diabetes. *J Peripher Nerv Syst* 2013;18:153-61.

29 Boyko EJ, Ahroni JH, Cohen V, Nelson KM, Heagerty PJ. Prediction of diabetic foot ulcer occurrence using commonly available clinical information: the Seattle Diabetic Foot Study. *Diabetes Care* 2006;29:1202-7.

30 Young MJ, Breddy JL, Veves A, Boulton AJ. The prediction of diabetic neuropathic foot ulceration using vibration perception thresholds. A prospective study. *Diabetes Care* 1994;17:557-60.

31 Malik RA, Tesfaye S, Newrick PG, Walker D, Rajbhandari SM, Siddique I, et al. Sural nerve pathology in diabetic patients with minimal but progressive neuropathy. *Diabetologia* 2005;48:578-85.

32 Thrainsdottir S, Malik RA, Rosen I, Jakobsson F, Bakhtadze E, Petersson J, et al. Sural nerve biopsy may predict future nerve dysfunction. *Acta Neurol Scand* 2009;120:38-46.

33 McArthur JC, Stocks EA, Hauer P, Cornblath DR, Griffin JW. Epidermal nerve fiber density: normative reference range and diagnostic efficiency. *Arch Neurol* 1998;55:1513-20.

34 Kennedy WR, Wendelschafer-Crabb G. Utility of skin biopsy in diabetic neuropathy. *Semin Neurol* 1996;16:163-71.

35 Smith AG, Ramachandran P, Tripp S, Singleton JR. Epidermal nerve innervation in impaired glucose tolerance and diabetes-associated neuropathy. *Neurology* 2001;57:1701-4.

36 Sumner CJ, Sheth S, Griffin JW, Cornblath DR, Polydefkis M. The spectrum of neuropathy in diabetes and impaired glucose tolerance. *Neurology* 2003;60:108-11.

37 Myers MI, Peltier AC, Li J. Evaluating dermal myelinated nerve fibers in skin biopsy. *Muscle Nerve* 2013;47:1-11.

38 Provitera V, Nolano M, Pagano A, Caporaso G, Stancanelli A, Santoro L. Myelinated nerve endings in human skin. *Muscle Nerve* 2007;35:767-75.

39 Myers MI, Peltier AC. Uses of skin biopsy for sensory and autonomic nerve assessment. *Curr Neurol Neurosci Rep* 2013;13:323l.

40 Feldman EL, Stevens MJ, Thomas PK, Brown MB, Canal N, Greene DA. A practical two-step quantitative clinical and electrophysiological assessment for the diagnosis and staging of diabetic neuropathy. *Diabetes Care* 1994;17:1281-9.

41 Cornblath DR, Chaudhry V, Carter K, Lee D, Seysedadr M, Miernicki M, et al. Total neuropathy score: validation and reliability study. *Neurology* 1999;53:1660-4.

42 Dyck PJ, Davies JL, Litchy WJ, O'Brien PC. Longitudinal assessment of diabetic polyneuropathy using a composite score in the Rochester Diabetic Neuropathy Study cohort. *Neurology* 1997;49:229-39.

43 Singleton JR, Bixby B, Russell JW, Feldman EL, Peltier A, Goldstein J, et al. The Utah early neuropathy scale: a sensitive clinical scale for early sensory predominant neuropathy. *J Peripher Nerv Syst* 2008;13:218-27.

44 Herman WH, Pop-Busui R, Braffett BH, Martin CL, Cleary PA, Albers JW, et al. Use of the Michigan neuropathy screening instrument as a measure of distal symmetrical peripheral neuropathy in type 1 diabetes: results from the Diabetes Control and Complications Trial/ Epidemiology of Diabetes Interventions and Complications. *Diabet Med* 2012;29:937-44.

45 Shy ME, Frohman EM, So YT, Arezzo JC, Cornblath DR, Giuliani MJ, et al. Quantitative sensory testing: report of the therapeutics and technology assessment subcommittee of the American Academy of Neurology. *Neurology* 2003;60:898-904.

46 Freeman R, Chase KP, Risk MR. Quantitative sensory testing cannot differentiate simulated sensory loss from sensory neuropathy. *Neurology* 2003;60:465-70.

47 Low PA, Denq JC, Opfer-Gehrking TL, Dyck PJ, O'Brien PC, Slezak JM. Effect of age and gender on sudomotor and cardiovagal function and blood pressure response to tilt in normal subjects. *Muscle Nerve* 1997;20:1561-8.

48 Gibbons CH, Illigens BM, Centi J, Freeman R. QDIRT: quantitative direct and indirect test of sudomotor function. *Neurology* 2008;70:2299-304.

49 Casellini CM, Parson HK, Richardson MS, Nevoret ML, Vinik AI. Sudoscan, a noninvasive tool for detecting diabetic small fiber neuropathy and autonomic dysfunction. *Diabetes Technol Ther* 2013;15:948-53.

50 Illigens BM, Siepmann T, Roofeh J, Gibbons CH. Laser Doppler imaging in the detection of peripheral neuropathy. *Autonom Neurosci* 2013;177:286-90.

51 Green AQ, Krishnan S, Finucane FM, Rayman G. Altered C-fiber function as an indicator of early peripheral neuropathy in individuals with impaired glucose tolerance. *Diabetes Care* 2010;33:174-6.

52 Vickrey BG, Hays RD, Beckstrand M. Development of a health-related quality of life measure for peripheral neuropathy. *Neurorehabil Neural Repair* 2000;14:93-104.

53 Smith SC, Lamping DL, Maclaine GD. Measuring health-related quality of life in diabetic peripheral neuropathy: a systematic review. *Diabetes Res Clin Pract* 2012;96:261-70.

54 Boyd A, Casselini C, Vinik E, Vinik A. Quality of life and objective measures of diabetic neuropathy in a prospective placebo-controlled trial of ruboxistaurin and topiramate. *J Diabetes Sci Technol* 2011;5:714-22.

55 Benbow SJ, Wallymahmed ME, MacFarlane IA. Diabetic peripheral neuropathy and quality of life. *QJM* 1998;91:733-7.

56 Pop-Busui R, Herman WH, Feldman EL, Low PA, Martin CL, Cleary PA, et al. DCCT and EDIC studies in type 1 diabetes: lessons for diabetic neuropathy regarding metabolic memory and natural history. *Curr Diabetes Rep* 2010;10:276-82.

57 The Diabetes Control and Complications Trial Research Group. The effect of intensive treatment of diabetes on the development and progression of long-term complications in insulin-dependent diabetes mellitus. *N Engl J Med* 1993;329:977-86.

58 Valdivia Valdivia JM, Weinand M, Maloney CT Jr, Blount AL, Dellon AL. Surgical treatment of superimposed, lower extremity, peripheral nerve entrapments with diabetic and idiopathic neuropathy. *Ann Plast Surg* 2013;70:675-9.

59 Callaghan BC, Hur J, Feldman EL. Diabetic neuropathy: one disease or two? *Curr Opin Neurol* 2012;25:536-41.

60 Callaghan BC, Little AA, Feldman EL, Hughes RA. Enhanced glucose control for preventing and treating diabetic neuropathy. *Cochrane Database Syst Rev* 2012;6:CD007543.

61 Chaudhry V, Russell J, Belzberg A. Decompressive surgery of lower limbs for symmetrical diabetic peripheral neuropathy. *Cochrane Database Syst Rev* 2008;3:CD006152.

62 Thomsen NO, Cederlund R, Rosen I, Bjork J, Dahlin LB. Clinical outcomes of surgical release among diabetic patients with carpal tunnel syndrome: prospective follow-up with matched controls. *J Hand Surg* 2009;34:1177-87.

63 Dellon AL. Treatment of symptomatic diabetic neuropathy by surgical decompression of multiple peripheral nerves. *Plast Reconstruct Surg* 1992;89:689-97; discussion 698-9.

64 Afilalo M, Morlion B. Efficacy of tapentadol ER for managing moderate to severe chronic pain. *Pain Phys* 2013;16:27-40.

65 Sills GJ. The mechanisms of action of gabapentin and pregabalin. *Curr Opin Pharmacol* 2006;6:108-13.

66 Finnerup NB, Otto M, McQuay HJ, Jensen TS, Sindrup SH. Algorithm for neuropathic pain treatment: an evidence based proposal. *Pain* 2005;118:289-305.

67 Raskin P, Donofrio PD, Rosenthal NR, Hewitt DJ, Jordan DM, Xiang J, et al. Topiramate vs placebo in painful diabetic neuropathy: analgesic and metabolic effects. *Neurology* 2004;63:865-73.

68 Wiffen PJ, Derry S, Lunn MP, Moore RA. Topiramate for neuropathic pain and fibromyalgia in adults. *Cochrane Database Syst Rev* 2013;8:CD008314.

69 Eisenberg E, Lurie Y, Braker C, Daoud D, Ishay A. Lamotrigine reduces painful diabetic neuropathy: a randomized, controlled study. *Neurology* 2001;57:505-9.

70 Eisenberg E, River Y, Shifrin A, Krivoy N. Antiepileptic drugs in the treatment of neuropathic pain. *Drugs* 2007;67:1265-89.

71 Zhou M, Chen N, He L, Yang M, Zhu C, Wu F. Oxcarbazepine for neuropathic pain. *Cochrane Database Syst Rev* 2013;3:CD007963.

72 Gill D, Derry S, Wiffen PJ, Moore RA. Valproic acid and sodium valproate for neuropathic pain and fibromyalgia in adults. *Cochrane Database Syst Rev* 2011;10:CD009183.

73 Pergolizzi JV Jr, Raffa RB, Taylor R Jr, Rodriguez G, Nalamachu S, Langley P. A review of duloxetine 60 mg once-daily dosing for the management of diabetic peripheral neuropathic pain, fibromyalgia, and chronic musculoskeletal pain due to chronic osteoarthritis pain and low back pain. *Pain Pract* 2013;13:239-52.

74 Rowbotham MC, Goli V, Kunz NR, Lei D. Venlafaxine extended release in the treatment of painful diabetic neuropathy: a double-blind, placebo-controlled study. *Pain* 2004;110:697-706.

75 Spallone V, Lacerenza M, Rossi A, Sicuteri R, Marchettini P. Painful diabetic polyneuropathy: approach to diagnosis and management. *Clin J Pain* 2012;28:726-43.

76 Han T, Bai J, Liu W, Hu Y. A systematic review and meta-analysis of alpha-lipoic acid in the treatment of diabetic peripheral neuropathy. *Eur J Endocrinol* 2012;167:465-71.

77 Vallianou N, Evangelopoulos A, Koutalas P. Alpha-lipoic acid and diabetic neuropathy. *Rev Diabet Studies* 2009;6:230-6.

78 Ohnari K, Uozumi T, Tsuji S. [Occupation and carpal tunnel syndrome.] *Brain Nerve* 2007;59:1247-52.

79 Ziegler D, Ametov A, Barinov A, Dyck PJ, Gurieva I, Low PA, et al. Oral treatment with alpha-lipoic acid improves symptomatic diabetic polyneuropathy: the SYDNEY 2 trial. *Diabetes Care* 2006;29:2365-70.

80 Ziegler D, Low PA, Litchy WJ, Boulton AJ, Vinik AI, Freeman R, et al. Efficacy and safety of antioxidant treatment with alpha-lipoic acid over 4 years in diabetic polyneuropathy: the NATHAN 1 trial. *Diabetes Care* 2011;34:2054-60.

81 Webster LR, Peppin JF, Murphy FT, Tobias JK, Vanhove GF. Tolerability of NGX-4010, a capsaicin 8% patch, in conjunction with three topical anesthetic formulations for the treatment of neuropathic pain. *J Pain Res* 2012;5:7-13.

82 Zur E. Topical treatment of neuropathic pain using compounded medications. *Clin J Pain* 2014;30:73-91.

83 Smith AG, Russell J, Feldman EL, Goldstein J, Peltier A, Smith S, et al. Lifestyle intervention for pre-diabetic neuropathy. *Diabetes Care* 2006;29:1294-9.

84 Kluding PM, Pasnoor M, Singh R, Jernigan S, Farmer K, Rucker J, et al. The effect of exercise on neuropathic symptoms, nerve function, and cutaneous innervation in people with diabetic peripheral neuropathy. *J Diabetes Complications* 2012;26:424-9.

85 Gossrau G, Wahner M, Kuschke M, Konrad B, Reichmann H, Wiedemann B, et al. Microcurrent transcutaneous electric nerve stimulation in painful diabetic neuropathy: a randomized placebo-controlled study. *Pain Med* 2011;12:953-60.

86 Dworkin RH, O'Connor AB, Kent J, Mackey SC, Raja SN, Stacey BR, et al. Interventional management of neuropathic pain: NeuPSIG recommendations. *Pain* 2013;154:2249-61.

87 Bosi E, Bax G, Scionti L, Spallone V, Tesfaye S, Valensi P, et al. Frequency-modulated electromagnetic neural stimulation (FREMS) as a treatment for symptomatic diabetic neuropathy: results from a double-blind, randomised, multicentre, long-term, placebo-controlled clinical trial. *Diabetologia* 2013;56:467-75.

88 Callaghan BC, Cheng HT, Stables CL, Smith AL, Feldman EL. Diabetic neuropathy: clinical manifestations and current treatments. *Lancet Neurol* 2012;11:521-34.

89 Young BA, Von Korff M, Heckbert SR, Ludman EJ, Rutter C, Lin EH, et al. Association of major depression and mortality in Stage 5 diabetic chronic kidney disease. *Gen Hosp Psychiatry* 2010;32:119-24.

90 Finnerup NB, Sindrup SH, Jensen TS. The evidence for pharmacological treatment of neuropathic pain. *Pain* 2010;150:573-81.

91 American Diabetes Association. Standards of medical care in diabetes—2013. *Diabetes Care* 2013;36(suppl 1):S11-66.

92 International Diabetes Federation. IDF diabetes atlas. Secondary IDF diabetes atlas. 2009. www.idf.org/diabetesatlas/europe.

93 Farrar JT, Berlin JA, Strom BL. Clinically important changes in acute pain outcome measures: a validation study. *J Pain Symptom Manage* 2003;25:406-11.

94 Tesfaye S, Vileikyte L, Rayman G, Sindrup S, Perkins B, Baconja M, et al. Painful diabetic peripheral neuropathy: consensus recommendations on diagnosis, assessment and management. *Diabetes Metab Res Rev* 2011; published online 21 June.

95 Daousi C, MacFarlane IA, Woodward A, Nurmikko TJ, Bundred PE, Benbow SJ. Chronic painful peripheral neuropathy in an urban community: a controlled comparison of people with and without diabetes. *Diabet Med* 2004;21:976-82.

96 Agrawal Y, Carey JP, Della Santina CC, Schubert MC, Minor LB. Diabetes, vestibular dysfunction, and falls: analyses from the National Health and Nutrition Examination Survey. *Otol Neurotol* 2010;31:1445-50.

97 Margolis DJ, Malay DS, Hoffstad OJ, Leonard CE, MaCurdy T, Lopez de Nava K, et al. Incidence of diabetic foot ulcer and lower extremity amputation among medicare beneficiaries, 2006-2008. Secondary Incidence of diabetic foot ulcer and lower extremity amputation among medicare beneficiaries, 2006-2008. 2011. www.ncbi.nlm.nih.gov/books/NBK65149/.

98 Tesfaye S, Chaturvedi N, Eaton SE, Ward JD, Manes C, Ionescu-Tirgoviste C, et al. Vascular risk factors and diabetic neuropathy. *N Engl J Med* 2005;352:341-50.

99 Sands ML, Shetterly SM, Franklin GM, Hamman RF. Incidence of distal symmetric (sensory) neuropathy in NIDDM. The San Luis Valley Diabetes Study. *Diabetes Care* 1997;20:322-9.

100 Adler AI, Boyko EJ, Ahroni JH, Stensel V, Forsberg RC, Smith DG. Risk factors for diabetic peripheral sensory neuropathy. Results of the Seattle Prospective Diabetic Foot Study. *Diabetes Care* 1997;20:1162-7.

101 Reinstatler L, Qi YP, Williamson RS, Garn JV, Oakley GP Jr. Association of biochemical B(1)(2) deficiency with metformin therapy and vitamin B(1)(2) supplements: the National Health and Nutrition Examination Survey, 1999-2006. *Diabetes Care* 2012;35:327-33.

102 Van Steenbergen-Weijenburg KM, van Puffelen AL, Horn EK, Nuyen J, van Dam PS, van Benthem TB, et al. More co-morbid depression in patients with Type 2 diabetes with multiple complications. An observational study at a specialized outpatient clinic. *Diabet Med* 2011;28:86-9.

103 Williams LH, Rutter CM, Katon WJ, Reiber GE, Ciechanowski P, Heckbert SR, et al. Depression and incident diabetic foot ulcers: a prospective cohort study. *Am J Med* 2010;123:748-54.

104 Heckbert SR, Rutter CM, Oliver M, Williams LH, Ciechanowski P, Lin EH, et al. Depression in relation to long-term control of glycemia, blood pressure, and lipids in patients with diabetes. *J Gen Intern Med* 2010;25:524-9.

105 Linn T, Ortac K, Laube H, Federlin K. Intensive therapy in adult insulin-dependent diabetes mellitus is associated with improved insulin sensitivity and reserve: a randomized, controlled, prospective study over 5 years in newly diagnosed patients. *Metabolism* 1996;45:1508-13.

106 Azad N, Emanuele NV, Abraira C, Henderson WG, Colwell J, Levin SR, et al. The effects of intensive glycemic control on neuropathy in the VA cooperative study on type II diabetes mellitus (VA CSDM). *J Diabetes Complications* 1999;13:307-13.

107 Duckworth W, Abraira C, Moritz T, Reda D, Emanuele N, Reaven PD, et al. Glucose control and vascular complications in veterans with type 2 diabetes. *N Engl J Med* 2009;360:129-39.

108 Ismail-Beigi F, Craven T, Banerji MA, Basile J, Calles J, Cohen RM, et al. Effect of intensive treatment of hyperglycaemia on microvascular outcomes in type 2 diabetes: an analysis of the ACCORD randomised trial. *Lancet* 2010;376:419-30.

109 Tovi J, Svanborg E, Nilsson BY, Engfeldt P. Diabetic neuropathy in elderly type 2 diabetic patients: effects of insulin treatment. *Acta Neurol Scand* 1998;98:346-53.

110 Chattopadhyay M, Mata M, Fink DJ. Continuous delta-opioid receptor activation reduces neuronal voltage-gated sodium channel (NaV1.7) levels through activation of protein kinase C in painful diabetic neuropathy. *J Neurosci* 2008;28:6652-8.

111 Costa LA, Canani LH, Lisboa HR, Tres GS, Gross JL. Aggregation of features of the metabolic syndrome is associated with increased prevalence of chronic complications in Type 2 diabetes. *Diabet Med* 2004;21:252-5.

112 Metascreen Writing Committee; Bonadonna R, Cucinotta D, Fedele D, Riccardi G, Tiengo A. The metabolic syndrome is a risk indicator of microvascular and macrovascular complications in diabetes: results from Metascreen, a multicenter diabetes clinic-based survey. *Diabetes Care* 2006;29:2701-7.

113 Vincent AM, Calabek B, Roberts L, Feldman EL. Biology of diabetic neuropathy. *Handbook Clin Neurol* 2013;115:591-606.

114 Vincent AM, Callaghan BC, Smith AL, Feldman EL. Diabetic neuropathy: cellular mechanisms as therapeutic targets. *Nat Rev Neurol* 2011;7:573-83.

115 Bierhaus A, Fleming T, Stoyanov S, Leffler A, Babes A, Neacsu C, et al. Methylglyoxal modification of Nav1.8 facilitates nociceptive neuron firing and causes hyperalgesia in diabetic neuropathy. *Nat Med* 2012;18:926-33.

116 Galloway C, Chattopadhyay M. Increases in inflammatory mediators in DRG implicate in the pathogenesis of painful neuropathy in type 2 diabetes. *Cytokine* 2013;63:1-5.

117 Callaghan B, Feldman E. The metabolic syndrome and neuropathy: therapeutic challenges and opportunities. *Ann Neurol* 2013;74:397-403.

Fibromyalgia

Anisur Rahman, professor[1], Martin Underwood, director[2], Dawn Carnes, senior research fellow[3]

[1]Department of Rheumatology, University College London, London WC1E 6JF, UK

[2]Warwick Clinical Trials Unit, University of Warwick, Coventry, UK

[3]Centre for Primary Care and Public Health, Barts and the London School of Medicine and Dentistry, London, UK

Correspondence to: A Rahman anisur.rahman@ucl.ac.uk

Cite this as: *BMJ* 2014;348:g1224

DOI: 10.1136/bmj.g1224

http://www.bmj.com/content/348/bmj.g1224

Most doctors—particularly rheumatologists, pain specialists, and general practitioners—are familiar with patients who describe chronic pain all over the body, which is associated with a range of other symptoms including poor sleep, fatigue, and depression. This complex of symptoms is sometimes referred to as fibromyalgia. Management of patients with this condition is often complex and challenging. The diagnosis of fibromyalgia has long been controversial, with some experts questioning whether it exists as a separate entity.[1] However, the symptoms and distress experienced by patients with fibromyalgia are real. The causes of fibromyalgia are incompletely understood, and optimal management is compromised by the limited evidence base for the available treatments. This article reviews current thinking about what fibromyalgia is, whether it is a useful diagnosis to make, and which drugs and non-drug treatments can be used to treat it.

What is fibromyalgia and how common is it?

In general medical practice, fibromyalgia is diagnosed in patients with chronic widespread pain and multiple muscular tender points on examination or associated symptoms of fatigue, unrefreshing sleep, or cognitive dysfunction (or a combination thereof). Many patients have both tender points and associated symptoms.

Chronic widespread pain is defined in epidemiological studies as pain for at least three months, affecting both sides of the body, both above and below the waist.[2 3] Epidemiological evidence from several countries shows that it is a common problem, present in about 10% of the population.[3 4] Not all of these people have fibromyalgia. The population prevalence of fibromyalgia was first measured as about 2% using consensus classification criteria for fibromyalgia published by the American College of Rheumatology (ACR) in 1990.[2 3 4 5] These criteria (sensitivity 88.4%, specificity 81.1%) were simple—fibromyalgia could be diagnosed in a patient with chronic widespread pain if at least 11 of 18 specific sites on the body surface were tender to digital palpation. However, the tender point test is hard to standardise, some healthy people also have tender points, and these criteria take no account of a history of symptoms commonly seen in fibromyalgia, such as sleep disturbance and tiredness.

For the general clinician, alternative criteria produced by the ACR in 2010 may be more useful. These criteria do not require palpation of tender points. Instead patients are assessed by the widespread pain index—which divides the body into 19 regions and scores how many regions are reported as painful—and a symptom severity score that assesses severity of fatigue, unrefreshing sleep, and cognitive symptoms. The widespread pain index and symptom severity scores have been combined into a single questionnaire with a maximum score of 31,[6 7] which can be completed by self report. Two recently published population surveys using this 31 point questionnaire found a population prevalence for fibromyalgia of 2.1% in Germany[8] and 6.4% in Minnesota, USA.[7] In the German study, a cut-off questionnaire score of 12-13 was statistically best at distinguishing those who fulfilled the ACR 2010 criteria from those who did not, but there was no sharp division of clinical features between populations above and below this score.[8] The authors concluded that patients with fibromyalgia are not a separate discrete group but instead constitute the upper end of a continuous spectrum of polysymptomatic distress within the population.[8]

Figure 1 summarises the way in which clinical features can be used to diagnose fibromyalgia by general clinicians or specialists.

Who gets fibromyalgia?

Fibromyalgia has often been considered to affect mostly women. The Minnesota population survey found that 7.7% of women and 4.9% of men fulfilled ACR 2010 criteria for fibromyalgia, but a parallel medical records study in the same population found that only 27% of these people had been diagnosed with the condition.[7] Strikingly, the prevalence of medically diagnosed fibromyalgia was 2% in women but only 0.15% in men, a difference inconsistent with the true population prevalence figures.[7] Similarly, although most patients diagnosed in clinics are young or middle aged, population surveys show clearly that the prevalence rises steadily with age, with a maximum prevalence in the over 60s.[3 7] Perhaps older people with chronic widespread pain are diagnosed with osteoarthritis rather than fibromyalgia. Fibromyalgia is not restricted to developed countries. A large study in Bangladesh (n=5211)

SUMMARY POINTS

- Symptoms of fibromyalgia are chronic widespread pain associated with unrefreshing sleep and tiredness
- Fibromyalgia is not a diagnosis of exclusion and often occurs in patients with other conditions, such as inflammatory arthritis and osteoarthritis
- No clear pathophysiological mechanism for fibromyalgia has been established, but evidence suggests that there is an abnormality in central pain processing
- Diagnosing fibromyalgia can allow the patient's polysymptomatic distress to be explained, thereby reducing fear and doubt
- Fibromyalgia has no cure, but a range of drug and non-drug treatments can reduce symptoms and their impact on the patient's life
- Trial evidence for all forms of treatment in fibromyalgia generally shows only small to moderate average effects

involving door-to-door surveys with a 99% response rate found fibromyalgia (ACR 1990 criteria) in 4.4% of people in a rural village, 3.2% in a poor city area, and 3.3% in a wealthy urban area.[5] These figures are similar to those seen in Western countries using the same diagnostic criteria.[3 7]

What causes fibromyalgia?

We do not know exactly what causes fibromyalgia. Patients have no consistent structural or functional abnormalities in the muscle tissue, but pain processing mechanisms in the central nervous system are dysfunctional.[9] A recent review described amplification of afferent pain signals within the spinal cord as a key mechanism underlying the development of chronic pain in rheumatic diseases including (but not restricted to) fibromyalgia.[10] Psychological and social factors can contribute to this central amplification mechanism, and population studies have shown an association of such factors with the initiation and persistence of fibromyalgia.[11] However, equivalent levels of psychosocial stress are not associated with the development of fibromyalgia in all people and a genetic component is probably involved. A genome-wide linkage study of people from 116 American families with multiple cases of fibromyalgia reported that siblings of patients with fibromyalgia have a 13.6-fold (95% confidence interval 10.0 to 18.5) increased risk of developing the condition compared with the general population.[12] A single region on chromosome 17 was significantly linked to fibromyalgia in this population ($P<0.001$).[12]

An experimental model of pain in which the upper limb was exposed to cold water and the degree of pain experienced was measured on a visual analogue scale found that patients with fibromyalgia experienced 50% more pain at the same level of painful stimulus than healthy controls or patients with low back pain ($P<0.001$). It also found that pain inhibition pathways did not operate as effectively in the fibromyalgia group.[13] It has been argued that this defective inhibition arises from an altered balance between excitatory (such as glutamate, aspartate, substance P) and inhibitory (serotonin, noradrenaline (norepinephrine), γ aminobutyric acid) neurotransmitters in the spinal cord.[10] Cerebrospinal fluid (CSF) samples from patients with fibromyalgia were reported to contain higher concentrations of substance P,[14] but lower levels of serotonin, noradrenaline, and dopamine metabolites,[15] than samples from healthy controls. Many of the drugs that have been the subject of clinical trials in fibromyalgia were chosen because they affect these neurotransmitters.

Functional magnetic resonance imaging studies of patients with fibromyalgia have shown abnormal signalling in areas of the brain involved in processing pain and emotions, such as the amygdala, thalamus, and insula.[9 10] More recently, magnetic resonance spectroscopy was used to show increased glutamate and glutamine in the right amygdala in 30 patients with fibromyalgia compared with healthy controls, but no correlation was found between these increases and clinical features of fibromyalgia.[16]

Although these changes in cerebrospinal fluid biochemistry and cerebral signalling are associated with fibromyalgia, it is unclear whether the association is causative.

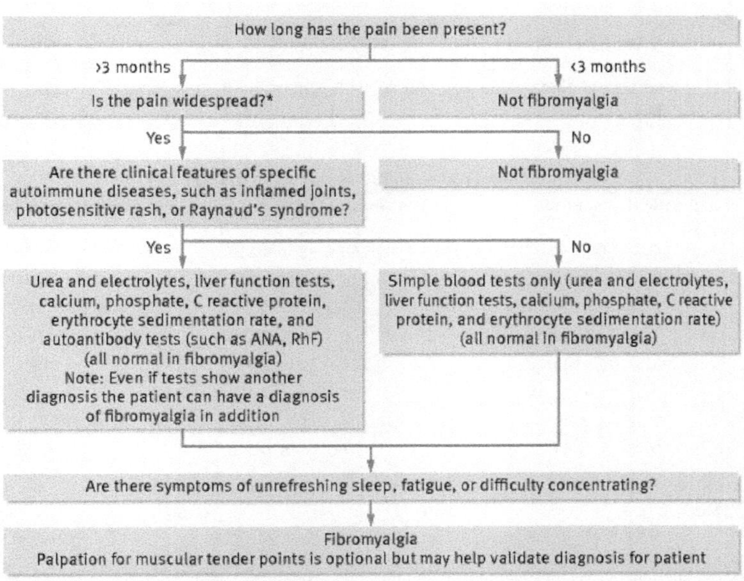

Fig 1 Flow chart for diagnosis of fibromyalgia. ANA=antinuclear antibodies; RhF=rheumatoid factor.
*Widespread pain defined as pain both above and below the waist and on both sides of the body

Why and how should fibromyalgia be diagnosed?

Some specialists have argued that a diagnosis of fibromyalgia is unhelpful because it overmedicalises this complex of distressing, medically unexplained symptoms.[1] But in our experience, many patients find the diagnosis helpful, especially when combined with a common sense explanation of the link between poor sleep, tiredness, and pain. Such a diagnosis can reassure patients that they do not have another, more severe illness, such as inflammatory arthritis or cancer, thereby halting a cycle of repeated normal investigations in search of a diagnosis. This allows patients to move forward and find ways of reducing the symptoms' impact on their lives. Two population studies reviewing the medical records of 2260 patients with fibromyalgia identified from the UK General Practice Research Database showed that rates of visits to the GP, prescriptions, and diagnosis related procedures fell in the three years after the diagnosis of fibromyalgia, leading to cost savings of £66.21 (€79.74; $107.84) per six months per patient.[17 18]

No blood tests or imaging modalities are useful for diagnosing fibromyalgia. C reactive protein concentrations and the erythrocyte sedimentation rate are not usually raised (unlike in inflammatory arthritis), and joint radiographs are usually normal (unlike in osteoarthritis). The diagnosis of fibromyalgia is made purely on a clinical basis. Some clinicians test tenderness at the 18 sites specified in the ACR 1990 criteria. This is quick and easy to do and provides the patient with objective evidence that the diagnosis is valid. However, 25% of patients diagnosed as having fibromyalgia do not have 11 tender points.[19] The 31 point questionnaire developed from the ACR 2010 criteria is not used routinely,[6 7] although it is useful to ask patients whether they have unrefreshing sleep, tiredness, or reduced ability to think and remember clearly (sometimes called "fibrofog"). In patients with chronic widespread pain, these symptoms strongly suggest fibromyalgia.

Fibromyalgia is not a diagnosis of exclusion and can occur together with other diseases. A population based study using the 31 point self report questionnaire found that 17% of 845 patients with osteoarthritis, 21% of 5210 with rheumatoid arthritis, and 37% of 439 with systemic lupus erythematosus fulfil the ACR 2010 criteria for fibromyalgia.[6] It is therefore advisable to examine patients for signs of these conditions before ascribing all their symptoms to fibromyalgia and to carry out a simple screen including full blood count, basic biochemistry, and inflammatory markers. Thyroid function tests and vitamin D levels may be helpful in some cases, but request autoantibodies only if the history and examination suggest that specific autoimmune rheumatic diseases—such as rheumatoid arthritis, systemic lupus erythematosus, or systemic sclerosis—should be excluded. This is because tests such as antinuclear antibody and rheumatoid factor are often positive in healthy people. For example, 13.3% of healthy adults are positive for antinuclear antibody at a titre of 1:80.[20] Positive autoantibody tests in patients with fibromyalgia but no features of autoimmune disease may be misleading. Assessment of clinical features such as tender joints in inflammatory arthritis may be complicated by coexisting fibromyalgia.[10] The diagnosis of fibromyalgia in the presence of an inflammatory arthritis usually requires specialist advice. It is important to remember that fibromyalgia can develop in a patient who already has another diagnosis (such as rheumatoid arthritis), and this may be a reason for apparently inadequate reduction of pain in response to treatment of the pre-existing disorder.

SOURCES AND SELECTION CRITERIA

We used recommendations from three current guidelines: those from the Canadian Pain Society, the Association of Scientific Medical Societies in Germany (AWMF, 2012; English version www.awmf.org/leitlinien/detail/ll/041-004.html), and the European League Against Rheumatism (EULAR, 2008). These were supplemented by data from current Cochrane reviews and a PubMed search for systematic reviews of drug treatment for fibromyalgia. We focused on drugs with a licence for use in the treatment of fibromyalgia in one or more major jurisdiction or drugs that are in widespread use for other indications.

In summary, consider fibromyalgia in a patient who has chronic widespread pain that is not fully explained by any other illness (such as cancer or inflammatory arthritis), especially if the pain is out of proportion to physical signs on examination or is associated with sleep disturbance, fatigue, or muscular tender points. Referral to a specialist is not necessary for the diagnosis of fibromyalgia,[21] but it should be considered if the diagnosis is uncertain—for example, if there is also joint swelling, rash, or Raynaud's phenomenon, which may suggest autoimmune diseases.

Treatment of fibromyalgia

Several outcome domains are of interest to patients—for example, pain, fatigue, and overall quality of life. All reported outcomes should be considered when interpreting the effects reported in systematic reviews of randomised controlled trials (RCTs). Tables 1-4 summarise the available data. For continuous outcome measures, to allow comparison across domains and between outcome measures standardised mean differences (SMD=between group difference/standard deviation at baseline) are reported. SMDs of 0.2, 0.5, and 0.8 indicate small, medium, and large effect sizes, respectively.[22]

What is the role of non-drug treatments?

Non-drug treatments can be physical or psychological (including education). Physical therapies include active (exercise) and passive approaches (joint manipulation and massage).

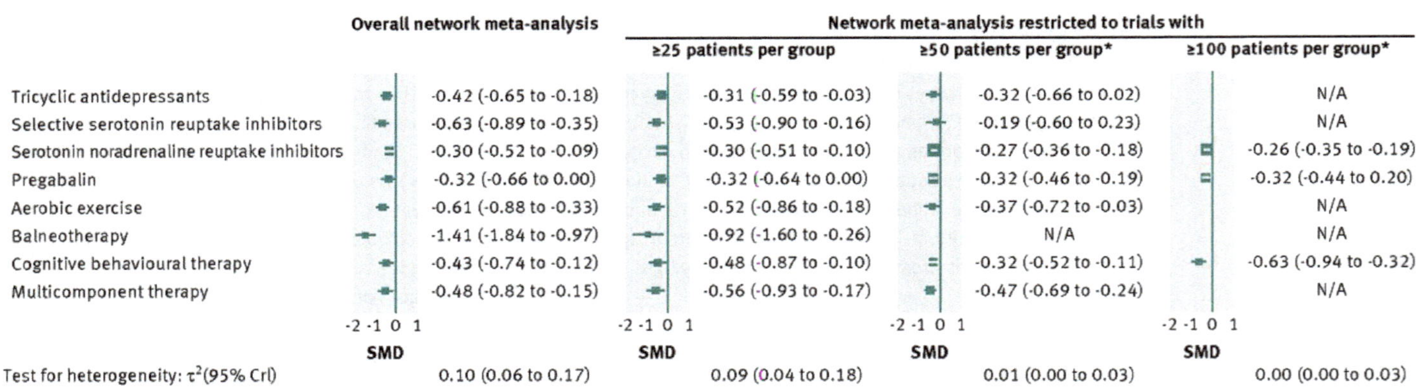

Fig 2 Comparative effect of interventions for pain in a network meta-analysis of trials of treatment of fibromyalgia. Reproduced, with permission, from *Annals of Rheumatic Diseases*.[24] 95% CrI=95% credibility interval; N/A=not available; SMD=standardised mean difference

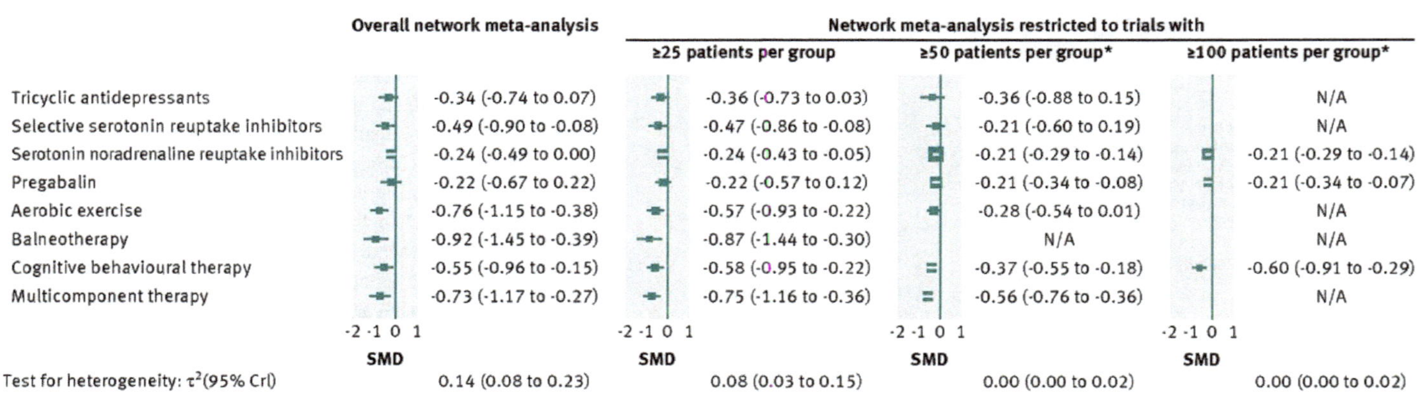

Fig 3 Comparative effect of different interventions for quality of life in a network meta-analysis of trials of treatment of fibromyalgia. Reproduced, with permission, from *Annals of Rheumatic Diseases*.[24] 95% CrI=95% credibility interval; N/A=not available; SMD=standardised mean difference

Physical therapies (active)

Exercise is commonly recommended in fibromyalgia,[35] and there is strong and moderate evidence to recommend specific types. A Cochrane systematic review of 34 studies that assessed the effects of exercise in fibromyalgia found that regular aerobic exercise (at least 20 min/day, 2-3 times a week for at least 2.5 weeks) improves wellbeing, aerobic capacity, tenderness, and pain compared with no aerobic exercise.[24] Strength training can also reduce pain and tenderness and improve wellbeing, although the quality of evidence is lower than for aerobic exercise (table 1).

Physical therapies (passive)

A systematic review and two clinical management papers provide moderate evidence for the effectiveness of balneotherapy (heated pool or spa treatments, with or without exercise).[24 35 36 37] Other passive therapies include manipulation, massage, electrotherapy and the use of ultrasound. These are often delivered by physiotherapists, osteopaths, or chiropractors. There is only weak evidence to support their use, partly because the data tend to come from small or pilot trials (table 1).[23 24 35]

Acupuncture

A Cochrane systematic review of nine trials provides evidence of low to moderate effectiveness of acupuncture.[25] It found that electro-acupuncture and manual acupuncture were no better than sham acupuncture for any outcome except stiffness at one month (six studies assessed as moderate quality, n=286). One study of moderate quality (n=58) that compared standard treatment with adjunctive acupuncture therapy found that acupuncture reduced pain in the short term (absolute reduction of 30%, range 21-39%). Four studies found no evidence for long term effectiveness for acupuncture versus control treatment after six months.[25] Acupuncture seemed safe and few adverse events were reported, but the risks are uncertain owing to the small number of participants in the trials.

Psychological therapies

In addition to exercise, guidelines for fibromyalgia recommend education and psychological and behavioural therapy. Education usually explains the nature of the condition and the underlying theory about the pain mechanisms involved in fibromyalgia. Education can provide the basis for psychological therapies, which are typically behaviourally based, such as cognitive behavioural therapy (CBT). CBT for pain management deals with the link between pain, thoughts (mood), and behaviour (negative coping strategies).[38]

There is strong and consistent evidence of the effectiveness of education for patients and carers (which usually includes advice on exercise), and most treatment programmes include some sort of education about fibromyalgia. Most studies cited used groups to deliver the education, and this may be an important element in the educational impact.[36 39]

Living and coping with fibromyalgia over a long period can have detrimental psychological effects. Mood can modulate pain perception.[38] One systematic review looked at 23 studies that included CBT as a treatment for fibromyalgia. Although the quality of evidence was low, it found that CBT was superior to control, with small benefits in reduction of pain (SMD 0.29, 0.17 to 0.49), negative mood (SMD 0.33, 0.17 to 0.49), and disability (SMD 0.30, 0.08 to 0.51) at the end of treatment. Improvements were maintained in the longer term (table 1).

Pain management and self management courses generally contain elements of education about fibromyalgia, exercise, and CBT, which are the three main non-drug treatments that are consistently effective for fibromyalgia.[40] A systematic review also provides strong evidence that combining these components and delivering multicomponent interventions (for example, those that include at least an exercise, education, and psychological component) has beneficial short term effects on key fibromyalgia symptoms.[27] CBT can be used to challenge negative or unhelpful thinking, thus

Table 1 Standardised effect sizes of non-drug treatments for fibromyalgia reported in systematic reviews

Intervention	Outcome	Standardised mean difference (95% CI)
Aerobic exercise (4 studies, n=223)[23]	Pain	0.81 (0.15 to 1.47)
Aerobic exercise (network meta-analysis)[24]	Pain	0.61 (0.33 to 0.88)*
Aerobic exercise (4 studies, n=253)[23]	Physical function	0.66 (0.41 to 0.92)
Aerobic exercise (5 studies, n=273)[23]	Depression	0.54 (0.14 to 0.94)
Aerobic exercise(network meta-analysis)[24]	Quality of life	0.76 (0.38 to 1.15)*
Strength training (2 studies, n=47)[23]	Physical function	0.52 (−0.07 to 1.10)
Strength training (2 studies, n=47)[23]	Global wellbeing	1.43 (0.76 to 2.10)
Balneotherapy (network meta-analysis)[24]	Pain	1.41 (0.12 to 0.74)
Balneotherapy (network meta-analysis)[24]	Quality of life	0.92 (0.39 to 1.45)
Acupuncture *v* sham control (2 studies, n=145)[25]	Pain	0.12 (−0.28 to 0.52)
Acupuncture *v* sham control (2 studies, n=145)[25]	Global wellbeing at 6 months	−0.03 (−0.87 to 0.81)
Acupuncture *v* sham control (2 studies, n=145)[25]	Sleep at 6 months	−0.09 (−0.44 to 0.26)
Acupuncture *v* sham control (2 studies, n=145)[25]	Fatigue at 6 months	−0.04 (−0.59 to 0.52)
Cognitive behavioural therapy (14 studies, n=893)[26]	Pain (long term)	0.40 (0.17 to 0.62)
Cognitive behavioural therapy (12 studies, n=792)[26]	Negative mood (long term)	0.43 (0.11 to 0.75)
Cognitive behavioural therapy (6 studies, n=429)[26]	Fatigue (long term)	0.46 (0.15 to 0.77)
Cognitive behavioural therapy (10 studies, n=735)[26]	Disability (long term)	0.52 (0.18 to 0.86)
Cognitive behavioural therapy (network meta-analysis)[24]	Pain	0.43 (0.12 to 0.43)*
Cognitive behavioural therapy (network meta-analysis)[24]	Quality of life	0.55 (0.15 to 0.96)*
Multicomponent therapy (network meta-analysis)[24]	Pain	0.48 (0.12 to 0.74)*
Multicomponent therapy (network meta-analysis)[24]	Quality of life	0.73 (0.27 to 1.17)*
Multicomponent therapy (5 studies, n=261)[27]	Pain	0.37 (0.13 to 0.62)
Multicomponent therapy (3 studies, n=162)[27]	Fatigue	0.85 (0.20 to 1.5)
Multicomponent therapy (4 studies, n=234)[27]	Depressive symptoms	0.67 (0.26 to 1.08)

**95% credibility interval rather than 95% confidence interval.*

enhancing the effects of other interventions—for example, by countering fear that exercise will worsen pain.

There is also moderate evidence from a systematic review and a summation of reviews of the benefit of mind-body therapies, including hypnotherapy, biofeedback, and stress reduction.[35]

How effective are drugs in the treatment of fibromyalgia?

Drugs for fibromyalgia include analgesics, opioids, and antidepressants. Some drugs, such as pregabalin, gabapentin, and serotonin and noradrenaline reuptake inhibitors (for example, milnacipran and duloxetine), alter levels or the function of neurotransmitters. Different drugs may be more or less effective for different manifestations of the disorder. The choice of drug should be discussed with the patient and should target the most troublesome symptoms while taking into account any possible adverse events.[41] Multiple drugs are sometimes needed.[41]

Drugs for fibromyalgia may have apparent benefits and harms that are independent of their pharmacological action. One systematic review that pooled data from the control arms of RCTs conducted for licensing purposes found that 19% (17.4% to 19.9%) of patients had at least a 50% reduction in pain but that 11% (9.9% to 11.9%) stopped treatment owing to adverse events.[42] Similar findings are seen in the control arms of drug trials in other diseases.

Analgesics

Direct data to support the use of paracetamol or non-steroidal anti-inflammatory drugs (NSAIDs) in fibromyalgia are limited.[37] In a population survey of 1799 patients with rheumatic diseases, including fibromyalgia, 60% reported preferring NSAIDs to paracetamol and 14% preferred paracetamol to NSAIDs.[43] Any decision to advise NSAIDs or paracetamol needs to take account of patient preference, comorbidities, and adverse effects.[37 41]

Opioids

The only opioid with evidence for effectiveness in fibromyalgia is tramadol (and tramadol combined with paracetamol). For tramadol on its own, the evidence is restricted to one crossover trial (n=12), which compared a single dose of intravenous tramadol with placebo over a two hour follow-up period.[44] There is only one RCT (n=315) of tramadol combined with paracetamol and this found a benefit on pain at three months (table 2).[45] Tramadol may have an additional analgesic effect through enhancing serotonin release and inhibiting noradrenaline reuptake.[28 30] Although widely prescribed in primary care, there is no evidence to support the use of preparations containing weak opioids, such as codeine or dihydrocodeine, for fibromyalgia. Use of potent opioids should be avoided because of the risk of producing iatrogenic addiction.[41] Opioids do not have a specific UK product licence for use in fibromyalgia but are licensed for the treatment of pain, including the pain of fibromyalgia. The *BNF* classifies tramadol as a strong opioid, whereas Canadian fibromyalgia guidelines draw a distinction between tramadol and potent opioids.[41]

Antidepressant drugs

Many systematic reviews of RCTs show that antidepressants are effective in the treatment of fibromyalgia.[32 41] One review found pooled SMDs, compared with placebo, of 0.43 (0.30 to 0.55) for pain, 0.13 (0.01 to 0.26) for fatigue, 0.32 (0.18 to 0.46) for sleep, 0.26 (0.12 to 0.39) for depressed mood, and 0.31 (0.20 to 0.42) for quality of life (table 3).[32] However, in the UK, none of these drugs is licensed for use in fibromyalgia.

A network meta-analysis of RCTs found that tricyclic antidepressants reduced pain (SMD 0.42, 0.18 to 0.65) but did not significantly affect quality of life (SMD 0.34, −0.07 to 0.74).[24] Another network meta-analysis found that the relative risk for a 30% reduction in pain from tricyclic

Table 2 Relative risk of improvement with drugs for fibromyalgia reported in systematic reviews

Intervention	Outcome	RR (95% CI)*
Analgesics		
Tramadol + paracetamol (network meta-analysis)[28]	Pain	RR30: 1.62 (1.16 to 2.36)
Tramadol + paracetamol (network meta-analysis)[28]	Pain	RR50: 1.91 (1.23 to 3.07)
Antidepressants		
Tricyclic antidepressants (network meta-analysis)[28]	Pain	RR30: 1.18 (0.41 to 2.98)
Amitriptyline[29]	Pain	RR: 2.9 (1.7 to 4.9)†
Fluoxetine (network meta-analysis)[28]	Pain	RR30: 1.84 (1.15 to 3.15)‡
Duloxetine (network meta-analysis)[28]	Pain	RR30: 1.64 (1.32 to 2.04)‡
Duloxetine (network meta-analysis)[28]	Pain	RR50: 1.82 (1.32 to 2.50)‡
Duloxetine (5 studies, n=1894)[30]	Pain	RR30: 1.33 (1.18 to 1.51)
Duloxetine (5 studies, n=1884)[30]	Pain	RR50: 1.59 (1.35 to 1.88)
Milnacipran (5 studies, n=4110)[30]	Pain	RR30: 1.38 (1.25 to 1.51)
Milnacipran (5 studies, n=4110)[30]	Pain	RR50: 1.44 (1.28 to 1.62)
Antiepileptics		
Gabapentin (1 study, n=150)[31]	Pain	RR30: 1.23 (0.65 to 2.33)
Gabapentin (1 study, n=150)[31]	Pain	RR50: 1.6 (1.01 to 2.53)§
Gabapentin (network meta-analysis)[28]	Pain	RR30: 1.65 (1.11 to 2.39)§
Pregabalin (5 studies, n=3259)[31]	Pain	RR30: 1.37 (1.22 to 1.53)
Pregabalin 300 mg (network meta-analysis)	Pain	RR30: 1.36 (1.14 to 1.64)‡
Pregabalin (5 studies, n=3259)[31]	Pain	RR50: 1.59 (1.33 to 1.90)
Pregabalin 300 mg (network meta-analysis)[28]	Pain	RR50: 1.29 (0.89 to 1.89)‡
Pregabalin (5 studies, n=3183)[31]	Global impression of change: much/very much improved	RR: 1.23 (1.33 to 1.55)

**RR=Relative risk of improvement (95% confidence interval); RR30=relative risk of 30% improvement (95% credible interval); RR50=relative risk of 50% improvement (95% credible interval).*

†Effect size not specified.

‡95% credible interval.

§Pooled analysis all studies; dose range 150-600 mg/day.

antidepressants was 1.18 (95% credible interval 0.41 to 2.98).[28] For amitriptyline alone one meta-analysis found a 2.9 (95% confidence interval 1.7 to 4.9) relative risk for an unspecified pain reduction.[29] A network meta-analysis of RCTs found that, compared with placebo, selective serotonin reuptake inhibitors had an SMD of 0.63 (0.35 to 0.89) for pain and 0.49 (0.08 to 0.90) for quality of life.[24] Another network meta-analysis found that the relative risk for a 30% improvement in pain was 1.84 (95% credible interval 1.15 to 3.15) for fluoxetine and 1.64 (95% credible interval 1.32 to 2.04[28]) for duloxetine. A systematic review found that the SMD for duloxetine was 0.32 (95% confidence interval 0.22 to 0.41) for pain, 0.12 (0.02 to 0.23) for fatigue, 0.24 (0.12 to 0.37) for sleep problems, and 0.26 (0.16 to 0.37) for depression (table 3).[30] The same systematic review found that the SMD for milnacipran was 0.20 (0.13 to 0.26) for pain, 0.14 (0.08 to 0.21) for fatigue, −0.02 (−0.10 to 0.05) for sleep problems, and 0.11 (0.04 to 0.17) for depression (table 3).[30] Use of amitriptyline, fluoxetine, paroxetine, duloxetine, milnacipran, and moclobemide (a monamine oxidase inhibitor) is supported by guideline recommendations.[37 41] Moclobemide should probably be avoided owing to a high incidence of adverse events. Milnacipran is not marketed in the UK. Duloxetine is not licensed for use in fibromyalgia in the UK. Both duloxetine and milnacipran have US Food and Drug Administration approval for use in fibromyalgia, whereas in Canada only duloxetine is approved.[41]

Anticonvulsant drugs

Several systematic reviews of multiple RCTs show that the second generation anticonvulsant pregabalin is effective in the treatment of fibromyalgia.[31 34] A review of trials of pregabalin (150-600 mg/day) versus placebo found an SMD for pain of 0.28 (0.20 to 0.35), for fatigue 0.17 (0.09 to 0.25), and for sleep problems and anxiety 0.35 (0.27 to 0.43).[31] The risk ratio for a 50% pain reduction was 1.59 (1.33 to 1.90).[31] A network meta-analysis found that when compared with placebo, pregabalin 300 mg had a relative risk for 30% improvement in pain of 1.36 (95% credible interval 1.14 to 1.64).[28] A third review found the number needed to treat

Table 3 Standardised effect sizes of drugs for fibromyalgia reported in systematic reviews

Intervention	Outcome	Standardised mean difference (95% CI)
Antidepressants		
Antidepressants (22 studies, n=2296)[32]	Pain	0.43 (0.30 to 0.55)
Antidepressants (14 studies, n=1435)[32]	Fatigue	0.13 (0.01 to 0.26)
Antidepressants (13 studies, n=1006)[32]	Sleep	0.32 (0.18 to 0.46)
Antidepressants (10 studies, n=887)[32]	Depressed mood	0.26 (0.12 to 0.39)
Antidepressants (12 studies, n=1766)[32]	Quality of life	0.31 (0.20 to 0.42)
Tricyclic antidepressants (network meta-analysis)[24]	Pain	0.42 (0.18 to 0.65)
Tricyclic antidepressants (network meta-analysis)[24]	Quality of life	0.34 (−0.07 to 0.74)
SSRIs (network meta-analysis)[24]	Pain	0.63 (0.35 to 0.89)
SSRIs (network meta-analysis)[24]	Quality of life	0.49 (0.08 to 0.90)
SNRIs (network meta-analysis)[24]	Pain	0.30 (0.09 to 0.25)
SNRIs (network meta-analysis)[24]	Quality of life	0.24 (0.00 to 0.49)
Duloxetine (5 studies, n=1925)[30]	Pain	0.32 (0.22 to 0.41)
Duloxetine (4 studies, n=1568)[30]	Fatigue	0.12 (0.02 to 0.23)
Duloxetine (2 studies, n=996)[30]	Sleep problems	0.24 (0.12 to 0.37)
Duloxetine (5 studies, n=1570)[30]	Depression	0.26 (0.16 to 0.37)
Milacipran (5 studies, n=4087)[30]	Pain	0.20 (0.13 to 0.26)
Milnacipran (5 studies, n=4088)[30]	Fatigue	0.14 (0.08 to 0.21)
Milnacipran (4 studies, n=3085)[30]	Sleep problems	−0.02 (−0.10 to 0.05)
Milnacipran (5 studies, n=4088)[30]	Depression	0.11 (0.04 to 0.17)
Antiepileptics		
Gabapentin (1 study, n =119)[31]	Pain	0.49 (0.13 to 0.86)
Gabapentin (1 study, n =119)[31]	Sleep problems	0.71 (0.34 to 1.08)
Gabapentin (1 study, n=119)[31]	Depression	0.53 (0.16 to 0.89)
Gabapentin (1 study, n=119)[31]	Health related quality of life	0.66 (0.29 to 1.03)
Pregabalin (5 studies, n=3252)* [31]	Pain	0.28 (0.20 to 0.35)
Pregabalin (5 studies, n=3195)* [31]	Fatigue	0.17 (0.09 to 0.25)
Pregabalin (5 studies, n=3193)* [31]	Sleep problems	0.35 (0.27 to 0.43)
Pregabalin (5 studies, n=3212)* [31]	Depression	0.09 (0.01 to 0.16)
Pregabalin (4 studies, n=2724)* [31]	Health related quality of life	0.17 (0.09 to 0.26)

**Pooled analysis all studies; dose range 150-600 mg/day.*

Table 4 Absolute effect sizes of drugs for fibromyalgia reported in systematic reviews

Intervention	Outcome	NNT (95% CI)*
Antidepressants		
Duloxetine (60 mg, 2 studies, n=528)[33]	Pain	NNT30=6 (3 to 12)
Duloxetine (60 mg, 2 studies, n=528)[33]	Pain	NNT50=8 (4 to 21)
Antiepileptics		
Gabapentin (1 study, n=150)[34]	Pain	NNT30=5.4 (2.9 to 31)
Pregabalin (300 mg, 4 studies, n=1374)[34]	Pain	NNT30=9.2 (6.3 to 17)
Pregabalin (300 mg, 4 studies, n=1374)[34]	Pain	NNT50=14 (9.0 to 33)
Pregabalin (300 mg, 4 studies, n=1354)[34]	Global impression change: very good or excellent	NNT=11 (7.3 to 26)
Pregabalin (300 mg, 4 studies, n=1354)[34]	Global impression change: excellent	NNT=16 (9.9 to 37)

**NNT=number needed to treat for a benefit; NNT30/50=NNT for a 30%/50% improvement; CI=confidence interval.*

with pregabalin 300 mg for a 30% reduction in pain intensity was 9.2 (95% confidence interval 6.3 to 17) and for a very good or excellent change the number needed to treat was 11 (7.3 to 26).[34]

A systematic review found one trial comparing gabapentin to placebo (n=150); compared with placebo the relative risk for a 30% improvement from gabapentin was 1.60 (1.01 to 2.53).[31]

Neither pregabalin nor gabapentin has a licence for use in fibromyalgia in the UK. Pregabalin is approved for treating fibromyalgia in the US and Canada. Guideline recommendations support the use of pregabalin or gabapentin.[37 41]

Other drugs

Many other drugs have been suggested for use in fibromyalgia. However, these drugs are used in specialist settings only and reviewing them is beyond the scope of this article

How strong is the evidence from clinical trials in fibromyalgia?

Most trials include a large proportion of women and white patients.[24] In addition, many trials have extensive exclusion factors, including psychiatric illness and chronic physical illness.[24] Thus, many patients with fibromyalgia seen in routine clinical practice may not be represented in the trial data. Because follow-up is typically short, it is not possible to comment on the risks and benefits of drug treatment beyond six months. Substantially more participants contribute to meta-analyses of different drugs than to meta-analyses of non-drug interventions. Typically, the published effect sizes of drug treatments on pain and quality of life for people living with fibromyalgia are small to moderate.[24]

The authors of a network meta-analysis concluded that the benefits of drug treatments were of questionable clinical value and that there was only limited evidence for non-drug treatments.[24] Once trials with fewer than 50 subjects per arm are excluded there is only evidence of effectiveness for one serotonin noradrenaline reuptake inhibitor (duloxetine) and pregabalin (for both pain and quality of life). Figures 2 and 3 summarise the results of this network analysis.

It may be misleading to describe effect sizes as small, moderate, large, however, because this may not relate to the individual patient. Expressing effectiveness as number needed to treat to obtain a specified outcome may be more useful clinically.[46] Clinicians and patients also need to recognise that in many cases treatment will be ineffective. If no worthwhile effect is seen after an adequate trial of a drug, it should be stopped and an alternative drug tried.[47] In the absence of any evidence for what may be an adequate trial we suggest four weeks at the full recommended dose (or the highest dose the patient can tolerate). The dose will need to be titrated upwards from a low starting point in many patients.

Tables 2-4 provide a summary of effect sizes and numbers needed to treat for several drugs commonly used in fibromyalgia.

AR is supported by the National Institute for Health Research University College London Hospitals Biomedical Research Centre. MU's contribution benefited from facilities funded through Birmingham Science City Translational Medicine Clinical Research and Infrastructure Trials Platform, with support from Advantage West Midlands.

ADDITIONAL EDUCATIONAL RESOURCES

Resources for healthcare professionals

- Arthritis Research UK (www.arthritisresearchuk.org/arthritis-information/conditions/fibromyalgia.aspx)—Useful leaflet on fibromyalgia; can be helpful to show this to patients during the consultation
- Canadian national guidelines (http://fmguidelines.ca)—Canadian guidelines for the diagnosis and management of fibromyalgia
- German guidelines (www.awmf.org/leitlinien/detail/ll/041-004.html)—German guidelines for fibromyalgia (including English version)

Resources for patients

- Arthritis Research UK (www.arthritisresearchuk.org/arthritis-information/conditions/fibromyalgia.aspx)—Useful leaflet on fibromyalgia available in paper form or on the web

TIPS FOR NON-SPECIALISTS

- Fibromyalgia often occurs in patients with an existing condition such as inflammatory arthritis or osteoarthritis. In such patients, if the degree of pain is not explained by the known diagnosis, consider whether there may also be an element of fibromyalgia
- It is important to explain that the aim of treatment is not to cure fibromyalgia but to reduce symptoms and improve quality of life. Some pain is likely to persist despite treatment
- In patients with fibromyalgia, individual drugs are often ineffective or cause side effects so it is important to consider a change in drug or a switch to non-drug approaches, such as cognitive behavioural therapy or exercise

QUESTIONS FOR FUTURE RESEARCH

- Why is fibromyalgia diagnosed so much more often in women than in men?
- Is the combination of drugs with cognitive behavioural therapy or exercise (or both) more effective than treatment with either modality alone?
- Which abnormalities of central pain processing are most important in patients with fibromyalgia and can understanding this lead to better treatment strategies?

Contributors: All three authors wrote the text and agreed the final version of the manuscript. MU wrote the section on drug treatments and created tables 2-4. DC wrote the section on non-drug treatments and created table 1. AR had the idea for the review, recruited the other authors, wrote the other sections, and is guarantor.

Competing interests: We have read and understood the BMJ Group policy on declaration of interests and declare the following interests: None.

Provenance and peer review: Commissioned; externally peer reviewed.

1 Wolfe F. Fibromyalgia wars. *J Rheumatol* 2009;36:671-8.
2 Wolfe F, Smythe HA, Yunus MB, Bennett RM, Bombardier C, Goldenberg DL, et al. The American College of Rheumatology 1990 criteria for the classification of fibromyalgia. report of the multicenter criteria committee. *Arthritis Rheum* 1990;33:160-72.
3 Wolfe F, Ross K, Anderson J, Russell IJ, Hebert L. The prevalence and characteristics of fibromyalgia in the general population. *Arthritis Rheum* 1995;38:19-28.
4 Croft P, Rigby AS, Boswell R, Schollum J, Silman A. The prevalence of chronic widespread pain in the general population. *J Rheumatol* 1993;20(4):710-3.
5 Haq SA, Darmawan J, Islam MN, Uddin MZ, Das BB, Rahman F, et al. Prevalence of rheumatic diseases and associated outcomes in rural and urban communities in Bangladesh: a COPCORD study. *J Rheumatol* 2005;32:348-53.

6 Wolfe F, Clauw DJ, Fitzcharles MA, Goldenberg DL, Hauser W, Katz RS, et al. Fibromyalgia criteria and severity scales for clinical and epidemiological studies: a modification of the ACR preliminary diagnostic criteria for fibromyalgia. *J Rheumatol* 2011;38:1113-22.
7 Vincent A, Lahr BD, Wolfe F, Clauw DJ, Whipple MO, Oh TH, et al. Prevalence of fibromyalgia: a population-based study in Olmsted County, Minnesota, utilizing the Rochester epidemiology project. *Arthritis Care Res* 2013;65:786-92.
8 Wolfe F, Brahler E, Hinz A, Hauser W. Fibromyalgia prevalence, somatic symptom reporting, and the dimensionality of polysymptomatic distress: results from a survey of the general population. *Arthritis Care Res* 2013;65:777-85.
9 Ablin J, Neumann L, Buskila D. Pathogenesis of fibromyalgia–a review. *Joint Bone Spine* 2008;75:273-9.
10 Phillips K, Clauw DJ. Central pain mechanisms in the rheumatic diseases: future directions. *Arthritis Rheum* 2013;65:291-302.
11 McBeth J, Macfarlane GJ, Benjamin S, Silman AJ. Features of somatization predict the onset of chronic widespread pain: results of a large population-based study. *Arthritis Rheum* 2001;44:940-6.
12 Arnold LM, Fan J, Russell IJ, Yunus MB, Khan MA, Kushner I, et al. The fibromyalgia family study: a genome-wide linkage scan study. *Arthritis Rheum* 2013;65:1122-8.
13 Julien N, Goffaux P, Arsenault P, Marchand S. Widespread pain in fibromyalgia is related to a deficit of endogenous pain inhibition. *Pain* 2005;114:295-302.
14 Russell IJ, Orr MD, Littman B, Vipraio GA, Alboukrek D, Michalek JE, et al. Elevated cerebrospinal fluid levels of substance P in patients with the fibromyalgia syndrome. *Arthritis Rheum* 1994;37:1593-601.
15 Russell IJ, Vaeroy H, Javors M, Nyberg F. Cerebrospinal fluid biogenic amine metabolites in fibromyalgia/fibrositis syndrome and rheumatoid arthritis. *Arthritis Rheum* 1992;35:550-6.
16 Valdes M, Collado A, Bargallo N, Vazquez M, Rami L, Gomez E, et al. Increased glutamate/glutamine compounds in the brains of patients with fibromyalgia: a magnetic resonance spectroscopy study. *Arthritis Rheum* 2010;62:1829-36.
17 Annemans L, Wessely S, Spaepen E, Caekelbergh K, Caubere JP, Le Lay K, et al. Health economic consequences related to the diagnosis of fibromyalgia syndrome. *Arthritis Rheum* 2008;58:895-902.
18 Hughes G, Martinez C, Myon E, Taieb C, Wessely S. The impact of a diagnosis of fibromyalgia on health care resource use by primary care patients in the UK: an observational study based on clinical practice. *Arthritis Rheum* 2006;54:177-83.
19 Wolfe F, Clauw DJ, Fitzcharles MA, Goldenberg DL, Katz RS, Mease P, et al. The American College of Rheumatology preliminary diagnostic criteria for fibromyalgia and measurement of symptom severity. *Arthritis Care Res* 2010;62:600-10.
20 Tan EM, Feltkamp TE, Smolen JS, Butcher B, Dawkins R, Fritzler MJ, et al. Range of antinuclear antibodies in "healthy" individuals. *Arthritis Rheum* 1997;40:1601-11.
21 Ferrari R, Russell AS. A questionnaire using the modified 2010 American College of Rheumatology criteria for fibromyalgia: specificity and sensitivity in clinical practice. *J Rheumatol* 2013;40:1590-5.
22 Cohen J. Statistical power analysis for the behavioral sciences. Laurence Earlsbaum Associates, 1988.
23 Busch AJ, Barber KA, Overend TJ, Peloso PM, Schachter CL. Exercise for treating fibromyalgia syndrome. *Cochrane Database Syst Rev* 2007;4:CD003786.
24 Nuesch E, Hauser W, Bernardy K, Barth J, Juni P. Comparative efficacy of pharmacological and non-pharmacological interventions in fibromyalgia syndrome: network meta-analysis. *Ann Rheum Dis* 2013;72:955-62.
25 Deare JC, Zheng Z, Xue CC, Liu JP, Shang J, Scott SW, et al. Acupuncture for treating fibromyalgia. *Cochrane Database Syst Rev* 2013;5:CD007070.
26 Bernardy K, Klose P, Busch AJ, Choy EH, Hauser W. Cognitive behavioural therapies for fibromyalgia. *Cochrane Database Syst Rev* 2013;9:CD009796.
27 Hauser W, Bernardy K, Arnold B, Offenbacher M, Schiltenwolf M, et al. Efficacy of multicomponent treatment in fibromyalgia syndrome: a meta-analysis of randomized controlled clinical trials. *Arthritis Rheum* 2009;61:216-24.
28 Roskell NS, Beard SM, Zhao Y, Le TK. A meta-analysis of pain response in the treatment of fibromyalgia. *Pain Pract* 2011;11:516-27.
29 Moore RA, Derry S, Aldington D, Cole P, Wiffen PJ. Amitriptyline for neuropathic pain and fibromyalgia in adults. *Cochrane Database Syst Rev* 2012;12:CD008242.
30 Hauser W, Urrutia G, Tort S, Uceyler N, Walitt B. Serotonin and noradrenaline reuptake inhibitors (SNRIs) for fibromyalgia syndrome. *Cochrane Database Syst Rev* 2013;1:CD010292.
31 Uceyler N, Sommer C, Walitt B, Hauser W. Anticonvulsants for fibromyalgia. *Cochrane Database Syst Rev* 2013;10:CD010782.
32 Hauser W, Bernardy K, Uceyler N, Sommer C. Treatment of fibromyalgia syndrome with antidepressants: a meta-analysis. *JAMA* 2009;301:198-209.
33 Lunn MP, Hughes RA, Wiffen PJ. Duloxetine for treating painful neuropathy, chronic pain or fibromyalgia. *Cochrane Database Syst Rev* 2014;1:CD007115.
34 Wiffen PJ, Derry S, Moore RA, Aldington D, Cole P, Rice AS, et al. Antiepileptic drugs for neuropathic pain and fibromyalgia–an overview of Cochrane reviews. *Cochrane Database Syst Rev* 2013;11:CD010567.
35 Hauser W, Thieme K, Turk DC. Guidelines on the management of fibromyalgia syndrome–a systematic review. *Eur J Pain* 2010;14:5-10.
36 Goldenberg DL, Burckhardt C, Crofford L. Management of fibromyalgia syndrome. *JAMA* 2004;292:2388-95.
37 Carville SF, Arendt-Nielsen S, Bliddal H, Blotman F, Branco JC, Buskila D, et al. EULAR evidence-based recommendations for the management of fibromyalgia syndrome. *Ann Rheum Dis* 2008;67:536-41.
38 Beck JS. Cognitive therapy. Guildford Press, 1995.
39 Burckhardt CS, Goldenberg DL, Crofford LJ, Gerwin RD, Gowans S, Jackson K, et al. Guideline for the management of fibromyalgia syndrome. Pain in adults and children. American Pain Society, 2005.
40 Cedraschi C, Desmeules J, Rapiti E, Baumgartner E, Cohen P, Finckh A, et al. Fibromyalgia: a randomised, controlled trial of a treatment programme based on self management. *Ann Rheum Dis* 2004;63:290-6.
41 Fitzcharles MA, Ste-Marie PA, Goldenberg DL, Pereira JX, Abbey S, Choiniere M, et al. Canadian guidelines for the diagnosis and management of fibromyalgia syndrome, 2012, 2012. www.canadianpainsociety.ca/pdf/Fibromyalgia_Guidelines_2012.pdf.
42 Hauser W, Sarzi-Puttini P, Tolle TR, Wolfe F. Placebo and nocebo responses in randomised controlled trials of drugs applying for approval for fibromyalgia syndrome treatment: systematic review and meta-analysis. *Clin Exp Rheumatol* 2012;30(6 suppl 74):78-87.
43 Wolfe F, Zhao S, Lane N. Preference for nonsteroidal antiinflammatory drugs over acetaminophen by rheumatic disease patients: a survey of 1799 patients with osteoarthritis, rheumatoid arthritis, and fibromyalgia. *Arthritis Rheum* 2000;43:378-85.
44 Biasi G, Manca S, Manganelli S, Marcolongo R. Tramadol in the fibromyalgia syndrome: a controlled clinical trial versus placebo. *Int J Clin Pharmacol Res* 1998;18:13-9.
45 Bennett RM, Kamin M, Karim R, Rosenthal N. Tramadol and acetaminophen combination tablets in the treatment of fibromyalgia pain: a double-blind, randomized, placebo-controlled study. *Am J Med* 2003;114:537-45.
46 Froud R, Underwood M, Carnes D, Eldridge S. Clinicians' perceptions of reporting methods for back pain trials: a qualitative study. *Br J Gen Pract* 2012;62:e151-9.
47 Moore A, Derry S, Eccleston C, Kalso E. Expect analgesic failure; pursue analgesic success. *BMJ* 2013;346:f2690.

Complex regional pain syndrome

Stephen Bruehl, professor

Department of Anesthesiology, Vanderbilt University School of Medicine, Nashville, TN 37212, USA

Correspondence to: S Bruehl Stephen.Bruehl@vanderbilt.edu

Cite this as: *BMJ* 2015;350:h2730

DOI: 10.1136/bmj.h2730

http://www.bmj.com/content/351/bmj.h2730

ABSTRACT

Complex regional pain syndrome is a chronic pain condition characterized by autonomic and inflammatory features. It occurs acutely in about 7% of patients who have limb fractures, limb surgery, or other injuries. Many cases resolve within the first year, with a smaller subset progressing to the chronic form. This transition is often paralleled by a change from "warm complex regional pain syndrome," with inflammatory characteristics dominant, to "cold complex regional pain syndrome" in which autonomic features dominate. Multiple peripheral and central mechanisms seem to be involved, the relative contributions of which may differ between individuals and over time. Possible contributors include peripheral and central sensitization, autonomic changes and sympatho-afferent coupling, inflammatory and immune alterations, brain changes, and genetic and psychological factors. The syndrome is diagnosed purely on the basis of clinical signs and symptoms. Effective management of the chronic form of the syndrome is often challenging. Few high quality randomized controlled trials are available to support the efficacy of the most commonly used interventions. Reviews of available randomized trials suggest that physical and occupational therapy (including graded motor imagery and mirror therapy), bisphosphonates, calcitonin, subanesthetic intravenous ketamine, free radical scavengers, oral corticosteroids, and spinal cord stimulation may be effective treatments. Multidisciplinary clinical care, which centers around functionally focused therapies is recommended. Other interventions are used to facilitate engagement in functional therapies and to improve quality of life.

Introduction

Complex regional pain syndrome (CRPS) is a chronic pain condition characterized by spontaneous and evoked regional pain, usually beginning in a distal extremity, that is disproportionate in magnitude or duration to the typical course of pain after similar tissue trauma.[1]

CRPS is distinguished from other chronic pain conditions by the presence of signs indicating prominent autonomic and inflammatory changes in the region of pain. In its most severe form, patients present with a limb displaying extreme hyperalgesia and allodynia (normally non-painful stimuli such as touch or cold are experienced as painful); obvious changes to skin color, skin temperature, and sweating relative to the unaffected side; edema and altered patterns of hair, skin, or nail growth in the affected region; reduced strength; tremors; and dystonia.[2] Altered body perception and proprioception may also be present, reflected in reduced limb positioning accuracy, delays in recognizing limb laterality, abnormal referred sensations and tactile perception, and altered subjective mental representations of the affected limb.[3 4 5 6 7 8] The syndrome is often associated with serious impairments in activities of daily living and ability to function.[9 10 11 12]

First recognized as a distinct pain condition during the American civil war,[13] CRPS has been known since that time by various names, including reflex neurovascular dystrophy, neuroalgodystrophy, shoulder-hand syndrome, reflex sympathetic dystrophy, and causalgia.

The dramatic nature of its presentation, limited understanding of its mechanisms, and frequent lack of response to intervention has led to clinical confusion and misunderstanding in the past. Research into CRPS and consequently understanding of the condition have grown extensively in the past 20 years, although understanding remains incomplete. Even now, the simple question of whether complex regional pain syndrome should be classified as a neuropathic pain condition remains a subject of debate among experts in the area.[14 15]

As currently conceptualized, CRPS is subdivided into type I and type II on the basis of absence or presence, respectively, of clinical signs of major peripheral nerve injury (such as nerve conduction study abnormalities). Despite this clinical distinction, core diagnostic features are identical across both subtypes, which adds to the confusion about the role of neuropathic mechanisms.

This review summarizes the current state of knowledge about CRPS, including its epidemiology, pathophysiological mechanisms, diagnosis, natural course, prevention, and treatment. Although complete understanding of the syndrome remains a work in progress, this review aims to dispel some misunderstandings that have continued despite recent advances.

Incidence

Two questions about the incidence of CRPS are of interest. The first is how commonly the condition occurs in the general population, and the second is how commonly it occurs after injuries that are known to trigger it.

Incidence in the general population

Two retrospective population based studies have assessed the incidence of CRPS in the general population. Both found that it is three to four times more common in women than in men, more commonly affects the upper limbs, and peaks in incidence at 50-70 years of age.[16 17] Estimates from both studies reflect the 1994 International Association for the Study of Pain (IASP) diagnostic criteria for CRPS.[18] In a study conducted in the United States, incidence rates of CRPS type I and CRPS type II were reported as 5.46 per 100 000 person years and 0.82 per 100 000 person years, respectively.[16] A population study in the Netherlands reported an incidence of CRPS type I and type II combined (based on clinician diagnoses of CRPS confirmed against 1994 IASP criteria in 93% of cases) of 26.2 cases per 100 000 person years[17]—more than four times higher than that noted in the US sample.

More specific diagnostic criteria were adopted in 2012 as the new international standard for the diagnosis of CRPS by the IASP (box 1),[1] and these criteria have been shown to reduce CRPS diagnostic rates by about 50%.[17 19 20] The earlier estimates may therefore provide an upper limit of the incidence of CRPS as currently defined in the general population. The US Food and Drug Administration and the European Medicines Agency have granted CRPS an orphan disease designation on the basis of their determination that fewer than 200000 people in the US and fewer than 154000 people in the European Union are affected each year.[21 22]

Incidence after injury

In the general population, CRPS seems to occur most often after fracture (>40% of CRPS cases in two population based studies[16 17]), although sprains, contusions, crush injuries, and surgery are also known triggers.[2] The best information on the incidence of CRPS after injury comes from two large prospective studies of fracture patients (n=596; n=1549).[23 24] Using the most restrictive research version of the 2012 IASP criteria,[25] the incidence of CRPS was 3.8-7.0% within four months of fracture.[23 24]

A slightly higher incidence (8.3%) was reported in a large (n=301) prospective study of patients undergoing carpal tunnel release.[26] In summary, only a minority of people develop CRPS even after the most common precipitating event—fracture. The fact that some people develop CRPS and others with similar injuries do not underlies the importance of understanding the pathophysiological mechanisms of CRPS.

Sources and selection criteria

The PubMed database was searched from 1985 to 1 October 2014 using the terms "complex regional pain syndrome", "reflex sympathetic dystrophy", "causalgia", "CRPS", and "RSD". Bibliographies of articles were also searched for other relevant studies. A selective narrative review is provided below that does not incorporate a systematic quality assessment of the literature. Studies presented below are those that the author judged to be representative of the highest methodological quality (for example, prospective studies) or most relevant to the topics discussed.

Pathophysiology

In contrast to past attempts to reduce CRPS to a single mechanism (such as sympathetically maintained pain),[27] it is now generally agreed that the syndrome is caused by a multifactorial process involving both peripheral and central mechanisms.[28 29] Although there is evidence for a role of each of the mechanisms below in the development or expression of CRPS (box 2), little is known experimentally about how these mechanisms might interact to produce CRPS. Given the diversity of presentations seen in CRPS, the relative contributions of different mechanisms probably differ across individual patients and even within patients over time. The figure provides a speculative model of interacting mechanisms involved in the development of CRPS.

Factors related to the initiating injury

Although CRPS is reported to occur without clear antecedent injury (or no specific injury that is recalled by the patient) in a small number of cases, most cases occur after known tissue injury. One key mechanistic question that is still debated is: what aspects of the initiating injury trigger the development of CRPS?

One important trigger seems to be the extent to which a proinflammatory and immunological response is elicited by the initiating injury. Evidence from animal fracture models of CRPS type I suggest that changes after injury, such as B cell activation and increased interleukin 1β (IL-1β) and substance P signaling, are crucial for the development of CRPS.[53 54 55]

A recent human study suggests that after injury persistently raised concentrations of osteoprotegerin, an osteoclastogenesis inhibitory factor, may also have a role in determining whether tissue injury resolves normally or evolves into CRPS.[104] On the basis of findings in a different animal model of CRPS type I,[35] ischemic reperfusion injury and related microvascular disease in deep tissues after injury have also been suggested as triggers for the onset of CRPS.[36] These processes have been shown to produce similar inflammatory responses and clinical characteristics (allodynia, hyperalgesia, edema, and altered vasoconstriction) to those seen in acute CRPS.[35 37]

It has also been suggested that nerve injury itself may trigger CRPS. A clinical distinction is made between CRPS type I and CRPS type II, with CRPS type II being distinguished by evidence of peripheral nerve injury. Nonetheless, similar injuries can trigger both CRPS subtypes, and the nature of

BOX 1 CURRENT INTERNATIONAL ASSOCIATION FOR THE STUDY OF PAIN CLINICAL DIAGNOSTIC CRITERIA FOR COMPLEX REGIONAL PAIN SYNDROME[1]

- Continuing pain, which is disproportionate to any inciting event
- Must report at least one symptom in three of the four following categories*:
  - Sensory: Reports of hyperalgesia and/or allodynia
  - Vasomotor: Reports of temperature asymmetry and/or skin color changes and/or skin color asymmetry
  - Sudomotor/edema: Reports of edema and/or sweating changes and/or sweating asymmetry
  - Motor/trophic: Reports of decreased range of motion and/or motor dysfunction (weakness, tremor, dystonia) and/or trophic changes (hair, nails, skin)
- Must display at least one sign at time of evaluation in two or more of the following categories*:
  - Sensory: Evidence of hyperalgesia (to pinprick) and/or allodynia (to light touch or deep somatic pressure, or joint movement)
  - Vasomotor: Evidence of temperature asymmetry and/or skin color changes and/or asymmetry
  - Sudomotor/edema: Evidence of edema and/or sweating changes and/or sweating asymmetry
  - Motor/trophic: Evidence of decreased range of motion and/or motor dysfunction (weakness, tremor, dystonia) and/or trophic changes (hair, nails, skin)
- There is no other diagnosis that better explains the signs and symptoms

**For research settings in which it is desirable to maximize specificity, a more stringent research diagnostic decision rule requires all four of the symptom categories and at least two of the sign categories to be positive for diagnostic criteria to be met.*

BOX 2 POSSIBLE MECHANISMS INVOLVED IN COMPLEX REGIONAL PAIN SYNDROME

- Nerve injury[31 32 33 34]
- Ischemic reperfusion injury or oxidative stress[35 36 37 38 39 40]
- Central sensitization[41 42 43]
- Peripheral sensitization[44 45]
- Altered sympathetic nervous system function or sympatho-afferent coupling[46 47 48 49 50 51 52]
- Inflammatory and immune related factors[53 54 55 56 57 58 59 60 61 62 63 64 65 66 67 68 69 70 71 72 73 74 75 76 77]
- Brain changes[78 79 80 81 82 83 84 85 86 87 88 89]
- Genetic factors[90 91 92]
- Psychological factors and disuse[93 94 95 96 97 98 99 100 101 102 103]

these injuries (for example, fractures, crush injuries, and surgery) could all plausibly be associated with some degree of nerve injury. Some studies report decreased C-fiber and A-δ fiber density in the affected limbs of patients with CRPS type I,[31 32 33] although others report that such changes were seen in only a subset (20%) of these patients.[34] These last findings suggest that such changes may reflect an occasional consequence or correlate of CRPS type I rather than a consistent cause.

Central and peripheral nociceptive sensitization

After tissue or nerve injury, the nervous system adapts in a manner that enhances responsiveness to pain and increases inflammation; this protects the injured area and leads to avoidance of activities that might cause further injury. These changes occur in both the peripheral and central nervous systems. Within the central nervous system, ongoing noxious input after tissue injury triggers central sensitization—an increase in the excitability of nociceptive neurons in the spinal cord that increase responsiveness to pain.[41] A role for central sensitization in CRPS is indicated by findings that the limb affected by CRPS (relative to unaffected limbs) exhibits increased temporal summation—a laboratory derived objective index believed to reflect central sensitization.[42 43] In the periphery, injury produces local changes to primary afferent fibers that increase background firing of nociceptors, increase firing in response to normally painful stimuli, and decrease the nociceptive firing threshold for thermal and mechanical stimuli.[44 45] Peripheral and central sensitization are mediated by the release of inflammatory mediators (such as bradykinin) and pronociceptive neuropeptides (such as substance P). In addition, proinflammatory cytokines also contribute to peripheral sensitization,[44] and the excitatory amino acid glutamate has a role in central sensitization through its activation of spinal N-methyl-D-aspartate (NMDA) receptors.[41 105] Both peripheral and central sensitization can contribute to some of the characteristic features of CRPS, including spontaneous pain, hyperalgesia, and allodynia.[41 44]

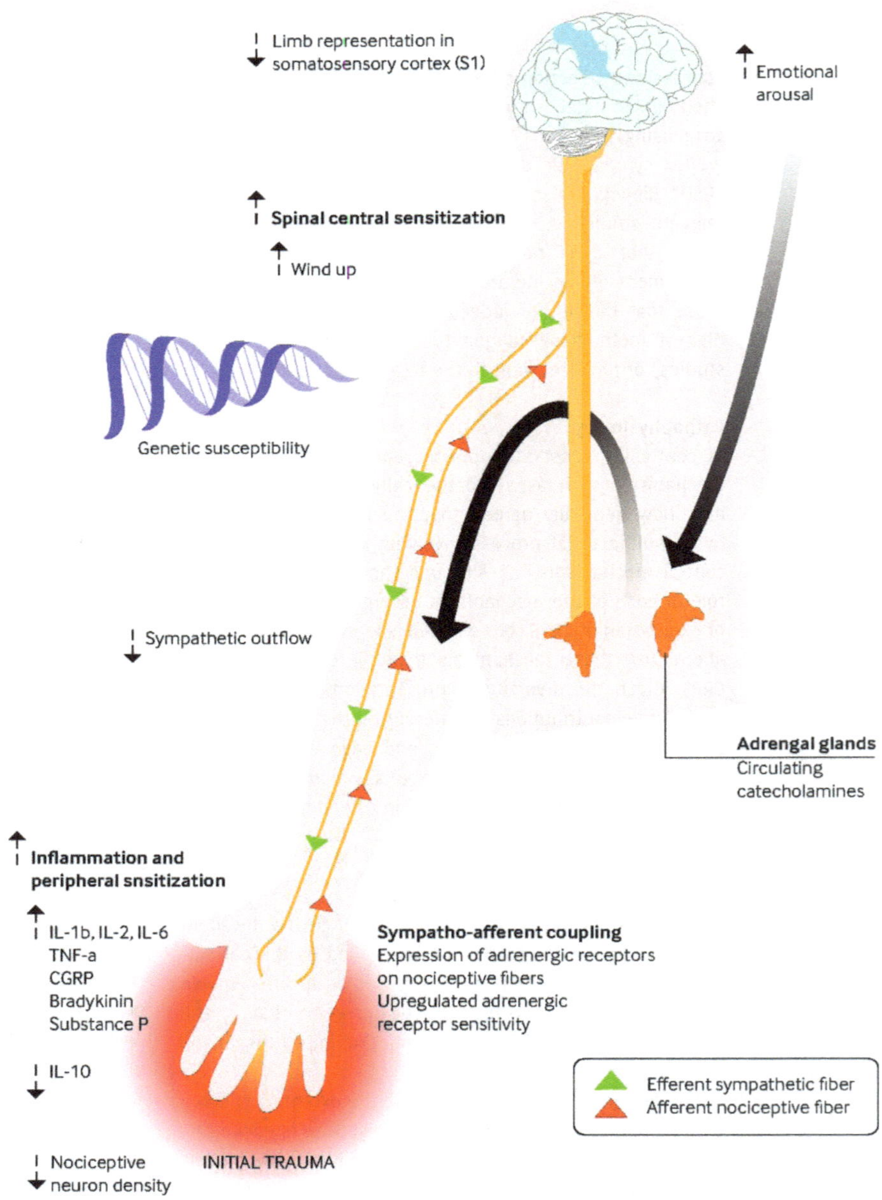

Speculative model of interacting mechanisms involved in the development of complex regional pain syndrome. CGRP=calcitonin gene related peptide; CRPS=complex regional pain syndrome; IL=interleukin; SNS=sympathetic nervous system; TNF=tumor necrosis factor. Adapted, with permission, from Bruehl[30]

Altered sympathetic nervous system function and sympatho-afferent coupling

Other nervous system changes after injury that may also contribute to CRPS are altered function of the sympathetic nervous system and possible sympatho-afferent coupling. It has long been assumed that the sympathetic nervous system plays a key role in CRPS—the most common older label for CRPS type I was "reflex sympathetic dystrophy." Because patients with chronic CRPS commonly present with a cold and sweaty limb, it was assumed that excessive sympathetic nervous system outflow was involved, and this was the rationale for using sympathetic ganglion blocks to reduce the symptoms of CRPS. However, a prospective study in patients early after fracture indicates that patients with reduced sympathetic nervous system outflow after injury are the ones at greatest risk of developing subsequent CRPS symptoms, with these changes noted to be bilateral despite unilateral injury.[46]

Other relevant nervous system changes after injury are more localized. One study found that within days after nerve injury, nociceptive fibers in the affected area, even when not directly injured, displayed increased firing in the presence of sympathetic nervous system activity.[106] Similar injuries have been shown to result in the expression of catecholamine receptors on nociceptive fibers,[47 48] leading to a situation in which sympathetic nervous system outflow or circulating catecholamines (released in response to pain or stress) might directly trigger firing of nociceptors (thus producing pain). This phenomenon is referred to as sympatho-afferent coupling.

Although this phenomenon has been directly observed in humans (through single nerve fiber recordings) in only a single case report,[49] it has been indirectly observed in several well controlled CRPS studies, suggesting it may play a role in the syndrome at least with regard to determining its severity.[50 51 52] Mechanisms by which reductions in function of the sympathetic nervous system after injury might eventually transform in many patients into a clinical picture more consistent with exaggerated sympathetic responses (reduced skin temperature, dusky skin color, increased sweating) are incompletely understood.

Inflammatory and immune related factors

Recent research has focused on the role of inflammatory and immune related mechanisms in CRPS, and animal models of CRPS type I also support a role for inflammatory mechanisms.[53 55] Evidence of the involvement of inflammatory mechanisms, especially in the acute phase, comes from studies documenting raised concentrations of proinflammatory neuropeptides and mediators (substance P, calcitonin gene related peptide, bradykinin) and cytokines (IL-1β, IL-2, and IL-6, and tumor necrosis factor α (TNF- α) in the systemic circulation, cerebrospinal fluid, and affected limbs of patients with CRPS.[56 57 58 59 60 61 62 63 64 65] These substances increase plasma extravasation (leading to edema), can produce vasodilation (leading to a warm red appearance in the affected area), and may increase hair growth and sweating.[66 67] Thus inflammatory mechanisms can induce several key clinical features of CRPS. There is evidence that the sympathetic nervous system is involved in facilitating inflammation after injury.[107 108] These findings show in principle that the various mechanisms that independently contribute to CRPS may interact.

Inflammation can be elicited not only enzymatically through the cyclo-oxygenase pathway, but also non-enzymatically through an oxidative stress pathway.[109 110] The ischemic reperfusion injury animal model described previously that reproduces many features of CRPS type I activates this oxidative stress pathway,[35 37] and pharmacological interventions that reduce oxidative stress in this model also reduce CRPS related symptoms.[35 38 39] Consistent with these animal data, at least one study indicates that indirect markers of oxidative stress are raised in patients with CRPS relative to healthy controls,[40] and this mechanism is the target of some CRPS interventions.

Although they did not specifically assess CRPS, several studies in patients undergoing limb surgery indicate that the use of a tourniquet (versus no tourniquet use) is associated with significantly greater pain and edema (up to six weeks after surgery); both of these features are characteristic of early CRPS.[111 112 113] Extended tourniquet use is known to be associated with ischemic reperfusion injury and raised oxidative stress.[35 114]

Immune related mechanisms are also probably involved in CRPS. For example, in a mouse model of CRPS type I, CRPS-like features including hyperalgesia and skin temperature changes emerge after limb fracture, but depletion of CD20+ B cells limits the development of these changes.[54] In humans, increased numbers of proinflammatory monocytes (CD14+ CD16+) and mast cells have been reported in patients with CRPS compared with healthy controls.[68 69 70] Altered innate immune responses (impaired neutrophil activity) have also been reported in patients with CRPS.[71]

Recent work suggests that antibodies from people with CRPS may be capable of transferring the condition to previously unaffected individuals, also supporting a role for immune mechanisms. IgG from patients with CRPS and a comparison group of healthy controls was given to mice that underwent a mild tissue injury.[72] Mice that received IgG from patients with CRPS, but not those that received IgG from controls, developed significant hyperalgesia and edema, both of which are characteristic of CRPS. Similar work found that IgG from patients with CRPS when injected into mice in the absence of any injury induced motor changes, another key characteristic of CRPS.[73] Data such as these have led to the suggestion that in some patients CRPS might be an expression of autoimmune processes.[74] This autoimmune model is further supported by the presence of autoantibodies directed against autonomic nervous system structures, including β2 adrenergic and muscarinic type 2 receptors, in a subset of patients with CRPS.[75 76 77]

Brain changes

Brain imaging studies over the past decade suggest that several brain changes are associated with CRPS. Two studies indicate that endogenous pain inhibitory pathways (opioid mediated) in the brain are impaired in patients with CRPS, with greater impairments associated with greater severity of pain.[78 79] For CRPS of the upper limb, reduced representation of the affected limb in both primary and secondary somatosensory cortices has also been consistently noted,[80 81 82 83] a finding supported by a recent meta-analysis.[84] However, new data suggest a surprising source for these effects—an increase in the somatosensory representation of the *unaffected* limb in patients with CRPS.[85]

Meta-analysis indicates that not only are there somatosensory changes in CRPS, but also motor changes, specifically disinhibition of the primary motor cortex.[86] Beyond changes in brain function, structural changes have also been noted—patients with CRPS showed reduced gray matter volume compared with healthy controls in brain regions underlying the affective component of pain (insula and cingulate cortex).[87]

Evidence suggests that the altered somatosensory representation in patients with CRPS can normalize with successful treatment.[88 89] In light of the similar normalization of specific brain changes (such as reduced gray matter volume) seen with successful treatment of other forms of chronic pain,[115 116] at least some of the brain changes in CRPS are likely to be an effect rather than a cause. Nonetheless, these changes seem to be related to symptom expression in some cases, as indicated by findings that clinical pain intensity in patients with CRPS is associated with the extent of some of the observed brain changes.[81 82 83]

Genetic factors

The role of genetic factors in CRPS is poorly understood. Studies that directly examined genetic associations with CRPS have identified several potential candidate polymorphisms, including those in genes encoding α1a adrenoceptors[90] and the HLA system (HLA-DQ8, HLA-B62).[91 92] The influences of the HLA system may be more prominent in patients with CRPS who have dystonia.[91 92] The identification of genetic influences in CRPS is made difficult by the heterogeneous phenotypic presentations related to different contributing mechanisms, as well as the need for large samples of a rare condition to produce conclusive findings.

Psychological factors

Psychological factors were assumed for many years to be involved in the development of CRPS partly because of clinical impressions that these patients were psychologically different from other patients with chronic pain. However, many studies suggest that patients with CRPS are not psychologically different from other patients with chronic pain and that psychological factors alone do not cause CRPS.[117] Comorbid axis I psychiatric disorders, mainly major depression, are common in patients with CRPS (24-49% of patients in various studies),[118 119 120] although their prevalence does not seem to be higher than in other chronic pain conditions.[119] Recent work suggests that patients with CRPS—particularly those with greater depression levels, higher pain intensity, and more functional impairments—have an increased risk of suicide.[118]

Evidence exists that psychological factors such as anxiety, depression, and anger expression may have a greater impact on pain in patients with CRPS than in those without.[93 94 95] This might be due to the effects of psychological distress on sympathetic nervous system arousal and catecholamine release and the potential impact of sympatho-afferent coupling on CRPS pain.[30]

In addition, prospective studies suggest that increased psychological distress in conjunction with physical injury might affect the later development of CRPS, or at least the condition's severity. In older patients undergoing total knee arthroplasty (n=77), greater increases in the extent of depressive symptoms from before surgery to one month after surgery predicted greater severity of CRPS symptoms at six month and 12 month follow-up.[96] Similar effects were seen for early increases in anxiety after surgery as a predictor of the severity of CRPS at six months.[96] In addition, preoperative anxiety significantly predicted the presence of a CRPS-like syndrome at one month after surgery, but not at three or six month follow-up.[97]

Similarly, in patients with an upper extremity fracture (n=50), higher anxiety (but not depression) two days after fracture predicted significantly higher risk of a diagnosis of CRPS at two to four month follow-up.[98] However, a larger prospective study of early post-fracture patients (n=596) found that none of the psychological variables assessed, including depression, predicted CRPS status at three month follow-up.[99] Nonetheless, the possible influence of anxiety on CRPS outcomes was not examined in this last study, leaving it unclear whether anxiety may contribute to the risk and severity of CRPS after injury.

Learnt disuse of the affected limb can also be considered a psychological factor, because it is typically the behavioral result of a desire to avoid pain, often driven by fear of future pain exacerbations.[100 101] Although expert opinion has long held that avoiding disuse and reactivating the affected limb are cornerstones of treatment,[121] only limited research supports this opinion. Results of one controlled human experimental study, however, do highlight the potential importance of disuse for CRPS. Among healthy people without CRPS (n=30), 28 days of upper limb casting in the absence of any injury resulted in pain with joint movement and several clinical features associated with CRPS, including hyperalgesia, hair growth changes (in a subset only), and skin temperature changes.[102]

The importance of disuse in the development of CRPS is also supported by recent animal work.[103] In a rat limb fracture model of CRPS type I, immobilization alone (casting) elicited the same increases in expression of inflammatory mediators (IL-1β, IL-6, TNF-α) and similar clinical changes (allodynia, temperature changes, and edema) as those elicited by limb fracture with casting.[103] Results such as these highlight the importance of early mobilization of the affected limb after injury to help prevent the development of chronic CRPS.

Natural course of CRPS

Clinical experience indicates that outcomes in patients with CRPS in tertiary pain care settings are often inadequate even with aggressive pain interventions. However, there are also reports suggesting high rates of resolution.[16] These discrepancies might be due to a substantial number of cases resolving with limited or no specific intervention early in the course of the condition, with a smaller subset of more persistent cases being seen in tertiary care pain clinics. A recent systematic review found some evidence to support this idea.[122]

Acute CRPS

The most convincing evidence would come from studies of untreated patients with CRPS because confounding with treatment effects would not influence the results. One study looked at the natural course of untreated CRPS.[123] Thirty patients with post-traumatic CRPS were followed without treatment for an average of 13 months after diagnosis; three patients were withdrawn from the study to be given treatment, and CRPS resolved over the course of the study in 26 of the 30 patients.[123] Some may be skeptical of this extraordinarily high rate of CRPS resolution, yet other studies support relatively high, if not quite so dramatic, resolution rates for acute CRPS (operationally defined in this review as CRPS <1 year in duration). For example, in a prospective series of 60 consecutive patients with tibial fracture who underwent standard care, 14 of the 18 patients diagnosed with CRPS at bone union were free of CRPS at one year follow-up.[124] Neither of the studies above used the 1994 or current IASP diagnostic criteria, which may have influenced the results. However, the US population study of CRPS described previously, which applied the 1994 IASP criteria, similarly found that 74% of diagnosed CRPS cases resolved with relatively conservative care.[16]

Chronic CRPS

In contrast to these findings for acute CRPS, the limited data on the natural course of well established chronic CRPS (operationally defined as CRPS of >1 year in duration) suggest much lower resolution rates even with specialty pain care.[125] In one large (n=102) retrospective longitudinal study of patients over an average six year follow-up period, 30% of patients reported resolution of chronic CRPS (diagnosed using the 1994 IASP criteria), 16% reported progressive deterioration, and the remaining 54% reported stable symptoms.[126]

These findings underscore the importance of understanding how patterns of CRPS change over time. One question is how quickly CRPS emerges after injury. Although such data are sparse, the mechanisms involved in the emergence of CRPS (such as injury related sympathetic nervous system changes, peripheral and central sensitization, inflammatory and immune responses to injury) suggest that the initial onset of symptoms should occur within the first few weeks of the initiating event.

A prospective study in a large sample of post-fracture patients found that CRPS was more commonly diagnosed at three months after cast removal than at cast removal, and that diagnosis rates decreased after three months.[23] This suggests that CRPS develops during a three to four month window after the initiating injury. The onset of CRPS symptoms after this three to four month window seems to be increasingly unlikely and difficult to explain mechanistically.

Delayed healing versus emerging CRPS

It is clinically accepted that early intervention in CRPS will lead to better outcomes, although there are few high quality data to support this view. The potential importance of early diagnosis and intervention raises the question of how to distinguish between normal but delayed healing versus emerging CRPS. In both cases, an inflammatory presentation (a warm, red, and hypersensitive limb) is common.[97] One potential discriminating factor is suggested by studies indicating that more severe pain early after fracture predicts those who will develop CRPS.[24] [127] This idea is supported by the finding that greater intensity of knee pain before surgery is a predictor of the development of CRPS after total knee arthroplasty.[97] Thus, a clinical rule of thumb might be that the greater the intensity of early pain and the longer a CRPS-like presentation persists, the more likely it is to be CRPS rather than delayed normal healing.

Warm and cold CRPS

Although not a formal diagnostic categorization, it is accepted that CRPS can be associated with two distinct presentations. "Warm CRPS" is associated with a warm, red, and edematous extremity, whereas "cold CRPS" presents with a cold, dusky, sweaty extremity. Acute CRPS is more often associated with a warm CRPS presentation, whereas chronic CRPS is more often characterized by a cold CRPS presentation,[128] although both subtypes can be seen in patients with CRPS of any duration.

Results of a retrospective longitudinal study reporting outcomes over an average eight year follow-up period suggest that CRPS is more likely to resolve in patients initially diagnosed with warm CRPS, the most common presentation in the acute CRPS phase, than in those initially diagnosed with cold CRPS.[129] Although there is no clear dividing line between acute and chronic CRPS, and these terms are inconsistently used in the literature, a recent prospective study of proinflammatory cytokines suggests that the inflammatory component that seems to underlie warm CRPS largely resolves within about 12 months of symptom onset, at least in patients on active treatment.[65]

This suggestion is supported by a recent report on patterns of cutaneous immune responses in patients with CRPS of different durations.[70] Local accumulation of mast cells was increased in CRPS of less than three months' duration but not in CRPS of longer than three months' duration.[70] Data regarding clinical features of CRPS also suggest that edema and warm or red skin, features caused by inflammatory processes, may become less prominent as the duration of CRPS increases.[2] [128] These findings parallel observations of a transition from warm CRPS to cold CRPS as the condition becomes more chronic. One cross sectional study suggests that sympatho-afferent coupling, which may contribute to the sympathetically maintained component of CRPS pain, may also diminish over time.[130] The prospective cytokine data above suggest that the transition from inflammatory warm CRPS to cold CRPS may start during the first year after injury, providing a possible marker for the transition from acute to chronic CRPS.

Traditional CPRS stages

CRPS often changes in character over time, but the changes are highly variable—no definitive sequence of stages occurs in all patients. For many years, clinical lore has held that there are three sequential stages of CRPS during which symptom patterns change in a consistent way.[131] Contrary to this idea, two studies using statistical pattern recognition techniques found that when patients are categorized by symptom patterns into three groups, there is no difference in pain duration between groups.[126] [132] Such findings argue more for CRPS subtypes rather than a uniform three stage sequential model.

CPRS spread

Data suggest that CRPS can spread outside of the originally affected limb,[133] although this is not a universal phenomenon. A population based epidemiological approach is needed to define how common such spreading is. However, available studies in this area are based on samples from pain clinics that may be biased by referral patterns. For example, clinics that specialize in treating patients with CRPS probably receive more referrals of patients with extensive spreading, so data from such clinics would overestimate the frequency of spreading. Given this caveat, a retrospective study in 185 patients with CRPS (from a clinic specializing in treating CRPS associated with movement disorders) found that 48% reported spreading to another limb.[134]

Studies of patterns of CRPS spread suggest that proximal spread from the initial distal site of CRPS is common,[135] although in some cases this may reflect secondary myofascial pain related to altered use of the limb. The largest systematic study of CRPS spreading (n=185) suggests that contralateral spread is most common (mirror image spread), followed by ipsilateral spread (for example, hand to foot), or diagonal spread.[134] All four limbs were affected in more than 29% of cases in this study. The two most common spreading patterns (ipsilateral and contralateral) developed on average 19 months or more after the initial onset of symptoms,[134] although another study suggests that spreading may occur earlier.[135] Depending on the pattern of spread, Van Rijn and colleagues' results indicated that 37-91% of cases of spreading CRPS occurred in the context of a second trauma.[134] Mechanisms of spreading are not well understood. However, research in patients with unilateral CRPS found evidence of bilateral facilitated neurogenic inflammation,[136] bone demineralization,[137] impaired sympathetic nervous system function,[46] brain changes,[138 139] and systemically circulating autoantibodies against autonomic structures.[76 77] This suggests that bilateral systemic alterations in unilateral CRPS could contribute to later contralateral spread.

Diagnosis

Because the pathophysiological mechanisms of CRPS are not fully understood, mechanism based diagnosis is not yet feasible. Therefore, the diagnosis of CRPS is based solely on clinical signs and symptoms. The fact that objective tests are not needed for diagnosis is directly related to the lack of definitive pathophysiological mechanisms in CRPS that could serve as a gold standard against which such tests could be referenced.

Additional objective testing (thermography, triple phase bone scan, quantitative sudomotor axon reflex test, or a trial sympathetic ganglion block) is not necessary to make the diagnosis, but in some cases may be used to support a clinical diagnosis. Because bone changes are not currently part of the diagnostic criteria used to define CRPS,[1] the value of a triple phase bone scan to support a diagnosis of CRPS is questionable. During the diagnostic process, objective medical tests may be needed to rule out other conditions that could account for the signs and symptoms that would otherwise be used to support a diagnosis of CRPS, given that CRPS is explicitly a diagnosis of exclusion (see criterion 4 in box 1). For example, duplex ultrasound testing might be used to rule out a deep vein thrombosis as the cause of pain, hypersensitivity, edema, and skin temperature changes in one limb.

In the past, the diagnosis of CRPS (known by various names) was inconsistent and based on multiple competing diagnostic criteria, none of which was widely accepted.[140 141 142 143] In 1994 the IASP published consensus based diagnostic criteria for CRPS that it was hoped would become the internationally accepted standard for both research and clinical care.[18] Subsequent validation research found problems with lack of specificity and potential overdiagnosis using these criteria,[2 25 144 145] prompting an international effort to develop and validate CRPS diagnostic criteria with high sensitivity but better specificity.[25] The resulting criteria (often referred to as the Budapest criteria) became the official IASP diagnostic criteria for CRPS in 2012.[1] Although the new criteria retained the sensitivity of the 1994 criteria (0.99 *v* 1.00), the new criteria are notably more specific (0.68) than the 1994 criteria (0.41), thereby reducing false positive diagnoses.[25]

Unlike the 1994 IASP criteria, a clinical diagnosis of CRPS using the 2012 IASP criteria (box 1) requires the presence of both subjective symptom reports and objective signs on clinical examination. Because objective signs are now needed to make a diagnosis and CRPS related autonomic features (color and temperature changes) may be labile, evaluation of diagnostic criteria over several clinic visits may in some cases help ensure accurate diagnosis. The 2012 IASP criteria include an alternative, more stringent, decision rule for the diagnosis of CRPS in research settings that requires symptoms in all four symptom categories and at least two of four sign categories. These research criteria result in even greater diagnostic specificity (0.79) to enhance homogeneity of research samples (fewer false positive diagnoses).[25]

Treatment

Although data suggest that many acute cases of CRPS may resolve with conservative medical care, expert opinion is that chronic CRPS is a challenging and complex biopsychosocial condition. Chronic CRPS is most likely to respond to comprehensive, integrated multidisciplinary treatment that includes medical, psychological, and physical and occupational therapy components.[121] While this view is supported by clinical experience in patients with CRPS and numerous clinical trials of such programs in other types of chronic pain,[146] no randomized controlled trials (RCTs) of multidisciplinary care have been performed specifically in patients with CRPS.

Within an evidence based medicine approach, it would be preferable to use outcome data from RCTs to guide the management of CRPS as much as possible. It is beyond the scope of this article to provide a thorough review and evaluation of the CRPS treatment literature, and readers are referred to several systematic reviews and meta-analyses.[147 148 149 150 151 152 153 154 155 156 157] However, the results of two more recent reviews are described below.[150 153] Although the number of clinical trials in CRPS has been increasing in recent years,[154] each of the reviews published between 1997 and 2013 has drawn two general conclusions:

- There is little support from high quality RCTs for many of the most common treatment approaches to CRPS
- More and better quality clinical trials are needed in CRPS.

A 2013 Cochrane review of treatment for CRPS found at least low quality evidence for the efficacy of bisphosphonates, calcitonin, subanesthetic intravenous ketamine, graded motor imagery and mirror therapy (specific physical therapy interventions, with mirror therapy effective particularly in acute post-stroke CRPS), and CRPS focused physical and occupational therapy.[153] It also found low and medium quality evidence, respectively, that sympathetic ganglion blockade with local anesthetics and intravenous regional blocks with guanethidine are ineffective. Evidence was deemed insufficient to draw conclusions for other interventions.

There is moderate overlap between this Cochrane review and results of a systematic review published by a consortium of CRPS experts in the Netherlands.[150] This review found at least some evidence for the efficacy of subanesthetic intravenous ketamine, free radical scavengers (topical dimethylsulfoxide, oral N-acetylcysteine, or oral vitamin C for prevention), oral corticosteroids, bisphosphonates, calcium channel blockers, intravenous ketanserine, surgical sympathectomy, spinal cord stimulation, and physical and occupational therapy.

Both reviews found that physical and occupational therapy, bisphosphonates, and subanesthetic ketamine might be effective, and there was some agreement that sympathetic blocks are probably ineffective. Of those treatments likely to be effective, functional therapies are described by experts as the cornerstone of CRPS treatment,[121] for reasons that are not entirely clear bisphosphonates are not routinely used, and ketamine is generally considered to be an experimental therapy and can be associated with serious side effects.

There is clearly a disconnect between clinical practice and the evidence base. This is underscored by the second review, which concludes that many standard treatments in clinical practice have no supporting evidence (absence of RCTs or negative trials) for efficacy in CRPS, including opioid analgesics, antidepressants, anticonvulsants, sympathetic ganglion blockade, or epidural sympathetic blockade using local anesthetics.[150]

In the absence of sufficient high quality evidence from RCTs to support treatment decisions, the clinical care of patients with CRPS must be guided by the collective experience of other clinicians, as reflected in standard practice (acknowledging that there may be regional biases towards particular treatments). It should be emphasized that clinical acceptance as part of standard care does not necessarily imply efficacy, unless also supported by RCTs. The table summarizes the treatments used in CRPS.

CRPS experts, even those who use more invasive interventional techniques, broadly agree that effective treatment should be functionally focused, centering around physical and occupational therapy designed to normalize use of the affected limb and mitigate problems related to disuse.[121] Best evidence suggests that mirror therapy and graded motor imagery should be included in these functional therapy protocols,[153 158] although a more recent trial of graded motor imagery in routine clinical practice (n=35) did not replicate the pain reducing effects seen in more highly controlled trials.[159] Limited research suggests that inclusion of an exposure therapy component to target fear of pain and fear of using the affected limb may also help.[160 161] Despite some evidence for their utility, the specific approaches above are not yet routinely included in functional therapy for CRPS except at specialty treatment centers.

HOW PATIENTS WERE INVOLVED IN THE CREATION OF THIS ARTICLE

The perspective of patients with complex regional pain syndrome (CRPS) was incorporated into the final article on the basis of comments made on an initial draft by a patient with CRPS and James Broatch, executive vice president/director of the Reflex Sympathetic Dystrophy Syndrome Association (RSDSA). The RSDSA is the primary CRPS patient advocacy organization in the United States.

Drug treatment

An initial trial of oral corticosteroids is often used in patients with acute phase CRPS to dampen the large inflammatory component believed to be common in the acute phase. Dosages of 30-40 mg per day of oral prednisolone for two weeks followed by a tapering period have been reported to be effective in acute CRPS.[162 163]

Other drugs commonly used in standard CRPS care include anticonvulsants (for example, gabapentin) and analgesic antidepressants (for example, duloxetine). One RCT suggests that gabapentin may have a small effect on pain in CRPS, with a somewhat larger effect on sensory deficits.[164]

The search strategy described above found no RCTs of the effects of antidepressants specifically in CRPS. Transdermal lidocaine patches applied to the affected area are a common component of early treatment, although no RCTs have evaluated their efficacy in CRPS. Each of these treatments is palliative rather than curative. Opioid analgesics are sometimes used if additional pain control is needed to facilitate engagement in functional therapies and resumption of more normal daily activities. Only one small RCT of opioid analgesics has included patients with CRPS (seven of 43 patients in the sample), with overall results indicating no significant analgesic effects of sustained release morphine (90 mg/day) over eight days.[165]

Ganglion blocks

In addition to oral and transdermal agents, if sympathetic ganglion blocks (stellate ganglion, lumbar sympathetic) have not already been used, and an initial trial indicates they provide sufficient relief to improve participation in

Summary of treatments for complex regional pain syndrome (CRPS)

Treatment	Category	Supporting RCT status
Multidisciplinary treatment	Standard	None
Physical and occupational therapy	Standard	Positive[150 153]
Oral corticosteroids (for acute CRPS)	Standard	Positive[150 162]
Anticonvulsants	Standard	Equivocal[164]
Analgesic antidepressants	Standard	None
Transdermal lidocaine	Standard	None
Opioids	Standard	None
Sympathetic nervous system blocks	Standard	Negative[150 153]
Spinal cord stimulation	Standard	Positive (<5 year efficacy)[167 168]
Pain focused psychological therapy	Standard	None
Graded motor imagery or mirror therapy	Uncommon	Positive[153 158]
Calcitonin	Uncommon	Positive[153]
Vitamin C (prevention after injury)	Uncommon	Positive[150 171-174 176]
Topical dimethylsulfoxide (DMSO)	Uncommon	Positive (warm CRPS)[150]
Oral N-acetylcysteine	Uncommon	Positive (cold CRPS)[150]
Bisphosphonates	Emerging	Positive[150 153 181-184]
Subanesthetic intravenous ketamine	Emerging	Positive[150 153 186 187]
Intravenous immunoglobulin	Emerging	Positive[189]
Oral tadalafil	Emerging	Positive[190]
Intrathecal baclofen (CRPS + dystonia)	Emerging	Positive[191]
Low dose oral naltrexone	Emerging	None

RCT=randomized controlled trial.

functional therapies, a series of several blocks at weekly intervals is often used. Sympathetic blocks have not been shown to have significant efficacy in patients with CRPS overall.[153] However, clinical experience and one small randomized trial (n=7) suggest that in some patients they may provide additional pain relief beyond the duration of action of the local anesthetics used (≥3 days[166]). There is no evidence that sympathetic blocks are curative for any patients.

Spinal cord stimulation

If after an extended trial (longer if CRPS is more acute) the above approach has not improved the patient's condition, it is common to move on to a trial of spinal cord stimulation. If this trial is successful, which it was in two thirds of patients (n=24/36) in the only RCT in these patients,[167] permanent implantation will follow, with continued emphasis on achieving improved function and normalizing daily activities. The one RCT of spinal cord stimulation in patients with CRPS (n=36 spinal cord stimulation; n=18 physical therapy) suggests it may be effective for pain reduction (but not necessarily functional improvement) for several years, but that efficacy is no greater than physical therapy alone five years after implantation.[167 168 169]

Psychological interventions

Given the psychosocial complexity of CRPS, it is generally agreed that inclusion of pain focused cognitive behavioral therapy is beneficial as part of standard care for chronic CRPS.[121 170] However, no RCT evidence is available specifically in patients with CRPS to support this belief.

Can CRPS be prevented?

Vitamin C

In the absence of efficacious treatments for CRPS, it would be preferable to prevent CRPS from developing. Several RCTs have been published on the use of vitamin C for the prevention of CRPS after limb fracture or surgery.[171 172 173 174 175] This treatment is based on the known antioxidant effects of vitamin C that could theoretically reduce the inflammatory mechanisms (related to oxidative stress) that are thought to contribute to acute CRPS. A meta-analysis of the first four published studies on this topic suggested that vitamin C significantly reduced the likelihood of CRPS developing after limb fracture or surgery (risk ratio 0.22, 0.12 to 0.39; n=616 for the vitamin C; n=449 for control),[176] with 500 mg vitamin C recommended daily for at least 45 days after injury or surgery. However, a recent large RCT (n=336) that used this protocol for the prevention of post-fracture CRPS found that vitamin C was associated with an increased incidence of CRPS at six weeks after fracture relative to placebo, with no effect at subsequent time points.[175] The potential utility of vitamin C in the prevention of CRPS is therefore unclear.

Ischemic reperfusion injury

Another potential means of prevention also relates to the possible role of oxidative stress (particularly in relation to ischemic reperfusion injury) in the development of CRPS. During limb surgery procedures, such as total knee arthroplasty, a tourniquet is routinely applied to the surgical limb to reduce blood loss, sometimes for as long as two hours. Given that ischemic reperfusion injury can occur on removal of the tourniquet, with its severity related to the duration of ischemia, minimizing the duration of tourniquet use during such procedures could potentially reduce the incidence of CRPS.

CRPS in children

Although clinical lore suggests that CRPS presents differently in children than in adults, there is no empirical evidence on such differences and this assumption has been questioned.[177] CRPS is currently diagnosed in children using the same 2012 IASP criteria that are used in adults. Two detailed clinical evaluation studies (n=20; n=42) suggest that the same objective signs are seen in children and adolescents with CRPS as are seen in adults, including allodynia and hyperalgesia, edema, skin color and temperature changes, and motor changes.[178 179]

Data from more than 100 children and adolescents with CRPS meeting the 2012 IASP diagnostic criteria indicated that these children exhibited more functional impairments and disability than those with other forms of chronic pain, consistent with the high levels of impairment often noted in adult patients with CRPS.[180] A longitudinal study of patients (n=42) diagnosed as having CRPS in childhood found that on follow-up in adulthood an average of 12 years later, 52% still experienced pain, with 36% having documented recurrences of CRPS.[179] This suggests that in many cases of childhood CRPS there may be no sustained recovery. These longitudinal data contrast with the common clinical assumption, not yet supported by high quality trials, that children with CRPS respond more favorably to conservative functionally focused care than do adults, in many cases with complete resolution of the condition.[177]

Emerging treatments

Several treatments for CRPS are emerging that go beyond the current standard of clinical care. The best supported of these is treatment with bisphosphonates, which several small RCTs suggest may be effective for CRPS.[181 182 183 184] The mechanistic relevance of treatment with bisphosphonates, which inhibit osteoclast activity, is suggested by recent work supporting a role for impaired bone metabolism in CRPS.[104] A definitive RCT of bisphosphonates is currently under way (ClinicalTrials.gov identifier: NCT02402530).

Other placebo controlled studies suggest that topical ketamine or a series of daily subanesthetic ketamine infusions may be useful in otherwise treatment resistant patients,[185 186 187] although liver injury has been noted with repeated ketamine infusions in some patients.[188] Additional experimental CRPS treatments supported by small RCTs include intravenous immunoglobulin (n=13),[189] oral tadalafil (n=24),[190] and intrathecal baclofen for CRPS related dystonia (n=36),[191] although high complication rates were noted with this last intervention.

An RCT of low dose naltrexone (an opioid antagonist) for CRPS is also currently ongoing. This intervention is based on the hypothetical ability of naltrexone to reduce glial inflammation by blocking Toll-like receptor 4, case reports suggesting efficacy in CRPS,[192] and positive results of a small RCT (n=31) in patients with fibromyalgia.[193]

Guidelines

Although several guidelines for the management of CRPS have been published over the past 20 years, evolving research and approaches to CRPS management make it particularly important to use the most recently developed

RESEARCH QUESTIONS

- How do the individual mechanisms shown to be associated with complex regional pain syndrome (CRPS) interact to produce the full syndrome?
- Do different subtypes of CRPS exist that reflect different underlying mechanisms?
- Can clinical signs and symptoms be clearly tied to underlying mechanisms?
- Do different CRPS subtypes, signs, and symptom patterns and different mechanisms predict differential responsiveness to specific treatments?

guidelines. General treatment guidelines have been published by groups in the Netherlands,[150] UK,[194] Germany,[195] and the US.[148] Guidelines with a specific focus on interventional pain procedures, which cover interventional approaches in greater detail than in the general treatment guidelines, are also available.[157] Although the emphasis of the guidelines differs, a relatively high degree of overlap exists across the general treatment guidelines. Some regional differences are apparent, however, with US guidelines providing little information on the antioxidant agents (such as dimethylsulfoxide) that are recommended treatments in the Dutch and German guidelines.[148 150 195] In addition, specific criteria (if any) used for systematically evaluating efficacy data differ across guidelines, which can lead to different recommendations being made. For example, guidelines that focus on interventional procedures have more positive conclusions about the efficacy of sympathetic nervous system blocks and recommend these in routine treatment,[157] whereas other guidelines have more negative conclusions about these blocks.[150] Such differences highlight the need to consider clinical biases that may affect the interpretation of CRPS guidelines.

Conclusion

Although CRPS is uncommon in the general population, it occurs in 4-7% of patients who have a limb fracture or limb surgery. In many cases, acute CRPS that is typically associated with a warm, red, and edematous presentation resolves with limited intervention. In a subset of patients, CRPS becomes chronic, often accompanied by a transition to a cold, dusky, and sweaty presentation. Initial symptoms typically emerge within weeks of injury, and the transition from acute to chronic CRPS usually occurs within the first year. Multiple mechanisms underlie CRPS, both peripheral and central, and these may differ across patients and even within patients over time. CRPS should be diagnosed on clinical grounds using the 2012 IASP diagnostic criteria.

Inadequate data are available to guide CRPS treatment solely on the basis of RCTs, although trials suggest that the most commonly used intervention (sympathetic blocks) is probably ineffective for the average patient. Support for the efficacy of spinal cord stimulation in CRPS derives from a single RCT. There is some evidence for the efficacy of physical and occupational therapy, bisphosphonates, subanesthetic ketamine, free radical scavengers, and corticosteroids (for acute CRPS). Analgesic antidepressants, anticonvulsants, and transdermal lidocaine are thought to be effective clinically, although their efficacy in CRPS has not been evaluated adequately in RCTs. It is clinically accepted that standard care should emphasize functional therapies that target disuse. Pharmacological, interventional, and psychological techniques are also used because they facilitate participation in functional therapies and ideally enhance quality of life. The number of clinical trials of CRPS specific interventions is growing, raising hope that more effective treatments may eventually emerge.

Competing interests: I have read and understood BMJ policy on declaration of interests and declare the following interests: I have received consulting fees from Eli Lilly, Grunenthal GmbH, and Thar Pharmaceuticals for assistance in the design of clinical trials of complex regional pain syndrome.

Provenance and peer review: Commissioned; externally peer reviewed.

1 International Association for the Study of Pain. Classification of chronic pain. 2nd edition (revised). www.iasp-pain.org/files/Content/ContentFolders/Publications2/ClassificationofChronicPain/Part_II-A.pdf.
2 Harden RN, Bruehl S, Galer BS, et al. Complex regional pain syndrome: are the IASP diagnostic criteria valid and sufficiently comprehensive? Pain1999;83:211-9.
3 Förderreuther S, Sailer U, Straube A. Impaired self-perception of the hand in complex regional pain syndrome (CRPS). Pain2004;110:756-61.
4 Lewis JS, Kersten P, McCabe CS, et al. Body perception disturbance: a contribution to pain in complex regional pain syndrome (CRPS). Pain2007;133:111-9.
5 Lewis JS, Kersten P, McPherson KM, et al. Wherever is my arm? Impaired upper limb position accuracy in complex regional pain syndrome. Pain2010;149:463-9.
6 Moseley GL. Why do people with complex regional pain syndrome take longer to recognize their affected hand? Neurology2004;62:2182-6.
7 McCabe CS, Haigh RC, Halligan PW, et al. Referred sensations in patients with complex regional pain syndrome type 1. Rheumatology (Oxford)2003;42:1067-73.
8 Cohen H, McCabe C, Harris N, et al. Clinical evidence of parietal cortex dysfunction and correlation with extent of allodynia in CRPS type 1. Eur J Pain.2013;17:527-38.
9 Geertzen JH, Dijkstra PU, van Sonderen EL, et al. Relationship between impairments, disability and handicap in reflex sympathetic dystrophy patients: a long-term follow-up study. Clin Rehabil1998;12:402-12.
10 Schasfoort FC, Bussmann JB, Zandbergen AM, et al. Impact of upper limb complex regional pain syndrome type 1 on everyday life measured with a novel upper limb-activity monitor. Pain2003;101:79-88.
11 Sharma A, Agarwal S, Broatch J, et al. A web-based cross-sectional epidemiological survey of complex regional pain syndrome. Reg Anesth Pain Med2009;34:110-5.
12 Van Velzen GA, Perez RS, van Gestel MA, et al. Health-related quality of life in 975 patients with complex regional pain syndrome type 1. Pain2014;155:629-34.
13 Mitchell SW, Morehouse GR, Keen WW. Gunshot wounds and other injuries of nerves. J B Lippincott, 1864.
14 Jensen TS, Baron R, Haanpää M, et al. A new definition of neuropathic pain. Pain2011;152:2204-5.
15 Oaklander AL, Wilson PR, Moskovitz PA, et al. Response to "A new definition of neuropathic pain." Pain2012;153:934-5.
16 Sandroni P, Benrud-Larson LM, McClelland RL, et al. Complex regional pain syndrome type I: incidence and prevalence in Olmsted county, a population-based study. Pain2003;103:199-207.
17 De Mos M, de Bruijn AG, Huygen FJ, et al. The incidence of complex regional pain syndrome: a population-based study. Pain2007;129:12-20.
18 Merskey H, Bogduk N. Classification of chronic pain: descriptions of chronic pain syndromes and definitions of pain terms. 2nd ed. IASP Press, 1994.
19 De Boer RD, Marinus J, van Hilten JJ, et al. Distribution of signs and symptoms of complex regional pain syndrome type I in patients meeting the diagnostic criteria of the International Association for the Study of Pain. Eur J Pain2011;15:830.e1-8.
20 Perez RS, Collins S, Marinus J, et al. Diagnostic criteria for CRPS I: differences between patient profiles using three different diagnostic sets. Eur J Pain2007;11:895-902.
21 European Medicines Agency. Public summary of opinion on orphan designation: zoledronic acid for the treatment of complex regional pain syndrome. 2013. www.ema.europa.eu/ema/index.jsp?curl=pages/medicines/human/orphans/2013/10/human_orphan_001271.jsp&mid=WC0b01ac058001d12b.
22 US Food and Drug Administration. Orphan drug designations and approvals. Neridronate. 2013. www.accessdata.fda.gov/scripts/opdlisting/oopd/OOPD_Results_2.cfm?Index_Number=372412.
23 Beerthuizen A, Stronks DL, Van't Spijker A, et al. Demographic and medical parameters in the development of complex regional pain syndrome type 1 (CRPS1): prospective study on 596 patients with a fracture. Pain2012;153:1187-92.
24 Moseley GL, Herbert RD, Parsons T, et al. Intense pain soon after wrist fracture strongly predicts who will develop complex regional pain syndrome: prospective cohort study. J Pain2014;15:16-23.
25 Harden RN, Bruehl S, Perez RS, et al. Validation of proposed diagnostic criteria (the "Budapest criteria") for complex regional pain syndrome. Pain2010;150:268-74.

26 Da Costa VV, de Oliveira SB, Fernandes Mdo C, et al. Incidence of regional pain syndrome after carpal tunnel release. Is there a correlation with the anesthetic technique? Rev Bras Anestesiol2011;61:425-33.
27 Roberts WJ. A hypothesis on the physiological basis for causalgia and related pains. Pain1986;24:297-311.
28 Jänig W, Baron R. Complex regional pain syndrome is a disease of the central nervous system. Clin Auton Res2002;12:150-64.
29 Jänig W, Baron R. Complex regional pain syndrome: mystery explained? Lancet Neurol2003;2:687-97.
30 Bruehl S. An update on the pathophysiology of complex regional pain syndrome. Anesthesiology2010;113:713-25.
31 Oaklander AL, Fields HL. Is reflex sympathetic dystrophy/complex regional pain syndrome type I a small-fiber neuropathy? Ann Neurol2009;65:629-38.
32 Oaklander AL, Rissmiller JG, Gelman LB, et al. Evidence of focal small-fiber axonal degeneration in complex regional pain syndrome-I (reflex sympathetic dystrophy). Pain2006;120:235-43.
33 Albrecht PJ, Hines S, Eisenberg E, et al. Pathologic alterations of cutaneous innervation and vasculature in affected limbs from patients with complex regional pain syndrome. Pain2006;120:244-66.
34 Kharkar S, Venkatesh YS, Grothusen JR, et al. Skin biopsy in complex regional pain syndrome: case series and literature review. Pain Physician2012;15:255-66.
35 Coderre TJ, Xanthos DN, Francis L, et al. Chronic post-ischemia pain (CPIP): a novel animal model of complex regional pain syndrome-type I (CRPS-I; reflex sympathetic dystrophy) produced by prolonged hindpaw ischemia and reperfusion in the rat. Pain2004;112:94-105.
36 Coderre TJ, Bennett GJ. A hypothesis for the cause of complex regional pain syndrome-type I (reflex sympathetic dystrophy): pain due to deep-tissue microvascular pathology. Pain Med2010;11:1224-38.
37 Xanthos DN, Bennett GJ, Coderre TJ. Norepinephrine-induced nociception and vasoconstrictor hypersensitivity in rats with chronic post-ischemia pain. Pain2008;137:640-51.
38 De Mos M, Laferrière A, Millecamps M, et al. Role of NFkappaB in an animal model of complex regional pain syndrome-type I (CRPS-I). J Pain2009;10:1161-9.
39 Ross-Huot MC, Laferrière A, Khorashadi M, et al. Glycemia-dependent nuclear factor κB activation contributes to mechanical allodynia in rats with chronic postischemia pain. Anesthesiology2013;119:687-97.
40 Eisenberg E, Shtahl S, Geller R, et al. Serum and salivary oxidative analysis in complex regional pain syndrome. Pain2008;138:226-32.
41 Ji RR, Woolf CJ. Neuronal plasticity and signal transduction in nociceptive neurons: implications for the initiation and maintenance of pathological pain. Neurobiol Dis2001;8:1-10.
42 Sieweke N, Birklein F, Riedl B, et al. Patterns of hyperalgesia in complex regional pain syndrome. Pain1999;80:171-7.
43 Eisenberg E, Chistyakov AV, Yudashkin M, et al. Evidence for cortical hyperexcitability of the affected limb representation area in CRPS: a psychophysical and transcranial magnetic stimulation study. Pain2005;113:99-105.
44 Cheng JK, Ji RR. Intracellular signaling in primary sensory neurons and persistent pain. Neurochem Res2008;33:1970-8.
45 Couture R, Harrisson M, Vianna RM, et al. Kinin receptors in pain and inflammation. Eur J Pharmacol2001;429:161-76.
46 Schürmann M, Gradl G, Zaspel J, et al. Peripheral sympathetic function as a predictor of complex regional pain syndrome type I (CRPS I) in patients with radial fracture. Auton Neurosci2000;86:127-34.
47 Drummond ES, Dawson LF, Finch PM, et al. Increased expression of cutaneous α1-adrenoceptors after chronic constriction injury in rats. J Pain2014;15:188-96.
48 Drummond PD, Drummond ES, Dawson LF, et al. Upregulation of α1-adrenoceptors on cutaneous nerve fibres after partial sciatic nerve ligation and in complex regional pain syndrome type II. Pain2014;155:606-16.
49 Jørum E, Ørstavik K, Schmidt R, et al. Catecholamine-induced excitation of nociceptors in sympathetically maintained pain. Pain2007;127:296-301.
50 Drummond PD, Finch PM, Skipworth S, et al. Pain increases during sympathetic arousal in patients with complex regional pain syndrome. Neurol2001;57:1296-303.
51 Ali Z, Raja SN, Wesselmann U, et al. Intradermal injection of norepinephrine evokes pain in patients with sympathetically maintained pain. Pain2000;88:161-8.
52 Baron R, Schattschneider J, Binder A, et al. Relation between sympathetic vasoconstrictor activity and pain and hyperalgesia in complex regional pain syndromes: a case-control study. Lancet2002;359:1655-60.
53 Li WW, Sabsovich I, Guo TZ, et al. The role of enhanced cutaneous IL-1beta signaling in a rat tibia fracture model of complex regional pain syndrome. Pain2009;144:303-13.
54 Li WW, Guo TZ, Shi X, et al. Autoimmunity contributes to nociceptive sensitization in a mouse model of complex regional pain syndrome. Pain2014;155:2377-89.
55 Guo TZ, Offley SC, Boyd EA, et al. Substance P signaling contributes to the vascular and nociceptive abnormalities observed in a tibial fracture rat model of complex regional pain syndrome type I. Pain2004;108:95-107.
56 Schinkel C, Gaertner A, Zaspel J, et al. Inflammatory mediators are altered in the acute phase of posttraumatic complex regional pain syndrome. Clin J Pain2006;22:235-9.
57 Schinkel C, Scherens A, Köller M, et al. Systemic inflammatory mediators in post-traumatic complex regional pain syndrome (CRPS I)—longitudinal investigations and differences to control groups. Eur J Med Res2009;14:130-5.
58 Alexander GM, van Rijn MA, van Hilten JJ, et al. Changes in cerebrospinal fluid levels of pro-inflammatory cytokines in CRPS. Pain2005;116:213-9.
59 Maihöfner C, Handwerker HO, Neundörfer B, et al. Mechanical hyperalgesia in complex regional pain syndrome: a role for TNF-alpha? Neurology2005;65:311-3.
60 Uçeyler N, Eberle T, Rolke R, et al. Differential expression patterns of cytokines in complex regional pain syndrome. Pain2007;132:195-205.
61 Wesseldijk F, Huygen FJ, Heijmans-Antonissen C, et al. Six years follow-up of the levels of TNF-alpha and IL-6 in patients with complex regional pain syndrome type 1. Mediators Inflamm2008;2008:469439.
62 Wesseldijk F, Huygen FJ, Heijmans-Antonissen C, et al. Tumor necrosis factor-alpha and interleukin-6 are not correlated with the characteristics of complex regional pain syndrome type 1 in 66 patients. Eur J Pain2008;12:716-21.
63 Birklein F, Schmelz M, Schifter S, et al. The important role of neuropeptides in complex regional pain syndrome. Neurology2001;57:2179-84.
64 Blair SJ, Chinthagada M, Hoppenstehdt D, et al. Role of neuropeptides in pathogenesis of reflex sympathetic dystrophy. Acta Orthop Belg1998;64:448-51.
65 Lenz M, Uçeyler N, Frettlöh J, et al. Local cytokine changes in complex regional pain syndrome type I (CRPS I) resolve after 6 months. Pain2013;154:2142-9.
66 Birklein F, Schmelz M. Neuropeptides, neurogenic inflammation and complex regional pain syndrome (CRPS). Neurosci Lett2008;437:199-202.
67 Schlereth T, Dittmar JO, Seewald B, et al. Peripheral amplification of sweating—a role for calcitonin gene-related peptide. J Physiol2006;576:823-32.
68 Ritz BW, Alexander GM, Nogusa S, et al. Elevated blood levels of inflammatory monocytes (CD14+ CD16+) in patients with complex regional pain syndrome. Clin Exp Immunol2011;164:108-17.
69 Huygen FJ, Ramdhani N, van Toorenenbergen A, et al. Mast cells are involved in inflammatory reactions during complex regional pain syndrome type 1. Immunol Lett2004;91:147-54.
70 Birklein F, Drummond PD, Li W, et al. Activation of cutaneous immune responses in complex regional pain syndrome. J Pain2014;15:485-95.
71 Kaufmann I, Eisner C, Richter P, et al. Psychoneuroendocrine stress response may impair neutrophil function in complex regional pain syndrome. Clin Immunol2007;125:103-11.
72 Tékus V, Hajna Z, Borbély É, et al. A CRPS-IgG-transfer-trauma model reproducing inflammatory and positive sensory signs associated with complex regional pain syndrome. Pain2014;155:299-308.
73 Goebel A, Leite MI, Yang L, et al. The passive transfer of immunoglobulin G serum antibodies from patients with longstanding complex regional pain syndrome. Eur J Pain2011;15:504.e1-6.
74 Goebel A, Blaes F. Complex regional pain syndrome, prototype of a novel kind of autoimmune disease. Autoimmun Rev2013;12:682-6.
75 Blaes F, Schmitz K, Tschernatsch M, et al. Autoimmune etiology of complex regional pain syndrome (M Sudeck). Neurology2004;63:1734-6.
76 Kohr D, Singh P, Tschernatsch M, et al. Autoimmunity against the β2 adrenergic receptor and muscarinic-2 receptor in complex regional pain syndrome. Pain2011;152:2690-700.
77 Kohr D, Tschernatsch M, Schmitz K, et al. Autoantibodies in complex regional pain syndrome bind to a differentiation-dependent neuronal surface autoantigen. Pain2009;143:246-51.
78 Freund W, Wunderlich AP, Stuber G, et al. The role of periaqueductal gray and cingulate cortex during suppression of pain in complex regional pain syndrome. Clin J Pain2011;27:796-804.
79 Klega A, Eberle T, Buchholz HG, et al. Central opioidergic neurotransmission in complex regional pain syndrome. Neurology2010;75:129-36.
80 Juottonen K, Gockel M, Silén T, et al. Altered central sensorimotor processing in patients with complex regional pain syndrome. Pain2002;98:315-23.
81 Pleger B, Tegenthoff M, Schwenkreis P, et al. Mean sustained pain levels are linked to hemispherical side-to-side differences of primary somatosensory cortex in the complex regional pain syndrome I. Exp Brain Res2004;155:115-9.
82 Pleger B, Ragert P, Schwenkreis P, et al. Patterns of cortical reorganization parallel impaired tactile discrimination and pain intensity in complex regional pain syndrome. Neuroimage2006;32:503-10.
83 Maihöfner C, Handwerker HO, Neundörfer B, et al. Patterns of cortical reorganization in complex regional pain syndrome. Neurology2003;61:1707-15.
84 Di Pietro F, McAuley JH, Parkitny L, et al. Primary somatosensory cortex function in complex regional pain syndrome: a systematic review and meta-analysis. J Pain2013;14:1001-18.
85 Di Pietro F, Stanton TR, Moseley GL, et al. Interhemispheric somatosensory differences in chronic pain reflect abnormality of the healthy side. Hum Brain Mapp2015;36:508-18.
86 Di Pietro F, McAuley JH, Parkitny L, et al. Primary motor cortex function in complex regional pain syndrome: a systematic review and meta-analysis. J Pain2013;14:1270-88.

87 Barad MJ, Ueno T, Younger J, et al. Complex regional pain syndrome is associated with structural abnormalities in pain-related regions of the human brain. J Pain2014;15:197-203.
88 Maihöfner C, Handwerker HO, Neundörfer B, et al. Cortical reorganization during recovery from complex regional pain syndrome. Neurology2004;63:693-701.
89 Pleger B, Tegenthoff M, Ragert P, et al. Sensorimotor retuning in complex regional pain syndrome parallels pain reduction. Ann Neurol2005;57:425-9.
90 Herlyn P, Müller-Hilke B, Wendt M, et al. Frequencies of polymorphisms in cytokines, neurotransmitters and adrenergic receptors in patients with complex regional pain syndrome type I after distal radial fracture. Clin J Pain2010;26:175-81.
91 De Rooij AM, Florencia Gosso M, Haasnoot GW, et al. HLA-B62 and HLA-DQ8 are associated with complex regional pain syndrome with fixed dystonia. Pain2009;145:82-5.
92 Van Rooijen DE, Roelen DL, Verduijn W, et al. Genetic HLA associations in complex regional pain syndrome with and without dystonia. J Pain2012;13:784-9.
93 Bruehl S, Husfeldt B, Lubenow TR, et al. Psychological differences between reflex sympathetic dystrophy and non-RSD chronic pain patients. Pain1996;67:107-14.
94 Bruehl S, Chung OY, Burns JW. Differential effects of expressive anger regulation on chronic pain intensity in CRPS and non-CRPS limb pain patients. Pain2003;104:647-54.
95 Bean DJ, Johnson MH, Kydd RR. Relationships between psychological factors, pain, and disability in complex regional pain syndrome and low back pain. Clin J Pain2014;30:647-53.
96 Harden RN, Bruehl S, Perez RS, et al. Development of a severity score for CRPS. Pain2010;151:870-6.
97 Harden RN, Bruehl S, Stanos S, et al. Prospective examination of pain-related and psychological predictors of CRPS-like phenomena following total knee arthroplasty: a preliminary study. Pain2003;106:393-400.
98 Dilek B, Yemez B, Kizil R, et al. Anxious personality is a risk factor for developing complex regional pain syndrome type I. Rheumatol Int2012;32:915-20.
99 Beerthuizen A, Stronks DL, Huygen FJ, et al. The association between psychological factors and the development of complex regional pain syndrome type 1 (CRPS1)—a prospective multicenter study. Eur J Pain2011;15:971-5.
100 De Jong JR, Vlaeyen JW, de Gelder JM, et al. Pain-related fear, perceived harmfulness of activities, and functional limitations in complex regional pain syndrome type I. J Pain2011;12:1209-18.
101 Marinus J, Perez RS, van Eijs F, et al. The role of pain coping and kinesiophobia in patients with complex regional pain syndrome type 1 of the legs. Clin J Pain2013;29:563-9.
102 Terkelsen AJ, Bach FW, Jensen TS. Experimental forearm immobilization in humans induces cold and mechanical hyperalgesia. Anesthesiology2008;109:297-307.
103 Guo TZ, Wei T, Li WW, et al. Immobilization contributes to exaggerated neuropeptide signaling, inflammatory changes, and nociceptive sensitization after fracture in rats. J Pain2014;15:1033-45.
104 Krämer HH, Hofbauer LC, Szalay G, et al. Osteoprotegerin: a new biomarker for impaired bone metabolism in complex regional pain syndrome? Pain2014;155:889-95.
105 Wang H, Kohno T, Amaya F, et al. Bradykinin produces pain hypersensitivity by potentiating spinal cord glutamatergic synaptic transmission. J Neurosci2005;25:7986-92.
106 Sato J, Perl ER. Adrenergic excitation of cutaneous pain receptors induced by peripheral nerve injury. Science1991;251:1608-10.
107 Jänig W, Levine JD, Michaelis M. Interactions of sympathetic and primary afferent neurons following nerve injury and tissue trauma. Prog Brain Res1996;113:161-84.
108 Li W, Shi X, Wang L, et al. Epidermal adrenergic signaling contributes to inflammation and pain sensitization in a rat model of complex regional pain syndrome. Pain2013;154:1224-36.
109 Basu S. F2-isoprostanes in human health and diseases: from molecular mechanisms to clinical implications. Antioxid Redox Signal2008;10:1405-34.
110 Evans AR, Junger H, Southall MD, et al. Isoprostanes, novel eicosanoids that produce nociception and sensitize rat sensory neurons. J Pharmacol Exp Ther2000;293:912-20.
111 Konrad G, Markmiller M, Lenich A, et al. Tourniquets may increase postoperative swelling and pain after internal fixation of ankle fractures. Clin Orthop Relat Res2005;433:189-94.
112 Omeroğlu H, Günel U, Biçimoğlu A, et al. The relationship between the use of tourniquet and the intensity of postoperative pain in surgically treated malleolar fractures. Foot Ankle Int1997;18:798-802.
113 Omeroğlu H, Uçaner A, Tabak AY, et al. The effect of using a tourniquet on the intensity of postoperative pain in forearm fractures. A randomized study in 32 surgically treated patients. Int Orthop1998;22:369-73.
114 Horlocker TT, Hebl JR, Gali B, et al. Anesthetic, patient, and surgical risk factors for neurologic complications after prolonged total tourniquet time during total knee arthroplasty. Anesth Analg2006;102:950-5.
115 Rodriguez-Raecke R, Niemeier A, Ihle K, et al. Brain gray matter decrease in chronic pain is the consequence and not the cause of pain. J Neurosci2009;29:13746-50.
116 Rodriguez-Raecke R, Niemeier A, Ihle K, et al. Structural brain changes in chronic pain reflect probably neither damage nor atrophy. PLoS One2013;8:e54475.
117 Beerthuizen A, van't Spijker A, Huygen FJ, et al. Is there an association between psychological factors and the complex regional pain syndrome type 1 (CRPS1) in adults? A systematic review. Pain2009;145:52-9.
118 Lee DH, Noh EC, Kim YC, et el. Risk factors for suicidal ideation among patients with complex regional pain syndrome. Psychiatry Invest2014;11:32-8.
119 Monti DA, Herring CL, Schwartzman RJ, et al. Personality assessment of patients with complex regional pain syndrome type I. Clin J Pain1998;14:295-302.
120 Rommel O, Malin JP, Zenz M, et al. Quantitative sensory testing, neurophysiological and psychological examination in patients with complex regional pain syndrome and hemisensory deficits. Pain2001;93:279-93.
121 Stanton-Hicks MD, Burton AW, Bruehl SP, et al. An updated interdisciplinary clinical pathway for CRPS: report of an expert panel. Pain Pract2002;2:1-16.
122 Bean DJ, Johnson MH, Kydd RR. The outcome of complex regional pain syndrome type 1: a systematic review. J Pain2014;15:677-90.
123 Zyluk A. The natural history of post-traumatic reflex sympathetic dystrophy. J Hand Surg Br1998;23:20-3.
124 Sarangi PP, Ward AJ, Smith EJ, et al. Algodystrophy and osteoporosis after tibial fractures. J Bone Joint Surg Br1993;75:450-2.
125 Schwartzman RJ, Erwin KL, Alexander GM. The natural history of complex regional pain syndrome. Clin J Pain2009;25:273-80.
126 De Mos M, Huygen FJ, van der Hoeven-Borgman M, et al. Outcome of the complex regional pain syndrome. Clin J Pain2009;25:590-7.
127 Jellad A, Salah S, Ben Salah Frih Z. Complex regional pain syndrome type I: incidence and risk factors in patients with fracture of the distal radius. Arch Phys Med Rehabil2014;95:487-92.
128 Birklein F, Riedl B, Sieweke N, et al. Neurological findings in complex regional pain syndromes—analysis of 145 cases. Acta Neurol Scand2000;101:262-9.
129 Vaneker M, Wilder-Smith OH, Schrombges P, et al. Patients initially diagnosed as "warm" or "cold" CRPS 1 show differences in central sensory processing some eight years after diagnosis: a quantitative sensory testing study. Pain2005;115:204-11.
130 Schattschneider J, Binder A, Siebrecht D, et al. Complex regional pain syndromes: the influence of cutaneous and deep somatic sympathetic innervation on pain. Clin J Pain2006;22:240-4.
131 Bonica JJ. Causalgia and other reflex sympathetic dystrophies. In: Bonica JJ, ed. Management of pain. 2nd ed. Lea and Febiger 1990:220-43.
132 Bruehl S, Harden RN, Galer BS, et al. Complex regional pain syndrome: are there distinct subtypes and sequential stages of the syndrome? Pain2002;95:119-24.
133 Veldman PH, Goris RJ. Multiple reflex sympathetic dystrophy. Which patients are at risk for developing a recurrence of reflex sympathetic dystrophy in the same or another limb. Pain1996;64:463-6.
134 Van Rijn MA, Marinus J, Putter H, et al. Spreading of complex regional pain syndrome: not a random process. J Neural Transm2011;118:1301-9.
135 Maleki J, LeBel AA, Bennett GJ, et al. Patterns of spread in complex regional pain syndrome, type I (reflex sympathetic dystrophy). Pain2000;88:259-66.
136 Leis S, Weber M, Schmelz M, et al. Facilitated neurogenic inflammation in unaffected limbs of patients with complex regional pain syndrome. Neurosci Lett2004;359:163-6.
137 Karacan I, Aydin T, Ozaras N. Bone loss in the contralateral asymptomatic hand in patients with complex regional pain syndrome type 1. J Bone Miner Metab2004;22:44-7.
138 Lenz M, Höffken O, Stude P, et al. Bilateral somatosensory cortex disinhibition in complex regional pain syndrome type I. Neurology2011;77:1096-101.
139 Lebel A, Becerra L, Wallin D, et al. fMRI reveals distinct CNS processing during symptomatic and recovered complex regional pain syndrome in children. Brain2008;131:1854-79.
140 Blumberg H. A new clinical approach for diagnosing reflex sympathetic dystrophy. In: Bond MR, Charlton JE, Woolf CJ, eds. Proceedings of the VIth World Congress on Pain. Elsevier; 1991:399-407.
141 Gibbons JJ, Wilson PR. RSD score: criteria for the diagnosis of reflex sympathetic dystrophy and causalgia. Clin J Pain1992;8:260-3.
142 Veldman PH, Reynen HM, Arntz IE, et al. Signs and symptoms of reflex sympathetic dystrophy: prospective study of 829 patients. Lancet1993;342:1012-6.
143 Kozin F, Ryan LM, Carerra GF, et al. The reflex sympathetic dystrophy syndrome III: scintigraphic studies, further evidence for the therapeutic efficacy of systemic corticosteroids, and proposed diagnostic criteria. Am J Med1981;70:23-30.
144 Bruehl S, Harden RN, Galer BS, et al. External validation of IASP diagnostic criteria for complex regional pain syndrome and proposed research diagnostic criteria. International Association for the Study of Pain. Pain1999;81:147-54.
145 Galer BS, Bruehl S, Harden RN. IASP diagnostic criteria for complex regional pain syndrome: a preliminary empirical validation study. International Association for the Study of Pain. Clin J Pain1998;14:48-54.

146 Gatchel RJ, Okifuji A. Evidence-based scientific data documenting the treatment and cost-effectiveness of comprehensive pain programs for chronic nonmalignant pain. J Pain2006;7:779-93.
147 Kingery WS. A critical review of controlled clinical trials for peripheral neuropathic pain and complex regional pain syndromes. Pain1997;73:123-39.
148 Harden RN, Oaklander AL, Burton AW, et al; Reflex Sympathetic Dystrophy Syndrome Association. Complex regional pain syndrome: practical diagnostic and treatment guidelines, 4th ed. Pain Med2013;14:180-229.
149 Perez RS, Kwakkel G, Zuurmond WW, et al. Treatment of reflex sympathetic dystrophy (CRPS type 1): a research synthesis of 21 randomized clinical trials. J Pain Symptom Manage2001;21:511-26.
150 Perez RS, Zollinger PE, Dijkstra PU, et al. CRPS I task force. Evidence based guidelines for complex regional pain syndrome type 1. BMC Neurol2010;10:20.
151 Chung OY, Bruehl SP. Complex regional pain syndrome. Curr Treat Options Neurol2003;5:499-511.
152 Daly AE, Bialocerkowski AE. Does evidence support physiotherapy management of adult complex regional pain syndrome type one? A systematic review. Eur J Pain2009;13:339-53.
153 O'Connell NE, Wand BM, McAuley J, et al. Interventions for treating pain and disability in adults with complex regional pain syndrome. Cochrane Database Syst Rev2013;4:CD009416.
154 Cossins L, Okell RW, Cameron H, et al. Treatment of complex regional pain syndrome in adults: a systematic review of randomized controlled trials published from June 2000 to February 2012. Eur J Pain2013;17:158-73.
155 Stanton TR, Wand BM, Carr DB, et al. Local anaesthetic sympathetic blockade for complex regional pain syndrome. Cochrane Database Syst Rev2013;8:CD004598.
156 Straube S, Derry S, Moore RA, et al. Cervico-thoracic or lumbar sympathectomy for neuropathic pain and complex regional pain syndrome. Cochrane Database Syst Rev2013;9:CD002918.
157 Van Eijs F, Stanton-Hicks M, Van Zundert J, et al. Evidence-based interventional pain medicine according to clinical diagnoses. 16. Complex regional pain syndrome. Pain Pract2011;11:70-87.
158 Moseley GL. Graded motor imagery is effective for long-standing complex regional pain syndrome: a randomised controlled trial. Pain2004;108:192-8.
159 Johnson S, Hall J, Barnett S, et al. Using graded motor imagery for complex regional pain syndrome in clinical practice: failure to improve pain. Eur J Pain2012;16:550-61.
160 De Jong JR, Vlaeyen JW, van Eijsden M, et al. Reduction of pain-related fear and increased function and participation in work-related upper extremity pain (WRUEP): effects of exposure in vivo. Pain2012;153:2109-18.
161 Van de Meent H, Oerlemans M, Bruggeman A, et al. Safety of "pain exposure" physical therapy in patients with complex regional pain syndrome type 1. Pain2011;152:1431-8.
162 Kalita J, Vajpayee A, Misra UK. Comparison of prednisolone with piroxicam in complex regional pain syndrome following stroke: a randomized controlled trial. QJM2006;99:89-95.
163 Atalay NS, Ercidogan O, Akkaya N, et al. Prednisolone in complex regional pain syndrome. Pain Phys2014;17:179-85.
164 Van de Vusse AC, Stomp-van den Berg SG, Kessels AH, et al. Randomised controlled trial of gabapentin in complex regional pain syndrome type 1 (ISRCTN84121379). BMC Neurol2004;4:13.
165 Harke H, Gretenkort P, Ladleif HU, et al. The response of neuropathic pain and pain in complex regional pain syndrome I to carbamazepine and sustained-release morphine in patients pretreated with spinal cord stimulation: a double-blinded randomized study. Anesth Analg2001;92:488-95.
166 Price DD, Long S, Wilsey B, et al. Analysis of peak magnitude and duration of analgesia produced by local anesthetics injected into sympathetic ganglia of complex regional pain syndrome patients. Clin J Pain1998;14:216-26.
167 Kemler MA, Barendse GA, van Kleef M, et al. Spinal cord stimulation in patients with chronic reflex sympathetic dystrophy. N Engl J Med2000;343:618-24.
168 Kemler MA, de Vet HC, Barendse GA, et al. The effect of spinal cord stimulation in patients with chronic reflex sympathetic dystrophy: two years' follow-up of the randomized controlled trial. Ann Neurol2004;55:13-8.
169 Kemler MA, de Vet HC, Barendse GA, et al. Effect of spinal cord stimulation for chronic complex regional pain syndrome type I: five-year final follow-up of patients in a randomized controlled trial. J Neurosurg2008;108:292-8.
170 Bruehl S, Chung OY. Psychological and behavioral aspects of complex regional pain syndrome management. Clin J Pain2006;22:430-7.
171 Besse JL, Gadeyne S, Galand-Desmé S, et al. Effect of vitamin C on prevention of complex regional pain syndrome type I in foot and ankle surgery. Foot Ankle Surg2009;15:179-82.
172 Cazeneuve JF, Leborgne JM, Kermad K, et al. [Vitamin C and prevention of reflex sympathetic dystrophy following surgical management of distal radius fractures.] Acta Orthop Belg2002;68:481-4.
173 Zollinger PE, Tuinebreijer WE, Breederveld RS, et al. Can vitamin C prevent complex regional pain syndrome in patients with wrist fractures? A randomized, controlled, multicenter dose-response study. J Bone Joint Surg Am2007;89:1424-31.
174 Zollinger PE, Tuinebreijer WE, Kreis RW, et al. Effect of vitamin C on frequency of reflex sympathetic dystrophy in wrist fractures: a randomized trial. Lancet1999;354:2025-8.
175 Ekrol I, Duckworth AD, Ralston SH, et al. The influence of vitamin C on the outcome of distal radial fractures: a double-blind, randomized controlled trial. J Bone Joint Surg Am2014;96:1451-9.
176 Shibuya N, Humphers JM, Agarwal MR, et al. Efficacy and safety of high-dose vitamin C on complex regional pain syndrome in extremity trauma and surgery-systematic review and meta-analysis. J Foot Ankle Surg2013;52:62-6.
177 Stanton-Hicks M. Plasticity of complex regional pain syndrome (CRPS) in children. Pain Med2010;11:1216-23.
178 Meier PM, Alexander ME, Sethna NF, et al. Complex regional pain syndromes in children and adolescents: regional and systemic signs and symptoms and hemodynamic response to tilt table testing. Clin J Pain2006;22:399-406.
179 Tan EC, van de Sandt-Renkema N, Krabbe PF, et al. Quality of life in adults with childhood-onset of complex regional pain syndrome type I. Injury2009;40:901-4.
180 Logan DE, Williams SE, Carullo VP, et al. Children and adolescents with complex regional pain syndrome: more psychologically distressed than other children in pain? Pain Res Manag2013;18:87-93.
181 Varenna M, Adami S, Rossini M, et al. Treatment of complex regional pain syndrome type I with neridronate: a randomized, double-blind, placebo-controlled study. Rheumatology (Oxford)2013;52:534-42.
182 Varenna M, Zucchi F, Ghiringhelli D, et al. Intravenous clodronate in the treatment of reflex sympathetic dystrophy syndrome. A randomized, double blind, placebo controlled study. J Rheumatol2000;27:1477-83.
183 Robinson JN, Sandom J, Chapman PT. Efficacy of pamidronate in complex regional pain syndrome type I. Pain Med2004;5:276-80.
184 Manicourt DH, Brasseur JP, Boutsen Y, et al. Role of alendronate in therapy for posttraumatic complex regional pain syndrome type I of the lower extremity. Arthritis Rheum2004;50:3690-7.
185 Finch PM, Knudsen L, Drummond PD. Reduction of allodynia in patients with complex regional pain syndrome: a double-blind placebo-controlled trial of topical ketamine. Pain2009;146:18-25.
186 Schwartzman RJ, Alexander GM, Grothusen JR, et al. Outpatient intravenous ketamine for the treatment of complex regional pain syndrome: a double-blind placebo controlled study. Pain2009;147:107-15.
187 Sigtermans MJ, van Hilten JJ, Bauer MC, et al. Ketamine produces effective and long-term pain relief in patients with complex regional pain syndrome type 1. Pain2009;145:304-11.
188 Noppers IM, Niesters M, Aarts LP, et al. Drug-induced liver injury following a repeated course of ketamine treatment for chronic pain in CRPS type 1 patients: a report of 3 cases. Pain2011;152:2173-8.
189 Goebel A, Baranowski A, Maurer K, et al. Intravenous immunoglobulin treatment of the complex regional pain syndrome: a randomized trial. Ann Intern Med2010;152:152-8.
190 Groeneweg G, Huygen FJ, Niehof SP, et al. Effect of tadalafil on blood flow, pain, and function in chronic cold complex regional pain syndrome: a randomized controlled trial. BMC Musculoskelet Disord2008;9:143.
191 Van Rijn MA, Munts AG, Marinus J, et al. Intrathecal baclofen for dystonia of complex regional pain syndrome. Pain2009;143:41-7.
192 Chopra P, Cooper MS. Treatment of complex regional pain syndrome (CRPS) using low dose naltrexone (LDN). J Neuroimmune Pharmacol2013;8:470-6.
193 Younger J, Noor N, McCue R, et al. Low-dose naltrexone for the treatment of fibromyalgia: findings of a small, randomized, double-blind, placebo-controlled, counterbalanced, crossover trial assessing daily pain levels. Arthritis Rheum2013;65:529-38.
194 Turner-Stokes L, Goebel A; Guideline Development Group. Complex regional pain syndrome in adults: concise guidance. Clin Med2011;11:596-600.
195 Birklein F, Schlereth T. [Current aspects of the therapy of complex regional pain syndrome.] Nervenarzt2013;84:1436-44.

Polymyalgia rheumatica

Sarah L Mackie, clinical lecturer[1], Christian D Mallen, professor[2]

[1]National Institute for Health Research-Leeds Musculoskeletal Biomedical Research Unit, Leeds Institute of Rheumatic and Musculoskeletal Medicine, University of Leeds, Chapel Allerton Hospital, Leeds LS7 4SA, UK

[2]Arthritis Research UK Primary Care Centre, Keele University, Keele, UK

Correspondence to: S L Mackie s.l.mackie@leeds.ac.uk

Cite this as: *BMJ* 2013;347:f6937

DOI: 10.1136/bmj.f6937

http://www.bmj.com/content/347/bmj.f6937

Polymyalgia rheumatica causes pain and stiffness that is worst in the morning and particularly affects the shoulders and hips. It is a treatable cause of profound debility and functional impairment.[1] The condition usually presents to primary care and is the most common inflammatory musculoskeletal disease in older people, with an age adjusted incidence of about one in 1000 person years.[2] The lifetime risk has been estimated at 2.4% for women and 1.7% for men.[3] There is little trial based evidence to guide diagnosis and treatment. This review describes current ideas about best practice in the diagnosis and management of this disease, drawing on recent clinical guidelines[4] and highlighting some research priorities.

What is polymyalgia rheumatica?

The site of pathology is unclear and little is known about the causes and pathogenesis of this disease. The clinical diagnosis can be challenging owing to the lack of a specific diagnostic test. Various diagnostic and classification criteria have been proposed.[5 6 7 8 9] Classification criteria have recently been developed by the European League against Rheumatic Diseases and the American College of Rheumatology on the basis of a large prospective, international multicentre study and data driven consensus process. These are currently awaiting validation in an independent dataset (table 1).[10] These criteria are not intended for diagnostic use but are a useful starting point for describing core clinical features of the condition, which include bilateral shoulder and hip pain with an abnormal erythrocyte sedimentation rate (ESR) or C reactive protein (CRP).

What are the objective abnormalities in polymyalgia rheumatica?

Ultrasound studies with power Doppler enhancement suggest inflammation of intra-articular and extra-articular structures (synovitis and bursitis). Histological studies show the presence of macrophages and T cells in the synovium.[11] Some magnetic resonance imaging studies suggest greater involvement of extracapsular structures compared with that seen in rheumatoid arthritis.[12] Positron emission tomography/computed tomography and magnetic resonance imaging studies have also shown that some patients have widespread inflammation in areas where the disease is not clinically apparent, such as the aorta and proximal branches,[13] and between the vertebral spinous processes.[14]

SUMMARY POINTS

- Polymyalgic syndrome can be a presenting feature of a wide range of diseases, including giant cell arteritis and rheumatoid arthritis
- Look for other diseases before starting glucocorticoids (≤20 mg prednisolone or equivalent)
- Carefully document the speed, completeness, and nature of the response to initial glucocorticoid treatment
- Atypical features should prompt early specialist evaluation
- Monitor patients carefully for adverse effects of glucocorticoids and taper drugs on an individual basis

About 90% of patients have an increase in inflammatory markers, including ESR.[15] Plasma viscosity gives similar information to ESR but is less strongly influenced by factors such as anaemia, polycythaemia, sex, or age.[16 17 18 19] Fibrinogen levels strongly influence ESR and plasma viscosity in polymyalgia rheumatica; fibrinogen may be a more specific marker than ESR for disease activity in treated polymyalgia.[20] However, other factors, including immunoglobulin and lipid levels, also influence ESR and plasma viscosity and may contribute to interindividual variation in these blood test results. CRP may be more sensitive diagnostically than ESR[15]; CRP production is mainly driven by interleukin 6, which is typically raised in polymyalgia rheumatica. A small prospective study suggested that failure of interleukin 6 to fall with glucocorticoid treatment may predict relapses.[21] However, whether or not it is useful to measure interleukin 6 in clinical practice is unclear. It has been proposed that high interleukin 6 levels result in insufficient glucocorticoid production.[22] However, this does not completely explain how polymyalgia rheumatica develops and ultimately resolves.

There is no general agreement on how high inflammatory markers should be for a diagnosis of polymyalgia rheumatica. Cases with "normal" (within laboratory reference ranges for age and sex) inflammatory markers have been described but are particularly difficult to diagnose,[10 15] and British Society for Rheumatology (BSR) guidelines advise specialist evaluation if inflammatory markers are normal.[4]

Can polymyalgia rheumatica "overlap" with other rheumatological disorders?

Longitudinal studies suggest that polymyalgia rheumatica is a heterogeneous disorder, even after differential diagnoses have been excluded.[21] Features of the disease may be present in other inflammatory diseases, including rheumatoid arthritis (seropositive or seronegative), cranial giant cell arteritis, large vessel vasculitis, spondyloarthropathy,[23 24] and crystal arthropathies such as inflammation caused by calcium pyrophosphate crystals (pseudogout).[25] It has been proposed that ultrasound imaging of the shoulders, hips, and possibly the small joints might help in the diagnosis by identifying specific features of particular inflammatory diseases,[26] but further studies are needed to clarify its relevance to routine clinical practice, especially in primary care.

Association with giant cell arteritis

Giant cell arteritis is a systemic vasculitis that affects large and medium sized arteries. There has been debate about whether polymyalgia rheumatica and giant cell arteritis are distinct diseases.[27] Although the patient population at risk is similar,[2] observational incidence data from a large primary care based study suggest that the two diseases are diagnosed in the same patient 38 times more often than might be expected owing to chance.[2] Unlike polymyalgia rheumatica, which usually responds to an initial dose of 15-20 mg prednisolone, at least 30-40 mg prednisolone is needed initially in giant cell arteritis for effective symptom relief (for example, from temporal headache or jaw pain).

These doses are based on clinical experience and expert consensus.[28] Data from the pre-steroid era suggest that untreated giant cell arteritis commonly results in blindness, so formal dose ranging studies have not been done. High doses of glucocorticoids ($\geq$30 mg prednisolone) have additional ("non-genomic") cellular mechanisms of action compared with low and medium doses ($\leq$15 mg),[29] so the fact that both polymyalgia rheumatica and giant cell arteritis respond to glucocorticoids is not necessarily evidence of a shared disease pathway. Case series show that a subset of patients with polymyalgic syndrome have occult giant cell arteritis on biopsy or imaging,[30 31] but these findings are not universal.

Overlap with rheumatoid arthritis

Rheumatoid arthritis may present with a polymyalgic syndrome before synovitis is clinically detectable.[32] Consequently, some polymyalgia rheumatica cohorts contain a subset of patients who are later diagnosed as having rheumatoid arthritis.[10 33] The addition of anti-cyclic citrullinated peptide antibodies to the classification of rheumatoid arthritis might help to reduce this overlap[34]—these antibodies are rarely present in polymyalgia rheumatica.[35] In observational studies, patients with polymyalgia rheumatica seem to have a greater clinical and laboratory response to glucocorticoids than those with polymyalgic onset rheumatoid arthritis.[36]

Genetic heterogeneity

In contrast to the known association of giant cell arteritis with HLA-DRB1*04,[37] and of rheumatoid arthritis with subtypes of HLA-DRB1*01, HLA-DRB1*04, and HLA-DRB1*10 alleles,[38] polymyalgia rheumatica has no well replicated HLA-DRB1 association.[37] It is unclear whether a reported association of HLA-DRB1*04 with risk of relapse[39] is due to an overlap of polymyalgia rheumatica with subclinical giant cell arteritis or rheumatoid arthritis.[33 40] Rheumatoid arthritis associated HLA-DRB1 alleles were also associated with relapse in polymyalgia rheumatica.[41]

How is polymyalgia rheumatica diagnosed?

Once the diagnosis is suspected, BSR guidelines recommend a three step procedure (fig 1).[4] Each step is intended to increase the probability that the diagnosis is correct. In the presence of clinical features, supportive investigation results, and a rapid complete response to glucocorticoids, it is thought that a diagnosis of polymyalgia rheumatica can be confidently made in primary care.[4] However, this approach is based on expert consensus and has not been formally evaluated. Arguably, the most challenging step is the first one, which depends on clinical experience and expertise. Where all three features (classic clinical features, supportive investigation results, rapid complete response to glucocorticoids) are not unequivocally present, there are arguments for referring the patient for a specialist opinion.[4]

How can the classic clinical features of polymyalgia rheumatica be identified?

Classic features of polymyalgia are bilateral pain and stiffness in the shoulders and hips in older patients, most commonly those in their 70s and rarely below age 50.[2] Patients may not be able to "turn over in bed or get up from the toilet in the mornings." There is pronounced diurnal variation, with symptoms being worst on waking. Morning stiffness usually lasts for at least an hour.[5] Symptoms may begin suddenly, sometimes accompanied by "flu-like" features, although onset can be more insidious. Generalised restriction of movement results in profound functional impairment. Gait may be affected, although isometric muscle power is relatively intact. Inflammatory markers are typically raised, sometimes with an accompanying normocytic "anaemia of inflammation."[42]

However, other haematological abnormalities (including lymphopenia) should prompt suspicion of other diseases. Look for evidence of giant cell arteritis, such as headache, scalp tenderness, jaw claudication, visual disturbance, or abnormal temporal arteries; if present, urgent specialist referral is needed. Recent limb claudication may signal large vessel giant cell arteritis. Educate patients with suspected

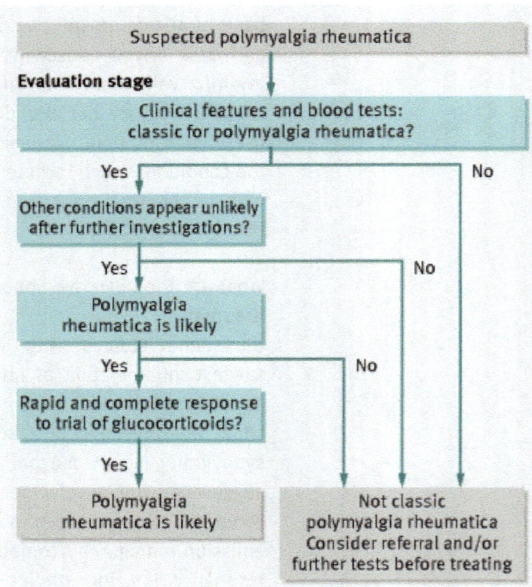

Fig 1 Summary of a three step procedure for evaluating suspected polymyalgia rheumatica; see British Society for Rheumatology guidelines for more detail[4]

Table 1 Scoring algorithm for provisional European League against Rheumatic Diseases and American College of Rheumatology classification criteria for polymyalgia rheumatica

Required criteria*	Points without ultrasound†	Points with ultrasound‡
Morning stiffness (duration >45 minutes)	2	2
Hip pain or limited range of motion	1	1
Absence of rheumatoid factor or anti-cyclic citrullinated peptide antibodies	2	2
Absence of other joint pain	1	1
Ultrasound: at least 1 abnormal§ shoulder and at least 1 abnormal¶ hip	–	1
Ultrasound: both shoulders abnormal§	–	1

Age $\geq$50 years, bilateral shoulder aching, and abnormal C reactive protein or erythrocyte sedimentation rate (or both).

†If total score $\geq$4, patient is categorised as having polymyalgia rheumatica.

‡If total score $\geq$5, patient is categorised as having polymyalgia rheumatica.

§Ultrasound evidence of glenohumeral synovitis or subacromial-subdeltoid bursitis.

¶Ultrasound evidence of coxofemoral synovitis or trochanteric bursitis.

polymyalgia rheumatica about the symptoms of giant cell arteritis and warn then to consult urgently if they develop.

There should be no lymphadenopathy or involvement of other organs including the nervous system, skin, hair, lung, gastrointestinal tract, or kidney. Consider alternative diagnoses if such clinical features are present. It is important to check for other causes of myopathy, including statin treatment or hypothyroidism (both of which are usually associated with raised creatine kinase).

Musculoskeletal ultrasound often identifies inflammation of structures around the shoulders and hips (subacromial bursitis, glenohumeral synovitis, trochanteric bursitis, hip synovitis).[43] However, these findings are not unique to polymyalgia rheumatica and quoted sensitivity and specificity estimates may be unreliable because of the case-control design of existing diagnostic accuracy studies. The usefulness of ultrasound has yet to be evaluated outside specialist settings. Ultrasound can be useful when diagnosis is uncertain or when overlap conditions (such as rheumatoid arthritis) are suspected. Table 2 provides details of selected differential diagnoses.

What further investigations are recommended before starting glucocorticoids?

There is currently no single diagnostic test for polymyalgia and investigation is largely aimed at excluding other explanations for the symptoms (table 2). BSR guidelines recommend measuring ESR, CRP, full blood count, liver and renal function tests, protein electrophoresis, rheumatoid factor (and anti-citrullinated peptide antibody if available), calcium, alkaline phosphatase, and thyroid function.[4] All of these tests, except for ESR and CRP, are done to exclude other conditions.

Actively look for clues about cancer or infection, especially if there are clinical risk factors (including personal or family history of cancer). Weight loss, fever, or very high inflammatory markers (ESR >100 is atypical for polymyalgia rheumatica) should prompt considerations of cancer, including myeloma and renal cell carcinoma, or occult infection, including endocarditis, osteomyelitis, and paraspinal infection. Microscopic haematuria is not a feature of polymyalgia rheumatica and may be a clue to other conditions.

When should glucocorticoids be started?

It is not known whether glucocorticoids modify the disease process itself or merely alleviate the symptoms of polymyalgia rheumatica. High quality randomised controlled trials of glucocorticoids versus other treatments have not been performed. Before starting glucocorticoids, screen for risk factors for glucocorticoid related adverse effects (such as diabetes, hypertension, peptic ulcer, osteoporosis, psychiatric comorbidity) and treat these appropriately.[4] These factors, together with the patient's weight,[44] may affect the initial choice of dose for a trial of glucocorticoids. In addition, counsel patients about potential adverse effects, which include the above risk factors as well as bruising, skin fragility, myopathy, and weight gain.

Symptoms of many non-polymyalgic disorders, including cancer, may initially respond to glucocorticoids, but lack of response can be a clue to other conditions such as solid tumours or osteoarthritis.[45] The diagnostic value of response to glucocorticoids becomes less specific as the dose increases. A typical starting dose is 15 mg prednisolone (or glucocorticoid equivalent), but some patients respond well to lower doses.[46] These recommendations are based on expert consensus because the studies informing them were largely observational, had various inclusion criteria, and were usually hospital based rather than community based. BSR guidelines recommend specialist evaluation in patients with an incomplete response to 20 mg prednisolone (defined as <70% self reported improvement in symptoms).[4] This is based on a pragmatic trade-off between the sensitivity and specificity of the diagnostic value of various doses of prednisolone, with a conservative approach being recommended as safest in primary care.

Where there is doubt, with the patient's agreement, some specialist practitioners use a "steroid sandwich" (alternating a week of vitamin C (or other placebo) with a week of prednisolone and evaluating the time course of symptomatic response).[47] In classic polymyalgia rheumatica, symptoms resolve within about three days and do not reappear unless the glucocorticoid dose is reduced or stopped. Inflammatory markers should normalise within two to four weeks and remain normal until the dose is reduced. These features would support a diagnosis of classic polymyalgia rheumatica.

Table 2 Selected differential diagnoses to consider in patients with polymyalgic symptoms*

Category	Example	Possible clues
Inflammatory rheumatological disorders	Rheumatoid arthritis (seropositive or seronegative) and other inflammatory arthritides eg spondyloarthropathy	Peripheral synovitis or sacroiliitis; insidious onset
	Calcium pyrophosphate deposition disease, atypical gout, single or multi-joint sepsis	Swollen joints; consider aspiration
	Giant cell arteritis, other vasculitis	Direct questioning, systems review
	Myositis, other myopathy (for example, statin related)	Creatine kinase
Non-inflammatory rheumatological disorders	Multiple mechanical joint pains (such as lower limb osteoarthritis plus subacromial impingement)	Examination; lack of improvement of symptoms over the day
Rare and important	Infections such as endocarditis, osteomyelitis, paraspinal infection, tuberculosis	Fevers, sweats, microscopic haematuria
	Cancer—for example, myeloma, lymphoma, renal cell carcinoma, carcinoma of prostate, others	Weight loss, monoclonal band (haematological), microscopic haematuria (renal cell carcinoma)
Endocrine	Hypothyroid myopathy	Creatine kinase
	Hyperparathyroidism	Calcium and phosphate concentrations
Neurological	Motor neurone disease	Wasting
	Parkinsonism	Physical signs
Occult fracture	Vertebral, sacral, or pelvic fracture (if present consider osteomalacia or other causes)	Pain on weight bearing

This is not an exhaustive list of the differential diagnoses of polymyalgic symptoms.

When and how should the glucocorticoid dose be tapered?

The dose is gradually tapered over months to years. In most case series the median time to stopping glucocorticoids is about two years,[48] but individuals vary greatly and few studies have been performed in primary care. No head to head trials have looked at the optimum rate of glucocorticoid tapering. Indeed rigid adherence to a tapering protocol may be unhelpful as many patients need to spend some time at a particular dose rather than aiming for a constant rate of reduction. Frequent, rapid changes in glucocorticoid dose are to be avoided where possible. The risks associated with glucocorticoids must be balanced against the risks of relapse, taking into account comorbidities (such as diabetes and hypertension) and the patient's priorities. Observational studies suggest that those with higher inflammatory markers before treatment are at higher risk of relapse[21 49 50 51 52 53] and need a longer duration of treatment.[48 54] Such studies also suggest that patients who need an initial dose of more than 20 mg prednisolone have a higher risk of relapse,[21] and that atypical features may be a predictor of prolonged glucocorticoid requirements (fig 2). In a retrospective study of 135 patients, 26% of patients initially thought to have polymyalgia rheumatica later received a different diagnosis (seronegative rheumatoid arthritis in half of them). These patients were younger, more often male, needed higher initial glucocorticoid doses, and were less able to reduce and stop glucocorticoids during follow-up.[55] In another observational study, patients who needed higher initial glucocorticoid doses were likely to need glucocorticoids for longer, and were also more likely to develop giant cell arteritis at a later date.[48]

There is no evidence that aggressively trying to reduce inflammatory markers improves prognosis in asymptomatic patients and it could mask a second disease. A composite score for monitoring disease activity—the "polymyalgia rheumatica activity score"—incorporates doctor and patient reported elements, as well as CRP concentrations,[56] but this score requires further validation and is seldom used outside research settings.

A degree of trial and error is involved in the tapering of glucocorticoids. Initially, the daily dose is usually reduced by 2.5 mg every two to four weeks, but, after reaching 10 mg daily, it is usually slowed to a mean 0.5-1.0 mg daily dose reduction per month. However, patients vary greatly, and alternate day dosing may be useful in those who cannot tolerate a full reduction in dose. Warn patients to expect a temporary increase in symptoms for about a week after each dose reduction. Prednisolone may need to be reduced very gradually once the dose gets down to 2.5-7.5 mg per day. This could be achieved by taking the reduced dose on certain days of the week only; giving an intramuscular glucocorticoid injection followed by a reduction of 2.5-5 mg daily two days later; and giving local glucocorticoid injection(s) to the most symptomatic area(s). These strategies are based on expert consensus (formal comparative studies have not been performed) and shared decision making is important.

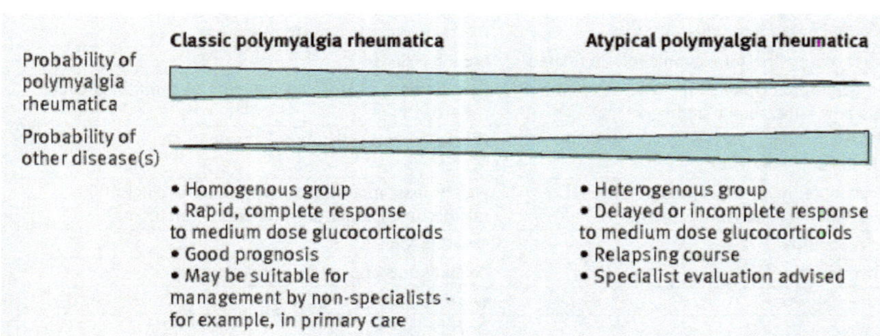

Fig 2 The clinical spectrum of polymyalgia from a diagnostic perspective. The triangles signify "greater" or "lesser" probability and are drawn on an arbitrary scale. There is no general agreement on what "atypical polymyalgia rheumatica" means, or at what point it becomes so atypical that it is no longer safe to make a diagnosis of polymyalgia rheumatica. These patients should probably be managed with input from a specialist

What if patients cannot tolerate glucocorticoid withdrawal even years later?

Some patients, often those with atypical polymyalgia or other rheumatological disorders, will require prolonged (>2 years) glucocorticoid treatment (fig 2). When referring for

QUESTIONS FOR FUTURE RESEARCH

- What is the anatomical basis of polymyalgia rheumatica and what causes it?
- Can we identify better biomarkers (including imaging tests) for diagnosing and monitoring the disease?
- Can we define a core set of robust outcome measures for future research studies in polymyalgia rheumatica, including assessment of the life impact and healthcare costs of the disease and its treatment?
- What are the optimum starting doses of glucocorticoids, best delivery methods, and optimum dose reduction strategies for different patients?
- What is the role of immunosuppressants such as methotrexate in this disease?

ADDITIONAL EDUCATIONAL RESOURCES

Resources for healthcare professionals

- Bird HA, Esselinckx W, Dixon AS, Mowat AG, Wood PH. An evaluation of criteria for polymyalgia rheumatica. *Ann Rheum Dis* 1979;38:434-9
- Weyand CM, Fulbright JW, Evans JM, Hunder GG, Goronzy JJ. Corticosteroid requirements in polymyalgia rheumatica. *Arch Intern Med* 1999;159:577-84
- Dasgupta B, Borg FA, Hassan N, Barraclough K, Bourke B, Fulcher J, et al. BSR and BHPR guidelines for the management of polymyalgia rheumatica. *Rheumatology (Oxford)* 2010;49:186-90
- Dasgupta B, Cimmino MA, Maradit-Kremers H, Schmidt WA, Schirmer M, Salvarani C, et al. 2012 provisional classification criteria for polymyalgia rheumatica: a European League Against Rheumatism/American College of Rheumatology collaborative initiative. *Ann Rheum Dis* 2012;71:484-92
- Hernández-Rodríguez J, Cid MC, López-Soto A, Espigol-Frigolé G, Bosch X. Treatment of polymyalgia rheumatica: a systematic review. *Arch Intern Med* 2009;169:1839-50

Resources for patients

- Polymyalgia rheumatica and giant cell arteritis UK (www.pmrgcauk.com/)—Provides information on polymyalgia rheumatica and giant cell arteritis, peer support from patients, and a telephone helpline
- Arthritis Research UK (www.arthritisresearchuk.org/arthritis-information/conditions/polymyalgia-rheumatica.aspx)—Provides written information on the diagnosis and treatment of polymyalgia rheumatica
- Patient.co.uk (www.patient.co.uk/health/polymyalgia-rheumatica)—Useful information on the diagnosis and treatment (and treatment side effects) of polymyalgia rheumatica

specialist advice, the records from the original presentation of polymyalgia rheumatica are helpful. Re-evaluation after temporarily forcing the dose of glucocorticoids down (with reminders about warning symptoms of giant cell arteritis) can also help diagnostically, because glucocorticoids can mask clinical and imaging features of other inflammatory diseases.

The pattern of disease activity is the first thing to consider in patients who require prolonged treatment with glucocorticoids. Are the symptoms truly inflammatory in nature, and what dose of glucocorticoids is needed for symptom relief? Case series suggest that it is unusual for polymyalgia rheumatica to require more than 10 mg prednisolone daily for more than a year. Other, non-inflammatory causes of musculoskeletal pain are common and could be exacerbated by glucocorticoid related weight gain or by physical deconditioning. Osteoarthritis of the spine, hip, or knee is often identified at this stage. If clinical features suggest subacromial or trochanteric bursitis, then local glucocorticoid injections can help. Even if the symptoms are truly inflammatory and responsive to glucocorticoids, a careful search for another inflammatory disease should be made.

Patients with ongoing or relapsing symptoms, a long duration of morning stiffness, raised inflammatory markers, and no other cause of inflammation may benefit from immunosuppressive treatments under specialist supervision. Although underpowered, randomised controlled trials of methotrexate found no convincing benefit in polymyalgia rheumatica, with confidence intervals of effect sizes close to the null.[57] Small trials of tumour necrosis factor antagonists also failed to show convincing benefit,[58 59] although again they were underpowered to detect small effect sizes or large effect sizes in small subgroups. Leflunomide and tocilizumab have been used in observational case reports and case series,[60 61] but randomised controlled trials have not been performed. Caution is needed when interpreting efficacy outcomes that depend on inflammatory markers, because some drugs (such as tocilizumab) may suppress CRP but have unknown effects on the underlying polymyalgic disease process.

What are the risks of long term glucocorticoids and how can they be reduced?

Patients with polymyalgia rheumatica are committed to months or years of glucocorticoid treatment, with a substantial risk of adverse effects.[62 63 64] Patients require regular monitoring for potential complications including diabetes and hypertension. Prophylaxis against other glucocorticoid related adverse effects (including gastrointestinal side effects and osteoporosis) should be considered.[64] Adequate calcium and vitamin D intake should be maintained and supplemented if appropriate. If assessment shows a high risk of osteoporotic fracture, a bisphosphonate is the usual first line of treatment.[65] Gastroprotection should be considered, particularly in older patients. Advice on physical activity—especially weight bearing activity—is important, and physiotherapy may be useful if there is deconditioning. A "steroid card" can be useful for patients on long term glucocorticoids.

In patients with mild or localised symptoms, or a high risk of adverse effects from glucocorticoids, intramuscular or periarticular injections of glucocorticoid may be tried, as suggested by a single small trial.[66] Non-steroidal anti-inflammatory drugs have been used,[64] although anecdotal evidence suggests these drugs have a lesser effect than glucocorticoids and a greater risk of gastrointestinal side effects, especially in older people.

ONGOING RESEARCH

- Keele PMR study (www.keele.ac.uk/pmr): an observational cohort study of patients with newly diagnosed polymyalgia rheumatica in primary care
- ADDRESS-PMR: diagnostic accuracy study of ultrasound in patients with suspected polymyalgia rheumatica
- Study of tocilizumab to treat polymyalgia rheumatica: NCT01396317
- TENOR: Tocilizumab Effect iN pOlymyalgia Rheumatica: NCT01713842
- Study on the efficacy and safety of Lodotra (delayed release prednisolone) compared with immediate release prednisone in patients with polymyalgia rheumatica: NCT01821040

TIPS FOR NON-SPECIALISTS

- Do not start glucocorticoids until all relevant investigations have been completed
- Have a low threshold for specialist referral of patients without classic symptoms Document findings carefully, including atypical features; these notes may be invaluable later if the patient is unable to stop glucocorticoids
- Give the patient written information including symptoms of giant cell arteritis, such as headache, scalp tenderness, jaw claudication, visual disturbance, or abnormal temporal arteries
- Once the diagnosis is made, treat the patient not the blood test results
- Try to avoid frequent large changes in glucocorticoid dose
- Remember that older patients may develop a second disease
- Evaluate for comorbidities early on and prescribe bone prophylaxis early

SOURCES AND SELECTION CRITERIA

We searched Medline, Embase, Cochrane Collaboration, and ClinicalTrials.gov using the word "polymyalgia". All study types were included owing to the limited amount of literature available.

What is the prognosis in polymyalgia rheumatica?

Information on prognosis is limited, especially in community settings. Men have a better prognosis than women. Case series and small secondary care based prospective cohorts show wide variations in the duration of glucocorticoid treatment.[21] In some patients, glucocorticoids can be reduced easily and stopped within a year, with no recurrence in symptoms. Others tend to relapse on dose reduction, until the disease seems to "burn itself out" after a few years. A few patients need to be treated for many years, for reasons that are not well understood. Higher inflammatory markers are associated with longer duration of treatment and more relapses. However, it is unclear how much this results from the underlying disease and how much from an over-reliance on blood tests for monitoring disease activity. Tailored treatment and a consistent approach from one well informed doctor can promote shared decision making and reduce the anxiety experienced by many patients with this disease. Patient support groups can play a vital role

Thanks to Colin Pease (Leeds Teaching Hospitals NHS Trust) and Jeremy Wyatt (University of Leeds) for their comments on the draft of this manuscript.

Contributors: Both authors planned and drafted the manuscript, commented on further drafts, and approved the final version. SLM was commissioned to write the article and is guarantor.

Competing interests: We have read and understood the BMJ Group policy on declaration of interests and declare: Both authors received no support for the submitted work. SLM is funded by a National Institute for Health Research (NIHR) clinician scientist fellowship to improve diagnosis of patients with polymyalgia rheumatica (ADDRESS-PMR study). SLM was funded to attend EULAR conferences by Pfizer (2007) and Napp Pharmaceuticals (2011). In 2011 SLM received an honorarium from AstraZeneca for giving educational talks to three local general practices. SLM is a member of a group producing clinical practice recommendations for management of polymyalgia rheumatica on behalf of the American College for Rheumatology and European League against Rheumatic Diseases recommendations/guidelines, and a member of the group updating the British Society of Rheumatology guidelines for diagnosis and management of polymyalgia rheumatica. She had no part in writing the original BSR guidelines, and the views represented here are not necessarily those of the guidelines groups concerned. CDM is funded by a clinician scientist fellowship from Arthritis Research UK and has no competing interests to declare (no financial relationships with any organisations that might have an interest in the submitted work in the previous three years; no other relationships or activities that could appear to have influenced the submitted work). The views expressed are those of the authors and not necessarily those of any of the abovementioned bodies, of the NHS, or of the Department of Health.

Provenance and peer review: Commissioned; externally peer reviewed.

1 Hutchings A, Hollywood J, Lamping DL, Pease CT, Chakravarty K, Silverman B, et al. Clinical outcomes, quality of life, and diagnostic uncertainty in the first year of polymyalgia rheumatica. *Arthritis Rheum* 2007;57:803-9.
2 Smeeth L, Cook C, Hall AJ. Incidence of diagnosed polymyalgia rheumatica and temporal arteritis in the United Kingdom, 1990-2001. *Ann Rheum Dis* 2006;65:1093-8.
3 Crowson CS, Matteson EL, Myasoedova E, Michet CJ, Ernste FC, Warrington KJ, et al. The lifetime risk of adult-onset rheumatoid arthritis and other inflammatory autoimmune rheumatic diseases. *Arthritis Rheum* 2011;63:633-9.
4 Dasgupta B, Borg FA, Hassan N, Barraclough K, Bourke B, Fulcher J, et al. BSR and BHPR guidelines for the management of polymyalgia rheumatica. *Rheumatology (Oxford)* 2010;49:186-90.
5 Bird HA, Esselinckx W, Dixon AS, Mowat AG, Wood PH. An evaluation of criteria for polymyalgia rheumatica. *Ann Rheum Dis* 1979;38:434-9.
6 Jones JG, Hazleman BL. Prognosis and management of polymyalgia rheumatica. *Ann Rheum Dis* 1981;40:1-5.
7 Chuang TY, Hunder GG, Ilstrup DM, Kurland LT. Polymyalgia rheumatica: a 10-year epidemiologic and clinical study. *Ann Intern Med* 1982;97:672-80.
8 Healey LA. Long-term follow-up of polymyalgia rheumatica: evidence for synovitis. *Semin Arthritis Rheum* 1984;13:322-8.
9 Nobunaga M, Yoshioka K, Yasuda M, Shingu M. Clinical studies of polymyalgia rheumatica. A proposal of diagnostic criteria. *Jpn J Med* 1989;28:452-6.
10 Dasgupta B, Cimmino MA, Maradit-Kremers H, Schmidt WA, Schirmer M, Salvarani C, et al. 2012 provisional classification criteria for polymyalgia rheumatica: a European League Against Rheumatism/American College of Rheumatology collaborative initiative. *Ann Rheum Dis* 2012;71:484-92.
11 Meliconi R, Pulsatelli L, Uguccioni M, Salvarani C, Macchioni P, Melchiorri C, et al. Leukocyte infiltration in synovial tissue from the shoulder of patients with polymyalgia rheumatica. Quantitative analysis and influence of corticosteroid treatment. *Arthritis Rheum* 1996;39:1199-207.
12 McGonagle D, Pease C, Marzo-Ortega H, O'Connor P, Gibbon W, Emery P. Comparison of extracapsular changes by magnetic resonance imaging in patients with rheumatoid arthritis and polymyalgia rheumatica. *J Rheumatol* 2001;28:1837-41.
13 Blockmans D, De Ceuninck L, Vanderschueren S, Knockaert D, Mortelmans L, Bobbaers H. Repetitive 18-fluorodeoxyglucose positron emission tomography in isolated polymyalgia rheumatica: a prospective study in 35 patients. *Rheumatology (Oxford)* 2007;46:672-7.
14 Salvarani C, Barozzi L, Cantini F, Niccoli L, Boiardi L, Valentino M, et al. Cervical interspinous bursitis in active polymyalgia rheumatica. *Ann Rheum Dis* 2008;67:758-61.
15 Cantini F, Salvarani C, Olivieri I, Macchioni L, Ranzi A, Niccoli L, et al. Erythrocyte sedimentation rate and C-reactive protein in the evaluation of disease activity and severity in polymyalgia rheumatica: a prospective follow-up study. *Semin Arthritis Rheum* 2000;30:17-24.
16 Zacharski LR. The erythrocyte sedimentation rate. *Br J Hosp Med* 1976;16:53-62.
17 Hutchinson RM, Eastham RD. A comparison of the erythrocyte sedimentation rate and plasma viscosity in detecting changes in plasma proteins. *J Clin Pathol* 1977;30:345-9.
18 Kanfer EJ, Nicol BA. Haemoglobin concentration and erythrocyte sedimentation rate in primary care patients. *J R Soc Med* 1997;90:16-8.
19 Késmárky G, Kenyeres P, Rábai M, Tóth K. Plasma viscosity: a forgotten variable. *Clin Hemorheol Microcirc* 2008;39:243-6.
20 McCarthy EM, MacMullan PA, Al-Mudhaffer S, Madigan A, Donnelly S, McCarthy CJ, et al. Plasma fibrinogen is an accurate marker of disease activity in patients with polymyalgia rheumatica. *Rheumatology (Oxford)* 2013;52:465-71.
21 Weyand CM, Fulbright JW, Evans JM, Hunder GG, Goronzy JJ. Corticosteroid requirements in polymyalgia rheumatica. *Arch Intern Med* 1999;159:577-84.
22 Straub RH, Glück T, Cutolo M, Georgi J, Helmke K, Schölmerich J, et al. The adrenal steroid status in relation to inflammatory cytokines (interleukin-6 and tumour necrosis factor) in polymyalgia rheumatica. *Rheumatology (Oxford)* 2000;39:624-31.
23 Olivieri I, Garcia-Porrua C, Padula A, Cantini F, Salvarani C, Gonzalez-Gay MA. Late onset undifferentiated spondyloarthritis presenting with polymyalgia rheumatica features: description of seven cases. *Rheumatol Int* 2007;27:927-33.
24 Aydeniz A, Altındağ O, Oğüt E, Gürsoy S. Late onset spondyloarthropathy mimicking polymyalgia rheumatica. *Rheumatol Int* 2012;32:1357-8.
25 Pego-Reigosa JM, Rodriguez-Rodriguez M, Hurtado-Hernandez Z, Gromaz-Martin J, Taboas-Rodriguez D, Millan-Cachinero C, et al. Calcium pyrophosphate deposition disease mimicking polymyalgia rheumatica: a prospective follow-up study of predictive factors for this condition in patients presenting with polymyalgia symptoms. *Arthritis Rheum* 2005;53:931-8.
26 Falsetti P, Acciai C, Volpe A, Lenzi L. Ultrasonography in early assessment of elderly patients with polymyalgic symptoms: a role in predicting diagnostic outcome? *Scand J Rheumatol* 2011;40:57-63.
27 Cantini F, Niccoli L, Storri L, Nannini C, Olivieri I, Padula A, et al. Are polymyalgia rheumatica and giant cell arteritis the same disease? *Semin Arthritis Rheum* 2004;33:294-301.
28 Dasgupta B, Borg FA, Hassan N, Alexander L, Barraclough K, Bourke B, et al. BSR and BHPR guidelines for the management of giant cell arteritis. *Rheumatology (Oxford)* 2010;49:1594-7.
29 Strehl C, Spies CM, Buttgereit F. Pharmacodynamics of glucocorticoids. *Clin Exp Rheumatol* 2011;29(suppl 68):S13-8.
30 Fauchald P, Rygvold O, Oystese B. Temporal arteritis and polymyalgia rheumatica. Clinical and biopsy findings. *Ann Intern Med* 1972;77:845-52.
31 Camellino D, Cimmino MA. Imaging of polymyalgia rheumatica: indications on its pathogenesis, diagnosis and prognosis. *Rheumatology (Oxford)* 2012;51:77-86.
32 Caporali R, Montecucco C, Epis O, Bobbio-Pallavicini F, Maio T, Cimmino MA. Presenting features of polymyalgia rheumatica (PMR) and rheumatoid arthritis with PMR-like onset: a prospective study. *Ann Rheum Dis* 2001;60:1021-4.
33 Pease CT, Haugeberg G, Morgan AW, Montague B, Hensor EM, Bhakta BB. Diagnosing late onset rheumatoid arthritis, polymyalgia rheumatica, and temporal arteritis in patients presenting with polymyalgic symptoms. A prospective longterm evaluation. *J Rheumatol* 2005;32:1043-6.
34 Aletaha D, Neogi T, Silman AJ, Funovits J, Felson DT, Bingham CO 3rd, et al. 2010 rheumatoid arthritis classification criteria: an American College of Rheumatology/European League Against Rheumatism collaborative initiative. *Ann Rheum Dis* 2010;69:1580-8.
35 Lopez-Hoyos M, Ruiz de Alegria C, Blanco R, Crespo J, Peña M, Rodriguez-Valverde V, et al. Clinical utility of anti-CCP antibodies in the differential diagnosis of elderly-onset rheumatoid arthritis and polymyalgia rheumatica. *Rheumatology (Oxford)* 2004;43:655-7.
36 Belloli L, Massarotti M, Marasini B. Polymyalgia rheumatica and elderly onset rheumatoid arthritis. *J Clin Rheumatol* 2008;14:59.
37 González-Gay MA, Amoli MM, Garcia-Porrua C, Ollier WE. Genetic markers of disease susceptibility and severity in giant cell arteritis and polymyalgia rheumatica. *Semin Arthritis Rheum* 2003;33:38-48.
38 Gregersen PK, Silver J, Winchester RJ. The shared epitope hypothesis. An approach to understanding the molecular genetics of susceptibility to rheumatoid arthritis. *Arthritis Rheum* 1987;30:1205-13.
39 González-Gay MA, García-Porrúa C, Vázquez-Caruncho M, Dababneh A, Hajeer A, Ollier WE. The spectrum of polymyalgia rheumatica in northwestern Spain: incidence and analysis of variables associated with relapse in a 10 year study. *J Rheumatol* 1999;26:1326-32.
40 Gonzalez-Gay MA, Hajeer AH, Dababneh A, Makki R, Garcia-Porrua C, Thomson W, et al. Seronegative rheumatoid arthritis in elderly and polymyalgia rheumatica have similar patterns of HLA association. *J Rheumatol* 2001;28:122-5.
41 Salvarani C, Boiardi L, Mantovani V, Ranzi A, Cantini F, Olivieri I, et al. HLA-DRB1 alleles associated with polymyalgia rheumatica in northern Italy: correlation with disease severity. *Ann Rheum Dis* 1999;58:303-8.
42 Ganz T, Nemeth E. Iron sequestration and anemia of inflammation. *Semin Hematol* 2009;46:387-93.
43 Sakellariou G, Iagnocco A, Riente L, Ceccarelli F, Carli L, Di Geso L, et al. Ultrasound imaging for the rheumatologist XLIII. Ultrasonographic evaluation of shoulders and hips in patients with polymyalgia rheumatica: a systematic literature review. *Clin Exp Rheumatol* 2013;31:1-7.

44 Cimmino MA, Parodi M, Montecucco C, Caporali R. The correct prednisone starting dose in polymyalgia rheumatica is related to body weight but not to disease severity. *BMC Musculoskelet Disord* 2011;12:94.

45 Gonzalez-Gay MA, Garcia-Porrua C, Salvarani C, Olivieri I, Hunder GG. The spectrum of conditions mimicking polymyalgia rheumatica in northwestern Spain. *J Rheumatol* 2000;27:2179-84.

46 Kyle V, Hazleman BL. Treatment of polymyalgia rheumatica and giant cell arteritis. I. Steroid regimens in the first two months. *Ann Rheum Dis* 1989;48:658-61.

47 Quick V, Kirwan JR. Our approach to the diagnosis and treatment of polymyalgia rheumatica and giant cell (temporal) arteritis. *J R Coll Physicians Edinb* 2012;42:341-9.

48 Mackie SL, Hensor EM, Haugeberg G, Bhakta B, Pease CT. Can the prognosis of polymyalgia rheumatica be predicted at disease onset? Results from a 5-year prospective study. *Rheumatology (Oxford)* 2010;49:716-22.

49 Salvarani C, Macchioni PL, Tartoni PL, Rossi F, Baricchi R, Castri C, et al. Polymyalgia rheumatica and giant cell arteritis: a 5-year epidemiologic and clinical study in Reggio Emilia, Italy. *Clin Exp Rheumatol* 1987;5:205-15.

50 Pountain G, Hazleman B. Erythrocyte sedimentation rate (ESR) at presentation is a prognostic indicator for duration of treatment in polymyalgia rheumatica (PMR). *Br J Rheumatol* 1997;36:508-9.

51 Dolan AL, Moniz C, Dasgupta B, Li F, Mackintosh C, Todd P, et al. Effects of inflammation and treatment on bone turnover and bone mass in polymyalgia rheumatica. *Arthritis Rheum* 1997;40:2022-9.

52 González-Gay MA, Rodríguez-Valverde V, Blanco R, Fernández-Sueiro JL, Armona J, Figueroa M, et al. Polymyalgia rheumatica without significantly increased erythrocyte sedimentation rate. A more benign syndrome. *Arch Intern Med* 1997;157:317-20.

53 Myklebust G, Gran JT. Prednisolone maintenance dose in relation to starting dose in the treatment of polymyalgia rheumatica and temporal arteritis. A prospective two-year study in 273 patients. *Scand J Rheumatol* 2001;30:260-7.

54 Narváez J, Nolla-Solé JM, Clavaguera MT, Valverde-García J, Roig-Escofet D. Longterm therapy in polymyalgia rheumatica: effect of coexistent temporal arteritis. *J Rheumatol* 1999;26:1945-52.

55 Do-Nguyen D, Inderjeeth CA, Edelman J, Cheah P. Retrospective analysis of the clinical course of patients treated for polymyalgia. *Open Access Rheumatol: Res Rev* 2013;5:33-41.

56 Leeb BF, Bird HA. A disease activity score for polymyalgia rheumatica. *Ann Rheum Dis* 2004;63:1279-83.

57 Caporali R, Cimmino RA, Ferracioli G, Gerli R, Klersy C, Salvarani C, et al; Systemic Vasculitis Study Group of the Italian Society for Rheumatology. Prednisone plus methotrexate for polymyalgia rheumatica: a randomized, double-blind, placebo-controlled trial. *Ann Intern Med* 2004;141:493-500.

58 Salvarani C, Macchioni P, Manzini C, Paolazzi G, Trotta A, Manganelli P, et al. Infliximab plus prednisone or placebo plus prednisone for the initial treatment of polymyalgia rheumatica: a randomized trial. *Ann Intern Med* 2007;146:631-9.

59 Kreiner F, Galbo H. Effect of etanercept in polymyalgia rheumatica: a randomized controlled trial. *Arthritis Res Ther* 2010;12:R176.

60 Adizie T, Christidis D, Dharmapaliah C, Borg F, Dasgupta B. Efficacy and tolerability of leflunomide in difficult-to-treat polymyalgia rheumatica and giant cell arteritis: a case series. *Int J Clin Pract* 2012;66:906-9.

61 Macchioni P, Boiardi L, Catanoso M, Pulsatelli L, Pipitone N, Meliconi R, et al. Tocilizumab for polymyalgia rheumatica: report of two cases and review of the literature. *Semin Arthritis Rheum* 2013; published online 20 Feb.

62 Hoes JN, Jacobs JW, Verstappen SM, Bijlsma JW, Van der Heijden GJ. Adverse events of low- to medium-dose oral glucocorticoids in inflammatory diseases: a meta-analysis. *Ann Rheum Dis* 2009;68:1833-8.

63 Mazzantini M, Torre C, Miccoli M, Baggiani A, Talarico R, Bombardieri S, et al. Adverse events during longterm low-dose glucocorticoid treatment of polymyalgia rheumatica: a retrospective study. *J Rheumatol* 2012;39:552-7.

64 National Institute for Health and Care Excellence. Osteoporosis—prevention of fragility fractures. 2013. http://cks.nice.org.uk/osteoporosis-prevention-of-fragility-fractures.

65 Dasgupta B, Dolan AL, Panayi GS, Fernandes L. An initially double-blind controlled 96 week trial of depot methylprednisolone against oral prednisolone in the treatment of polymyalgia rheumatica. *Br J Rheumatol* 1998;37:189-95.

66 Gabriel SE, Sunku J, Salvarani C, O'Fallon WM, Hunder GG. Adverse outcomes of antiinflammatory therapy among patients with polymyalgia rheumatica. *Arthritis Rheum* 1997;40:1873-8.

Temporomandibular disorders

Justin Durham, NIHR clinician scientist, senior lecturer[1], Toby R O Newton-John, senior lecturer, clinical psychology[2], Joanna M Zakrzewska, professor[3]

[1]Centre for Oral Health Research & Institute of Health and Society, Newcastle University, Newcastle, UK

[2]Graduate School of Health, University of Technology, Sydney, NSW, Australia

[3]Facial Pain Unit, Eastman Dental Hospital, UCLH NHS Foundation Trust, London, UK

Correspondence to: J Durham, Level 5—School of Dental Sciences, Newcastle University, Newcastle NE2 4BW, UK justin.durham@ncl.ac.uk

Cite this as: *BMJ* 2015;350:h1154

DOI: 10.1136/bmj.h1154

http://www.bmj.com/content/350/bmj.h1154

After odontogenic pain, temporomandibular disorders (TMDs) are one of the most common causes of pain in the mouth and face and also have the potential to produce persisting (chronic) pain.[1 2] Chronic or persistent (myogenous) TMDs can be associated with other chronic pain conditions,[3] including migraine, fibromyalgia, and widespread pain.[4 5 6 7 8] They are also known to be comorbid with bruxism, depression, irritable bowel syndrome, and chronic fatigue.[6 9 10] With or without these comorbidities, TMDs are recognised to have a considerable impact on quality of life.[11 12 13 14 15 16 17]

Early diagnosis and explanation followed by management is likely to be key to improving prognosis and reducing the impact of this group of conditions on quality of life.[11 18] The purpose of this review is to give non-specialists an overview of the diagnosis and management of TMDs.

What are TMDs?

Some of the signs and symptoms suggestive of TMDs were identified back in the 1930s by Costen, who incorrectly attributed them to changes in occlusion (bite of the teeth).[19] Over the next 80 years the terminology has changed and been revised several times[20 21 22] until the collective term temporomandibular disorders has been accepted.[23 24 25 26] The most widely accepted definition is "a group of musculoskeletal . . . conditions that involve the temporomandibular joints (TMJs), the masticatory muscles and all associated tissues."[27] A new expanded taxonomy is now available defining the various subtypes of disorder or disease incorporated in this group.[28]

How common are TMDs and who gets them?

Data from a US large and ongoing prospective cohort study (OPPERA)[29] suggest that the incidence of first onset painful TMDs is 3-4% per annum. Among the population studied (adults aged 18-44) for first onset of painful TMDs there seemed to be only a slight preponderance for women to be affected more than men (imputed hazard ratio 1.3, $P>0.05$) and an increasing incidence with age: 18-24 age band 2.5%, 25-34 age band 3.7%, and 35-44 age band 4.5%.[30] The probability of first onset TMDs is also strongly associated with concurrent headaches and body pain.[31 32] The prevalence of painful TMDs in adolescents is still a matter of debate,[33] with some estimates reaching 25%, but in developed countries it is estimated to be between 2% and 6%.[34 35 36] In adults aged more than 45 the prevalence of painful TMDs is likely to lie in the range of 2-7%,[37] although estimates vary and those aged over 45 are more likely to display objective signs of TMDs but be asymptomatic.[38]

Among all incident cases in the OPPERA study, pain occurred as a singular episode in 12%, recurrent episode in 65%, and persistent episode in 19%. Pain was most commonly reported in both the joint and the muscles of mastication (arthralgia with myalgia: 73% of the incident cases); the next most common presentation was myalgia alone (23% of incident cases).[30] OPPERA and other US data suggest there is a disproportionate increase in healthcare utilisation with TMDs.[32 39] The reasons behind this are not fully explained, but ongoing research[40] in the United Kingdom seeking to determine the effectiveness and efficacy of care pathways for orofacial pain (http://research.ncl.ac.uk/deepstudy) may help to explain this from a UK context in due course.

What causes TMDs?

The causes and underlying pathophysiology of TMDs have been the subject of much debate and some controversy over the years.[26 41] It is suggested that the cause is likely to be both multifactorial and biopsychosocial, consisting of initiating, predisposing, and perpetuating factors, for example, macro-trauma or micro-trauma, linked to a failure to heal appropriately because of the underlying psychosocial profile of the patient, failed treatment, or genotype.[41 42 43] Evidence is now emerging for factors involved in the complex multifactorial pathophysiology of TMDs relating to both genotype and phenotype.[44 45]

In recent years major advances have occurred in the knowledge of the underlying pathophysiology of TMDs. It is suggested that women with an oestrogen receptor polymorphism have twice and three times the odds of developing a non-painful or painful TMD, respectively, compared with women without the polymorphism.[46] Several studies suggest the pain of TMDs to be potentially mediated by several different mechanisms: central sensitisation, through neuroplasticity and calcitonin gene related peptide,[47 48 49 50 51] and differing haplotypes of the gene encoding catecholamine-O-methyltransferase, which produce less activity of this enzyme.[52 53] Some of the neural abnormalities detected in chronic TMDs are in the trigeminal and limbic systems,[54] and cortical activity may be changed such that cognitive and emotional tasks are harder to perform.[55]

Further to this genetic polymorphisms in the folate and oxidative metabolic pathways may be associated with oxidative stress and be implicated in degenerative joint disease.[56 57 58] Such disease has also been associated with a metalloproteinase gene polymorphism.[59]

Clearly there may be further advances in the coming years, but what is truly exciting are the potential advances in identifying targets for treatment, such as calcitonin gene related peptide and β adrenergic receptors. β Adrenergic receptors have already been shown in a proof of concept trial to be of benefit if targeted by treatment.[60]

THE BOTTOM LINE

- TMDs represent a range of conditions with multifactorial complex pathophysiology, which are common up to the age of 40 years
- TMDs can present as a continuous or episodic pain of varying intensity around and in the ears radiating up to the temple or down the mandible to the neck
- Persistent (chronic) TMDs can be associated with other chronic pain conditions
- Early management with education and counselling is highly effective
- More complex patients or those with persistent TMDs require a biopsychosocial approach delivered by a multidisciplinary pain team

What are the clinical features?

TMDs can present with any or all of the following signs and symptoms: pain in the temporomandibular joint or muscles of mastication (figures 1 and 2), which may radiate or refer to local or distant structures; clicking, popping, or crepitus of the temporomandibular joint on any of its movements with or without locking of the joint; headache limited to the temporal region[61]; and otalgia or tinnitus, or both in the absence of aural disease. The correlation between self reported severity of pain and pathological changes in the joints or muscles is poor.[26]

The table summarises the 12 most common TMDs and the most salient points of their history and examination findings. Some patients present principally with a self reported painless clicking (disc displacement with reduction) and are mistakenly concerned that this indicates damage. Others report episodic painful (closed) locking, an inability to open the mouth wide (disc displacement with reduction with intermittent limited opening), persistent closed lock (disc displacement without reduction with limited opening), or repeated dislocation of the temporomandibular joint, which are all clearly of functional importance.

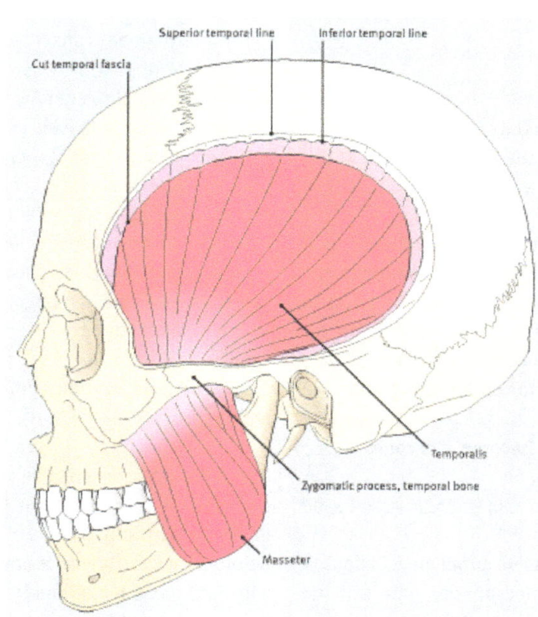

Fig 1 Surface anatomy of temporalis and masseter muscles. Adapted from Standring 2008[113]

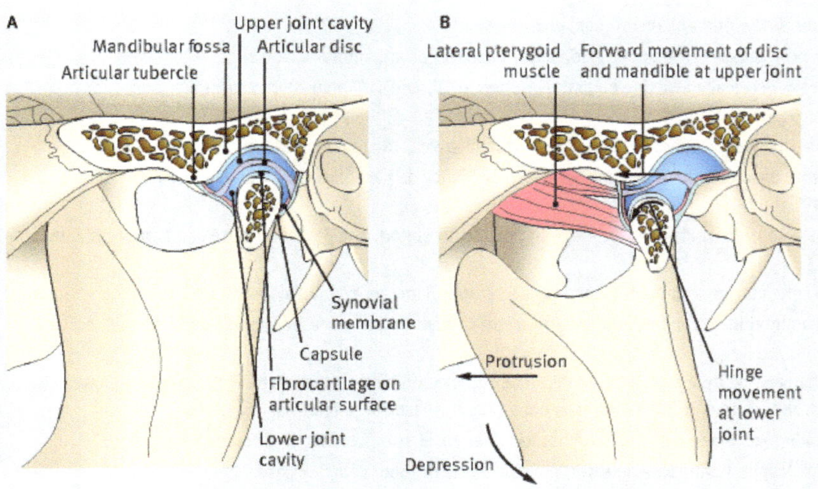

Fig 2 Surface anatomy of temporomandibular joint. Mouth closed (left) and mouth open (right). Adapted from Drake et al 2005[114]

How are TMDs diagnosed?

Over the past two decades progress in revising and validating the diagnostic criteria for TMDs has been considerable.[62 63 64 65 66 67 68 69 70 71 72 73 74] In their validated and revised form these criteria, originally known as the RDC/TMD (Research Diagnostic Criteria for TMD),[62] are now known as the DC/TMD (Diagnostic Criteria for TMD).[75] They provide a standard and operationalised manner in which to examine the temporomandibular joint and its associated structures (axis 1) physically and to screen for psychosocial comorbidity (axis 2).

A simple method to screen for painful TMDs (as a physical entity) is to use a six item self complete questionnaire developed in tandem with the Diagnostic Criteria for TMD.[76] When used in a facial pain clinic this method has 99% sensitivity and 98% specificity for painful TMDs and may be of utility in busy general medical practices. The questionnaire is freely available on the RDC/TMD consortium's website (www.rdc-tmdinternational.org/OtherInstruments/TMDPainScreener.aspx). A score of 3 or more is indicative of a positive screening for TMDs. Alternatively the questions posed could be incorporated into a standard clinical history for orofacial pain.

Axis 1

The physical axis of the DC/TMD, axis 1, defines 38 different types of TMDs of which 12 types present most commonly (table).[75] As this is a summary table the list is not exhaustive. We believe that the easiest way to recall these 12 separate TMDs is to subdivide them into four main categories or groups: myalgia, arthralgia, intra-articular disorders, and headache attributable to TMDs. Full details on DC/TMD diagnostic algorithms and their sensitivity and specificity (where determined) are available in an open access publication[75] and on the RDC/TMD consortium's website (table).

The concept of eliciting pain that is "familiar" by provocation underpins the new revised and validated diagnostic criteria for TMD.[75] Familiar pain is the process of recreating the patients' symptoms during an examination and confirming with them that this is what they experience. The following features on examination should raise suspicion of, but do not formally confirm or exclude, a diagnosis of painful TMD: provocation of familiar pain through palpation

SOURCES AND SELECTION CRITERIA

We conducted a systematic search of Medline (1966 to 5 August 2014), PROSPERO, and Cochrane libraries for systematic reviews relating to interventions for TMDs. For systematic reviews in Medline we used the search strategy suggested by BMJ Clinical Evidence search strategy. We searched PROSPERO and Cochrane libraries using their own search engines with the terms "temporomandibular", "temporomandibular disorder", "temporomandibular joint", and "pain dysfunction syndrome". The supplementary table summarises the most recent and relevant systematic reviews. It excludes older systematic reviews that duplicate more recent ones unless they are within a five year period and offer contradictory evidence. All Cochrane reviews identified are contained within the summary table.

of masseter and or temporalis (fig 1), through palpation of the temporomandibular joint (fig 2), or by putting the joint through its normal range of movements.

Of note in the diagnostic algorithm of the DC/TMD is the rationalised, limited, use of either plain or computed imaging (employing ionising radiation), which is outlined on the consortium's website (table). Generally, imaging is only performed if clinical examination indicates a functional problem. Great care should be taken when explaining the results of any imaging to patients as the use of words such as "degenerative" may cause great concern and consequently affect patients' behaviour.

Axis 2

Axis 2 of the DC/TMD can be used in a shortened form (a brief screening axis for psychosocial comorbidity) or in its full form (a comprehensive axis for psychosocial comorbidity). The instruments comprising axis 2 are available in full on the consortium's website. Axis 2's focus on psychosocial comorbidity is because this is known to impact on prognosis and treatment outcome.[5 45 77]

What are the red flags?

Box 1 outlines some of the red flags that may mimic a TMD,[78 79 80 81] although this is not an exhaustive list. These red flags can act as signposts for conditions to consider in differential diagnoses.

Specialties that will help in the case of relevant oral and maxillofacial red flag symptoms include oral medicine, oral and maxillofacial surgery, and oral surgery. Referral to ear, nose, and throat surgeons should be considered for worrisome signs in these areas and referral to a headache neurologist should be considered for upper face pain.

What makes TMDs more likely to become a chronic musculoskeletal pain?

Box 2 describes the factors that are more likely to be associated with chronic pain.[83 84 85 86 87]

For patients with a noted affective problem in addition to the pain or where there is a preoccupation with somatic symptoms and experiences, referral to a clinical psychologist or psychiatrist is an important adjunctive pain management option.[89]

Convincing evidence shows that psychosocial factors are influential in the development of general chronic pain states[90] and of TMD specifically.[5 45 77]

Importantly, research has shown that a chronic pain trajectory can be modified. People with acute TMDs identified as being at high risk of chronic TMDs have been shown to benefit considerably from early psychological intervention.[91] This suggests that although mood disorder, pain catastrophising, somatic preoccupation, and poor coping skills may predispose people with acute TMDs to develop long term problems, intervening with appropriate psychological input before these problems become entrenched can be of great value.

What is the management?

The recurring theme in the systematic reviews examined for this review (see supplementary table) is that well designed pragmatic randomised controlled trials using standardised and patient based outcome measures in TMD are urgently needed.

An international consensus reached in 1995 and revised slightly in 2010[27 92] was that reversible, conservative treatments should generally form the first line intervention for TMDs. This is based on data that suggest between 75% and 90% of patients with TMDs will respond to these simpler, potentially less costly, and much less invasive techniques.[93] After an initial diagnosis of acute TMD the first approach to management should be a careful explanation of the (provisional) diagnosis alongside education about the condition and its largely benign course. This can be supplemented by advice on appropriate, time limited, simple analgesic use and altered dietary consistency for acute exacerbations plus information on self management techniques.

Reversible and conservative treatments

Education—education about the condition and reassurance of its benign and usually non-progressive nature can be helpful. Lack of, or uncertainty in, diagnosis for patients with TMD has a major impact on their quality of life and can lead to care pathways that are not efficacious and possibly compound or worsen symptoms.[11 12 94] Health professionals should seek to explain a clear (provisional) diagnosis to

BOX 1 RED FLAGS THAT MAY MIMIC TMDS

- History of malignancy—potential for a new primary, recurrence, or metastases
- Presence of lymphadenopathy or neck masses—consider a neoplastic, infective, or autoimmune cause
- Sensory or motor function changes (specifically focusing on cranial nerves V, VII, and VIII)—consider intracranial causes, or malignancy affecting the nerve's peripheral branches
- Recurrent epistaxis, purulent nasal drainage, or anosmia—consider nasopharyngeal carcinoma or chronic sinusitis
- Trismus especially if history of using paan or betel nut—consider oral malignancy as part of differential diagnoses and think about employing the "Trismus checklist"[82]
- Unexplained pyrexia or weight loss—consider malignant tumours, immunosuppression, and infective causes as part of differential diagnoses
- First episode in over 50s, unilateral headache accompanied by jaw claudication, and general malaise—consider temporal arteritis
- Facial asymmetry or masses (uncommon in TMD unless there is masseteric hypertrophy)—consider neoplastic, infective, or inflammatory causes
- Occlusal changes (bite of teeth changes) as determined by dentist that do not predate the start of the TMD—consider growth disturbance of condyle, neoplasia, rheumatoid arthritis, and traumatic causes as part of differential diagnoses
- Ipsilateral objective change in hearing—consider acoustic neuroma, or other ear disease as part of differential diagnoses
- Persisting or worsening symptoms despite treatment—consider a misdiagnosis or more complex case
- History of recent head and neck trauma
- Paroxysmal unilateral lancinating pain with or without autonomic features—more likely to be associated with trigeminal neuralgia or one of the trigeminal autonomic cephalagias

patients at the earliest opportunity and then signpost helpful information and supportive organisations. Providing diagrams to increase knowledge of the anatomy are useful. Education would be the starting point for management of any patient with a suspected TMD. Useful resources to help with this are signposted in the additional educational resources box.

Self management (or self care) techniques—specific suggestions for self management and for physiotherapy are given in the recently published primary care guidance for TMDs (www.rcseng.ac.uk/fds/publications-clinical-guidelines/clinical_guidelines/documents/temporomandibular-disorders-guideline-2013). Simple generic advice around sleep hygiene, caffeine consumption, and avoidance of parafunctional activities such as daytime clenching, nail biting, or excessive chewing of gum can be helpful. This advice along with suggestions on relaxation techniques such as diaphragmatic breathing, and local measures for pain relief such as the use of covered ice or warm flannels to painful areas can be of benefit for some patients.

Physiotherapy and acupuncture—there is limited evidence to suggest that physiotherapeutic modalities such as massage or targeted exercises may help provide short term relief for acute TMDs, although the results of a Cochrane systematic review (see supplementary table) are awaited. A systematic review on acupuncture suggests that it may reduce pain intensity and specifically help with masseteric tenderness (see supplementary table).

Cognitive behavioural therapy—such treatment is considered the ideal psychological treatment for chronic pain.[95] Cognitive behavioural treatment for pain is an active, structured, collaborative therapy, which aims to teach patients the most adaptive ways of coping with their pain. Techniques might include dealing with pain related anxieties, behavioural activation plans, management of pain flare-ups, sleep hygiene, and optimal communication strategies with family members. The evidence for cognitive behavioural treatment in relation to TMDs indicates important long term improvements in pain intensity and mood, and reductions in activity limitation due to pain.[96 97] Cognitive behavioural treatment does not seem to reduce pain on muscle palpation.

Splints—"mouth guards" in either a soft polyethylene or a hard acrylic that provide full coverage of all the upper or lower teeth worn, can be worn at night in those who grind or clench their teeth. Mouth guards help to protect tooth substance and may also provide an element of biofeedback.

Simple analgesia—non-steroidal anti-inflammatory drugs can be used, being mindful of gastrointestinal side effects from continual use and drug overuse headache.

Other drug interventions—more "advanced" approaches include the use of neuromodulatory agents for persistent pain, which would all come under off-label prescribing. A small number of published trials support the use of gabapentin, benzodiazepines, amitriptyline, and propranolol for the management of pain of a myogenous origin.[60 98 99 100] Botulinum toxin applied to the muscles of mastication has been the subject of a small number of randomised controlled trials of varying quality and with the potential for type II errors.[101 102 103 104] Considering the results of these various studies as a whole the evidence at present is at best equivocal for the use of botulinum toxin

BOX 2 FACTORS ASSOCIATED WITH PAIN FROM TMDS BECOMING CHRONIC

- Females with myogenous TMD
- Increasing age at presentation
- Graded chronic pain scale[88] score of 3 or 4
- Higher pain intensity
- Higher pain interference
- More widespread non-specific symptoms (or higher number of pain locations)
- Concurrent psychiatric diagnosis or mood disturbance (depression, anxiety, anger)

Summary of salient history and examination findings for 12 most common (numbers in parentheses) temporomandibular disorders[62]

Category	Subcategory	Summary history and examination findings
Myalgia (1): history positive for both of following: pain in jaw, temple, in ear, or in front of ear; pain modified with jaw movement, function, or parafunction. Examination: pain in masseter or temporalis produced by palpation or maximum assisted or unassisted opening	Local myalgia (2); myofascial pain (3); myofascial pain with referral (4)	Pain local to palpation; pain within body of muscle; pain spreads outside the body muscle
Arthralgia (5): history as for myalgia		Pain in temporomandibular joint region produced by one of: palpation or assisted or unassisted jaw movements
Intra-articular disorders	Disc displacements: with reduction (6); with reduction with intermittent locking (7); without reduction with limited opening (8); without reduction without limited opening (9)	Click, pop, snap: on open and close (1 out of 3 movements), or one of opening and closing plus a lateral movement; as above but history of lock does not matter how long; history: decreased mouth opening and inability to eat or interference with eating. Examination: maximum assisted opening <40 mm; history as above but maximum assisted opening >40 mm
	Degenerative joint disease (10)	Crepitus in any movement, with relatively little pain
	Subluxation (11)	History: lock open and self manipulation to achieve closure
Headache attributable to temporomandibular disorder (12)*		History: headache in temple and modified with jaw movement, function, or parafunction. Examination: familiar headache with palpation temporalis or with jaw movements

**As determined in the Diagnostic Criteria for TMD. The Diagnostic Criteria for TMD definition differs slightly from that described in international classification of headache disorders, version 3.*

in myogenous TMDs, but there is still a need for a definitive and appropriately powered randomised controlled trial.[105] Some concerns are emerging from a small scale study about the potential osteopenic effects on the temporomandibular joint of repeatedly administered botulinum toxin to the muscles of mastication over a long period.[106]

Irreversible approaches

The American Association for Dental Research has also issued a statement to recommend strongly that unless there are "specific and justifiable indications," irreversible approaches should not be used as primary management for TMDs.[27]

Orthodontics and occlusal equilibration—systematic reviews of irreversible approaches such as orthodontics and occlusal equilibration (careful grinding of the natural teeth to achieve a more "harmonious" bite) show these approaches lack evidence to support their use in the management of TMDs.[107 108]

Surgical interventions—these are only indicated in a small number of cases and only if there is an intra-articular disorder, degenerative joint disease, or other evident disease affecting the temporomandibular joint.[96]

Why is psychological management of TMDs important?

TMDs, as with other causes of pain, are best conceptualised in biopsychosocial terms.[109] The patient's beliefs, expectations, emotional state, family environment, and cultural background can all play a role in the onset, development, and maintenance of persistent pain. The axis 2 classification of the DC/TMD explicitly recognises the importance of psychological and social aspects of pain by assessing not just pain intensity but also depressed mood, anxiety, pain related disability, parafunctional behaviours, and a variety of associated comorbidities. The DC/TMD also helps to perform a basic ("screening") or a "comprehensive" assessment of the patient's psychosocial status and can be used to inform referrals for specialised psychological input.

In addition to cognitive behavioural therapy, there is limited evidence for a range of other psychologically based interventions for TMDs, including electromyographic biofeedback, stress management, and hypnosis.[96 97] In the past, referral for psychological therapy has tended to be the last resort, once all biological treatments have been exhausted and present treatment "failed." As a result of this type of approach patients may interpret the referral to a psychologist as an indication that their medical or dental practitioner has given up on them, or that their pain is considered to be "psychological" and somehow not genuine.[110] Making time for adequate explanation of the multidisciplinary nature of complex pain treatment as early as possible in the diagnosis and management process is generally time well spent.

Having laid the groundwork that chronic pain is best managed using a team approach (which includes the patient as an active member of the team), the literature relating to facilitating the engagement of patients in biopsychosocial intervention offers several useful suggestions.[111] As always, the quality of patient-provider communication is important, with empathy for the patient's pain experience particularly relevant.[112] The use of patient centered communication skills, promoting patient self efficacy, and providing positive feedback on patient's coping efforts can all enhance patient motivation to engage in self management approaches.[111]

TIPS FOR NON-SPECIALISTS

- Problems associated with TMDs are common and associated with pain and sometimes clicking and locking
- Consider either liaision with the patient's dental practitioner, or use of a simple screening questionnaire if confirmation of clinical diagnosis is required
- It is important to exclude temporal arteritis, especially if the patient is older than 50 years
- Reassurance, explanation, and non-steroidal anti-inflammatory drugs used early in the history of the disorder are highly effective
- Management of both comorbid migraine and TMDs may help improve outcome
- In patients with other chronic pains and depression, consider referral to specialist centres for biopsychosocial management

ADDITIONAL EDUCATIONAL RESOURCES

Resources for healthcare professionals

- Research Diagnostic Criteria for TMD consortium network (www.rdc-tmdinternational.org/OtherResources/TrainingReliability/RDCExaminerTraining.aspx)—contains all instruments and parts of the DC/TMD
- Davies S, Al-Ani Z. The three minute examination of the articulatory system. Video in the E-Den (on e-lfh) session on "Assessing the articulatory system." (http://portal.e-lfh.org.uk/)—e-learning for healthcare (requires registration and working within the National Health Service)
- Royal College of Surgeons of England guidance on Primary care management of TMD (www.rcseng.ac.uk/fds/publications-clinical-guidelines/clinical_guidelines)
- Open access diagnosis and treatment of non-dental facial pain on Cardiff pain community (www.paincommunitycentre.org/article/diagnosis-and-treatment-non-dental-facial-pain)—e-learning on facial pain

Resources for patients

- American Academy of Orofacial Pain (www.aaop.org/content.aspx?page_id=22&club_id=508439&module_id=108085)—patient leaflets
- European Federation of International Association for the Study of Pain chapters (www.efic.org/index.asp?sub=F8AMLHLAP9216P&topicsid=314#view)—patient leaflets
- International Association for the Study of Pain (www.iasp-pain.org/Advocacy/Content.aspx?ItemNumber=1078&navItemNumber=580)— healthcare providers leaflets
- National Institute for Health and Care Excellence. Clinical knowledge summary on TMDs (http://cks.nice.org.uk/tmj-disorders)—practical guidance for the diagnosis and management of TMD
- National Institute for Health (www.nidcr.nih.gov/oralhealth/topics/tmj/tmjdisorders.htm)—general information on TMD for patients
- Temporomandibular Joint Association (www.tmj.org)—patient advocacy agency in United States

A further communication problem for clinicians relates to patients wanting to pursue treatment options that are risky, ill advised, or dangerous, such as an irreversible intervention where there is no objective clinical evidence to support its use. These requests are best understood as reflecting the patient's desperation in living with intractable pain. In response, clinicians should firstly empathise with the difficulty of the patient's situation, but provide a clear, evidence based explanation as to the inadvisability of the treatment. Encouraging patients to refrain from falling into the trap of seeking "quick fixes" for complex problems and assisting and supporting them to develop and expand their own coping resources, offers a better long term solution.

Contributors: JD and JMZ conceived and designed the article. JD drafted the manuscript. TNJ contributed the psychological aspects. All authors approved the final version of the manuscript and are the guarantors.

Competing interests: We have read and understood the BMJ policy on declaration of interests and declare the following: JMZ is part funded by UCL/UCLHT, which received a proportion of funding from the Department of Health's NIHR Biomedical Research Centre funding scheme; JD is funded by a NIHR clinician scientist award (NIHR-CS-011-003). The views expressed in this publication are those of the authors and not necessarily those of the National Health Service, the National Institute for Health Research, or the Department of Health in the United Kingdom.

Provenance and peer review: Commissioned; externally peer reviewed.

1 Dworkin SF, Massoth DL. Temporomandibular disorders and chronic pain: disease or illness? *J Prosthet Dent* 1994;72:29-38.
2 Lipton JA, Ship JA, Larach-Robinson D. Estimated prevalence and distribution of reported orofacial pain in the United States. *J Am Dent Assoc* 1993;124:115-21.
3 Plesh O, Adams SH, Gansky SA. Temporomandibular joint and muscle disorder-type pain and comorbid pains in a national US sample. *J Orofac Pain* 2011;25:190-8.
4 Velly AM, Look JO, Schiffman E, Lenton PA, Kang W, Messner RP, et al. The effect of fibromyalgia and widespread pain on the clinically significant temporomandibular muscle and joint pain disorders—a prospective 18-month cohort study. *J Pain* 2010;11:1155-64.
5 Velly AM, Look JO, Carlson C, Lenton PA, Kang W, Holcroft CA, et al. The effect of catastrophizing and depression on chronic pain—a prospective cohort study of temporomandibular muscle and joint pain disorders. *Pain* 2011;152:2377-83.
6 Aggarwal VR, McBeth J, Zakrzewska JM, Lunt M, Macfarlane GJ. The epidemiology of chronic syndromes that are frequently unexplained: do they have common associated factors? *Int J Epidemiol* 2006;35:468-76.
7 Ballegaard V, Thede-Schmidt-Hansen P, Svensson P, Jensen R. Are headache and temporomandibular disorders related? A blinded study. *Cephalalgia* 2008;28:832-41.
8 Goncalves DA, Bigal ME, Jales LC, Camparis CM, Speciali JG. Headache and symptoms of temporomandibular disorder: an epidemiological study. *Headache* 2010;50:231-41.
9 Fernandes G, Franco AL, Goncalves DA, Speciali JG, Bigal ME, Camparis CM. Temporomandibular disorders, sleep bruxism, and primary headaches are mutually associated. *J Orofac Pain* 2013;27:14-20.
10 Hoffmann RG, Kotchen JM, Kotchen TA, Cowley T, Dasgupta M, Cowley AWJ. Temporomandibular disorders and associated clinical comorbidities. *Clin J Pain* 2011;27:268-74.
11 Durham J, Steele JG, Wassell RW, Exley C. Living with uncertainty: temporomandibular disorders. *J Dent Res* 2010;89:827-30.
12 Durham J, Steele J, Moufti MA, Wassell R, Robinson P, Exley C. Temporomandibular disorder patients' journey through care. *Community Dent Oral Epidemiol* 2011;39:532-41.
13 Durham J, Steele JG, Wassell RW, Exley C, Meechan JG, Allen PF, et al. Creating a patient-based condition-specific outcome measure for Temporomandibular Disorders (TMDs): Oral Health Impact Profile for TMDs (OHIP-TMDs). *J Oral Rehabil* 2011;38:871-83.
14 Moufti MA, Wassell RW, Meechan JG, Allen PF, John MT, Steele JG. The oral health impact profile: ranking of items for temporomandibular disorders. *Eur J Oral Sci* 2011;119:169-74.
15 Reissmann DR, John MT, Schierz O, Wassell RW. Functional and psychosocial impact related to specific temporomandibular disorder diagnoses. *J Dent* 2007;35:643-50.
16 Reissmann DR, John MT, Wassell RW, Hinz A. Psychosocial profiles of diagnostic subgroups of temporomandibular disorder patients. *Eur J Oral Sci* 2008;116:237-44.
17 Dahlstrom L, Carlsson GE. Temporomandibular disorders and oral health-related quality of life. A systematic review. *Acta Odontol Scand* 2010;68:80-5.
18 Durham J, Breckons M, Araujo-Soares V, Exley C, Steele J, Vale L. Developing Effective and Efficient care pathways in chronic Pain: DEEP study protocol. *BMC Oral Health* 2014;14:6.
19 Costen JB. A syndrome of ear and sinus symptoms based on disturbed function of the tempromandibular joint. *Ann Otol Rhinol Laryngol* 1934;43:1-15.
20 Gray RJ, Davies SJ, Quayle AA. A clinical approach to temporomandibular disorders. 1. Classification and functional anatomy. *Br Dent J* 1994;176:429-35.
21 Madland G, Feinmann C, Newman S. Factors associated with anxiety and depression in facial arthromyalgia. *Pain* 2000;84:225-32.
22 Shore NA. Occlusal equilibration and temporomandibular joint dysfunction. Lippincott, 1959.
23 Laskin DM. Temporomandibular disorders: a term past its time? *J Am Dent Assoc* 2008;139:124-8.
24 McNeill C. Temporomandibular disorders. Guidelines for classification, assessment and management. Quintessence, 1990.
25 Bell WE. Clinical management of temporomandibular disorders. Year Book Medical Publishers, 1982.
26 Cairns B, List T, Michelotti A, Ohrbach R, Svensson P. JOR-CORE recommendations on rehabilitation of temporomandibular disorders. *J Oral Rehabil* 2010;37:481-9.
27 Greene CS. Managing the care of patients with temporomandibular disorders: a new guideline for care. *J Am Dent Assoc* 2010;141:1086-8.
28 Peck CC, Goulet JP, Lobbezoo F, Schiffman EL, Alstergren P, Anderson GC, et al. Expanding the taxonomy of the diagnostic criteria for temporomandibular disorders. *J Oral Rehabil* 2014;41:2-23.
29 Dworkin SF. The OPPERA study: act one. *J Pain* 2011;12:T1-3.
30 Slade GD, Bair E, Greenspan JD, Dubner R, Fillingim RB, Diatchenko L, et al. Signs and symptoms of first-onset TMD and sociodemographic predictors of its development: the OPPERA prospective cohort study. *J Pain* 2013;14:T20-32.e1.
31 Sanders AE, Slade GD, Bair E, Fillingim RB, Knott C, Dubner R, et al. General health status and incidence of first-onset temporomandibular disorder: the OPPERA prospective cohort study. *J Pain* 2013;14:T51-62.
32 Slade GD, Sanders AE, Bair E, Brownstein N, Dampier D, Knott C, et al. Preclinical episodes of orofacial pain symptoms and their association with health care behaviors in the OPPERA prospective cohort study. *Pain* 2013;154:750-60.
33 Fernandes G, van Selms MK, Goncalves DA, Lobbezoo F, Camparis CM. Factors associated with temporomandibular disorders pain in adolescents. *J Oral Rehabil* 2015;42:113-9.
34 LeResche L, Mancl LA, Drangsholt MT, Huang G, Von Korff M. Predictors of onset of facial pain and temporomandibular disorders in early adolescence. *Pain* 2007;129:269-78.
35 List T, Wahlund K, Wenneberg B, Dworkin SF. TMD in children and adolescents: prevalence of pain, gender differences, and perceived treatment need. *J Orofac Pain* 1999;13:9-20.
36 Nilsson IM. Reliability, validity, incidence and impact of temporormandibular pain disorders in adolescents. *Swed Dent J Suppl* 2007;(183):7-86.
37 Isong U, Gansky SA, Plesh O. Temporomandibular joint and muscle disorder-type pain in U.S. adults: the National Health Interview Survey. *J Orofac Pain* 2008;22:317-22.
38 Schmitter M, Rammelsberg P, Hassel A. The prevalence of signs and symptoms of temporomandibular disorders in very old subjects. *J Oral Rehabil* 2005;32:467-73.
39 White BA, Williams LA, Leben JR. Health care utilization and cost among health maintenance organization members with temporomandibular disorders. *J Orofac Pain* 2001;15:158-69.
40 Durham J, Breckons M, Araujo-Soares V, Exley C, Steele J, Vale L. Developing Effective and Efficient care pathways in chronic Pain: DEEP study protocol. *BMC Oral Health* 2014;14:6.
41 McNeill C. Management of temporomandibular disorders: concepts and controversies. *J Prosthet Dent* 1997;77:510-22.
42 Suvinen TI, Reade PC, Kemppainen P, Kononen M, Dworkin SF. Review of aetiological concepts of temporomandibular pain disorders: towards a biopsychosocial model for integration of physical disorder factors with psychological and psychosocial illness impact factors. *Eur J Pain* 2005;9:613-33.
43 Svensson P. Temporomandibular disorders—a tough case to break! *Scand J Pain* 2014;2:70-1.
44 Meloto CB, Serrano PO, Ribeiro-DaSilva MC, Rizzatti-Barbosa CM. Genomics and the new perspectives for temporomandibular disorders. *Arch Oral Biol* 2011;56:1181-91.
45 Fillingim RB, Ohrbach R, Greenspan JD, Knott C, Diatchenko L, Dubner R, et al. Psychological factors associated with development of TMD: the OPPERA prospective cohort study. *J Pain* 2013;14:T75-90.
46 Ribeiro-Dasilva MC, Peres Line SR, Leme Godoy dos Santos MC, Arthuri MT, Hou W, Fillingim RB, et al. Estrogen receptor-alpha polymorphisms and predisposition to TMJ disorder. *J Pain* 2009;10:527-33.
47 Woolf CJ. Central sensitization: implications for the diagnosis and treatment of pain. *Pain* 2011;152:S2-15.
48 Cady RJ, Glenn JR, Smith KM, Durham PL. Calcitonin gene-related peptide promotes cellular changes in trigeminal neurons and glia implicated in peripheral and central sensitization. *Mol Pain* 2011;7:94.
49 Kopp S. Neuroendocrine, immune, and local responses related to temporomandibular disorders. *J Orofac Pain* 2001;15:9-28.
50 Sato J, Segami N, Kaneyama K, Yoshimura H, Fujimura K, Yoshitake Y. Relationship of calcitonin gene-related peptide in synovial tissues and temporomandibular joint pain in humans. *Oral Surg Oral Med Oral Pathol Oral Radiol Endod* 2004;98:533-40.
51 Appelgren A, Appelgren B, Kopp S, Lundeberg T, Theodorsson E. Neuropeptides in the arthritic TMJ and symptoms and signs from the stomatognathic system with special consideration to rheumatoid arthritis. *J Orofac Pain* 1995;9:215-25.
52 Diatchenko L, Slade GD, Nackley AG, Bhalang K, Sigurdsson A, Belfer I, et al. Genetic basis for individual variations in pain perception and the development of a chronic pain condition. *Hum Mol Genet* 2005;14:135-43.
53 Diatchenko L, Nackley AG, Slade GD, Fillingim RB, Maixner W. Idiopathic pain disorders—pathways of vulnerability. *Pain* 2006;123:226-30.
54 Younger JW, Shen YF, Goddard G, Mackey SC. Chronic myofascial temporomandibular pain is associated with neural abnormalities in the trigeminal and limbic systems. *Pain* 2010;149:222-8.

55 Weissman-Fogel I, Moayedi M, Tenenbaum HC, Goldberg MB, Freeman BV, Davis KD. Abnormal cortical activity in patients with temporomandibular disorder evoked by cognitive and emotional tasks. *Pain* 2011;152:384-96.

56 Aneiros-Guerrero A, Lendinez AM, Palomares AR, Perez-Nevot B, Aguado L, Mayor-Olea A, et al. Genetic polymorphisms in folate pathway enzymes, DRD4 and GSTM1 are related to temporomandibular disorder. *BMC Med Genet* 2011;12:75.

57 Milam SB, Zardeneta G, Schmitz JP. Oxidative stress and degenerative temporomandibular joint disease: a proposed hypothesis. *J Oral Maxillofac Surg* 1998;56:214-23.

58 Milam SB. Pathogenesis of degenerative temporomandibular joint arthritides. *Odontology* 2005;93:7-15.

59 Planello AC, Campos MI, Meloto CB, Secolin R, Rizatti-Barbosa CM, Line SR, et al. Association of matrix metalloproteinase gene polymorphism with temporomandibular joint degeneration. *Eur J Oral Sci* 2011;119:1-6.

60 Light KC, Bragdon EE, Grewen KM, Brownley KA, Girdler SS, Maixner W. Adrenergic dysregulation and pain with and without acute beta-blockade in women with fibromyalgia and temporomandibular disorder. *J Pain* 2009;10:542-52.

61 Schiffman E, Ohrbach R, List T, Anderson G, Jensen R, John MT, et al. Diagnostic criteria for headache attributed to temporomandibular disorders. *Cephalalgia* 2012;32:683-92.

62 Dworkin SF, LeResche L. Research Diagnostic Criteria for Temporomandibular Disorders: review, criteria, examinations and specifications, critique. *J Craniomandib Disord* 1992;6:301-55.

63 Ahmad M, Hollender L, Anderson Q, Kartha K, Ohrbach R, Truelove EL, et al. Research Diagnostic Criteria for Temporomandibular Disorders (RDC/TMD): development of image analysis criteria and examiner reliability for image analysis. *Oral Surg Oral Med Oral Pathol Oral Radiol Endod* 2009;107:844-60.

64 Anderson GC, Gonzalez YM, Ohrbach R, Truelove EL, Sommers E, Look JO, et al. The Research Diagnostic Criteria for Temporomandibular Disorders. VI: future directions. *J Orofac Pain* 2010;24:79-88.

65 Dworkin SF. Research Diagnostic Criteria for Temporomandibular Disorders: current status & future relevance. *J Oral Rehabil* 2010;37:734-43.

66 Lobbezoo F, Visscher CM, Naeije M. Some remarks on the RDC/TMD validation project: report of an IADR/Toronto-2008 workshop discussion. *J Oral Rehabil* 2010;37:779-83.

67 Look JO, John MT, Tai F, Huggins KH, Lenton PA, Truelove EL, et al. The Research Diagnostic Criteria For Temporomandibular Disorders. II: reliability of Axis I diagnoses and selected clinical measures. *J Orofac Pain* 2010;24:25-34.

68 Look JO, Schiffman EL, Truelove EL, Ahmad M. Reliability and validity of Axis I of the Research Diagnostic Criteria for Temporomandibular Disorders (RDC/TMD) with proposed revisions. *J Oral Rehabil* 2010;37:744-59.

69 Ohrbach R. Assessment and further development of RDC/TMD Axis II biobehavioural instruments: a research programme progress report. *J Oral Rehabil* 2010;37:784-98.

70 Ohrbach R, Turner JA, Sherman JJ, Mancl LA, Truelove EL, Schiffman EL, et al. The Research Diagnostic Criteria for Temporomandibular Disorders. IV: evaluation of psychometric properties of the Axis II measures. *J Orofac Pain* 2010;24:48-62.

71 Schiffman EL, Ohrbach R, Truelove EL, Tai F, Anderson GC, Pan W, et al. The Research Diagnostic Criteria for Temporomandibular Disorders. V: methods used to establish and validate revised Axis I diagnostic algorithms. *J Orofac Pain* 2010;24:63-78.

72 Schiffman EL, Truelove EL, Ohrbach R, Anderson GC, John MT, List T, et al. The Research Diagnostic Criteria for Temporomandibular Disorders. I: overview and methodology for assessment of validity. *J Orofac Pain* 2010;24:7-24.

73 Truelove E, Pan W, Look JO, Mancl LA, Ohrbach RK, Velly AM, et al. The Research Diagnostic Criteria for Temporomandibular Disorders. III: validity of Axis I diagnoses. *J Orofac Pain* 2010;24:35-47.

74 Visscher C, Lobbezoo F, Naeije M. The RDC/TMD validation project: an important or a final step towards a revised version of the RDc/TMD? *J Orofac Pain* 2010;24:234-5.

75 Schiffman E, Ohrbach R, Truelove E, Look J, Anderson G, Goulet JP, et al. Diagnostic Criteria for Temporomandibular Disorders (DC/TMD) for clinical and research applications: recommendations of the International RDC/TMD Consortium Network and Orofacial Pain Special Interest Group. *J Oral Facial Pain Headache* 2014;28:6-27.

76 Gonzalez YM, Schiffman E, Gordon SM, Seago B, Truelove EL, Slade G, et al. Development of a brief and effective temporomandibular disorder pain screening questionnaire: reliability and validity. *J Am Dent Assoc* 2011;142:1183-91.

77 Litt MD, Porto FB. Determinants of pain treatment response and nonresponse: identification of TMD patient subgroups. *J Pain* 2013;14:1502-13.

78 Durham J. Acute presentations of chronic orofacial pain conditions. In: Greenwood M, Corbett I, eds. Dental emergencies. Wiley-Blackwell, 2012.

79 Epstein JB, Jones CK. Presenting signs and symptoms of nasopharyngeal carcinoma. *Oral Surg Oral Med Oral Pathol* 1993;75:32-6.

80 Siccoli MM, Bassetti CL, Sandor PS. Facial pain: clinical differential diagnosis. *Lancet Neurol* 2006;5:257-67.

81 Durham J, Aggarwal VA, Davies SJ, Harrison SD, Jagger RG, Leeson R, et al. Temporomandibular Disorders (TMDs): an update and management guidance for primary care from the UK Specialist Interest Group in Orofacial Pain and TMDs (USOT). 2013. www.rcseng.ac.uk/fds/publications-clinical-guidelines/clinical_guidelines.

82 Beddis HP, Davies SJ, Budenberg A, Horner K, Pemberton MN. Temporomandibular disorders, trismus and malignancy: development of a checklist to improve patient safety. *Br Dent J* 2014;217:351-5.

83 Epker J, Gatchel RJ, Ellis E. A model for predicting chronic TMD: practical application in clinical settings. *J Am Dent Assoc* 1999;130:1470-5.

84 Garofalo JP, Gatchel RJ, Wesley AL, Ellis E 3rd. Predicting chronicity in acute temporomandibular joint disorders using the research diagnostic criteria. *J Am Dent Assoc* 1998;129:438-47.

85 Slade GD, Bair E, By K, Mulkey F, Baraian C, Rothwell R, et al. Study methods, recruitment, sociodemographic findings, and demographic representativeness in the OPPERA study. *J Pain* 2011;12:T12-26.

86 Von Korff M, Dunn KM. Chronic pain reconsidered. *Pain* 2008;138:267-76.

87 Wright AR, Gatchel RJ, Wildenstein L, Riggs R, Buschang P, Ellis E. Biopsychosocial differences between high-risk and low-risk patients with acute TMD-related pain. *J Am Dent Assoc* 2004;135:474-83.

88 Von Korff M, Ormel J, Keefe FJ, Dworkin SF. Grading the severity of chronic pain. *Pain* 1992;50:133-49.

89 Turp JC, Jokstad A, Motschall E, Schindler HJ, Windecker-Getaz I, Ettlin DA. Is there a superiority of multimodal as opposed to simple therapy in patients with temporomandibular disorders? A qualitative systematic review of the literature. [Erratum appears in *Clin Oral Implants Res* 2008;19:326-8.] *Clin Oral Implants Res* 2007;18(Suppl 3):138-50.

90 Phillips K, Clauw DJ. Central pain mechanisms in chronic pain states—maybe it is all in their head. *Best Pract Res Clin Rheumatol* 2011;25:141-54.

91 Gatchel RJ, Stowell AW, Wildenstein L, Riggs R, Ellis E. Efficacy of an early intervention for patients with acute temporomandibular disorder-related pain: a one-year outcome study. *J Am Dent Assoc* 2006;137:339-47.

92 Albino JEN. Management of temporomandibular disorders. National Institutes of Health Technology Assessment Conference Statement. *J Am Dent Assoc* 1996;127:1595-606.

93 Greene CS. The etiology of temporomandibular disorders: implications for treatment. *J Orofac Pain* 2001;15:93-105; discussion 106.

94 Beecroft EV, Durham J, Thomson P. Retrospective examination of the healthcare 'journey' of chronic orofacial pain patients referred to oral and maxillofacial surgery. *Br Dent J* 2013;214:E12.

95 Ehde DM, Dillworth TM, Turner JA. Cognitive-behavioral therapy for individuals with chronic pain: efficacy, innovations, and directions for research. *Am Psychol* 2014;69:153-66.

96 List T, Axelsson S. Management of TMD: evidence from systematic reviews and meta-analyses. *J Oral Rehabil* 2010;37:430-51.

97 Aggarwal VR, Lovell K, Peters S, Javidi H, Joughin A, Goldthorpe J. Psychosocial interventions for the management of chronic orofacial pain. *Cochrane Database Syst Rev* 2011;11:CD008456.

98 Kimos P, Biggs C, Mah J, Heo G, Rashiq S, Thie NM, et al. Analgesic action of gabapentin on chronic pain in the masticatory muscles: a randomized controlled trial. *Pain* 2007;127:151-60.

99 Rizzatti-Barbosa CM, Nogueira MT, de Andrade ED, Ambrosano GM, de Barbosa JR. Clinical evaluation of amitriptyline for the control of chronic pain caused by temporomandibular joint disorders. *Cranio* 2003;21:221-5.

100 Sharav Y, Singer E, Schmidt E, Dionne RA, Dubner R. The analgesic effect of amitriptyline on chronic facial pain. *Pain* 1987;31:199-209.

101 Kurtoglu C, Gur OH, Kurkcu M, Sertdemir Y, Guler-Uysal F, Uysal H. Effect of botulinum toxin-A in myofascial pain patients with or without functional disc displacement. *J Oral Maxillofac Surg* 2008;66:1644-51.

102 Ernberg M, Hedenberg-Magnusson B, List T, Svensson P. Efficacy of botulinum toxin type A for treatment of persistent myofascial TMD pain: a randomized, controlled, double-blind multicenter study. *Pain* 2011;152:1988-96.

103 Guarda-Nardini L, Manfredini D, Salamone M, Salmaso L, Tonello S, Ferronato G. Efficacy of botulinum toxin in treating myofascial pain in bruxers: a controlled placebo pilot study. *Cranio* 2008;26:126-35.

104 Nixdorf DR, Heo G, Major PW. Randomized controlled trial of botulinum toxin A for chronic myogenous orofacial pain. *Pain* 2002;99:465-73.

105 Laskin DM. Botulinum toxin A in the treatment of myofascial pain and dysfunction: the case against its use. *J Oral Maxillofac Surg* 2012;70:1240-2.

106 Raphael KG, Tadinada A, Bradshaw JM, Janal MN, Sirois DA, Chan KC, et al. Osteopenic consequences of botulinum toxin injections in the masticatory muscles: a pilot study. *J Oral Rehabil* 2014;41:555-63.

107 Koh H, Robinson PG. Occlusal adjustment for treating and preventing temporomandibular joint disorders. *Cochrane Database Syst Rev* 2003;1:CD003812.

108 Luther F, Layton S, McDonald F. Orthodontics for treating temporomandibular joint (TMJ) disorders. *Cochrane Database Syst Rev* 2010;7:CD006541.

109 Palla S. Biopsychosocial pain model crippled? *J Orofac Pain* 2011;25:289-90.

110 Cohen M, Quintner J, Buchanan D, Nielsen M, Guy L. Stigmatization of patients with chronic pain: the extinction of empathy. *Pain Med* 2011;12:1637-43.

111 Dorflinger L, Kerns RD, Auerbach SM. Providers' roles in enhancing patients' adherence to pain self management. *Transl Behav Med* 2013;3:39-46.

112 Vowles KE, Thompson M. The patient-provider relationship in chronic pain. *Curr Pain Headache Rep* 2012;16:133-8.

113 Standring S. Gray's anatomy: the anatomical basis of clinical practice, 40th edn. Fig 31.11. Churchill Livingstone, 2008;538.

114 Drake RL, Vogl W, Mitchell AWM. Gray's anatomy for students. Fig 8.128 A & B. Churchill Livingstone, 2005;874.

Management of chronic pain in older adults

M Carrington Reid, associate professor of medicine[1], Christopher Eccleston, director[2], Karl Pillemer, professor of human development and of gerontology in medicine[3]

[1]Division of Geriatrics and Palliative Medicine, Weill Cornell Medical College, New York, NY 10065, USA

[2]Centre for Pain Research, University of Bath, Bath, UK

[3]Department of Human Development, Cornell University, Ithaca, NY, USA

Correspondence to: M C Reid mcr2004@med.cornell.edu

Cite this as: *BMJ* 2015;350:h532

DOI: 10.1136/bmj.h532

http://www.bmj.com/content/350/bmj.h532

Chronic pain is one of the most common conditions encountered by healthcare professionals, particularly among older (≥65 years) patients.[1] Pain is associated with substantial disability from reduced mobility, avoidance of activity, falls, depression and anxiety, sleep impairment, and isolation.[1 2 3] Its negative effects extend beyond the patient, to disrupt both family and social relationships. Chronic pain poses a significant economic burden on society.[1] Prevalence rates for pain are expected to increase as populations continue to age—by 2035 an estimated one quarter of the population in the European Union will be 65 or older—thereby increasing the public health impact of pain. Healthcare providers, irrespective of specialty, should develop competencies to assess and manage chronic pain in their older patients. In this review we summarize recent evidence on the assessment and management of pain in older patients. Evidence is taken from systematic reviews, meta-analyses, individual trials, and clinical guidelines.

What is chronic pain and how is it caused?

Although no universally accepted definition exists for chronic pain, it is often defined as pain that persists beyond the expected time of healing (typically 12 weeks) and may or may not be associated with an identifiable cause or actual tissue damage.[3 4] Musculoskeletal disorders are common in later life, and increasingly common are painful neuropathies from diabetes, herpes zoster, chemotherapy, and surgery. Other types of pain are also prevalent among older adults, including pain due to cancer as well as cancer treatments.[5 6] Pain is also common in the advanced stages of many chronic diseases, including congestive heart failure, end stage renal disease, and chronic obstructive pulmonary disease.[7] Furthermore, millions of joint repair and replacement surgeries are performed annually, and an important minority of patients undergoing these procedures report chronic pain despite surgery.[8] Finally, vertebral compression fractures are highly prevalent and cause substantial pain and discomfort, particularly among older women.[9] Box 1 lists other common diseases where pain is a major symptom.

Who gets it?

Chronic pain in later life is a worldwide problem. In one nationwide survey of older adults (n=7601) in the United States, 52.8% reported experiencing bothersome pain in the preceding month.[10] Similar findings have been reported in studies conducted in Europe, Asia, and Australia[11 12 13] and in both developed and less developed countries.[14] Risk factors include advancing age, female sex, lower socioeconomic status, lower educational level, obesity, tobacco use, history of injury, history of a physically strenuous job, childhood trauma, and depression or anxiety.

Factors predicting poor outcomes (that is, higher pain scores, disability, depression) among people with chronic pain include higher levels of pain severity and disability, longer duration of pain, multiple pain sites, history of anxiety or depression, maladaptive coping strategies (for example, worry, avoidance), and low social support at the time of diagnosis. In one study of older adults (n=403) with musculoskeletal pain, three brief items assessed at the initial clinical encounter—degree of interference from pain, pain in multiple body sites, and duration of pain—predicted lack of patient improvement at six months and helped general practitioners predict this outcome above clinical judgment alone.[15] Simple risk stratification approaches like this could help to tailor care.

How are older patients with chronic pain assessed?

A comprehensive pain assessment can increase the likelihood of identifying a specific diagnosis for the pain, guide selection of treatments most likely to benefit the patient, and identify targets for intervention (for example,

THE BOTTOM LINE

- Chronic pain in later life is a worldwide problem
- All older adults with chronic pain should undergo a comprehensive geriatric pain assessment
- A comprehensive assessment can guide selection of treatments most likely to benefit the patient and identify targets for intervention besides pain relief
- A multimodal approach that includes both drug and non-drug modalities for pain is recommended
- Given the limited reach of cognitive behavioral and exercise approaches to manage pain in later life, patients should be encouraged to engage in and adopt these techniques
- Involve and engage family members and paid caregivers and seek out other resources that can help to reinforce adherence to treatment and maintain gains from treatment

BOX 1 DISEASES ASSOCIATED WITH CHRONIC PAIN IN LATER LIFE, BY SYSTEM OR SPECIALTY

- *Dermatology*—pressure or ischemic ulcers, burns, scleroderma
- *Gastrointestinal*—constipation, irritable bowel disease, diverticulitis, inflammatory bowel disease
- *Cardiovascular*—advanced heart disease, peripheral vascular disease
- *Pulmonary*—advanced chronic obstructive pulmonary disease, pleurisy
- *Rheumatology*—osteoarthritis, rheumatoid arthritis, gout, pseudogout, polymyalgia rheumatica, spinal stenosis and other low back syndromes, myofascial syndromes, osteoporotic related fractures
- *Endocrine*—diabetic neuropathy, Paget's disease
- *Nephrology*—chronic cystitis, end stage renal disease
- *Immune*—herpes zoster, post-herpetic neuralgia, HIV/AIDs neuropathy
- *Neurology*—headache, peripheral neuropathies, compressive neuropathies, radiculopathies, Parkinson's disease, post-stroke pain
- *Oncology*—cancer
- *Miscellaneous*—depression, tendonitis, bursitis

unrealistic treatment goals) besides pain relief. Office based assessment can be challenging, however, because of constraints on time. Having patients complete parts of the assessment before the visit (or in the office over multiple visits) can be helpful.

Clinicians often struggle with the question of how comprehensive the assessment needs to be to establish a specific cause of pain. Unfortunately the literature provides little guidance on this but does indicate that a specific cause is not found in a large number of patients, despite comprehensive evaluation. Potential benefits to identifying a cause of pain include earlier initiation of an appropriate treatment and providing reassurance as patients often worry about the cause of their pain. These putative benefits must be weighed against the risks of extensive investigations, which often uncover incidental findings, are expensive, and can increase patient worry.

History

Chronic pain is more than just a sensory event; it has affective (emotional responses to pain), cognitive (attitudes and beliefs about pain), behavioral (for example, behaviors manifested in response to pain by patients and their family members or caregivers), as well as sensory components (for example, quality, location, temporal pattern). Assessing for the presence and severity of pain captures only a small part of the pain experience. All older patients with chronic pain should undergo a comprehensive pain assessment (box 2 outlines the key elements).

Box 3 lists these and other core elements of the assessment along with sample questions that can be employed during the interview. Additional guidance about assessment approaches can be found in UK and US guidelines[17 18] and in an international consensus report on this topic.[19]

Examination

A physical examination should be conducted, focusing on the musculoskeletal (is there evidence of inflammation?) and neurologic (is there evidence of weakness or neuropathy?) systems. Because many older adults with chronic pain report the presence of weakness, it is important to distinguish pain induced weakness from true motor weakness. This can be done by documenting abnormal results from nerve conduction studies or by treating pain successfully and seeing if the muscle weakness improves. Tackling physical functioning and risk of falls is critically important, given that pain is associated with these outcomes. This part of the assessment should include self report and performance based measures such as gait speed, timed up and go test, balance. The results provide a baseline against which the functional impact of treatment can be evaluated.

Imaging

Diagnostic imaging is often overused and does not indicate better care.[20] In one study of Portuguese adults (n=5094) more than half of all respondents with chronic pain reported undergoing a diagnostic imaging procedure in the previous six months.[21] Such imaging often uncovers incidental findings, leading to more testing, costs, and worry for patients. An additional concern is the low correlation between pathologic findings identified by imaging and the extent to which patients report experiencing pain.[22] Many patients with major disease identified by imaging report no pain, whereas others without major disease often report severe pain.[22] Diagnostic imaging is appropriate when the history or physical examination identifies abnormalities that suggest a specific diagnosis for the pain. Imaging procedures should also be strongly considered in the presence of "red flags," to include worsening pain in patients with a history of cancer, risk factors for infection (injecting drug use, immunosuppressive therapy), and worrisome constitutional signs or symptoms such as unexplained weight loss, fever, or loss of appetite.

Assessing pain in older patients with major cognitive impairment

Patients with limited verbal or cognitive abilities require modified approaches to assessment. A hierarchy of techniques is recommended, the first including an attempt to obtain self report data followed by a search for potential causes of the pain, observing patient behavior (for example, facial expressions, vocalizations, guarding), obtaining proxy data from family members or caregivers who know the patient well and can report on whether changes in behavior or activity are very different from baseline, and conducting an analgesic trial to see whether the behavior resolves with treatment.[23] Several tools for behavioral pain assessment have been developed to assess for pain in non-verbal patients and are reviewed elsewhere.[19 23]

BOX 2 KEY ELEMENTS OF A COMPREHENSIVE PAIN ASSESSMENT

- *Administering standardized pain assessment tools*—this can provide additional information above and beyond what is generated by the interview and physical examination. Table 1 includes measures that are for the most part simple, brief, and appropriate for being self administered. The brief pain inventory-short form and the geriatric pain measure are recommended for routine use in practice because they are easy to complete, have been successfully used in studies of older adults, and assess multiple salient dimensions of the pain experience. It is important to employ assessments that older patients can do without difficulty and to use the same tools at each visit to assess for change in a given outcome over time
- *Ascertaining the impact of chronic pain on functioning*—for example, activities of daily living, social functioning, sleep
- *Identifying attitudes and beliefs about pain, as well as treatment goals and expectations*—many older patients endorse beliefs that operate as important barriers to engagement with and adherence to treatment. Older patients' goals may or may not be the same as the healthcare provider's goals. In addition, patients may have unrealistic (for example, expect complete pain relief) or negative (for example, treatments will not help) expectations that can serve as targets for intervention[16]
- *Gathering data from family members and paid caregivers*—gathering information from third parties about an older patient's response to pain and the impact it has at home may be essential, particularly when patients cannot provide this information because of difficulties with communication as a consequence of stroke or advanced dementia
- *Identifying resources to include family members, other caregivers, and faith communities, when appropriate*—these can provide emotional or instrumental support and help to reinforce engagement with and adherence to treatment
- *Reviewing comorbidities and drugs*—some chronic conditions might be made worse by starting a particular analgesic agent and some drugs may constitute a contraindication to initiating a specific analgesic trial

BOX 3 ELEMENTS OF A COMPREHENSIVE GERIATRIC PAIN ASSESSMENT

Sensory
- Please tell me all of the places you experience pain or discomfort. What does it feel like? What words come to mind?
- Is your pain or discomfort with you all of the time or does it come and go? How long has it been present? What makes it better, what makes it worse?

Emotional impact
- Has pain affected your mood, sense of wellbeing, energy level?
- Are you worried about your pain or what may be causing it?

Functional impact
- Has pain affected your ability to do every day activities? To do things you enjoy?
- How about relating with others? If so, how?

Sleep
- Has pain affected your sleep?
- Do you have trouble falling asleep or need to take drugs to help you sleep on account of your pain?

Attitudes and beliefs
- Do you have any thoughts or opinions about experiencing pain at this point in your life that you believe would be important for me to know?
- Do you have any thoughts or opinions about specific pain treatments that you believe would be important for me to know?

Coping styles
- What things do you do to help you cope with your pain? This could be listening to your favorite music, praying, sitting still, or isolating yourself from others

Treatment expectations and goals
- What do you think is likely to happen with the treatment I have recommended?
- What are the most important things you hope will happen as a result of the treatment?

Resources
- Is there anyone at home or in the community that you can turn to for help and support when your pain is really bad?

Table 1 Standardized tools for pain assessment

Measure (No of items)	Domains assessed
Multidimensional measures:	
Brief pain inventory-short form (n=9)[w1]	Sensory (intensity, location); pain related interference or disability; treatments, degree of relief provided by treatments; affect
Geriatric pain measure (n=24)[w2]	Sensory (intensity, temporal pattern); pain related interference or disability; affect
Pain disability index (n=7)[w3]	Pain related interference or disability
Short-form McGill pain questionnaire (n=15)[w4]	Sensory; exacerbating or ameliorating factors; affect
PROMIS* pain interference, behavior, intensity items[w5]	Pain related interference or disability; pain behaviors; pain intensity
WOMAC (n=24)[w6]	Sensory (intensity); pain related interference or disability; joint stiffness
Roland Morris disability questionnaire† (n=24)[w7]	Pain related interference or disability; affect
Unidimensional measures:	
Numeric rating scale (n=1)[w8]	Sensory (intensity)
Verbal rating scale (n=1)[w9]	Sensory (severity)
Visual analog scale (n=1)[w9]	Sensory (intensity)
Faces pain scale (n=1)[w10]	Sensory (intensity)
LANSS pain scale (n=7)[w11]	Sensory (assessment of possible neuropathic pain)
DN4 (n=4)[w12]	Sensory (assessment of possible neuropathic pain)

WOMAC=Western Ontario and McMaster Universities osteoarthritis index; LANSS=Leeds assessment of neuropathic symptoms and signs; DN4=Douleur Neuropathique 4 questions.

**Available in long and short form versions: long version for pain interference has 40 items; there are five short form versions for pain interference where the number of questions varies from 4 to 8; long form version for pain behavior has 39 items, short form version has 7. PROMIS pain intensity measure has three items.*

†Originally developed as tool to measure perceived disability in patients with back pain. Increasingly used to measure perceived disability due to pain from any cause.

What is the approach to management?

Management of pain in later life can be complex; problems with both nociceptive and neuropathic pain are common and often coexist. Nociceptive pain arises from actual or threatened damage to non-neural tissue through activation of nociceptors, whereas neuropathic pain occurs as a consequence of abnormalities in the central or peripheral somatosensory nervous system.[4] Management is further complicated by age related physiologic changes, which lead to altered drug absorption and decreased renal excretion, sensory and cognitive impairments, polypharmacy, and multimorbidity, particularly chronic conditions such as disorders of gait and balance, and kidney, lung, and cardiovascular disease.[16] Other barriers to management include a limited evidence base to guide decisions, physician concerns about the potential for treatment related harm, as well as older adults' beliefs about pain and treatments for the pain. However, it is important to note that these barriers are not universally present in older adults; an important tenet of geriatric medicine is that chronologic age does not equal biologic age.

Chronic pain in older patients most often occurs in the setting of multiple comorbidities, limiting treatment options. A comprehensive management approach should deal with common sequelae such as depression, isolation, and physical disability, and include both drug and non-drug treatments. UK and US guidelines on the management of pain in later life strongly endorse this approach.[2 3] Recent data provide support for multimodal treatment approaches. In one randomized clinical trial (n=454) of overweight or obese older adults with osteoarthritis of the knee, intensive weight reduction combined with exercise training produced significant improvements in pain, functional status, and physical performance over an 18 month period when compared with exercise only (and diet only) control groups.[24]

In terms of care delivery, collaborative approaches have proved efficacy in the primary care setting.[25 26 27] One recent randomized clinical trial involving older primary care patients (n=250) with chronic musculoskeletal pain found that a telephone based collaborative care management intervention delivered by a nurse care manager, physician pain specialist, and the patient's primary care provider led to improved patient outcomes at 12 months, largely through optimizing non-opioid analgesics by using a stepped care approach.[25] Given the complexities of managing most older patients with chronic pain, a multidisciplinary approach that includes physician, nursing, and social work perspectives is strongly recommended.

SOURCES AND SELECTION CRITERIA

We searched Medline, Embase, and the Cochrane Database of Systematic Reviews using the search terms "chronic pain", "older adults", "prevalence", "diagnosis", and "treatment". We specifically focused on identifying and reviewing systematic reviews, meta-analyses, high quality randomized controlled trials, and clinical guidelines published during the past five years whenever possible.

Social aspects of management

Clinicians are advised to take family responses and dynamics into account when formulating treatment plans. Older patients' chronic pain often affects their close relatives and caregivers.

Spouses typically play an important role in caring for older patients, often times delivering emotional and instrumental support. However, when an older spouse experiences chronic pain, problems of communication and commitment to the marriage can occur.

Therapeutic interventions directed at patients with chronic pain increasingly involve the family, most often by including relatives in cognitive behavior therapy (CBT) or self management training. Although evidence is mixed, several well conducted, randomized trials suggest that spousal participation in the treatment process can yield measurable benefits for patients, including enhanced emotional wellbeing and reduced pain levels.[28 29]

Home visits

We are not aware of any literature that has examined the value of home visits for older adults with chronic pain. Despite a lack of evidence supporting the use of home visits, clinicians should consider them on a case by case basis because of several potential benefits, which include clarifying reasons for non-adherence to drug and behavioral interventions, gathering proxy data that may not be available during an office visit, and preventing the use of old prescription drugs often stored by patients. Perhaps the most important benefit is a strengthening of the doctor-patient relationship. From the physician's perspective,

Table 2 Guideline recommendations for drug management of chronic pain

Analgesic class	Recommendation*	Safety concerns	Quality of evidence†
Paracetamol (acetaminophen)	Use for mild to moderate pain	Liver toxicity a concern at higher doses, particularly from unintentional overdose	High
Oral NSAIDs	Use for shortest time possible; may be appropriate when other treatments have failed	Selective and non-selective NSAIDs associated with adverse gastrointestinal, renal, and cardiovascular side effects	High
Topical NSAIDs	Use as alternative to oral NSAIDs, particularly when pain is localized	Safety of topical NSAIDs in patients receiving anticoagulation or with renal impairment remains unknown	Moderate
Tramadol	Consider for use in patients who do not respond to paracetamol/ NSAIDs	Increased risk of seizures or serotonin syndrome when used with antidepressants; side effect profile similar to that of opioids	Not reported
Opioids	Use for moderate to severe pain or with substantial impairments in functioning or quality of life and when other treatments have been unsuccessful	Side effects limit use (constipation, sedation, nausea)	Low
Tricyclic antidepressants	Avoid tertiary tricyclics (for example, amitriptyline) because of concerns over adverse side effects; consider trial of secondary amine (nortriptyline) for neuropathic pain	Side effects limit use, electrocardiographic monitoring required owing to risk of QTc prolongation; serum level monitoring also recommended	Moderate
Anticonvulsants (for example, pregabalin, gabapentin)	Use for neuropathic pain	Side effects limit use (for example, sedation, peripheral edema); dose adjustment necessary in those with renal impairment	Moderate

NSAIDs=non-steroidal anti-inflammatory drugs.
**Recommendations present in both UK and US guidelines.[2 3]*
†Quality of evidence ratings are from the 2009 American Geriatrics Society guideline.

QUESTIONS FOR FUTURE RESEARCH

- What are the implications of ethnic and cultural diversity on the experience of pain among older people, and the effectiveness of interventions?
- What are the best ways to measure outcomes in geriatric pain research, including both observable and subjective dimensions?
- Can access to psychological therapies be improved by training non-psychologists in delivering them and by using mhealth and ehealth solutions?
- What effect does pain have on cognitive ability and motivation in older people, and how can this be best managed with cognitive behavioral therapy?
- How can the evidence base in trials of pharmacologic, physical, and psychological treatments be improved for older people?
- Should the inclusion of older people in the design of novel interventions be mandatory?
- What evidence based approaches work best to maximize treatment adherence?

observing the patient's environment often offers intangible but valuable insights into the patient's condition. From the patient's perspective, most feel enormously supported by a physician who cares enough to make a home visit.

What drug interventions are available?

Table 2 summarizes current UK and US guideline recommendations,[2] [3] highlights key safety concerns about analgesics, and provides guidance on specific drug treatments for both nociceptive and neuropathic pain disorders. The use of drug combinations often results in enhanced analgesic effectiveness, with lower toxicity than is seen with the use of a single agent at higher doses, and is encouraged.[30]

Paracetamol

Because of its favourable safety profile, paracetamol (acetaminophen) is the preferred treatment for older patients with mild or moderate pain. In one meta-analysis of seven randomized controlled trials comparing paracetamol with placebo, paracetamol (up to 4 g daily) was found to be modestly effective in reducing pain, which decreased on average by 4 points on a scale of 0-100. The number needed to treat ranged from 4 to 16. Paracetamol did not improve physical function or stiffness when compared with placebo.[31] While it is not associated with significant cardiovascular, renal, or gastrointestinal effects,[3] unintentional overdose of paracetamol is an important cause of hepatotoxicity. Patients should be counseled to not exceed the maximum recommended daily dose.

Non-steroidal anti-inflammatory drugs

Oral non-steroidal anti-inflammatory drugs (NSAIDs) have established gastrointestinal, cardiovascular, and renal risks, which increase with age. Oral NSAIDs can be effective in some patients but are safest when used for pain flares (transient increases in pain that typically persist for hours to days). The current evidence base provides little guidance about the NSAID for safest use in this patient population. A network meta-analysis examined the cardiovascular safety of various NSAIDs and found that naproxen was the least harmful compared with other non-selective (for example, ibuprofen) and selective (for example, celecoxib) NSAIDs.[32] These data indicate that naproxen is most appropriate (compared with other NSAIDs) for patients with cardiovascular risk factors. Risk of renal and gastrointestinal injury must also be weighed, however, before initiating any trial involving NSAIDs. If a trial of an NSAID is undertaken, have the patient return to the office within two weeks to ask about treatment benefit and gastrointestintal side effects, check blood pressure, and carry out renal function tests.

Topical NSAIDs represent an alternative to oral NSAIDs, are generally well tolerated, and should be considered, especially for patients with localized pain.

Opioids

Opioids may be considered when an older patient's pain has not responded to other treatments or when major functional impairment persists despite treatment. The short term efficacy of opioid use (≤12 weeks) among older adults has been established.[33] In a retrospective cohort study of (n=133) older patients (mean age 82) newly started on an opioid because of pain due to chronic musculoskeletal conditions, reductions in pain were recorded in 66% of participants.[34] However, opioids were discontinued in 48% of the participants, mostly as a result of poorly tolerated side effects, including constipation, changes to mental status, and nausea. Given the established risks associated with opioid use,[35] the potential negative effects must be weighed against the consequences of untreated or partially treated pain. A recent systematic review found limited evidence in support of long term opioid treatment, and the risk for serious harm increased in line with opioid dose.[35] If an opioid trial is undertaken, it is important to closely monitor (that is, biweekly during the initiation and dose titration phase of treatment) whether treatment goals are being met. If not, the drug should be tapered and discontinued.

There is no evidence to support the use of one weak opioid (for example, hydrocodone, codeine) over another when the response to paracetamol or a NSAID is lacking. Selection of a specific opioid depends on the clinician's clinical experience and knowledge, the patient's previous experiences, and availability of the drug in local pharmacies. Strong opioids (for example, morphine, hydrocodone) should not be given to patients who have never used opioids. Efforts to reduce opioid related risks are particularly appropriate given dramatic increases in and complications associated with opioid use. These include the use of screening tools (for example, the screener and opioid assessment for people with pain, opioid risk tool) that can be used to assess risk for the likelihood of opioid misuse, as well as guide decisions about the extent of monitoring needed if an opioid trial is undertaken. Such monitoring might extend to the use of urine toxicology screens on a periodic basis. Before older patients are prescribed opioid analgesics, physicians should be satisfied with arrangements for safe storage of the drug, given the risk for drug diversion (that is, use of the drug for a purpose other than pain reduction). In terms of initiating a given opioid trial, no special dosing guidelines exist for older patients. Beginning at the lowest possible dose and titrating upwards based on tolerability and efficacy is recommended, given that age is associated with a greater incidence of treatment related adverse effects. This risk is increased by the presence of multiple comorbidities, polypharmacy, and physiologic vulnerability. Careful surveillance is necessary after beginning an analgesic trial. Frequent telephone or email contact is recommended to assess for and deal with any adverse effects.

What psychological interventions are available?

There is optimism about the role of psychological interventions as treatment for older patients with chronic pain.[36]

Cognitive behavioral therapy

The use of CBT is promising.[37] CBT is used to enhance patients' control over pain, based on the premise that an individual's beliefs, attitudes, and behaviors play a central role in the experience of pain. Standard CBT protocols instruct patients in the use of specific cognitive and behavioral techniques, teach them how certain thoughts, beliefs, attitudes, and emotions influence pain, and highlight the patient's own role in controlling and adapting to chronic pain. CBT techniques are underutilized, particularly among older adults with chronic pain. Few providers have been trained to deliver the protocols for pain, particularly in less developed countries.[38] Early innovation in remote therapy that makes use of communication technology may help to overcome this barrier. Although the quality of the early trials in this area is poor, the use of ehealth and mhealth technologies can improve access to treatments and could improve the treatments.[39] Particularly promising are efforts to train non-psychologists in CBT delivery and related therapies, which could increase the reach of these treatments.[40] In addition, two recent high quality trials broaden the scope of treatment to include sustainable self management practices in primary care.[41] [42] In one trial, investigators evaluated a CBT based self management program for use by older patients with chronic pain in primary care.[41] Significant improvements in distress from the pain, disability, and self efficacy were found in patients who received CBT training compared with an exercise only and wait list control group. Communicating with older patients—particularly those who are reluctant to try behavioral treatments—that using non-drug as well as drug treatments is the standard of care can be helpful. Routinely inquiring about and dealing with patient barriers to engagement with treatment (for example, belief that non-drug treatments are ineffective) is also recommended.

Self management programs

Self management programs merge physical, psychological, and social dimensions and adopt a largely educational approach, teaching patients specific strategies to reduce pain by changing their behavioral, cognitive, and emotional responses to pain and building self efficacy for managing pain and its sequelae. These programs combine education about pain and its consequences and training in relaxation and communication skills. Among the best known of these programs is the Arthritis Foundation self help program (http://patienteducation.stanford.edu/programs/asmp.html). Evidence about the value of self management programs for pain is mixed. Several reviews have reported positive treatment outcomes,[43] [44] whereas others have not.[45] [46] Despite the conflicting data, we believe it is reasonable to encourage patient participation in self management, and a clearer matching of tailored treatment content to specific outcomes.[47]

What rehabilitative and exercise approaches are available?

Exercise interventions for older adults with chronic pain are evidenced based, underutilized, and should be a core component of any long term treatment plan. Primary components include training in balance, flexibility, endurance, and strengthening, the mix of which should be tailored to best meet the needs of each patient. Clinicians can refer patients to physiotherapists to develop an exercise program. Physiotherapists can also reinforce related concepts to include coaching on risk of falls, balance training, body mechanics, and pacing. Simple physician advice to remain physically active despite pain, in the absence of a specific exercise routine, is ineffective.

Community based programs include the evidence based Arthritis Foundation exercise program (www.cdc.gov/arthritis/interventions/physical_activity.htm), which is delivered in a group format. Classes are held 1-3 times a week for eight weeks. Health or fitness trainers (such as exercise therapists) lead the groups, which focus on specific exercises appropriate for patients with arthritis or arthritis related diseases. In a recent uncontrolled study (n=110) of a group based exercise training program for older adults with arthritis, participation led to significant improvements in physical functioning.[48] Tai Chi and yoga programs should also be considered, with the caveat that the instructor should be properly qualified.[18] Exercise based programs are low cost and accessible in many communities.[49] Healthcare providers should familiarize themselves with these resources.

Practitioners should consider the preferences of individual patients when prescribing exercise, including the preferred location (for example, gym, home) as well as type of exercise. Older patients with chronic pain may not have access to facilities for exercise or may lack the motivation to engage. It is important to address these barriers or adherence will be low. In support of this approach is a randomized controlled trial of community dwelling older adults (n=56) with chronic pain.[50] In this study, participants randomized to an eight week group based exercise program that included motivational interviewing techniques delivered by a physiotherapist showed significant improvements in pain

ADDITIONAL EDUCATIONAL RESOURCES

Resources for healthcare professionals

- International Association for the Study of Pain (www.iasp-pain.org/)—Offers extensive resources for healthcare professionals, including listings of educational opportunities, resources on management and treatment, and clinical updates (many countries have affiliates of IASP)
- American Geriatrics Society (www.americangeriatrics.org/health_care_professionals/clinical_practice/clinical_guidelines_recommendations/2009/)—Provides resources and guidelines for clinicians in providing care to older adults with pain
- European Pain Federation (www.efic.org/)—Promotes research, education, clinical management, and professional practice on pain, with training and educational opportunities

Resources for patients

- British Pain Society (www.britishpainsociety.org/)—Provides extensive information for people with pain, including suggested readings, frequently asked questions, and free downloadable publications on various aspects of pain management
- American Chronic Pain Association (www.theacpa.org/)—Offers education and support for people in pain, including educational online resources and a network of support groups in the United States, United Kingdom, and other countries
- Arthritis Foundation (www.arthritis.org/)—Offers programs, practical tips, and education to help people to better manage arthritis related pain

intensity, self efficacy, anxiety level, and mobility compared with a group based activity control group.[50]

When should patients be referred to a pain specialist?

Practitioners should refer patients when pain is unresponsive (or poorly responsive) to standard treatments, a psychiatric condition (for example, active substance use disorder, excluding nicotine) or medical condition (for example, hepatic or renal dysfunction) would complicate management, there are concerns about misuse of opioids, and procedures (for example, nerve block) may help to clarify a diagnosis or are indicated for the treatment of a given pain disorder.

What is the role of mobile health technology?

Recent advances in mobile health technologies suggest these devices may play a role in the near future by facilitating the collection and transmission of information for the assessment of pain.[51 52] These devices could potentially improve patient care through more effective monitoring of treatment outcomes, enhanced patient-provider communication, and by providing new ways to deliver treatment.[51] For example, a recent SMS text message based social support intervention delivered by mobile phone was found to reduce pain and pain interference levels among patients with chronic pain.[52]

What limitations exist in the evidence base about treatment?

Although the number of well designed studies evaluating drug or non-drug treatments for older adults with chronic pain is growing, there are important limitations in the existing evidence base. Factors limiting the generalizability of findings include the use of various outcome measures, which make it difficult to compare across studies, short duration of most trials ($\leq$12 weeks), lack of diversity in study populations (inclusion of mostly white, non-Hispanic patients), and greater enrolment of young-old participants (with few participants aged $\geq$80) without major comorbidity. Questions about treatment adherence, as well as the long term safety and efficacy of these modalities in older populations remain inadequately defined. In terms of behavioral treatments, patient factors that positively (or negatively) impact treatment outcomes remain inadequately defined. Identifying optimal strategies for the delivery of behavioral treatment (for example, individual versus group based and online versus mobile health approaches) warrant further attention.[36]

Despite these knowledge gaps, we recommend that healthcare providers educate older patients about diverse treatment approaches and encourage their use, to include both drug and non-drug modalities, as a way of broadening their "pain management portfolio." Lack of evidence does not mean evidence of no effect; clinicians must make treatment decisions based on the interaction of individual needs and existing evidence. Given low rates of use of many non-drug management approaches in older patients, encouraging engagement in and adoption of these modalities, to include cognitive behavioral therapy and exercise is particularly recommended.

TIPS FOR NON-SPECIALISTS

- Pain is more than just a sensory event; assessing for the presence and severity of pain captures only a small part of the pain experience
- Diagnostic imaging is often overused and does not equal better care
- Consider specialist referral for older patients who have complicated psychiatric histories, debilitating pain, or pain that does not respond to customary treatments
- Use combinations of analgesic drugs to enhance analgesic effectiveness
- Non-drug approaches to include exercise and cognitive behavioral approaches are underutilized. Educate older patients about these approaches and identify local practitioners or agencies that provide them
- Implement surveillance plan to assess treatment efficacy, tolerability, and adherence with each new treatment

A PATIENT'S PERSPECTIVE

I have lived with chronic back pain for over 30 years. Early on I had surgery on my back that helped for maybe six months, but then the pain returned and has been with me ever since. It has affected my life in many ways: I don't have as much energy as I would like, I can only do housework for short periods before my back starts to hurt, and my kids only know me as a person with chronic back pain. I use different techniques to help me manage it. First off, having a supportive spouse and family is very important. I also find massage, which I get several times a week, to be incredibly helpful. I also go to the gym where I do stretches, walk on the treadmill, and do the exercise bike and elliptical for short periods (five minutes each) before my back starts to bother me. I do take pain medications; I will take ibuprofen for short periods. I also take hydrocodone when the pain is really bad but don't like taking it regularly because my mother had an addiction problem, which is a concern. I would say I have learned to live with the pain and won't let it defeat me. Sally Smith, New York City

Contributors: All authors conceived and designed the article, participated in its drafting and revision, and approved the final version. MCR is guarantor.

Competing interests: We have read and understood the BMJ policy on declaration of interests and declare that: MCR has received funding from the National Institute on Ageing (P30AG022845), the Agency for Healthcare Quality and Research (R01HS020648), Howard and Phyllis Schwartz Philanthropic Fund, and Endo Pharmaceuticals. KP has received research funding from the National Institute on Ageing (P30AG022845). CE has received a grant from the UK National Institute for Health Research Cochrane Program.

Patient consent obtained.

Provenance and peer review: Commissioned; externally peer reviewed.

1 Institute of Medicine (US) Committee on Advancing Pain Research, Care, and Education. Relieving pain in America: a blueprint for transforming prevention, care, education, and research. National Academies Press (US), 2011.
2 Abdulla A, Adams N, Bone M, Elliott AM, Gaffin J, Jones D, et al. Guidance on the management of pain in older people. *Age Ageing* 2013;42 (Suppl 1):1-57.
3 American Geriatrics Society Panel on Persistent Pain in Older Persons. Pharmacological management of persistent pain in older persons. *J Am Geriatr Soc* 2009;57:1331-46.
4 International Association for the Study of Pain. IASP taxonomy. 2012. www.iasp-pain.org/Taxonomy?navItemNumber=576.
5 Solano JP, Gomes B, Higginson IJ. A comparison of symptom prevalence in far advanced cancer, AIDS, heart disease, chronic obstructive pulmonary disease, and renal disease. *J Pain Symptom Manage* 2006;31:58-69.
6 Enck RE. Postsurgical chronic pain. *Am J Hosp Palliat Care* 2010;27:301-2.
7 Smith AK, Cenzer IS, Knight SJ, Puntillo KA, Widera E, Williams BA, et al. The epidemiology of pain in the last 2 years of life. *Ann Intern Med* 2010;153:563-9.
8 Wyldea V, Hewlett S, Learmonth ID. Persistent pain after joint replacement: prevalence, sensory qualities, and postoperative determinants. *Pain* 2011;152:457-76.
9 Cooper G, Lane JM, Lin J. Medscape: overview of osteoporotic compression fractures. 2013. www.emedicine.com/pmr/byname/nonoperative-treatment-of-osteoporotic-compression-fractures.htm.
10 Patel KV, Guralnik JM, Dansie EJ, Turk DC. Prevalence and impact of pain among older adults in the United States: findings from the 2011 National Health and Aging Trends Study. *Pain* 2013;154:2649-57.

11 Leadley RM, Armstrong N, Lee YC, Allen A, Kleijnen J. Chronic diseases in the European Union: the prevalence and health cost implications of chronic pain. *J Pain Palliat Care Pharmacother* 2012;26:310-25.

12 Henderson JV, Harrison CM, Britt HC, Bayram CF, Miller GC. Prevalence, causes, severity, impact, and management of chronic pain in Australian general practice patients. *Pain Med* 2013;14:1346-61.

13 Jackson T, Chen H, Iezzi T, Yee M, Chen F. Prevalence and correlates of chronic pain in a random population study of adults in Chongqing, China. *Clin J Pain* 2014;3:346-52.

14 Tsang A, Von Korff M, Lee S, Alonso J, Karam E, Angermeyer MC, et al. Common chronic pain conditions in developed and developing countries: gender and age differences and comorbidity with depression-anxiety disorders . *J Pain* 2008;9:883-91.

15 Mallen CD, Thomas E, Belcher J, Rathod T, Croft P, Peat G. Point-of-care prognosis for common musculoskeletal pain in older adults. *JAMA Intern Med* 2013;173:1119-25.

16 Makris UE, Abrams RC, Gurland B, Reid MC. Management of persistent pain in the older patient: a clinical review. *JAMA* 2014;312:825-36.

17 Royal College of Physicians, British Geriatrics Society, and British Pain Society. The assessment of pain in older people: national guidelines. Concise guidance to good practice series, No 8. Royal College of Physicians, Oct 2007.

18 American Geriatrics Society Panel on Persistent Pain in Older Persons. The management of persistent pain in older persons. *J Am Geriatr Soc* 2002;50(Suppl 6):205-24.

19 Hadjistavropoulos T, Herr K, Turk DC, Fine PG, Dworkin RH, Helme R, et al. An interdisciplinary expert consensus statement on assessment of pain in older persons. *Clin J Pain* 2007;23(Suppl 1):1-43.

20 Chou R, Qaseem A, Owens DK, Shekelle P. Clinical Guidelines Committee of the American College of Physicians. Diagnostic imaging for low back pain: advice for high-value health care from the American College of Physicians. *Ann Intern Med* 2011;154:181-9.

21 Azevedo LF, Costa-Pereira A, Mendonça L, Dias CC, Castro-Lopes JM. Chronic pain and health services utilization: is there overuse of diagnostic tests and inequalities in nonpharmacologic treatment methods utilization? *Med Care* 2013;51:859-69.

22 Dansie EJ, Turk DC. Assessment of patients with chronic pain. *Br J Anaesth* 2013;111:19-25.

23 Herr K, Coyne PJ, McCaffery M, Manworren R, Merkel S. Pain assessment in the patient unable to self-report: position statement with clinical practice recommendations. *Pain Manag Nurs* 2011;12:230-50.

24 Messier SP, Mihalko SL, Legault C, Miller GD, Nicklas BJ, DeVita P, et al. Effects of intensive diet and exercise on knee joint loads, inflammation, and clinical outcomes among overweight and obese adults with knee osteoarthritis: the IDEA randomized clinical trial. *JAMA* 2013;310:1263-73.

25 Kroenke K, Krebs EE, Wu J, Yu Z, Chumbler NR, Bair MJ. Telecare collaborative management of chronic pain in primary care: a randomized clinical trial. *JAMA* 2014;312:240-8.

26 Dobscha SK, Corson K, Perrin NA, Hanson GC, Leibowitz RQ, Doak MN, et al. Collaborative care for chronic pain in primary care: a cluster randomized trial. *JAMA* 2009;301:1242-52.

27 Lin EHB, Katon W, Von Korff M, Tang L, Williams JW Jr, Kroenke K, et al. Effect of improving depression care on pain and functional outcomes among older adults with arthritis: a randomized controlled trial. *JAMA* 2003;290:2428-9.

28 Keefe FJ, Blumenthal J, Baucom D, Affleck G, Waugh R, Caldwell DS, et al. Effects of spouse-assisted coping skills training and exercise training in patients with osteoarthritic knee pain: a randomized controlled study. *Pain* 2004;110:539-49.

29 Martire LM, Schulz R, Keefe FJ, Rudy TE, Starz TW. Couple-oriented education and support intervention for osteoarthritis: effects on spouses' support and responses to patient pain. *Fam Syst Health* 2008;26:185-95.

30 Gilron I, Bailey JM, Tu D, Holden RR, Weaver DF, Houlden RL. Morphine, gabapentin, or their combination for neuropathic pain. *N Engl J Med* 2005;352:1324-34.

31 Towheed TE, Maxwell L, Judd MG, Catton M, Hochberg MC, Wells G. Acetaminophen for osteoarthritis. *Cochrane Database Syst Rev* 2006;1:CD004257.

32 Trelle S, Reichenbach S, Wandel S, Hildebrand P, Tschannen B, Villiger PM, et al. Cardiovascular safety of non-steroidal anti-inflammatory drugs: network meta-analysis. *BMJ* 2011;342:c7086.

33 Papaleontiou M, Henderson CR Jr, Turner BJ, Moore AA, Olkhovskaya Y, Amanfo L, et al. Outcomes associated with opioid use in the treatment of chronic noncancer pain in older adults: a systematic review and meta-analysis. *J Am Geriatr Soc* 2010;58:1353-69.

34 Reid MC, Henderson CR Jr, Papaleontiou M, Amanfo L, Olkhovskaya Y, Moore AA, et al. Characteristics of older adults receiving opioids in primary care: treatment duration and outcomes. *Pain Med* 2010;11:1063-71.

35 Chou R, Turner JA, Devine EB, Hansen RN, Sullivan SD, Blazina I, et al. The effectiveness and risks of long-term opioid therapy for chronic pain: a systematic review for a National Institutes of Health pathways to prevention workshop. *Ann Intern Med* 2015; published online 13 Jan.

36 McGuire BE, Nicholas MK, Asghari A, Wood BM, Main CJ. The effectiveness of psychological treatments for chronic pain in older adults: cautious optimism and an agenda for research. *Curr Opin Psychiatry* 2014;27:380-4.

37 Lunde LH, Nordhus I, Pallesen S. The effectiveness of cognitive and behavioural treatment of chronic pain in the elderly: a quantitative review. *J Clin Psychol Med Settings* 2009;16:254-62.

38 Draguns JG. Cross-cultural and international extensions of evidence-based psychotherapy: toward more effective and sensitive psychological services everywhere. *Psychologia* 2013;56:74-88.

39 Eccleston C, Fisher E, Craig L, Duggan GB, Rosser BA, Keogh E. Psychological therapies (Internet-delivered) for the management of chronic pain in adults. *Cochrane Database Syst Rev* 2014;2:CD010152.

40 Riddle DL, Keefe FJ, Ang D, Khaled J, Dumenci L, Jensen MP, et al. A phase III randomized three-arm trial of physical therapist delivered pain coping skills training for patients with total knee arthroplasty: the KASTPain protocol. *BMC Musculoskelet Disord* 2012;13:149.

41 Nicholas MK, Asghari A, Blyth FM, Wood BM, Murray R, McCabe R, et al. Self-management intervention for chronic pain in older adults: a randomized controlled trial. *Pain* 2013;154:824-35.

42 Broderick JE, Keefe FJ, Bruckenthal P, Junghaenel DU, Schneider S, Schwartz JE, et al. Nurse practitioners can effectively deliver pain coping skills training to osteoarthritis patients with chronic pain: a randomized, controlled trial. *Pain* 2014;155:1743-54.

43 Reid MC, Papaleontiou M, Ong A, Breckman R, Wethington E, Pillemer K. Self-management strategies to reduce pain and improve function among older adults in community settings: a review of the evidence. *Pain Med* 2008;9:409-24.

44 Du S, Yuan C, Xiao X, Chu J, Qiu Y, Qian H. Self-management programs for chronic musculoskeletal pain conditions: a systematic review and meta-analysis. *Patient Educ Couns* 2011;85:e299-310.

45 Chodosh J, Morton SC, Mojica W, Maglione M, Suttorp MJ, Hilton L, et al. Meta-analysis: chronic disease self-management programs for older adults. *Ann Intern Med* 2005;143:427-38.

46 Warsi A, Wang PS, LaValley MP, Avorn J, Solomon DH. Self-management education programs in chronic disease. A systematic review and methodological critique of the literature. *Arch Intern Med* 2004;164:1641-9.

47 Morley S, Williams A, Eccleston C. Examining the evidence of psychological treatments for chronic pain: time for a paradigm shift? *Pain* 2012;154:1929-31.

48 Levy SS, Macera CA, Hootman JM, Coleman KJ, Lopez R, Nichols JF, et al. Evaluation of a multi-component group exercise program for adults with arthritis: Fitness and Exercise for People with Arthritis (FEPA). *Disabil Health J* 2012;5:305-11.

49 Tobias KR, Lama SD, Parker SJ, Henderson CR Jr, Nickerson AJ, Reid MC. Meeting the public health challenge of pain in later life: what role can senior centers play? *Pain Manag Nurs* 2014;15:760-7.

50 Tse MM, Vong SK, Tang SK. Motivational interviewing and exercise programme for community-dwelling older persons with chronic pain: a randomized controlled study. *J Clin Nurs* 2013;22:1843-56.

51 Richardson JE, Reid MC. The promises and pitfalls of leveraging mobile health technology for pain care. *Pain Med* 2013;14:1621-6.

52 Guillory J, Chang P, Henderson CR Jr, Shengelia R, Lama S, Warmington M, et al. Piloting a text message-based social support intervention for patients with chronic pain: establishing feasibility and preliminary efficacy. *Clin J Pain* 2015; published online 6 Jan.

BPP UNIVERSITY SCHOOL OF HEALTH BMJ

Cancer induced bone pain

Christopher M Kane, NIHR academic clinical fellow in palliative medicine[1], Peter Hoskin, professor of clinical oncology[2], Michael I Bennett, St Gemma's professor of palliative medicine[1]

[1]Academic Unit of Palliative Care, Leeds Institute of Health Sciences, School of Medicine, University of Leeds, Leeds, UK

[2]Mount Vernon Cancer Centre, Northwood, University College London, London, UK

Correspondence to: C M Kane Christopher.Kane@nhs.net

Cite this as: *BMJ* 2015;350:h315

DOI: 10.1136/bmj.h315

http://www.bmj.com/content/350/bmj.h315

Bone pain is the most common type of pain from cancer and is present in around one third of patients with bone metastases.[1 2] Based on postmortem studies of patients with advanced cancer and clinical knowledge of how often bone metastases result in pain, the incidence of cancer induced bone pain is estimated at 30 000 patients in the United Kingdom each year.[3 w1] Currently, improvements in cancer treatments mean that many patients are living with metastatic cancer for several years. The prevalence of cancer induced bone pain is therefore likely to be much greater than the annual incidence.[w1] Cancer induced bone pain is considered one of the most difficult pain conditions to treat because of its frequent association with weight bearing and movement. Not surprisingly, it has a major impact on patients' daily functioning and mood and can result in admission to hospital.[w2 w3]

Given the prevalence of cancer induced bone pain, it is likely that clinicians in primary or secondary care will be confronted by patients in pain crises. Recognising and initiating management of this specific pain state, as well as an awareness of the specialist treatments, is important for all clinicians.

What is cancer induced bone pain?

Cancer induced bone pain is a specific pain state with overlapping but distinct features of both inflammatory and neuropathic pain.[4] The most important changes are in bone homeostasis, with corresponding events in the peripheral and central nervous system.[5] In healthy bone, osteoclasts and osteoblasts are highly regulated to maintain balanced resorption and formation of bone respectively, through RANK-ligand (receptor activator of nuclear factor κ). In the presence of a bone metastasis, increased expression of RANK-ligand disrupts this relation leading to increased osteoclast activity and bone destruction. Cancer cells also stimulate local inflammatory mediators and create a highly acidic environment, which sensitises peripheral nerve endings within the bone marrow and bone matrix. When combined with the destruction of nerve endings through cancer invasion, the resulting pain is a mixture of ongoing inflammatory and neuropathic processes, which lead to a hyperexcitability state within the spinal cord. Patients experience this as constant pain, with high sensitivity to movement.[4]

Who gets cancer induced bone pain?

Cancer induced bone pain can occur anywhere that cancer has metastasised to bone. Cancers most often involved are those of the prostate, breast, and lung, as well as myeloma.[3] The most common sites of metastases are vertebrae, pelvis, long bones, and ribs.[3] At postmortem examination, up to 70% of patients who died of cancer will have bone metastases.[3] Bone metastases can be found in a wide range of places (figure). However, not all patients with bone metastases get pain; bone pain was identified in only a third of patients with bone metastases in one large prospective study.[1] It is not yet clear why some bone metastases cause pain and others do not.

What are the clinical features of cancer induced bone pain?

In a cross sectional survey in 2011 patients described their cancer induced bone pain as annoying, gnawing, aching, and nagging.[w4] The pain is commonly a mixture of steady background pain, as well as pain that is exacerbated by weight

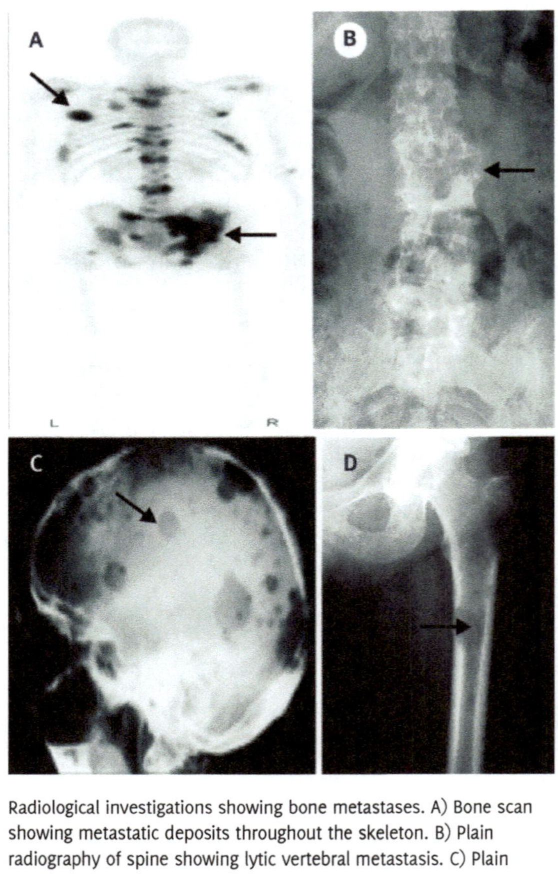

Radiological investigations showing bone metastases. A) Bone scan showing metastatic deposits throughout the skeleton. B) Plain radiography of spine showing lytic vertebral metastasis. C) Plain radiography of a skull showing multiple metastatic deposits. D) Plain radiography showing a lytic lesion of the upper shaft of the left femur

THE BOTTOM LINE

- Cancer induced bone pain is a common problem, which can be extremely debilitating to patients with an already limited life expectancy
- When treating cancer induced bone pain, maintenance of function should be given high priority alongside pain relief
- Early recognition, intervention with functional aids, and behaviour modification, combined with initial titration with analgesia (commonly, strong opioids) are important first steps for non-specialists
- The evidence for early referral for radiotherapy is strong, although bisphosphonates will have an important role for some patients
- Specialist support will be required if pain persists despite initial treatment with behaviour modification, commencement of a non-steroidal anti-inflammatory drug, and initial titration of a strong opioid

bearing or movement, called incident or episodic pain.[4] In a recent well conducted European-wide observational study of 1000 patients with cancer, 85.5% reported some form of incident pain episodes.[6] The presence of movement related pain has most impact on function and daily activity.[w4]

Cancer induced bone pain is most commonly experienced in the lower back, pelvis, long bones, and ribs. This can be the presenting feature of the cancer or highlight a recurrence in those previously treated. Therefore in patients with or without active cancer, persistent pain in these areas should alert clinicians to the possibility of bone metastases. Findings on examination are often non-specific with only some tenderness over the site of metastasis or pain specifically related to movement.

A bony metastasis can weaken bone sufficiently such that an innocuous movement, bump, or fall may result in a pathological fracture. Vertebral pain should always alert clinicians to the risk of spinal cord compression, especially in the presence of sensory disturbance, generalised leg weakness, or changes in bladder or bowel function. Even without "red flag" signs, a full neurological examination should be done in these patients, with a low threshold for a spinal magnetic resonance scan.[7] Even if suspicion is low, advice should be sought from the patient's oncologist; retrospective cohort studies have shown that being able to walk at the time of diagnosis of spinal cord compression is correlated with overall survival and the ability to walk after treatment. Early diagnosis and treatment of impending spinal cord compression can drastically improve quality of life for patients.[8 9]

Table 1 outlines the advantages and disadvantages of the various investigations for suspected cancer induced bone pain. Generalists may consider plain film radiography or computed tomography as initial investigations; other investigations are usually undertaken by specialists.

QUESTIONS FOR FUTURE RESEARCH

- Why do some bone metastases cause pain and others do not?
- What are the disease processes that are responsible for some bone metastases causing pain and others not, and are there any associations with cancer type?
- Are there specific phenotypes of cancer bone pain that might predict response to analgesia?
- What is the contribution of spinal hyperexcitability in the experience of bone pain, and how best can this be identified and managed?
- What non-drug treatments may offer patients benefit in managing movement related pain?

How is cancer induced bone pain initially managed?

The first steps in management are simple measures that can be initiated in non-specialist care, while referral for specialist treatments such as radiotherapy or bisphosphonates is awaited. In the following section we describe the evidence for each treatment that is commonly used for cancer induced bone pain. Consider specialist referral in any patient where pain persists despite these initial steps, those with rapidly increasing pain despite treatment or evidence of toxicity from opioids, and where pathological fracture or spinal cord compression are suspected.

Non-drug interventions

Important aspects of managing cancer induced bone pain are to support patient self management and encourage the use of non-drug measures. An observational study of 1000 European patients with cancer showed that in those who had pain on movement, many of whom had bone metastasis, 43% found consistent pain relief with non-drug measures, often reported as either rest or sleep.[6] Discussing behaviour modifications, such as avoiding strenuous movement, and referring patients for any appropriate movement aids (walking stick, Zimmer frame) or home adaptations (bath rails) can make important contributions to the maintenance of function and quality of life.

World Health Organization pain ladder

For cancer pain in general, the mainstay of treatment has been the World Health Organization's method for the relief of cancer pain, commonly known as the analgesic ladder.[10] Observational studies have shown that about 73% of patients achieved adequate analgesia by following these guidelines, leaving an important minority of patients with inadequately controlled pain despite receiving strong opioids.[11 12]

The first step of the WHO ladder is non-opioid analgesics, such as paracetamol and non-steroidal anti-inflammatory drugs. Although some patients find over the counter analgesics helpful, several systematic reviews that have examined the effectiveness of paracetamol for cancer pain showed that although it was well tolerated there was no significant benefit particularly when added to strong opioids.[13 14] Non-steroidal anti-inflammatory drugs are often perceived to be more efficacious in cancer induced bone pain than in other pain states, and this is a reasonable

Table 1 Advantages and disadvantages of investigations for bone metastases

Investigation	Advantages	Disadvantages
Plain film radiography	Universal availability; portable films possible, low cost	Low sensitivity: requires >50% cortical destruction to be visible
Computed tomography	More sensitive than plain radiography; best for ribs and pelvic and shoulder girdles; gives information about soft tissue; can be reconstructed in three planes	Access variable outside large hospitals; high cost
Technetium 99m bone scan	Available widely; whole skeleton assessed; intermediate cost	Relatively low sensitivity; reflects osteoblastic activity: non-specific
Magnetic resonance imaging	Optimal images of bone; high sensitivity; detects small metastases before bone damage occurs; optimal for cord compression; gives soft tissue and nerve images; whole body magnetic resonance imaging screens entire skeleton	Access limited; high cost
Fluorodeoxyglucose positron emission tomography	Similar sensitivity to technetium 99m for bone metastases; additional information about other organs	Access limited; high cost; limited specificity: false positives can occur
Fluorine positron emission tomography	Most sensitive detection of bone metastases	Limited experience, evidence, and access; high cost
Choline positron emission tomography	Sensitive for prostate cancer metastases	Access limited but increasing; high cost

assumption given the major inflammatory component. However, a well conducted systematic review in 2012 showed some benefit from adding non-steroidal anti-inflammatory drugs to strong opioids for cancer pain, although this evidence is limited and weak.[13] There are well reported concerns regarding adverse effects of non-steroidal anti-inflammatory drugs; however, this systematic review failed to show any additional harm of adding a non-steroidal anti-inflammatory drug to a strong opioid.[13] The studies did not perform subgroup analysis on cancer induced bone pain. Therefore the assertion that non-steroidal anti-inflammatory drugs are specifically beneficial in cancer induced bone pain cannot be supported.

The next step in the WHO ladder is the use of weak opioids, although a systematic review has only shown marginal benefits of tramadol and codeine in cancer pain, with significant nausea and vomiting associated with tramadol compared with placebo or when added to fentanyl. The authors in these studies did not report the specific proportion of patients with bone metastases.[w5] Therefore it is common to miss this step and start low dose strong opioids if non-opioid analgesia is ineffective.

Strong opioids

Strong opioids are the mainstay of treatment for background pain in patients with cancer induced bone pain. In the United Kingdom, the National Institute for Health and Care Excellence has published extensive guidance on initiating and managing strong opioids in palliative care.[15] This guidance is not specific to cancer induced bone pain, but the principles are directly relevant. Several relatively small randomised controlled trials found no difference between immediate release and sustained release morphine in terms of efficacy or side effects when treatment with opioids was initiated. Therefore this decision should be based on patient and clinician consensus.[16 w6-7]

Several different preparations and types of strong opioid are available. A network meta-analysis showed no important differences in efficacy between morphine and other strong opioids.[17] Based on one well conducted randomised controlled trial, about 75% of patients will achieve good pain control with strong opioids, resulting in a number needed to treat of 2.[18] Within this study, however, there was no subgroup analysis for cancer induced bone pain. Table 2 provides a summary of the numbers needed to treat for various treatments for cancer induced bone pain.

In the United Kingdom, morphine is recommended by NICE as the preferred opioid treatment in patients who can take oral drugs. When morphine was compared with oxycodone no difference was found in pain intensity or adverse effects.[17 18]

Transdermal opioids (fentanyl or buprenophine) are likely to be less constipating than morphine or oxycodone.[17] Specialist advice should be sought if pain control is inadequate after the initial titration of opioid analgesia, or treatment fails.[17]

Management of incident pain is less satisfactory. This is because pain manifests within five minutes, is often movement related, and subsides within 15 minutes in about half of patients with cancer induced bone pain.[w4] Timing drug treatment to coincide with this pain profile is challenging.

A meta-analysis of fast acting fentanyl preparations found them to be statistically superior over oral morphine in the treatment of incident pain.[19] When compared with oral morphine, however, the numbers needed to treat at 10 and 15 minutes after the drugs have been administered are 18 and 12, respectively.[20] This means that of 12 patients treated with fast acting fentanyl, only one would have gained benefit after 15 minutes of treatment that would not have done so had they been treated with morphine.[20] Given the additional cost of these preparations, current advice is to use immediate release morphine preparations as the preferred treatment and to try a fast acting fentanyl preparation if this treatment fails. Adverse events are difficult to quantify in these studies as patients are already taking regular background opioids. Constipation is a common side effect of opioid treatment and a laxative should be prescribed at the time treatment is started.[17]

Other drug interventions

Adjuvant drugs such as antidepressants and anticonvulsants may enhance analgesia from strong opioids and can target neuropathic pain mechanisms. A systematic review in 2011 examined the efficacy of these drugs for the treatment of cancer pain when added to opioids. A modest reduction

Table 2 Numbers needed to treat values for a meaningful clinical response* for various treatments in cancer induced bone pain

Intervention	Numbers needed to treat
Strong opioids for background pain	2
Fast acting fentanyl for incident pain (at 15 mins)	12
Radiotherapy (meaningful response)	2.8
Bisphosphonates (at 12 weeks)	7

**Defined as either 30% or 50% reduction in pain scores or an outcome of partial or complete response.*

SOURCES AND SELECTION CRITERIA

We searched Medline, Clinical Evidence, and the Cochrane Library using the terms "bone metastases", "pain", and "bone pain" and then combined these with the specific treatment terms individually. Where possible we have used systematic reviews but not referenced trials included in these reviews. We limited our search from 1990 to December 2014. We also searched the National Institute for Health and Care Excellence and the Scottish Intercollegiate Guidelines Network. In calculating the numbers needed to treat, we have assumed a conservative placebo response of 25%.

A PATIENT'S PERSPECTIVE

I was diagnosed with cancer on my wedding anniversary a year ago. I developed back pain, which felt exactly the same as sciatica; however, it wasn't getting any better. One Saturday it became so unbearable that I went to A and E and they diagnosed a water infection and sent me home with antibiotics. I saw my general practitioner and he sent me back to A and E where they did a scan and told me my kidney looked slightly inflamed. They said it would settle down in a few days with antibiotics. They called me back a few days later to tell me they'd found cancer in the bones in my back and my pelvis on the scan I'd had.

Since then the pain has been bad but it's the things that it stops me from doing that I get upset about. I can't swim or walk anymore and it really wears you down. It's affected my marriage so we now sleep in separate beds.

I've really appreciated the doctors' help but they don't understand that I don't just want to lie in bed all day, because the tablets have made me sleepy. I want to be able to do things and this is so important to me. I'd really like doctors to think about trying to make sure I'm able to do things still rather than just giving me tablets.

in pain scores was found in patients with a neuropathic element to their pain, but more adverse effects were reported. Benefit was seen within 4-8 days and did not improve beyond this. These conclusions are limited owing to the quality of the studies included in the review.[21] Although animal studies have suggested that gabapentin can have an important analgesic effect in cancer induced bone pain, there is no evidence confirming the efficacy of this class of drugs in humans.[w8]

Currently there is no evidence to support the use of steroids for cancer induced bone pain; two randomised controlled studies have shown no sustained benefit for cancer pain.[22 23]

Lidocaine (lignocaine) patches are not absorbed systemically and evidence to support their use for cancer induced bone pain is lacking.[w9 w10]

What further treatment options are available?

Once initial treatment has been started, further treatment options are available to maintain function and quality of life.

Radiotherapy

Radiotherapy has been shown to reduce pain significantly and is the most effective treatment that is specific for cancer induced bone pain. Therefore patients with confirmed cancer induced bone pain should be referred to a clinical oncologist as soon as possible. A well conducted systematic review comparing single dose radiotherapy with multiple doses found no important differences between treatments. Both approaches resulted in a meaningful improvement in pain for about 60% of patients (number needed to treat 2.8).[24 25] Within this group it was reported that approximately 25% would be pain-free. This means that a single dose of radiotherapy can be effective and without major burden for even very frail patients.

In a well conducted randomised trial of 850 patients, where most had had an initial response to radiotherapy but recurrence of pain, 28% experienced a further overall pain response at two months after re-irradiation. This was also associated with improved quality of life.[26 27]

Radioisotopes

Referral to oncology also provides the opportunity to review hormonal treatment and chemotherapy, as well as to consider radioisotope treatment. Some evidence, largely from studies in prostate cancer, indicates that radioisotopes may provide complete reduction in pain over one to six months, with no increase in analgesic use, but severe adverse effects (leucocytopenia and thrombocytopenia) are common.[w11]

WHAT TO DISCUSS WITH PATIENTS WHO ARE STARTING STRONG OPIOIDS

- Address concerns about addiction, tolerance, and side effects, being clear that prescription of strong opioids does not mean patients are in the last stage of life
- Give verbal and written advice on when and how to take opioids for both background and breakthrough pain
- Explain how long the pain relief should last and that patients' ability to drive may be impaired during initiation of treatment or when doses are increased
- Give advice on signs of toxicity, such as drowsiness, twitching, and hallucinations, and who to contact if any occur out of hours
- Provide drugs at the start of treatment, to deal with side effects such as constipation
- Offer regular review

Adapted from NICE clinical guideline 140 (http://guidance.nice.org.uk/CG140)

Bisphosphonates

Bisphosphonates such as pamidronate and zoledronate are used to reduce both pain and skeletal events in patients with bone metastases. They act by inhibiting osteoclast function. Globally they are used to prevent skeletal related events and reduce pain in breast, prostate, and lung cancer as well as multiple myeloma. In the United Kingdom NICE only recommends early treatment with bisphosphonates for bone pain associated with breast cancer.[28] NICE advise it can be used in lung and prostate cancer once palliative measures and radiotherapy have been given. Several well conducted randomised controlled trials have shown a persistent reduction in pain scores over years with bisphosphonates in patients with breast cancer, and although pain scores increase over time in studies in prostate cancer there is still a significant difference in favour of bisphosphonate compared with placebo.[29] In a large well conducted randomised controlled trial in which patients with bone pain from prostate cancer were randomised to a single infusion of 6 mg of the bisphosphonate ibandronate or a single 8Gy fraction of radiotherapy, overall response rates at four weeks were 49% and 53%, respectively. This non-significant difference was also similar at 12 weeks.[30] This suggests that radiotherapy and bisphosphonates are equally appropriate and effective interventions.

A Cochrane review from 2002 examined the effects of bisphosphonates on cancer induced bone pain and calculated numbers needed to treat of 11 at four weeks after infusion and 7 at 12 weeks after infusion.[31] This review concluded that although evidence supports the use of bisphosphonates they should not be considered as first line management, which is in keeping with the advice from NICE.[31] In patients with cancer induced bone pain from myeloma, a Cochrane review showed benefit from bisphosphonates in pain management.[32]

Denosumab

Denosumab is a novel agent that specifically inhibits RANK-ligand. Clinical trials have shown important benefits in reducing skeletal related events. One randomised controlled trial recruited patients with breast cancer with mild levels of pain. The median time for moderate or severe pain to develop in those receiving denosumab was significantly delayed when compared with bisphosphonate zolendronic acid, although there was no difference in the use of strong analgesics at the end of the study.[33]

Interventional procedures

If patients have ongoing complex cancer induced bone pain despite receiving opioids, radiotherapy, or bisphosphonates, referral to pain services should be considered. There is good evidence from a randomised controlled trial that implantable intrathecal devices lead to a reduction in pain and increased survival in patients taking high dose opiates for refractory pain.[w12]

Surgery

In patients with a good performance status, prophylactic surgery may be considered for relief of cancer induced bone pain. One randomised controlled trial showed that

ADDITIONAL EDUCATIONAL RESOURCES

Resources for healthcare professionals

- National Comprehensive Cancer Network (www.nccn.org)—Provides guidelines for the management of adult cancer pain and treatment of specific cancers (free with registration)
- European Society for Medical oncology (www.esmo.org)—Guidelines for pain management in cancer with access to a smartphone app
- National Institute for Health and Care Excellence (www.nice.org.uk)—Evidence based guidance for specific treatments and an online treatment algorithm for initiating strong opioids and managing side effects

Resources for patients

- Macmillan Cancer Support (www.macmillan.org.uk)—Provides information and help on cancer and the management of symptoms, including bone pain; provides links to local support groups in the United Kingdom
- Cancer Research UK (www.cancerresearchuk.org)—Contains information about cancer and the management of specific symptoms such as pain and includes a forum for patients to discuss their illness
- American Cancer Society (www.cancer.org)—Has general information about bone metastases, and enables patients to search for local support services in the United States

TIPS FOR NON-SPECIALISTS

- The focus of management should be maintenance of function
- Non-steroidal anti-inflammatory drugs may be helpful for some patients but most will require strong opioids
- Early referral for single fraction radiotherapy should be sought, even in relatively frail patients
- Referral for treatment with bisphosphonates can be helpful for some patients
- Consider early referral to specialist services in patients with refractory pain despite initial measures

percutaneous stabilisation in the long bones of leg can significantly reduce pain.[w13] Once a pathological fracture has occurred, however, orthopaedic intervention can stabilise the fracture.

Complementary therapies

Complementary therapies may be considered, but as yet they are supported by weak evidence. A Cochrane systematic review of acupuncture acknowledged that there were studies showing benefit in cancer pain, but that evidence was insufficient to recommend this as a treatment.[w14] Evidence was also insufficient to support TENS (transcutaneous electrical nerve stimulation), but one small feasibility randomised controlled trial in patients with cancer induced bone pain suggests that verbal rating scores of pain on movement are reduced with active TENS compared with sham TENS.[34 w15] Patients may appreciate non-drug measures that they can manage themselves and so TENS may be of value.

Contributors: CK conceived, drafted, and revised the paper and interviewed a patient to develop the patient's story. PH revised the paper and provided tables and images for inclusion. MIB conceived and revised the paper and calculated the numbers needed to treat. All authors approved the final manuscript. MIB is the guarantor.

Competing interests: We have read and understood the BMJ policy on declaration of interests and declare the following interests: none.

Provenance and peer review: Not commissioned; externally peer reviewed.

1 Grond S, Zech D, Diefenbach C, Radbruch L, Lehmann KA Assessment of cancer pain: a prospective evaluation in 2266 cancer patients referred to a pain service. *Pain* 1996;64:107-14.
2 Caraceni A, Portenoy RK. An international survey of cancer pain characteristics and syndromes. IASP Task Force on Cancer Pain. International Association for the Study of Pain. *Pain* 1999;82:263-74.
3 Coleman RE. Clinical features of metastatic bone disease and risk of skeletal morbidity. *Clin Cancer Res* 2006;12(20 Pt 2):6243s-49s.
4 Falk S, Dickenson AH. Pain and nociception: mechanisms of cancer-induced bone pain. *J Clin Oncol* 2014;32:1647-54.
5 Middlemiss T, Laird BJ, Fallon MT. Mechanisms of cancer-induced bone pain. *Clin Oncol* 2011;23:387-92.
6 Davies A, Buchanan A, Zeppetella G, Porta-Sales J, Likar R, Weismayr W, et al. Breakthrough cancer pain: an observational study of 1000 European oncology patients. *J Pain Symptom Manage* 2013;46:619-28.
7 White BD, Stirling AJ, Paterson E, Asquith-Coe K, Melder A. Diagnosis and management of patients at risk of or with metastatic spinal cord compression: summary of NICE guidance. *BMJ* 2008;337:a2538.
8 Chaichana KL, Woodworth GF, Sciubba DM, McGirt MJ, Witham TJ, Bydon A, et al Predictors of ambulatory function after decompressive surgery for metastatic epidural spinal cord compression. *Neurosurgery* 2008;62:683-92; discussion 83-92.
9 Brown PD, Stafford SL, Schild SE, Martenson JA, Schiff D. Metastatic spinal cord compression in patients with colorectal cancer. *J Neuro-oncol* 1999;44:175-80.
10 World Health Organization. Cancer pain relief. 2nd ed. WHO, 1996. http://whqlibdoc.who.int/publications/9241544821.pdf.
11 Zech DF, Grond S, Lynch J, Hertel D, Lehmann KA. Validation of World Health Organization guidelines for cancer pain relief: a 10-year prospective study. *Pain* 1995;63:65-76.
12 Bennet MI. What evidence do we have that the WHO analgesic ladder is effective in cancer pain? In: McQuay HJ, Moore R, Kalso E, eds. Systematic reviews in pain research; methodology refined. IASP Press, 2008.
13 Nabal M, Librada S, Redondo MJ, Pigni A, Brunelli C, Caraceni A. The role of paracetamol and nonsteroidal anti-inflammatory drugs in addition to WHO Step III opioids in the control of pain in advanced cancer. A systematic review of the literature. *Palliat Med* 2012;26:305-12.
14 McNicol E, Strassels SA, Goudas L, Lau J, Carr DB. NSAIDS or paracetamol, alone or combined with opioids, for cancer pain. *Cochrane Database Syst Rev* 2005;1:CD005180.
15 Bennett MI, Graham J, Schmidt-Hansen M, Prettyjohns M Arnold S. Prescribing strong opioids for pain in adult palliative care: summary of NICE guidance. *BMJ* 2012;344:e2806.
16 Klepstad P, Kaasa S, Jystad A, Hval B, Borchgrevink PC. Immediate- or sustained-release morphine for dose finding during start of morphine to cancer patients: a randomized, double-blind trial. *Pain* 2003;101:193-8.
17 National Institute for Health and Care Excellence. Opioids in palliative care. (Clinical guideline 140.) 2012. www.nice.org.uk/cg140.
18 Riley J, Branford R, Droney J, Gretton S, Sato H, Kennett A, et al. Morphine or oxycodone for cancer-related pain? A randomized, open-label, controlled trial. *J Pain Sympt Manage* 2014; published online 26 Jun. doi: 10.1016/j.jpainsymman.2014.05.021.
19 Jandhyala R, Fullarton JR, Bennett MI. Efficacy of rapid-onset oral fentanyl formulations vs. oral morphine for cancer-related breakthrough pain: a meta-analysis of comparative trials. J *Pain Sympt Manage* 2013;46:573-80.
20 Davis MP. Efficacy of rapid-onset oral fentanyl: what does it mean? *J Pain Sympt Manage* 2014;48:e2-3.
21 Bennett MI. Effectiveness of antiepileptic or antidepressant drugs when added to opioids for cancer pain: systematic review. *Palliat Med* 2011;25:553-9.
22 Yennurajalingam S, Frisbee-Hume S, Palmer JL, Delgado-Guay MO, Bull J, Phan AT, et al. Reduction of cancer-related fatigue with dexamethasone: a double-blind, randomized, placebo-controlled trial in patients with advanced cancer. *J Clin Oncol* 2013;31:3076-82.
23 Paulsen O, Klepstad P, Rosland JH, Aass N, Albert E, Fayers P, et al. Efficacy of methylprednisolone on pain, fatigue, and appetite loss in patients with advanced cancer using opioids: a randomized, placebo-controlled, double-blind trial. *J Clin Oncol* 2014;32:3221-8.
24 Dennis K, Makhani L, Zeng L, Lam H, Chow E. Single fraction conventional external beam radiation therapy for bone metastases: a systematic review of randomised controlled trials. *Radiother Oncol* 2013;106:5-14.
25 Chow E, Zeng L, Salvo N, Dennis K, Tsao M, Lutz S. Update on the systematic review of palliative radiotherapy trials for bone metastases. *Clin Oncol* 2012;24:112-24.
26 Chow E, Meyer RM, Chen BE, van der Linden YM, Roos D, Hartsell WF, et al. Impact of reirradiation of painful osseous metastases on quality of life and function: a secondary analysis of the NCIC CTG SC.20 randomized trial. *J Clin Oncol* 2014; published online 27 Oct.
27 Chow E, van der Linden YM, Roos D, Hartsell WF, Hoskin P, Wu JS et al. Single versus multiple fractions of repeat radiation for painful bone metastases: a randomised, controlled, non-inferiority trial. *Lancet Oncol* 2014;15:164-71.

28 National Institute for Health and Care Excellence Advancerd breast cancer. (Clinical guideline 81). 2014. www.nice.org.uk/guidance/cg81.

29 Gralow J, Tripathy D. Managing metastatic bone pain: the role of bisphosphonates. *J Pain Sympt Manage* 2007;33:462-72.

30 Hoskin P, Sundar S, Reczko K, Forsyth S, Mithal N, Sizer B et al. A Multicentre Randomised Trial of Ibandronate Compared to Single Dose Radiotherapy for Localised Metastatic Bone Pain in Prostate Cancer (RIB). *Eur J Cancer* 2011;47:6.

31 Wong R, Wiffen PJ. Bisphosphonates for the relief of pain secondary to bone metastases. *Cochrane Database Syst Rev* 2002;2:CD002068.

32 Mhaskar R, Redzepovic J, Wheatley K, Clark OA, Miladinovic B, Glasmacher A, et al. Bisphosphonates in multiple myeloma: a network meta-analysis. *Cochrane Database Syst Rev* 2012;5:CD003188.

33 Stopeck AT, Lipton A, Body JJ, et al. Denosumab compared with zoledronic acid for the treatment of bone metastases in patients with advanced breast cancer: a randomized, double-blind study. *J Clin Oncol* 2010;28:5132-9.

34 Hurlow A, Bennett MI, Robb KA, Johnson MI, Simpson KH, Oxberry SG Transcutaneous electric nerve stimulation (TENS) for cancer pain in adults. *Cochrane Database Syst Rev* 2012;3:CD006276.

More titles in The BMJ Series

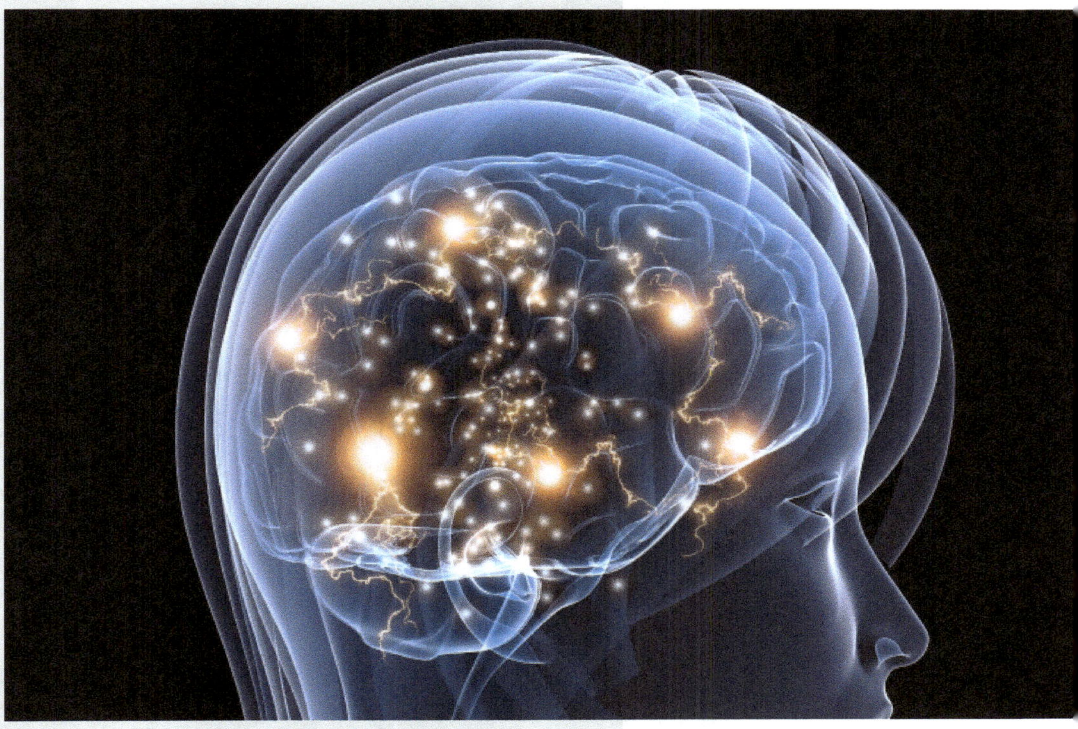

More titles from BPP School of Health

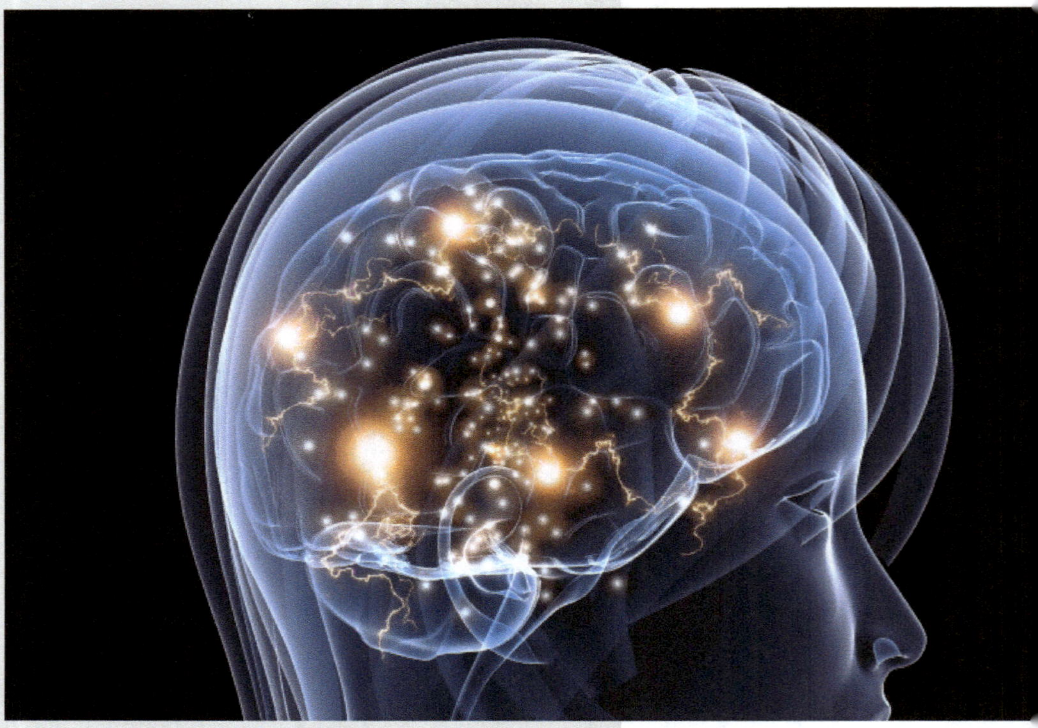

BPP UNIVERSITY SCHOOL OF HEALTH

More titles in The Progressing Your Medical Career Series

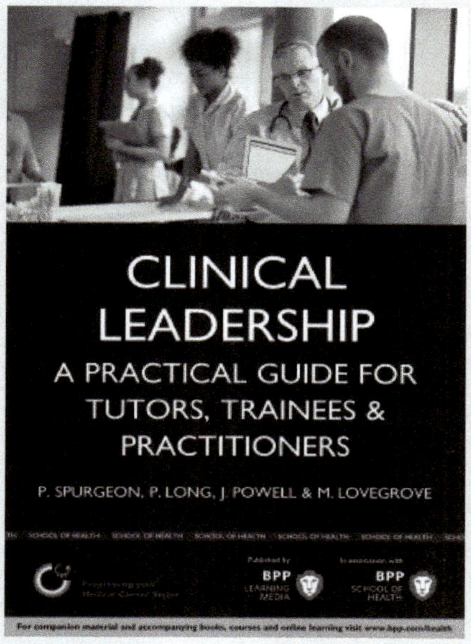

Are you a healthcare professional or student who wishes to acquire and develop your leadership and management skills? Do you recognise the role and influence of strong leadership and management in modern healthcare?

Clinical leadership is something in which all healthcare professionals can participate in, in terms of driving forward high quality care for their patients. In this up-to-date guide, the authors take you through the latest leadership and management thinking, and how this links in with the Clinical Leadership Competency Framework. As well as influencing undergraduate curricula this framework forms the basis of the leadership component of the curricula for all healthcare specialties, so a practical knowledge of it is essential for all healthcare professionals in training.

Using case studies and practical exercises to provide a strong work-based emphasis, this practical guide will enable you to build on your existing experiences to develop your leadership and management skills, and to develop strategies and approaches to improving care for your patients.

This book addresses:

- Why strong leadership and management are crucial to delivering high quality care;
- The theory and evidence behind the Clinical Leadership Competency Framework;
- The practical aspects of leadership learning in a wide range of clinical environments
- How clinical professionals and trainers can best facilitate leadership learning for their trainees and students within the clinical work-place.

Whether you are a student just starting out on your career, or an established healthcare professional wishing to develop yourself as a clinical leader, this practical, easy-to-use guide will give you the techniques and knowledge you require to excel.

£24.99

June 2015

Paperback

978-1-472727-83-1

BPP UNIVERSITY SCHOOL OF HEALTH

www.bpp.com/medical-series

BPP
UNIVERSITY
SCHOOL OF HEALTH

More titles in The Progressing Your Medical Career Series

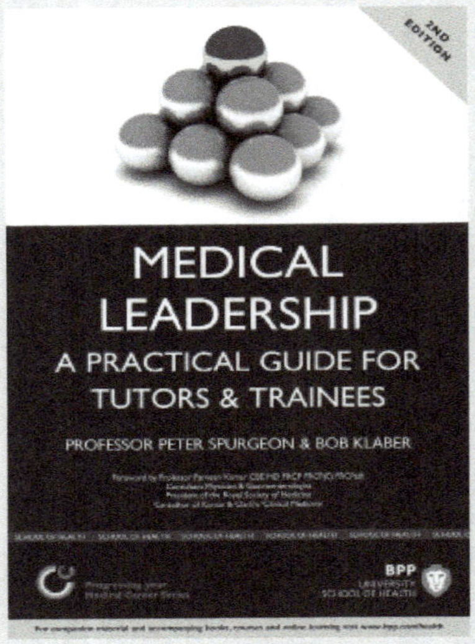

£19.99

April 2016

Paperback

9781-472745-59-0

Are you a doctor or medical student who wishes to acquire and develop your leadership and management skills? Do you recognise the role and influence of strong leadership and management in modern medicine?

Clinical leadership is something in which all doctors should have an important role in terms of driving forward high quality care for their patients. In this up-to-date guide Peter Spurgeon and Robert Klaber take you through the latest leadership and management thinking, and how this links in with the Medical Leadership Competency Framework. As well as influencing undergraduate curricula and some of the concepts underpinning revalidation, this framework forms the basis of the leadership component of the curricula for all medical specialties, so a practical knowledge of it is essential for all doctors in training.

Using case studies and practical exercises to provide a strong work-based emphasis, this practical guide will enable you to build on your existing experiences to develop your leadership and management skills, and to develop strategies and approaches to improving care for your patients.

This book addresses:

- Why strong leadership and management are crucial to delivering high quality care
- The theory and evidence behind the Medical Leadership Competency Framework
- The practical aspects of leadership learning in a wide range of clinical environments (eg handover, EM, ward etc)
- How Consultants and trainers can best facilitate leadership learning for their trainees and students within the clinical workplace

Whether you are a medical student just starting out on your career, or an established doctor wishing to develop yourself as a clinical leader, this practical, easy-to-use guide will give you the techniques and knowledge you require to excel.

BPP
UNIVERSITY
SCHOOL OF HEALTH

www.bpp.com/medical-series

More titles in The Progressing Your Medical Career Series

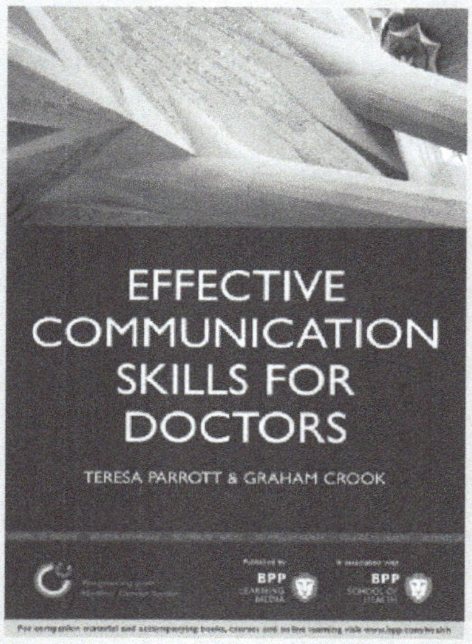

£19.99
September 2011
Paperback
978-1-445379-56-2

Would you like to know how to improve your communication skills? Are you looking for a clearly written book which explores all aspects of effective medical communication?

There is an urgent need to improve doctors' communication skills. Research has shown that poor communication can contribute to patient dissatisfaction, lack of compliance and increased medico-legal problems. Improved communication skills will impact positively on all of these areas.

The last fifteen years have seen unprecedented changes in medicine and the role of doctors. Effective communication skills are vital to these new roles. But communication is not just related to personality. Skills can be learned which can make your communication more effective, and help you to improve your relationships with patients, their families and fellow doctors.

This book shows how to learn those skills and outlines why we all need to communicate more effectively. Healthcare is increasingly a partnership. Change is happening at all levels, from government directives to patient expectations. Communication is a bridge between the wisdom of the past and the vision of the future.

Readers of this book can also gain free access to an online module which upon successful completion can download a certificate for their portfolio of learning/ Revalidation/ CPD records.

This easy-to-read guide will help medical students and doctors at all stages of their careers improve their communication within a hospital environment.

BPP UNIVERSITY SCHOOL OF HEALTH

www.bpp.com/medical-series

BPP UNIVERSITY SCHOOL OF HEALTH

More Titles in The Progressing Your Medical Career Series

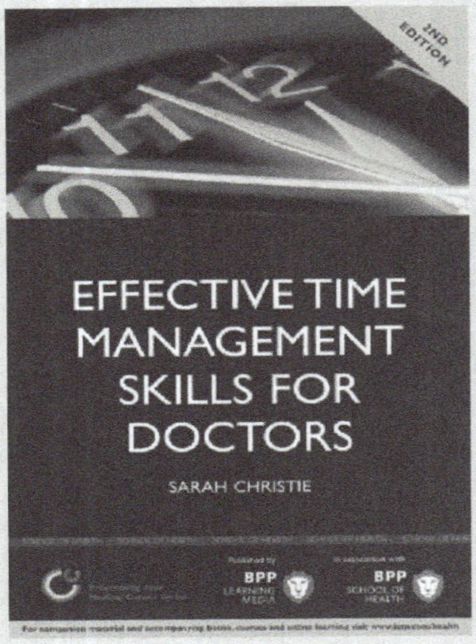

£19.99
October 2011
Paperback
978-1-906839-08-6

Do you find it difficult to achieve a work-life balance? Would you like to know how you can become more effective with the time you have?

With the introduction of the European Working Time Directive, which will severely limit the hours in the working week, it is more important than ever that doctors improve their personal effectiveness and time management skills. This interactive book will enable you to focus on what activities are needlessly taking up your time and what steps you can take to manage your time better.

By taking the time to read through, complete the exercises and follow the advice contained within this book you will begin to:

- Understand where your time is being needlessly wasted
- Discover how to be more assertive and learn how to say 'No'
- Set yourself priorities and stick to them
- Learn how to complete tasks more efficiently
- Plan better so you can spend more time doing the things you enjoy

In recent years, with the introduction of the NHS Plan and Lord Darzi's commitment to improve the quality of healthcare provision, there is a need for doctors to become more effective within their working environment. This book will offer you the chance to regain some clarity on how you actually spend your time and give you the impetus to ensure you achieve the tasks and goals which are important to you.

BPP UNIVERSITY SCHOOL OF HEALTH

www.bpp.com/medical-series

BPP UNIVERSITY SCHOOL OF HEALTH

More titles in The Progressing Your Medical Career Series

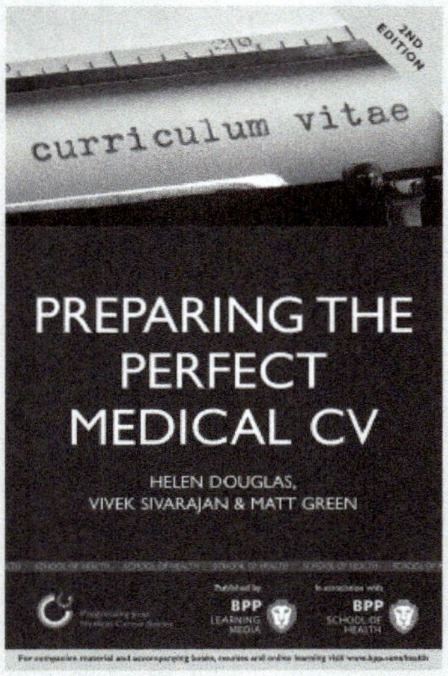

£19.99
October 2011
Paperback
978-1-445381-62-6

Are you unsure of how to structure your Medical CV? Would you like to know how to ensure you stand out from the crowd?

With competition for medical posts at an all time high it is vital that your Medical CV stands out over your fellow applicants. This comprehensive, unique and easy-to-read guide has been written with this in mind to help prospective medical students, current medical students and doctors of all grades prepare a Medical CV of the highest quality. Whether you are applying to medical school, currently completing your medical degree or a doctor progressing through your career (foundation doctor, specialty trainee in general practice, surgery or medicine, GP career grade or Consultant) this guide includes specific guidance for applicants at every level.

This time-saving and detailed guide:

- Explains what selection panels are looking for when reviewing applications at all levels.
- Discusses how to structure your Medical CV to ensure you stand out for the right reasons.
- Explores what information to include (and not to include) in your CV.
- Covers what to consider when maintaining a portfolio at every step of your career, including, for revalidation and relicensing purposes.
- Provides examples of high quality CVs to illustrate the above.

This unique guide will show you how to prepare your CV for every step of your medical career from pre-Medical School right through to Consultant level and should be a constant companion to ensure you secure your first choice post every time.

BPP UNIVERSITY SCHOOL OF HEALTH

www.bpp.com/medical-series